DID YOU KNOW . . .

- The healthiest populations in the world derive most of their calories from carbohydrates?
- Public health experts recommend that Americans should double their daily fiber intake?
- The USDA Dietary Guidelines have been moderated to allow more liberal intake of sugar—and that recent research shows sugar may have a calming effect on most people?

THE CARBOHYDRATE, FIBER, AND SUGAR COUNTER is packed with information on these essential elements of a healthy diet. While some nutrition guides focus on one or the other, no other book includes all three—your power triad for high-energy living and optimal health.

Annette B. Natow, Ph.D., R.D., and Jo-Ann Heslin, M.A., R.D., are the authors of twenty-five books on nutrition. Both are former faculty members of Adelphi University and the State University of New York, Downstate Medical Center. They are editors of the *Journal of Nutrition for the Elderly,* serve as editorial board members for the *Environmental Nutrition Newsletter,* and are contributors to magazines and journals.

Books by Annette B. Natow and Jo-Ann Heslin

THE
CARBOHYDRATE, FIBER, AND SUGAR
COUNTER

Annette B. Natow, Ph.D., R.D.
and **Jo-Ann Heslin, M.A., R.D.**

POCKET BOOKS
New York   London   Toronto   Sydney   Singapore

An *Original* Publication of POCKET BOOKS

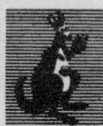

POCKET BOOKS, a division of Simon & Schuster Inc.
1230 Avenue of the Americas, New York, NY 10020

Copyright © 1999 by Annette Natow and Jo-Ann Heslin

ISBN: 0-671-02562-7

First Pocket Books printing October 1999

10 9 8 7 6

POCKET and colophon are registered trademarks of Simon & Schuster Inc.

Cover photo by FoodPix

Printed in the U.S.A.

To our families, who support us through every project: Harry, Allen, Irene, Sarah, Meryl, Marty, Laura, George, Emily, Steven, Joseph, Kristen and Karen.

ACKNOWLEDGMENTS

Without the tireless cooperation of Steven Natow, M.D., and Stephen Llano, *The Carbohydrate, Fiber, and Sugar Counter* would never have been completed. Our thanks also to all the food manufacturers who graciously shared their data, and a special thanks to our agent, Nancy Trichter, and to Jane Cavolina, our editor.

———————

"Most people can eat large amounts of carbohydrate food with ease. Thus bread, in which eight-tenths of the calories are in the form of carbohydrate, is the 'staff of life.' "

MARY SWARTZ ROSE, PH.D.
Feeding the Family
The Macmillan Company, 1919

INTRODUCTION

Only *The Carbohydrate, Fiber, and Sugar Counter* gives you the whole carbohydrate story with all the information you need to make the best food choices. Carbohydrates are favorites. We all seem to love potatoes, pasta, bread, tortillas, bagels and, of course, sweets. Americans get most of their calories from "carbs." You can see why when you add cereals and other grains, popcorn, rice, beans, vegetables, fruits, milk and milk products, all high in carbohydrates. Carbohydrates taste good and are good for you. The Dietary Guidelines, government advice for healthy eating, recommend that you choose a diet with plenty of grain products, vegetables and fruits. And the U.S. Department of Agriculture's (USDA) Food Guide Pyramid, which illustrates a healthy diet for Americans, has as its base and largest section the bread, cereals, grains and pasta group. Six to eleven servings are recommended daily. They are the foundation of healthy eating.

What are carbohydrates?

Carbohydrates (sugar, starch and fiber) are made in plants from carbon, hydrogen and oxygen. When you eat plants, or foods made from them, your body gets the energy it needs for fuel (calories). Many people believe that eating carbohydrates will make you fat. That's not true. In fact, there are only four calories in a gram of carbs. Compared to the other energy-yielding nutrients, fat and protein, carbohydrates have less than one half of the calories in fat and the same number of calories as protein. *Excess* calories, or more than your body needs, from any of these three energy sources—carbohydrate, fat or protein—will put on weight. It may surprise you to learn that many studies in the United States and other countries show that people who eat more sugar and other carbohydrates tend to weigh less than those who eat smaller amounts. Carbohydrates are a less efficient fuel than fat. Converting the carbohydrates you eat into stored body fat uses up 25 percent of the calories. Converting the fat you eat into stored body fat uses up only 3 percent of the fat calories.

How much carbohydrate should I get every day?

You need at least 100 grams of carbohydrate a day to meet the needs of your brain and other body tissues that do not easily use other fuels. Adequate carbohydrate will also reduce the amount of body protein that is broken down. Some carbohydrates are needed to help break down body fat and prevent the accumulation of ketones (formed when fat is broken down), which can upset the normal balance in the body.

Experts recommend that we get about 60 percent of our calories from carbohydrates. The Daily Values (DV), printed on food labels, suggest 300 grams of carbohydrate (1200 calories) in a 2,000-calorie diet, which is 60 percent of daily calories. Calorie intake each day varies depending on your body size and level of activity. The following table will help you choose your best intake.

DAILY INTAKE OF CARBOHYDRATE

Calories Eaten in a Day	Grams of Carbohydrate
1500	225
1800	270
2000	300
2500	375
3000	450

Do athletes need more carbohydrate?

Yes. Some long-distance runners, for instance, eat as much as 85 percent of their daily calories as carbohydrates. Most of us don't need that much. Active adults—runners, tennis players, swimmers—do benefit from high carbohydrate intake. Carbohydrates fuel muscles.

Glycogen is the form in which carbohydrate is stored in muscles. Excess carbohydrate is converted to glycogen and stored in the liver and muscles until needed. The amount stored is small, only enough to last for less than a day. These muscle stores can be increased by a combination of a high carbohydrate diet and exercise. Trained muscles store more glycogen.

FAST FACT

Americans are eating more cereal—60 percent more than in the late 1970s.

Can a person with diabetes eat carbohydrate foods?

People with diabetes do not handle carbohydrate normally. Either they cannot make enough insulin (the hormone needed to use most carbohydrates) or their bodies cannot use the insulin they do make.

There are two main types of diabetes: Type 1, also called insulin-dependent diabetes and Type 2, non-insulin dependent diabetes. (The name of Type 2 is misleading because one-third of the people with this kind of diabetes do use insulin.) Type 2 is more common, affecting about 14 million Americans—that is, 90 percent of all persons with diabetes.

In both types of diabetes, the goal is to keep blood sugar as close to normal as possible. This is done by keeping track of the amount of carbohydrate eaten each day. People with diabetes and their health care practitioners work out diet plans that include dietary carbohydrate levels based on usual intake, activity level, medication or amount of insulin used. In the past, people with diabetes were advised to avoid sugar. This is no longer considered necessary. All carbohydrates—sugar and starches—are broken down into glucose (sugar) in the body. The diabetic diet can include all types of carbohydrates as long as the amounts eaten fall within prescribed limits for each meal and snack.

Why do people count carbohydrates?

Many people count carbohydrates. You can do so to keep track of your carbohydrate and sugar intake in order to lose weight, if you are an athlete or if you have diabetes. *The Carbohydrate, Fiber, and Sugar Counter* will help you count carbohydrates by telling you how many grams of carbohydrate and sugar are in the foods you eat. Reasonable amounts of sugar and sugar-containing foods, such as cookies, can be included. Just be careful that sugary foods do not crowd out more healthy carbohydrate choices.

What is low blood sugar?

Low blood sugar (hypoglycemia) is a condition in which a person's blood sugar (glucose) falls below normal levels, causing symptoms such as sweating, trembling, agitation, rapid heartbeat, and hunger. These symptoms show that too little blood sugar is available to fuel the body cells. It can happen in people with diabetes who have taken too much insulin or have not eaten enough food. In persons who do not have diabetes, hypoglycemia may occur several hours after a meal. This is known as *reactive hypoglycemia*. Eating frequent small meals made up of high-protein foods, fewer carbohydrates and less sugar usually relieves the symptoms. To establish a diagnosis blood glucose tests have to be taken when the symptoms occur because many people mistakenly believe they are hypoglycemic.

What is glucose?

Glucose is the body's main fuel used to support movement, nerve function and temperature control. All carbohydrate foods—potatoes, apples, sugar, rice, pasta—are changed to glucose in the body. Every cell and almost all body fluids contain glucose; it is the way sugar travels in the blood. Plants store glucose as starch and we get glucose when we eat them. Grains, beans, peas, and potatoes are the main sources.

FAST FACT

The average American eats 142 pounds of sugar and corn syrup a year, along with 24 pounds of low-calorie sweeteners.

FAST FACT

The average American gets 16 percent of his or her calories from added sugars. Teens get 20 percent, mainly from sodas, cookies, cakes, and pastries. Teenage boys, on average, drink more than 575 cans of soda a year, while teenage girls drink more than 400 cans.

Is sugar bad for you?

Most people enjoy the sweet taste of sugar. Babies are born with a preference for sweets. Their first food, milk, contains milk sugar (lactose), which is slightly sweet. Sugar is not just a source of empty calories. It makes other foods taste better, so nutritious foods are more pleasant to eat. Adding small amounts of sugar to cereal makes it tastier, and a little chocolate syrup added to milk can encourage children to drink more milk.

While it is true that eating too many sugary foods can crowd more nutritious foods out of your diet, moderate amounts of sugar—12 to 15 percent of total calories—will not harm healthy people. Sugar does cause cavities, but what matters more is how often you eat sugary foods (and other carbohydrates) rather than the amount you eat. In the past, sugar was believed to cause many other health problems, including diabetes, hyperactivity, heart disease and even criminal behavior, but at present there is no evidence that sugar causes these problems. The evidence points to obesity, not sugar, as a major cause of diabetes. And sugar does not cause hyperactivity in children. Hyperactive behavior is more likely to occur in a stimulating situation like a birthday party where many sweets are eaten. Research shows that when sugar is eaten in everyday situations, it usually has a calming effect. The 1995 USDA Dietary Guidelines advise us to eat moderate amounts of sugar. This would be about 12 to 15 percent of total calories, as shown in the following table.

HEALTHY INTAKE OF SUGAR

Calories Eaten in a Day	12% of Calories (Grams of Sugar)	15% of Calories (Grams of Sugar)
1500	45	56
1800	54	68
2000	60	75
2500	75	94
3000	90	113

Isn't it healthier to eat very little sugar?

Not really. Grains, fruits, vegetables, milk, yogurt and other milk products contain natural sugars. To reduce sugar intake below 12 percent of your daily calories, you would have to cut down on these healthy foods. On the other hand, too much sugar is not good either. When you eat a lot of sugar from soda, sweetened fruit drinks, cake, cookies, candy and frozen desserts, you are substituting these sweetened foods for more nutritious choices. A moderate sugar intake is best—some from naturally sweet foods, like fruit and cereal, and some from foods with added sugar.

SUGAR BY ANY OTHER NAME

Brown sugar	Invert sugar
Corn syrup	Lactose
Dextrose	Maltose
Fructose	Maple syrup
Glucose	Molasses
High-fructose corn syrup	Raw sugar
Honey	Sucrose

Are honey and molasses better for you than sugar?

Since honey tastes good and is about twice as sweet as sugar, you can use less to sweeten your tea, but the real problem with honey is that it really isn't a good source of nutrients. Even if you ate an entire cup of honey you would get only tiny amounts of vitamins and minerals. The exception to this is vitamin B_{12}. One cup of honey will give you 50 percent of your daily need of this vitamin—along with 1,031 calories.

Molasses does contain some minerals—calcium, magnesium, potassium and iron. But don't count on it as a source because you probably eat very small amounts of it. One tablespoon of molasses contains only 41 milligrams of calcium, less than one twentieth of the amount needed daily.

Is raw sugar better for you than regular sugar?

Raw sugar is practically identical to regular white sugar. The only differences are its coarser shape, its tan color (from a tiny amount of added molasses), and its much higher cost.

What are sorbitol and mannitol?

Sorbitol and mannitol are sugar alcohols that are less sweet than sugar and are absorbed more slowly. They are used in foods such as cookies, gums and candies that are often labeled "sugar-free." They have just as many calories as regular sugar, but because they are not as sweet as sugar, larger amounts of the sugar alcohols have to be used. As a result, foods sweetened with sorbitol or mannitol are not useful for weight loss. Also, large amounts of either one can cause diarrhea.

FAST FACT

In prehistoric times, early man learned to stay away from poisonous plants, which often tasted bitter. It is believed that this is how people developed a preference for sweet foods, which were not as likely to be poisonous.

Your brain needs about 100 grams of glucose a day to function. This is one-third to one-half of all the carbohydrate eaten by the average person.

SUGAR SUBSTITUTES—ARTIFICIAL SWEETENERS

Acesulfame-K (Sweet One, Sunett)

Calorie-free and almost 200 times as sweet as sugar, acesulfame-K is used in desserts, confections and beverages, and it stays sweet when heated. The Food and Drug Administration (FDA) has found acesulfame-K to be safe for all people.

Aspartame (Equal, NutraSweet)

Aspartame is 200 times sweeter than sugar and contains only two calories in the amount equal in sweetness to one teaspoon of sugar. It is an all-purpose sweetener made from two amino acids (aspartic acid and phenylalanine). People with the inherited disorder PKU (phenylketonuria) are cautioned to limit their use of foods with the amino acid phenylalanine. The FDA requires foods containing aspartame to have a label stating that it contains phenylalanine.

Saccharin (Sweet 'n Low)

Saccharin is 400 times sweeter than sugar and provides no calories because it is not broken down in the body. Saccharin is often combined with other low-calorie sweeteners to mask its bitter aftertaste. It is possibly a carcinogen, but because of the small amounts used, the risk is minor. The

FDA requires foods containing saccharin to have the following label: "Use of this product may be hazardous to your health. This product contains saccharin, which has been determined to cause cancer in laboratory animals."

Sucralose (Splenda)

Although sucralose is the only low-calorie sweetener actually made from sugar, the body does not recognize it as sugar and it passes through the body unchanged. That is why it provides no calories. Six hundred times sweeter than sugar, sucralose is used in soda, gum, baked goods and frozen desserts.

What is fiber?

Fiber is the part of a plant that people cannot digest because they do not have the enzymes needed to break it down. Fiber is found in whole grains, fruits, vegetables, cereals, breads, bran and popcorn. Animal foods like meat, chicken, milk and cheese do not contain any fiber.

There are actually two types of fiber: soluble and insoluble. The first dissolves in water and the second doesn't. Both types fill you up, but each has special health benefits. Soluble fiber helps lower cholesterol. The best sources of soluble fiber are apples, barley, beans, carrots, grapefruit, oats, oranges, peas, rice bran and berries.

Insoluble fiber comes from the outer hard shell of grains. It bulks up one's stool, helping to prevent or relieve constipation. It is also believed to help prevent colon cancer. Bran, celery, green beans, green leafy vegetables, potato skins, flaxseed and whole grains are all good sources of insoluble fiber. Most food plants contain a mixture of both types of fiber.

FAST FACT

Because small amounts of soluble fiber can be digested by bacteria in the intestines, some vegetarians, who eat a lot of high-fiber foods, may get as much as 15 percent of their calories from fiber.

What is dietary fiber?

You see values for dietary fiber on food labels. This is the fiber that the body cannot digest. The Daily Value (DV) used on food labels recommends an intake of 25 to 30 grams of dietary fiber a day. To reach this level you would need to eat 3 to 5 servings of whole grain bread and cereals, 3 servings of fruit, and 3 servings of vegetables a day. Most Americans do not eat that much. The typical intake of adults in the United States is about 13 grams a day.

ADD FIBER TO YOUR SHOPPING LIST

Baked Beans	Fruits
Bean soup	Green peas
Berries	Oatmeal
Bran	Soy nuts
Brown rice	Vegetables
Canned beans	Whole grain bread, crackers
Chestnuts	Whole wheat English muffins, pasta,
Dried fruit	pita, pretzels, rolls

ADD SOME FIBER TO YOUR LIFE

- Eat whole fruits and vegetables instead of just drinking their juices.
- Enjoy the fiber-rich skin of fruits and vegetables like apples, pears, potatoes and kiwis.
- Choose whole grains more often: brown rice, oats, cracked wheat, and whole wheat spaghetti, cereal and bread

- Enjoy beans, lentils and split peas. They are frequently on menus and in salad bars.
- Try soybeans or one of its forms—soy nuts, tofu or tempeh—for an interesting food or snack.
- Try popular dried fruits, like raisins, or some of the more unusual kinds, like pineapple, mango and persimmon.
- Start adding fiber slowly so that your body can adjust to it. Don't go overboard. Excess fiber intake—over 50 grams a day—can displace other nutritious foods and may block the absorption of important minerals, such as iron, zinc, calcium and magnesium.
- Drink more fluids when adding fiber to your diet. Fiber acts like a sponge, absorbing large amounts of water. If fluid intake is low, constipation can result and, in some cases, cause an obstruction in the colon.
- Try to get fiber from your food. Fiber pills and supplements are usually not necessary and you will miss the chance to get all the other healthy substances found in high-fiber foods.

Fiber and Kids: Go Easy

Young children have very small stomachs and often eat only a small amount of food at each meal. Experts suggest that the daily fiber intake of children age three years and older should equal their age plus 5 grams. For example, nine-year-olds should eat 14 grams (9 + 5). If they eat more than this amount, other important nutritious foods can be crowded out of their diet. Research shows that over 50 percent of children under ten eat less fiber than they need. But remember: when you increase fiber intake, you should increase fluid intake as well.

Health Benefits of Fiber

- High-fiber foods absorb water, making you feel full with fewer calories.
- Fiber speeds food through the intestines, limiting the exposure of colon walls to cancer-causing substances.
- Fiber binds bile and carries it out of the body, lowering the risk of colon cancer.
- Fiber combines with fat in the intestines, reducing fat absorption.
- Fiber helps to prevent or relieve constipation by bulking up stools.
- Fiber lowers blood glucose levels in the blood, helping to control diabetes.
- Fiber reduces the risk of heart disease by lowering blood cholesterol levels.
- Because high-fiber foods tend to be low in fat and sugars, they can displace other higher calorie foods.

FAST FACT

Researchers at the USDA found that when the average woman doubles her daily fiber intake from 12 to 24 grams, she saves 90 calories a day.

PERSONALIZING YOUR CARBOHYDRATE INTAKE

Now that you know how important it is to eat enough carbohydrate and fiber along with moderate amounts of sugar, it's time to count up your daily intake on the sample worksheet on page xxvi. You don't have to reach your goal every day. Just try to increase total carbohydrate and fiber while keeping sugar intake moderate.

- You usually eat _____ calories a day
- From the chart "Daily Intake of Carbohydrate" on page xv you should aim for _____ grams of carb.

COUNT UP YOUR GRAMS OF CARBOHYDRATE, FIBER AND SUGAR

FOOD	AMOUNT	CALORIES	CARB	FIBER	SUGAR
Your goals		_____	25	_____	_____
BREAKFAST					
SNACK					
LUNCH					
SNACK					
DINNER					
SNACK					
TOTAL		_____	_____	_____	_____

- From the chart "Healthy Intake of Sugar" on page xix, select either 12% or 15% of your total calories as sugar. You should aim for _____ grams of sugar.
- Most adults should aim for 25 grams of fiber.

USING YOUR CARBOHYDRATE, FIBER, AND SUGAR COUNTER

This book lists the carbohydrate, fiber and sugar values of more than 15,000 foods. Now you can compare your favorite foods before you go out to shop or to eat. This will help you save time while making choices.

The Carbohydrate, Fiber, and Sugar Counter lists foods alphabetically. In each category, you will find nonbranded (generic) foods listed first, in alphabetical order, followed by an alphabetical listing of brand name foods. The nonbranded list will help you determine carbohydrate, fiber and sugar values when you do not find your favorite brand name food listed. It will also help you evaluate generic and store brands. Large categories are divided into subcategories such as canned, dried, fresh and frozen so that you can easily find what you are looking for. This section of the book is divided into two parts: Part One, Brand Name and Nonbranded Foods; Part Two, Restaurant and Take-Out Foods, which will help you estimate the carb, fiber and sugar in restaurant and homemade foods.

Most foods are listed alphabetically, but in some cases, foods are grouped by category. For example, chicken stir-fry and chicken salad are found under the category CHICKEN DISHES. Other group categories include:

ASIAN FOOD   (page 7)
    Includes all types of Asian foods except
       egg rolls and sushi

DEFINITIONS

as prep (as prepared): prepared according to package directions

home recipe: homemade dishes; those included can be used as a guide to the carbohydrate values of similar products you may prepare or take-out food you buy

lean and fat: meat with some fat on its edges that is not cut away before cooking; also used for poultry prepared with skin and fat as purchased

lean only: trimmed of all visible fat

shelf stable: prepared products found on the supermarket shelf that are ready to eat or be heated and do not require refrigeration

take-out: dishes that you purchase ready-to-eat; those included serve as a guide to the carb, fiber and sugar values of similar products you may purchase

ABBREVIATIONS

avg	=	average
diam	=	diameter
fl	=	fluid
frzn	=	frozen
g	=	gram
in	=	inch
lb	=	pound
lg	=	large
med	=	medium
mg	=	milligram
oz	=	ounce
pkg	=	package
prep	=	prepared
pt	=	pint
qt	=	quart
reg	=	regular
sec	=	second
serv	=	serving
sm	=	small
sq	=	square
tbsp	=	tablespoon
tr	=	trace
tsp	=	teaspoon
w/	=	with
w/o	=	without
<	=	less than

EQUIVALENT MEASURES

3 teaspoons	=	1 tablespoon
4 tablespoons	=	¼ cup
8 tablespoons	=	½ cup
12 tablespoons	=	¾ cup
16 tablespoons	=	1 cup
1000 milligrams	=	1 gram
28 grams	=	1 ounce

LIQUID MEASURES

2 tablespoons	=	1 ounce
2 ounces	=	¼ cup
4 ounces	=	½ cup
6 ounces	=	¾ cup
8 ounces	=	1 cup
2 cups	=	1 pint
4 cups	=	1 quart

DRY MEASURES

4 ounces	=	¼ pound
8 ounces	=	½ pound
12 ounces	=	¾ pound
16 ounces	=	1 pound

PART ONE

BRAND NAME

AND

NONBRANDED FOODS

Discrepancies in figures are due to rounding, product reformulation and reevaluation. Labeling law allows rounding of values. Because most of the data is analysis data, obtained directly from manufacturers and not from labels, in some cases our values may not be exactly the same as label information because they have not been rounded.

Carb, fiber and sugar values are given in grams (g).

A dash (—) indicates data not available.

FOOD	PORTION	CALS.	CARB.	SUG.	FIB.
ABALONE					
fresh fried	3 oz	161	9	—	—
ACEROLA					
fresh	1	2	tr	—	—
ACEROLA JUICE					
juice	1 cup	51	12	—	—
ADZUKI BEANS					
canned sweetened	1 cup	702	163	—	—
dried cooked	1 cup	294	57	—	—
yokan sliced	3¼ in slices	112	26	—	—
Eden					
Organic	½ cup (4.6 oz)	110	19	—	5
AKEE					
fresh	3½ oz	223	5	—	—
ALE					
(*see* BEER AND ALE, and MALT)					
ALFALFA					
sprouts	1 tbsp	1	tr	—	—
ALLIGATOR					
tail cooked	3½ oz	143	1	—	—
ALLSPICE					
ground	1 tsp	5	1	—	—
ALMONDS					
almond butter honey & cinnamon	1 tbsp	96	4	—	—
almond butter w/ salt	1 tbsp	101	3	—	—
almond paste	1 oz	127	12	—	—
jordan almonds	10 (1.4 oz)	190	28	24	1
oil roasted blanched	1 oz	174	5	—	3
toasted unblanched	1 oz	167	7	—	3
Planters					
Almonds	1 oz	170	5	1	3
Gold Measure Slivered	1 pkg (2 oz)	340	11	2	4
Honey Roasted	1 oz	160	7	4	2
AMARANTH					
(*see also* CEREAL, COOKIES)					
uncooked	1 cup (6.8 oz)	729	129	—	30
Arrowhead					
Seeds	¼ cup (1.6 oz)	170	29	0	3

FOOD	PORTION	CALS.	CARB.	SUG.	FIB.
Health Valley					
Fast Menu Amaranth With Garden Vegetables	7½ oz	140	16	—	8
ANASAZI BEANS					
Arrowhead					
Dried	¼ cup (1.5 oz)	150	27	0	9
ANGLERFISH					
raw	3½ oz	72	0	0	0
ANISE					
seed	1 tsp	7	1	—	—
ANTELOPE					
roasted	3 oz	127	0	0	0
APPLE					
CANNED					
White House					
Escalloped Apples	4 oz	120	28	—	1
Sliced	4 oz	55	15	—	1
Spiced Apple Rings	1 ring	25	6	—	tr
DRIED					
cooked w/ sugar	½ cup	116	29	—	—
Del Monte					
Sliced	⅓ cup (1.4 oz)	80	23	18	5
Sonoma					
Pieces	10-12 pieces (1.4 oz)	110	29	25	4
FRESH					
apple	1	81	21	—	3
w/o skin sliced	1 cup	62	16	—	2
Dole					
Apple	1	80	18	—	5
Tastee					
Candy Apple	1 (3 oz)	160	26	16	4
Caramel Apple	1 (3 oz)	160	26	16	4
FROZEN					
Stouffer's					
Escalloped	1 cup (6 oz)	180	37	30	3
APPLE JUICE					
juice	1 cup	116	29	—	tr
After The Fall					
Organic	1 bottle (10 oz)	110	28	23	—
Vermont Apple	1 bottle (10 oz)	110	27	23	—

FOOD	PORTION	CALS.	CARB.	SUG.	FIB.
After The Fall (CONT.)					
Vermont Apple	1 bottle (8 oz)	90	22	18	—
Vermont Harvest Moon Sparkling Apple Cider	8 fl oz	110	27	26	—
Everfresh					
Apple Juice	1 can (8 oz)	110	29	29	0
Hi-C					
Jammin' Apple	8 fl oz	130	31	31	—
Hood					
Select Cider	1 cup (8 oz)	120	30	30	—
Minute Maid					
Box	8.45 fl oz	120	29	29	—
Juices To Go	1 can (11.5 fl oz)	160	40	40	—
Juices To Go	1 bottle (10 fl oz)	140	35	34	—
Juices To Go	1 bottle (16 fl oz)	110	28	28	—
Naturals	8 fl oz	110	28	28	—
Mott's					
From Concentrate as prep	8 fl oz	120	29	23	0
Fruit Basket Cocktail as prep	8 fl oz	120	29	28	0
Natural	8 fl oz	120	29	23	0
Ocean Spray					
100% Juice	8 fl oz	110	28	28	0
Odwalla					
Live Apple	8 fl oz	140	34	32	0
Red Cheek					
From Concentrate	8 fl oz	120	29	23	0
Natural	8 fl oz	120	29	23	0
Seneca					
Clarified frzn, as prep	8 fl oz	120	30	—	0
Granny Smith frzn as prep	8 fl oz	120	30	—	0
Natural frzn as prep	8 fl oz	120	30	—	0
Tree Of Life					
East Coast Apple	8 fl oz	120	30	30	—
Tropicana					
Season's Best	8 fl oz	110	28	26	—
Season's Best	1 container (6 fl oz)	80	21	19	—
Season's Best	1 container (8 fl oz)	110	28	26	—
Season's Best	1 container (10 fl oz)	140	35	32	—
Season's Best	1 can (11.5 fl oz)	160	40	38	—
Season's Best	1 bottle (10 fl oz)	140	35	32	—
Season's Best	1 bottle (7 fl oz)	100	24	23	—

FOOD	PORTION	CALS.	CARB.	SUG.	FIB.
Veryfine					
100% Juice	1 bottle (10 oz)	150	38	38	0
Juice-Ups	8 fl oz	120	30	30	0
White House					
Juice	6 oz	90	22	—	0
APPLESAUCE					
sweetened	½ cup	97	25	—	2
unsweetened	½ cup	53	14	—	2
Mott's					
Chunky	5 oz	110	26	22	2
Cinnamon	5 oz	120	29	24	1
Fruit Snacks Apple Spice	4 oz	70	18	16	1
Fruit Snacks Cinnamon	4 oz	90	23	19	1
Fruit Snacks Sweetened	4 oz	90	22	18	1
Sweetened	5 oz	110	28	23	1
Seneca					
Cinnamon	½ cup	100	24	—	3
Golden Delicious	½ cup	100	24	—	3
McIntosh	½ cup	100	24	—	3
Natural	½ cup	60	15	—	3
Regular	½ cup	100	24	—	3
Tree Of Life					
Applesauce	½ cup (4.3 oz)	50	15	11	2
White House					
Chunky	4 oz	80	22	—	1
Cinnamon	4 oz	100	25	—	1
Natural Packed w/ Apple Juice	4 oz	60	14	—	1
Regular	4 oz	80	22	—	1
Unsweetened	4 oz	50	12	—	2
APRICOT JUICE					
nectar	1 cup	141	36	—	2
Del Monte					
Nectar	8 fl oz	140	35	28	1
Libby					
Nectar	1 can (11.5 fl oz)	220	52	44	—
APRICOTS					
CANNED					
Del Monte					
Halves Unpeeled In Heavy Syrup	½ cup (4.5 oz)	100	26	25	1
Halves Unpeeled Lite	½ cup (4.3 oz)	60	16	15	1

FOOD	PORTION	CALS.	CARB.	SUG.	FIB.
Libby					
Halves Unpeeled Lite	½ cup (4.4 oz)	60	13	11	1
DRIED					
halves	10	83	22	—	3
Del Monte					
Sun Dried	⅓ cup (1.4 oz)	80	25	19	6
Sonoma					
Dried	10 pieces (1.4 oz)	120	31	—	1
FRESH					
apricots	3	51	12	—	—

ARROWROOT

flour	1 cup (4.5 oz)	457	113	—	4

ARTICHOKE
CANNED

Progresso					
Hearts	2 pieces (2.9 oz)	35	6	1	1
Hearts Marinated	⅓ cup (3 oz)	160	6	1	1
FRESH					
boiled	1 med (4 oz)	60	13	—	—
hearts cooked	½ cup	42	9	—	—
Dole					
Large Whole	1	23	5	—	3

ARUGULA

raw	½ cup	2	tr	—	—

ASIAN FOOD
(*see also* DINNER, EGG ROLLS, PASTA, SUSHI)
CANNED

La Choy					
Bi-Pack Beef Pepper	¾ cup	80	10	—	2
Bi-Pack Chow Mein Chicken	¾ cup	80	8	—	1
Bi-Pack Chow Mein Pork	¾ cup	80	7	—	2
Bi-Pack Chow Mein Shrimp	¾ cup	70	6	—	1
Bi-Pack Sweet & Sour Chicken	¾ cup	120	18	—	2
Bi-Pack Teriyaki Chicken	¾ cup	85	8	—	1
Dinner Chow Mein Chicken	¾ pkg	300	29	—	2
Entree Beef Pepper Oriental	¾ cup	100	12	—	2
Entree Chow Mein Beef	¾ cup	40	5	—	2
Entree Chow Mein Chicken	¾ cup	70	2	—	4
Entree Chow Mein Meatless	¾ cup	25	5	—	2
Entree Chow Mein Shrimp	¾ cup	35	4	—	2

FOOD	PORTION	CALS.	CARB.	SUG.	FIB.
La Choy (CONT.)					
Entree Sweet & Sour Chicken	¾ cup	240	47	—	1
Entree Sweet & Sour Pork	¾ cup	250	48	—	1
FROZEN					
Banquet					
Chow Mein Chicken	1 pkg (9 oz)	400	28	3	3
Birds Eye					
Easy Recipe Meal Starter Oriental Stir Fry as prep	1 serv	280	30	9	2
Easy Recipe Meal Starter Spicy Asian	1 serv	280	30	22	2
Easy Recipe Meal Starter Teriyaki Stir Fry as prep	1 serv	280	30	14	2
Chun King					
Beef Pepper Steak	1 pkg (13 oz)	300	50	15	5
Chow Mein Chicken	1 pkg (13 oz)	370	45	6	4
Imperial Chicken	1 pkg (13 oz)	460	59	17	5
Sweet & Sour Pork	1 pkg (13 oz)	450	66	12	4
Walnut Chicken	1 pkg (13 oz)	460	56	15	5
Green Giant					
Create A Meal LoMein Stir Fry as prep	1¼ cups (10 oz)	320	35	9	4
Create A Meal Sweet & Sour Stir Fry as prep	1¼ cups (10 oz)	290	29	16	5
Create A Meal Szechuan Stir Fry as prep	1¼ cups (10 oz)	340	22	10	5
Create A Meal Teriyaki Stir Fry as prep	1¼ cups (10 oz)	240	18	10	4
Lean Cuisine					
Chicken Chow Mein With Rice	1 pkg (9 oz)	220	33	4	3
Chicken Oriental w/ Vegetables & Vermicelli	1 pkg (9 oz)	250	30	4	4
Oriental Style Dumplings	1 pkg (9 oz)	300	51	14	2
Teriyaki Stir Fry	1 pkg (10 oz)	290	48	9	4
Luigino's					
Chicken & Almonds With Rice	1 pkg (8 oz)	250	33	1	3
Chop Suey Pork With Rice	1 pkg (8.5 oz)	210	34	2	2
Lo Mein Chicken	1 pkg (8 oz)	320	35	1	3

FOOD	PORTION	CALS.	CARB.	SUG.	FIB.
Luigino's (CONT.)					
Lo Mein Shrimp	1 pkg (8 oz)	190	31	1	4
Oriental Beef & Peppers With Rice	1 pkg (8 oz)	230	38	1	2
Pasta Favorites					
Chicken Lo Mein	1 pkg (10.5 oz)	270	43	8	5
Rice Gourmet					
Chicken Teriyaki Rice Bowl	1 bowl (10.9 oz)	430	77	10	1
Stouffer's					
Chicken Chow Mein w/ Rice	1 pkg (10.6 oz)	260	40	3	3
Weight Watchers					
Smart Ones Chicken Chow Mein	1 pkg (9 oz)	200	34	5	3
Smart Ones Hunan Style Rice & Vegetables	1 pkg (10.34 oz)	250	39	6	8
Smart Ones King Pao Noodles & Vegetables	1 pkg (10 oz)	260	35	4	5
Smart Ones Spicy Szechaun Style Vegetables & Chicken	1 pkg (9 oz)	220	39	1	3
MIX					
La Choy					
Dinner Classics Egg Foo Young	2 patties + 3 oz sauce	170	20	—	1
Dinner Classics Pepper Steak	¾ cup	180	9	—	1
Dinner Classics Sweet & Sour	¾ cup	310	30	—	tr
ASPARAGUS					
CANNED					
Del Monte					
Salad Tips Tender Green	½ cup (4.4 oz)	20	3	0	1
Spears Cut Tender Green	½ cup (4.4 oz)	20	3	0	1
Spears Extra Long Tender Green	½ cup (4.4 oz)	20	3	0	1
Spears Tender Green	½ cup (4.4 oz)	20	3	0	1
Tips Tender Green	½ cup (4.4 oz)	20	3	0	1
Green Giant					
Cut Spears	½ cup (4.2 oz)	20	3	tr	1
Cut Spears 50% Less Sodium	½ cup (4.2 oz)	20	3	tr	1
Extra Long Spears	4.5 oz	20	3	tr	1

FOOD	PORTION	CALS.	CARB.	SUG.	FIB.
Green Giant (CONT.)					
Spears	4.5 oz	20	3	tr	1
LeSueur					
Spears Extra Large	4.5 oz	20	3	tr	1
Seneca					
Asparagus	½ cup	20	3	—	2
FRESH					
Dole					
Spears	5	18	2	—	2
FROZEN					
Big Valley					
Spears	5-6 (3 oz)	20	3	2	1
Green Giant					
Harvest Fresh Cuts	⅔ cup (3 oz)	25	4	tr	1
ATEMOYA					
fresh	½ cup	94	24	—	—
AVOCADO					
fresh	1	324	15	—	—
BACON					
(*see also* BACON SUBSTITUTES)					
breakfast strips cooked	3 strips	156	tr	—	0
gammon lean & fat grilled	4.2 oz	274	0	0	0
pan fried	3 strips	109	tr	—	0
Black Label					
Center Cut cooked	3 slices (0.5 oz)	70	0	0	0
Cooked	2 slices (0.5 oz)	80	0	0	0
Low Salt cooked	2 slices (0.5 oz)	80	0	0	0
Hormel					
Bacon Bits	1 tbsp (7 g)	30	0	0	0
Bacon Pieces	1 tbsp (7 g)	25	0	0	0
Microwave cooked	2 slices (0.5 oz)	70	0	0	0
Old Smokehouse					
Cooked	2 slices (0.5 oz)	80	0	0	0
Oscar Mayer					
Bacon Bits	1 tbsp (0.2 oz)	25	0	0	0
Bacon Pieces	1 tbsp (0.2 oz)	25	0	0	0
Center Cut cooked	2 slices (0.4 oz)	70	0	0	0
Cooked	2 slices (0.5 oz)	70	0	0	0
Lower Sodium cooked	2 slices (0.5 oz)	70	1	0	0
Thick Cut cooked	1 slice (0.4 oz)	60	0	0	0
Range Brand					
Cooked	2 slices (0.7 oz)	100	0	0	0

FOOD	PORTION	CALS.	CARB.	SUG.	FIB.
Red Label					
Cooked	2 slices (0.5 oz)	80	0	0	0

BACON SUBSTITUTES
Bac-Os

Pieces	1½ tbsp	30	2	0	0
Harvest Direct					
Bacon Bits	3.5 oz	320	24	—	17
Louis Rich					
Turkey Bacon	1 slice (0.5 oz)	35	0	0	0
Morningstar Farms					
Breakfast Strips	2 (0.5 oz)	60	2	0	tr
Worthington					
Stripples	2 strips (0.5 oz)	60	2	0	tr

BAGEL
FRESH

onion	1 (3½ in)	195	38	—	2
plain	1 (3½ in)	195	38	—	2
plain toasted	1 (3½ in)	195	38	—	2
poppy seed	1 (3½ in)	195	38	—	2
Alvarado St. Bakery					
Sprouted Wheat	1 (3.3 oz)	260	54	24	2
Sprouted Wheat Cinnamon/ Raisin	1 (3.3 oz)	280	59	28	3
Sprouted Wheat Onion/ Poppyseed	1 (3.3 oz)	320	66	8	2
Sprouted Wheat Sesame	1 (3.3 oz)	320	64	7	2

FROZEN
Amy's Organic

Cinnamon Raisin	1 (3.5 oz)	240	52	9	3
Plain	1 (3.5 oz)	230	48	2	2
Poppy Seed	1 (3.5 oz)	230	48	2	2
Sesame	1 (3.5 oz)	240	48	2	2
Lender's					
Cinnamon'N Raisin	1 (2.5 oz)	200	40	—	1
Onion	1 (2 oz)	160	31	—	1
Sara Lee					
Blueberry	1 (2.8 oz)	210	43	6	3
Cinnamon Raisin	1 (2.8 oz)	220	45	12	3
Egg	1 (2.8 oz)	210	44	7	2
Oat Bran	1 (2.8 oz)	210	42	7	3

FOOD	PORTION	CALS.	CARB.	SUG.	FIB.
Sara Lee (CONT.)					
Onion	1 (2.8 oz)	210	44	6	2
Plain	1 (2.8 oz)	210	43	3	2
Poppy Seed	1 (2.8 oz)	210	41	5	2
Sesame Seed	1 (2.8 oz)	210	42	5	2
Tree Of Life					
Onion	1 (3 oz)	210	44	3	0
Plain	1 (3 oz)	210	44	3	0
Poppy	1 (3 oz)	210	44	3	0
Raisin	1 (3 oz)	210	45	5	tr
Sesame	1 (3 oz)	210	44	3	0

BAKING POWDER
Calumet

Baking Powder	¼ tsp (1 g)	0	0	0	0
Watkins					
Baking Powder	¼ tsp (1 g)	0	0	0	0

BAKING SODA

baking soda	1 tsp	0	0	0	0

BALSAM PEAR

leafy tips cooked	½ cup	10	2	—	—
pods cooked	½ cup	12	3	—	—

BAMBOO SHOOTS
CANNED
Ka-Me

Sliced	½ cup (4.5 oz)	15	3	0	1
La Choy					
Sliced	¼ cup	6	1	—	tr
FRESH					
cooked	½ cup	15	2	—	—

BANANA

banana chips	1 oz	147	17	—	2
fresh	1	105	27	—	2
fresh mashed	1 cup	207	53	—	4
Dole					
Fresh	1	120	28	—	3
Rainforest Farms					
Slices Dried	5 slices (1.3 oz)	60	12	10	—

BANANA JUICE
Libby

Nectar	1 can (11.5 fl oz)	190	47	44	—

FOOD	PORTION	CALS.	CARB.	SUG.	FIB.
BARBECUE SAUCE					
(see also SAUCE)					
Healthy Choice					
Hickory	2 tbsp (1.1 oz)	26	6	2	tr
Hot & Spicy	2 tbsp (1.1 oz)	25	6	2	tr
Original	2 tbsp (1.1 oz)	25	6	2	tr
House Of Tsang					
Hong Kong	1 tbsp (0.6 oz)	10	2	1	0
Hunt's					
Barbeque	¼ cup (2.2 oz)	57	14	10	1
Bold Hickory	2 tbsp (1.2 oz)	47	11	9	1
Bold Original	2 tbsp (1.2 oz)	46	11	10	1
Hickory	2 tbsp (1.2 oz)	38	9	7	1
Hickory & Brown Sugar	2 tbsp (1.3 oz)	75	18	16	1
Honey Hickory	2 tbsp (1.2 oz)	38	9	7	1
Honey Mustard	2 tbsp (1.2 oz)	48	12	4	1
Hot & Spicy	2 tbsp (1.2 oz)	48	12	4	1
Light	2 tbsp (1.2 oz)	23	6	5	1
Mesquite Barbecue	2 tbsp (1.2 oz)	40	9	8	1
Mild	2 tbsp (1.2 oz)	41	10	7	1
Mild Dijon	2 tbsp (1.2 oz)	39	9	7	tr
Original	2 tbsp (1.2 oz)	39	9	8	1
Teriyaki	2 tbsp (1.2 oz)	46	11	10	1
Kraft					
Char-Grill	2 tbsp (1.3 oz)	60	13	11	0
Extra Rich Original	2 tbsp (1.2 oz)	50	12	10	0
Hickory Smoke	2 tbsp (1.2 oz)	40	9	7	0
Hickory Smoke Onion Bits	2 tbsp (1.2 oz)	45	11	9	0
Honey	2 tbsp (1.3 oz)	50	13	11	0
Honey Hickory	2 tbsp (1.3 oz)	60	14	12	0
Honey Mustard	2 tbsp (1.3 oz)	60	13	12	0
Hot	2 tbsp (1.2 oz)	40	9	7	0
Hot Hickory Smoke	2 tbsp (1.2 oz)	40	9	7	0
Kansas City Style	2 tbsp (1.2 oz)	50	11	9	0
Mesquite Smoke	2 tbsp (1.2 oz)	40	9	7	0
Molasses	2 tbsp (1.3 oz)	70	16	14	0
Onion Bits	2 tbsp (1.2 oz)	45	11	9	0
Original	2 tbsp (1.2 oz)	40	9	7	0
Roasted Garlic	2 tbsp (1.2 oz)	50	12	10	0
Spicy Honey	2 tbsp (1.3 oz)	60	14	13	0
Teriyaki	2 tbsp (1.3 oz)	60	12	10	0
Thick 'N Spicy Brown Sugar	2 tbsp (1.2 oz)	60	15	13	0

FOOD	PORTION	CALS.	CARB.	SUG.	FIB.
Kraft (CONT.)					
Thick 'N Spicy Hickory Bacon	2 tbsp (1.2 oz)	60	13	11	0
Thick 'N Spicy Hickory Smoke	2 tbsp (1.2 oz)	50	12	10	0
Thick 'N Spicy Honey	2 tbsp (1.3 oz)	60	13	11	0
Thick 'N Spicy Honey Mustard	2 tbsp (1.3 oz)	60	14	12	0
Thick'N Spicy Hickory Smoke	2 tbsp (1.2 oz)	50	12	10	0
Thick'N Spicy Honey	2 tbsp (1.2 oz)	60	13	11	0
Thick'N Spicy Kansas City Style	2 tbsp (1.3 oz)	60	14	12	0
Thick'N Spicy Mesquite Smoke	2 tbsp (1.2 oz)	50	12	10	0
Thick'N Spicy Original	2 tbsp (1.2 oz)	50	12	10	0
Lawry's					
Dijon Honey	¼ cup	203	27	—	tr
McIlhenny					
Sauce	2 tbsp (1.1 oz)	70	6	3	tr
Red Wing					
"K" Sauce	2 tbsp (1.2 oz)	45	9	8	0
Watkins					
Bold	2 tsp (0.4 oz)	25	5	4	0
Honey	2 tsp (0.4 oz)	25	6	5	0
Mesquite	2 tsp (0.4 oz)	25	5	5	0
Original	2 tsp (0.4 oz)	25	5	5	0
Smokehouse	2 tsp (0.4 oz)	25	5	5	0
BARLEY					
flour	1 cup (5.2 oz)	511	110	—	15
malt flour	1 cup (5.7 oz)	585	127	—	12
pearled cooked	1 cup (5.5 oz)	193	44	—	6
pearled uncooked	1 cup (7 oz)	704	155	—	31
Arrowhead					
Barley	¼ cup (1.7 oz)	170	37	tr	6
Hulless	¼ cup (1.6 oz)	140	35	0	6
Quaker					
Medium Pearled	¼ cup	172	36	—	5
Quick Pearled	¼ cup	172	36	—	5
Scotch					
Medium Pearled	¼ cup	172	36	—	5
Quick Pearled	¼ cup	172	36	—	5
BASIL					
fresh chopped	2 tbsp	1	tr	—	—

FOOD	PORTION	CALS.	CARB.	SUG.	FIB.
ground	1 tsp	4	1	—	—
leaves fresh	5	1	tr	—	—
Watkins					
Liquid Spice	1 tbsp (0.5 oz)	120	0	0	0

BASS

sea cooked	3 oz	105	0	0	0
striped baked	3 oz	105	0	0	0

BAY LEAF

crumbled	1 tsp	2	tr	—	—
Watkins					
Bay Leaves	¼ tsp (0.5 g)	0	0	0	0

BEAN SPROUTS

La Choy					
Bean Sprouts	⅔ cup	8	1	—	tr

BEANS

(*see also individual names*)

CANNED

FOOD	PORTION	CALS.	CARB.	SUG.	FIB.
baked beans plain	½ cup	118	26	—	10
baked beans vegetarian	½ cup	118	26	—	10
baked beans w/ franks	½ cup	182	20	—	9
baked beans w/ pork	½ cup	133	25	—	7
baked beans w/ pork & sweet sauce	½ cup	140	26	—	7
baked beans w/ pork & tomato sauce	½ cup	123	24	—	7
Allen					
Baked	½ cup (4.5 oz)	150	29	10	8
B&M					
99% Fat Free Baked Beans	½ cup (4.6 oz)	160	31	8	7
Baked With Honey	½ cup (4.7 oz)	170	30	7	8
Barbeque Baked Beans	½ cup (4.7 oz)	170	32	8	6
Brick Oven Baked	½ cup (4.6 oz)	180	32	10	7
Extra Hearty Baked	½ cup (4.6 oz)	190	36	14	8
Brown Beauty					
Mexican Beans With Jalapeno	½ cup (4.5 oz)	120	21	1	7
Bush's					
Baked	½ cup (4.6 oz)	150	29	5	7
Baked With Onions	½ cup (4.6 oz)	150	26	6	6
Homestyle Baked	½ cup (4.6 oz)	160	28	8	8
Vegetarian	½ cup (4.6 oz)	140	24	4	6

FOOD	PORTION	CALS.	CARB.	SUG.	FIB.
Chi-Chi's					
Refried	½ cup (4.2 oz)	100	18	1	4
Refried Beans Fat Free	½ cup (4.2 oz)	120	17	1	4
Refried Beans Vegetarian	½ cup (4.2 oz)	100	18	1	4
Crest Top					
Pork And Beans	½ cup (4.5 oz)	130	21	1	6
Eden					
Organic Baked w/ Sweet Sorghum & Organic Mustard	½ cup (4.6 oz)	150	27	6	7
Friend's					
Maple Baked	8 oz	240	52	—	11
Original Baked	½ cup (4.6 oz)	170	32	10	7
Gebhardt					
Chili	4 oz	115	21	—	5
Refried	4 oz	100	20	—	7
Refried Jalapeno	4 oz	115	19	—	7
Green Giant					
Pork And Beans w/ Tomato Sauce	½ cup (4.5 oz)	120	23	4	4
Spicy Chili	½ cup (4.5 oz)	110	20	1	5
Three Bean Salad	½ cup (4.2 oz)	90	20	10	4
Health Valley					
Boston Baked	7.5 oz	190	41	—	5
Boston Baked No Salt Added	7.5 oz	190	41	—	5
Fast Menu Honey Baked Organic Beans With Tofu Weiner	7.5 oz	150	15	—	16
Vegetarian With Miso	7.5 oz	180	38	—	5
Heartland					
Iron Kettle Baked	½ cup (4.6 oz)	150	29	13	5
Hormel					
Beans & Wieners	1 can (7.5 oz)	290	34	12	6
Hunt's					
Big John's Beans & Fixin's	½ cup (4.7 oz)	127	23	11	6
Pork & Beans	½ cup (4.5 oz)	130	28	16	4
Kid's Kitchen					
Microwave Meals Beans & Weiners	1 cup (7.5 oz)	310	37	13	8
McIlhenny					
Spicy	1 oz	7	1	1	1

FOOD	PORTION	CALS.	CARB.	SUG.	FIB.
Old El Paso					
Mexe-Beans	½ cup (4.6 oz)	110	19	0	7
Refried	½ cup (4.2 oz)	110	17	1	5
Refried Fat Free	½ cup (4.4 oz)	110	20	1	6
Refried Spicy	½ cup (4.3 oz)	140	22	1	6
Refried Vegetarian	½ cup (4.1 oz)	100	16	2	6
Refried With Cheese	½ cup (4.2 oz)	130	18	1	6
Refried With Green Chilies	½ cup (4.3 oz)	110	19	1	6
Refried With Sausage	½ cup (4.1 oz)	200	14	1	8
Rosarita					
Refried	4 oz	100	18	—	6
Refried Spicy	4 oz	100	19	—	6
Refried Vegetarian	4 oz	100	18	—	6
Refried With Bacon	4 oz	110	20	—	6
Refried With Green Chilies	4 oz	90	18	—	6
Refried With Nacho Cheese	4 oz	110	20	—	6
Refried With Onions	4 oz	110	21	—	6
Taco Bell					
Home Originals Fat Free Refried Beans	½ cup (4.6 oz)	110	21	1	6
Home Originals Fat Free Refried Beans w/ Mild Chilies	½ cup (4.5 oz)	110	20	tr	5
Home Originals Refried Beans	½ cup (4.7 oz)	140	23	1	7
Trappey					
Mexi-Beans With Jalapeno	½ cup (4.5 oz)	130	22	6	8
Pork And Beans	½ cup (4.5 oz)	110	21	3	7
Pork And Beans With Jalapeno	½ cup (4.5 oz)	130	24	9	6
Van Camp's					
Baked Beans Fat Free	½ cup (4.6 oz)	130	28	—	5
Baked Beans Premium	½ cup (4.6 oz)	140	29	—	5
Beanee Weenee	1 cup (9 oz)	320	35	—	8
Beanee Weenee Baked Flavor	1 cup (9 oz)	410	58	—	10
Beanee Weenee Barbeque	1 cup (9 oz)	340	43	—	8
Brown Sugar Beans	½ cup (4.6 oz)	170	31	—	6
Mexican Style Chili Beans	½ cup (4.6 oz)	110	21	—	8
Pork And Beans	½ cup (4.6 oz)	110	24	—	6
Vegetarian In Tomato Sauce	½ cup (4.6 oz)	110	23	—	5

FOOD	PORTION	CALS.	CARB.	SUG.	FIB.
Wagon Master					
Pork And Beans	½ cup (4.5 oz)	110	21	3	7
FROZEN					
Natural Touch					
Nine Bean Loaf	1 in slice (3 oz)	160	13	tr	5
MIX					
Melting Pot					
Terrazza Napoli Mixed Beans	1 cup	200	41	7	2

BEAR
simmered	3 oz	220	0	0	0

BEAVER
roasted	3 oz	140	0	0	0
simmered	3 oz	141	0	0	0

BEECHNUTS
dried	1 oz	164	10	—	—

BEEF
(*see also* BEEF DISHES, VEAL)

FOOD	PORTION	CALS.	CARB.	SUG.	FIB.
CANNED					
Armour					
Tripe	3 oz	90	0	0	0
Hormel					
Corned Beef	2 oz	120	0	0	0
Cubed Beef	½ cup (4.9 oz)	130	0	0	0
Potted Meat	4 tbsp (2 oz)	100	0	0	0
Treet					
50% Less Fat	2 oz	120	4	—	—
DRIED					
Hormel					
Pillow Pack	10 slices (1 oz)	45	0	0	0
Rough Cut					
Beef Steak Hot	1 pkg (1 oz)	70	2	2	0
Beef Steak Original	1 pkg (1 oz)	60	2	2	0
Beef Steak Peppered	1 pkg (1 oz)	60	2	1	0
FRESH					
bottom round lean & fat trim 0 in Choice roasted	3 oz	172	0	0	0
bottom round lean & fat trim 0 in Select braised	3 oz	171	0	0	0
bottom round lean & fat trim 0 in Select roasted	3 oz	150	0	0	0
bottom round lean & fat trim 0 in braised	3 oz	193	0	0	0

FOOD	PORTION	CALS.	CARB.	SUG.	FIB.
bottom round lean & fat trim ¼ in Choice braised	3 oz	241	0	0	0
bottom round lean & fat trim ¼ in Choice roasted	3 oz	221	0	0	0
bottom round lean & fat trim ¼ in Select braised	3 oz	220	0	0	0
bottom round lean & fat trim ¼ in Select roasted	3 oz	199	0	0	0
brisket flat half lean & fat trim 0 in braised	3 oz	183	0	0	0
brisket flat half lean & fat trim ¼ in braised	3 oz	309	0	0	0
brisket point half lean & fat trim 0 in braised	3 oz	304	0	0	0
brisket point half lean & fat trim ¼ in braised	3 oz	343	0	0	0
brisket whole lean & fat trim 0 in braised	3 oz	247	0	0	0
brisket whole lean & fat trim ¼ in braised	3 oz	327	0	0	0
chuck arm pot roast lean & fat trim 0 in braised	3 oz	238	0	0	0
chuck arm pot roast lean & fat trim ¼ in braised	3 oz	282	0	0	0
chuck blade roast lean & fat trim 0 in braised	3 oz	284	0	0	0
chuck blade roast lean & fat trim ¼ in braised	3 oz	293	0	0	0
corned beef brisket cooked	3 oz	213	tr	—	—
eye of round lean & fat trim 0 in Choice roasted	3 oz	153	0	0	0
eye of round lean & fat trim 0 in Select roasted	3 oz	137	0	0	0
eye of round lean & fat trim ¼ in Choice roasted	3 oz	205	0	0	0
eye of round lean & fat trim ¼ in Select roasted	3 oz	184	0	0	0
flank lean & fat trim 0 in braised	3 oz	224	0	0	0
flank lean & fat trim 0 in broiled	3 oz	192	0	0	0
ground extra lean broiled medium	3 oz	217	0	0	0
ground extra lean broiled well done	3 oz	225	0	0	0

FOOD	PORTION	CALS.	CARB.	SUG.	FIB.
ground extra lean fried medium	3 oz	216	0	0	0
ground extra lean fried well done	3 oz	224	0	0	0
ground extra lean raw	4 oz	265	0	0	0
ground lean broiled medium	3 oz	231	0	0	0
ground lean broiled well done	3 oz	238	0	0	0
ground regular broiled medium	3 oz	246	0	0	0
ground regular broiled well done	3 oz	248	0	0	0
ground low-fat w/ carrageenan raw	4 oz	160	tr	—	—
porterhouse steak lean & fat trim ¼ in Choice broiled	3 oz	260	0	0	0
porterhouse steak lean only trim ¼ in Prime broiled	3 oz	185	0	0	0
rib eye small end lean & fat trim 0 in Choice broiled	3 oz	261	0	0	0
rib large end lean & fat trim 0 in roasted	3 oz	300	0	0	0
rib large end lean & fat trim ¼ in broiled	3 oz	295	0	0	0
rib large end lean & fat trim ¼ in roasted	3 oz	310	0	0	0
rib small end lean & fat trim 0 in broiled	3 oz	252	0	0	0
rib small end lean & fat trim ¼ in broiled	3 oz	285	0	0	0
rib small end lean & fat trim ¼ in roasted	3 oz	295	0	0	0
rib whole lean & fat trim ¼ in Choice broiled	3 oz	306	0	0	0
rib whole lean & fat trim ¼ in Choice roasted	3 oz	320	0	0	0
rib whole lean & fat trim ¼ in Prime roasted	3 oz	348	0	0	0
rib whole lean & fat trim ¼ in Select broiled	3 oz	274	0	0	0
rib whole lean & fat trim ¼ in Select roasted	3 oz	286	0	0	0
shank crosscut lean & fat trim ¼ in Choice simmered	3 oz	224	0	0	0
short loin top loin lean & fat trim 0 in Choice broiled	3 oz	193	0	0	0

FOOD	PORTION	CALS.	CARB.	SUG.	FIB.
short loin top loin lean & fat trim 0 in Choice broiled	1 steak (5.4 oz)	353	0	0	0
short loin top loin lean & fat trim 0 in Select broiled	1 steak (5.4 oz)	309	0	0	0
short loin top loin lean & fat trim ¼ in Choice braised	3 oz	253	0	0	0
short loin top loin lean & fat trim ¼ in Choice broiled	1 steak (6.3 oz)	536	0	0	0
short loin top loin lean & fat trim ¼ in Prime broiled	1 steak (6.3 oz)	582	0	0	0
short loin top loin lean & fat trim ¼ in Select broiled	1 steak (6.3 oz)	473	0	0	0
short loin top loin lean only trim 0 in Choice broiled	1 steak (5.2 oz)	311	0	0	0
short loin top loin lean only trim ¼ in Choice broiled	1 steak (5.2 oz)	314	0	0	0
shortribs lean & fat Choice braised	3 oz	400	0	0	0
t-bone steak lean & fat trim ¼ in Choice broiled	3 oz	253	0	0	0
t-bone steak lean only trim ¼ in Choice broiled	3 oz	182	0	0	0
tenderloin lean & fat trim 0 in Select broiled	3 oz	194	0	0	0
tenderloin lean & fat trim ¼ in Choice broiled	3 oz	259	0	0	0
tenderloin lean & fat trim ¼ in Choice roasted	3 oz	288	0	0	0
tenderloin lean & fat trim ¼ in Choice broiled	3 oz	208	0	0	0
tenderloin lean & fat trim ¼ in Prime broiled	3 oz	270	0	0	0
tenderloin lean & fat trim ¼ in Select roasted	3 oz	275	0	0	0
tenderloin lean only trim 0 in Select broiled	3 oz	170	0	0	0
tenderloin lean only trim ¼ in Choice broiled	3 oz	188	0	0	0
tenderloin lean only trim ¼ in Select broiled	3 oz	169	0	0	0
tip round lean & fat trim 0 in Choice roasted	3 oz	170	0	0	0
tip round lean & fat trim 0 in Select roasted	3 oz	158	0	0	0

FOOD	PORTION	CALS.	CARB.	SUG.	FIB.
tip round lean & fat trim ¼ in Choice roasted	3 oz	210	0	0	0
tip round lean & fat trim ¼ in Prime roasted	3 oz	233	0	0	0
tip round lean & fat trim ¼ in Select roasted	3 oz	191	0	0	0
top round lean & fat trim 0 in Choice braised	3 oz	184	0	0	0
top round lean & fat trim 0 in Select braised	3 oz	170	0	0	0
top round lean & fat trim ¼ in Choice braised	3 oz	221	0	0	0
top round lean & fat trim ¼ in Choice broiled	3 oz	190	0	0	0
top round lean & fat trim ¼ in Choice fried	3 oz	235	0	0	0
top round lean & fat trim ¼ in Prime broiled	3 oz	195	0	0	0
top round lean & fat trim ¼ in Select braised	3 oz	199	0	0	0
top sirloin lean & fat trim 0 in Choice broiled	3 oz	194	0	0	0
top sirloin lean & fat trim 0 in Select broiled	3 oz	166	0	0	0
top sirloin lean & fat trim ¼ in Choice broiled	3 oz	228	0	0	0
top sirloin lean & fat trim ¼ in Choice fried	3 oz	277	0	0	0
top sirloin lean & fat trim ¼ in Select broiled	3 oz	208	0	0	0
tripe raw	4 oz	111	0	0	0
READY-TO-EAT					
Healthy Choice					
Deli-Thin Roast Beef	6 slices (2 oz)	60	1	1	0
Fresh-Trak Roast Beef	1 slice (1 oz)	30	0	0	0
Jordan's					
Healthy Trim 97% Fat Free Roast Beef Medium	1 slice (1 oz)	30	0	0	0
Healthy Trim 97% Fat Free Roast Beef Rare	1 slice (1 oz)	30	0	0	0

BEEF DISHES
CANNED
Dinty Moore

Meatball Stew	1 cup (8.4 oz)	250	17	3	2

FOOD	PORTION	CALS.	CARB.	SUG.	FIB.
Dinty Moore (CONT.)					
Sliced Potatoes & Beef	1 can (7.5 oz)	230	28	1	4
Stew	1 cup (8.3 oz)	230	16	3	2
Stew	1 cup (8.2 oz)	230	16	3	2
Hormel					
Beef Goulash	1 can (7.5 oz)	230	19	6	3
Roast Beef With Gravy	2 oz	60	1	0	0
Mary Kitchen					
Corned Beef Hash	1 cup (8.3 oz)	410	22	1	2
Roast Beef Hash	1 cup (8.3 oz)	390	22	1	2
Roast Turkey Hash	1 can (14.9 oz)	420	42	4	3
Sausage Hash	1 cup (8.3 oz)	410	23	1	2
FROZEN					
Hot Pocket					
Stuffed Sandwich Barbecue	1 (4.5 oz)	340	45	10	1
Stuffed Sandwich Beef & Cheddar	1 (4.5 oz)	360	36	5	tr
Stuffed Sandwich Beef Fajita	1 (4.5 oz)	360	39	3	5
Lean Pockets					
Stuffed Sandwich Beef & Broccoli	1 (4.5 oz)	250	37	5	7
Luigino's					
Creamed Sauce Shaved Cured Beef With Croutons	1 pkg (8 oz)	360	29	1	3
Egg Noodles Rich Gravy Swedish Meatballs	1 pkg (9 oz)	340	36	1	3
Egg Noodles Rich Gravy Swedish Meatballs	1 cup (7.5 oz)	280	30	1	3
Mrs. Paterson's					
Aussie Pie Philly Steak	1 (5.5 oz)	420	39	3	2
MIX					
Casbah					
Gyro as prep	1 patty (2 oz)	145	12	0	tr
Hamburger Helper					
BBQ Beef as prep	1 cup	320	37	8	1
Beef Pasta as prep	1 cup	270	26	2	tr
Beef Romanoff as prep	1 cup	280	27	4	0
Beef Stew as prep	1 cup	250	26	3	2
Beef Taco as prep	1 cup	310	31	4	1
Beef Teriyaki as prep	1 cup	290	34	5	2
Cheddar 'n Bacon as prep	1 cup	350	28	5	tr
Cheddar Melt as prep	1 cup	310	31	4	tr
Cheddar Spirals Reduced Sodium as prep	1 cup	320	27	5	1

FOOD	PORTION	CALS.	CARB.	SUG.	FIB.
Hamburger Helper (CONT.)					
Cheeseburger Macaroni as prep	1 cup	360	31	6	tr
Cheesy Italian as prep	1 cup	330	29	6	tr
Cheesy Shells as prep	1 cup	340	30	5	tr
Chili Macaroni as prep	1 cup	290	30	4	tr
Fettuccine Alfredo as prep	1 cup	310	26	5	1
Four Cheese Lasagne as prep	1 cup	330	31	6	0
Italian Herb Reduced Sodium as prep	1 cup	270	29	6	2
Italian Rigatoni as prep	1 cup	280	29	6	1
Lasagne as prep	1 cup	280	30	7	0
Meat Loaf as prep	1/6 loaf	270	11	3	0
Mushroom & Wild Rice as prep	1 cup	310	30	4	2
Nacho Cheese as prep	1 cup	320	30	5	tr
Pizza Pasta as prep	1 cup	290	31	5	0
Pizzabake as prep	1/6 pie	270	28	4	tr
Potatoes Au Gratin as prep	1 cup	290	24	5	2
Potatoes Stroganoff as prep	1 cup	270	25	2	2
Ravioli as prep	1 cup	280	30	5	1
Rice Oriental as prep	1 cup	310	35	4	0
Salisbury as prep	1 cup	270	26	2	tr
Southwestern Beef Reduced Sodium as prep	1 cup	300	32	6	2
Spaghetti as prep	1 cup	300	29	6	tr
Stroganoff as prep	1 cup	320	30	7	0
Swedish Meatballs as prep	1 cup	300	24	2	tr
Three Cheeses as prep	1 cup	340	32	5	tr
Zesty Italian as prep	1 cup	320	34	8	tr
Zesty Mexican as prep	1 cup	300	32	5	1
SHELF-STABLE					
Dinty Moore					
Microwave Cup Corned Beef Hash	1 pkg (7.5 oz)	350	19	1	2
Microwave Cup Hearty Burger Stew	1 pkg (7.5 oz)	240	19	5	3
Microwave Cup Stew	1 pkg (7.5 oz)	190	15	2	2
Hormel					
Microcup Meals Stew	1 cup (7.5 oz)	190	15	3	2
BEEFALO					
roasted	3 oz	160	0	0	0

FOOD	PORTION	CALS.	CARB.	SUG.	FIB.

BEER AND ALE

FOOD	PORTION	CALS.	CARB.	SUG.	FIB.
alcohol free beer	7 fl oz	50	11	5	—
ale brown	10 oz	77	8	—	0
ale pale	10 oz	88	12	—	0
lager	10 oz	80	4	—	0
pilsener lager beer	7 fl oz	85	13	2	—
stout	10 oz	102	6	—	0

BEETS
CANNED
Del Monte

FOOD	PORTION	CALS.	CARB.	SUG.	FIB.
Pickled Crinkle Style Sliced	½ cup (4.5 oz)	80	19	16	2
Sliced	½ cup (4.3 oz)	35	8	5	2
Whole	½ cup (4.3 oz)	35	8	5	2
Whole Tiny	½ cup (4.3 oz)	35	8	5	2

Green Giant

FOOD	PORTION	CALS.	CARB.	SUG.	FIB.
Harvard	⅓ cup (3.1 oz)	60	15	10	2
Sliced	½ cup (4.2 oz)	35	8	5	2
Sliced No Salt Added	½ cup (4.2 oz)	35	8	5	2
Whole	½ cup (4.2 oz)	35	8	5	2

LeSueur

FOOD	PORTION	CALS.	CARB.	SUG.	FIB.
Baby Whole	½ cup (4.3 oz)	35	8	5	2

Seneca

FOOD	PORTION	CALS.	CARB.	SUG.	FIB.
Cut	½ cup	35	9	—	2
Diced	½ cup	35	9	—	2
Harvard	½ cup	90	21	—	1
Pickled	2 tbsp	20	6	—	0
Pickled With Onions	2 tbsp	20	6	—	0
Sliced	½ cup	35	9	—	2
Whole	½ cup	35	9	—	2

BEVERAGES

(*see* BEER AND ALE, CHAMPAGNE, COFFEE, DRINK MIXERS, FRUIT DRINKS, ICED TEA, LIQUOR/LIQUEUR, MALT, MILKSHAKE, MINERAL/BOTTLED WATER, SODA, SPORTS DRINKS, TEA/HERBAL TEA, WINE, WINE COOLER)

BISCUIT
FROZEN
Jimmy Dean

FOOD	PORTION	CALS.	CARB.	SUG.	FIB.
Chicken Twin	2 (3.2 oz)	280	32	3	2
Sausage Twin	2 (3.4 oz)	330	25	3	2
Steak Twin	2 (3.2 oz)	270	26	3	2

Rudy's Farm

FOOD	PORTION	CALS.	CARB.	SUG.	FIB.
Ham Twin	2 (3 oz)	160	23	2	1
Sausage & Cheese Twin	2 (3 oz)	290	22	2	1

FOOD	PORTION	CALS.	CARB.	SUG.	FIB.
Rudy's Farm (CONT.)					
Sausage Twin	2 (2.7 oz)	296	22	2	1
HOME RECIPE					
oatcakes	2 (4 oz)	115	16	—	1
MIX					
buttermilk	1 (2 oz)	191	28	—	1
plain	1 (2 oz)	191	28	—	1
Arrowhead					
Biscuit Mix	¼ cup (1.2 oz)	120	23	4	3
Bisquick					
Reduced Fat	⅓ cup (1.4 oz)	150	28	2	1
Health Valley					
Buttermilk Biscuit Mix not prep	1 oz	100	20	—	3
Jiffy					
As prep	1	150	30	—	2
Biscuit	¼ cup (1.1 oz)	130	22	tr	1
Buttermilk as prep	1	170	29	2	tr
REFRIGERATED					
buttermilk	1 (1 oz)	98	14	—	—
Roman Meal					
Biscuit	2 (2.4 oz)	180	34	—	1
Honey Nut Oat Bran	1 (1.5 oz)	131	21	—	1
BISON					
roasted	3 oz	122	0	0	0
BLACK BEANS					
CANNED					
Allen					
Seasoned	½ cup (4.5 oz)	120	20	3	7
Eden					
Organic	½ cup (4.6 oz)	100	18	—	6
Organic w/ Ginger & Lemon	½ cup (4.6 oz)	120	21	1	7
Green Giant					
Black Beans	½ cup (4.5 oz)	50	18	tr	5
Health Valley					
Fast Menu Organic Black Beans With Tofu Weiners	7.5 oz	150	20	—	15
Fast Menu Western Black Beans With Garden Vegetable	7.5 oz	160	14	—	14
Old El Paso					
Black Beans	½ cup (4.6 oz)	100	17	0	7

FOOD	PORTION	CALS.	CARB.	SUG.	FIB.
Old El Paso (CONT.)					
Refried	½ cup (4.2 oz)	120	18	2	6
Progresso					
Black Beans	½ cup (4.6 oz)	100	17	0	7
Trappey					
Seasoned	½ cup (4.5 oz)	120	20	3	7
MIX					
Mahatma					
Black Beans & Rice	1 cup	200	39	1	6
BLACKBERRIES					
canned in heavy syrup	½ cup	118	30	—	—
fresh	½ cup	37	9	—	3
Allen-Wolco					
Canned	½ cup (5.3 oz)	60	13	3	9
Big Valley					
Frozen	⅔ cup (4.9 oz)	70	15	8	4
BLACKBERRY JUICE					
Kool-Aid					
Scary Blackberry Ghoul-Aid Drink as prep w/ sugar	1 serv (8 oz)	100	25	25	0
BLACKEYE PEAS					
CANNED					
Allen					
Blackeye Peas	½ cup (4.5 oz)	110	18	0	4
Fresh Shell	½ cup (4.4 oz)	120	21	tr	6
With Bacon	½ cup (4.5 oz)	105	20	tr	5
With Snaps	½ cup (4.4 oz)	120	20	0	5
Dorman					
Fresh Shell	½ cup (4.4 oz)	120	21	tr	6
East Texas Fair					
Blackeye Peas	½ cup (4.5 oz)	110	18	0	4
Fresh Shell	½ cup (4.4 oz)	120	21	tr	6
With Snaps	½ cup (4.4 oz)	120	20	0	5
Green Giant					
Blackeye Peas	½ cup (4.4 oz)	90	16	tr	3
Homefolks					
Fresh Shell	½ cup (4.4 oz)	120	21	tr	6
With Jalapeno	½ cup (4.4 oz)	120	20	0	5
With Snaps	½ cup (4.4 oz)	120	20	0	5
Sunshine					
With Bacon	½ cup (4.5 oz)	105	20	tr	5
Trappey					
With Bacon	½ cup (4.5 oz)	120	19	3	5

FOOD	PORTION	CALS.	CARB.	SUG.	FIB.
Trappey (CONT.)					
With Bacon & Jalapeno	½ cup (4.4 oz)	110	19	2	5
DRIED					
cooked	1 cup	198	36	—	16
Hurst					
HamBeens California	1 serv	120	22	1	¬
w/ Ham					
FROZEN					
Birds Eye					
Blackeye Peas	½ cup (2.8 oz)	110	21	1	4
Fresh Like	3.5 oz	138	24	—	1

BLINTZE

FOOD	PORTION	CALS.	CARB.	SUG.	FIB.
Empire					
Apple	2 (4.4 oz)	220	36	12	5
Blueberry	2 (4.4 oz)	190	36	12	2
Cheese	2 (4.4 oz)	200	29	8	3
Cherry	2 (4.4 oz)	200	38	10	3
Potato	2 (4.4 oz)	190	32	0	3

BLUEBERRIES

FOOD	PORTION	CALS.	CARB.	SUG.	FIB.
Big Valley					
Frozen	¾ cup (4.9 oz)	70	12	8	4
Sonoma					
Dried	¼ cup (1.3 oz)	140	33	17	5

BLUEBERRY JUICE

FOOD	PORTION	CALS.	CARB.	SUG.	FIB.
After The Fall					
Maine Coast	1 cup (8 oz)	90	25	19	0

BLUEFIN

FOOD	PORTION	CALS.	CARB.	SUG.	FIB.
fillet baked	4.1 oz	186	0	0	0

BLUEFISH

FOOD	PORTION	CALS.	CARB.	SUG.	FIB.
fresh baked	3 oz	135	0	0	0

BOAR

FOOD	PORTION	CALS.	CARB.	SUG.	FIB.
wild roasted	3 oz	136	0	0	0

BOK CHOY

FOOD	PORTION	CALS.	CARB.	SUG.	FIB.
Dole					
Shredded	½ cup	5	1	—	

BONIATO

FOOD	PORTION	CALS.	CARB.	SUG.	FIB.
fresh	½ cup	90	20	—	—

BORAGE

FOOD	PORTION	CALS.	CARB.	SUG.	FIB.
fresh chopped cooked	3½ oz	25	4	—	–

FOOD	PORTION	CALS.	CARB.	SUG.	FIB.
BOTTLED WATER					
(*see* MINERAL/BOTTLED WATER)					
BRAINS					
beef pan-fried	3 oz	167	0	0	0
beef simmered	3 oz	136	0	0	0
lamb braised	3 oz	124	0	0	0
lamb fried	3 oz	232	0	0	0
pork braised	3 oz	117	0	0	0
veal braised	3 oz	115	0	0	0
veal fried	3 oz	181	0	0	0
Armour					
Pork Brains In Milk Gravy	⅔ cup (5.5 oz)	150	10	—	—
BRAN					
corn	1 cup (2.7 oz)	170	65	—	65
oat	½ cup (1.6 oz)	116	31	—	7
oat cooked	½ cup (3.8 oz)	44	13	—	3
rice	½ cup (2.1 oz)	187	29	—	12
wheat	½ cup (2 oz)	63	19	—	12
Arrowhead					
Oat Bran	⅓ cup (1.4 oz)	150	23	0	7
Wheat Bran	¼ cup (0.6 oz)	30	7	0	6
Good Shepherd					
Wheat Bran	1 oz	80	18	—	3
H-O					
Super Bran	⅓ cup	110	18	—	3
Health Valley					
Fast Menu Oat Bran Pilaf With Garden Vegetables	7.5 oz	210	30	—	15
Hodgson Mill					
Oat	¼ cup (1.3 oz)	120	23	0	6
Wheat	¼ cup (0.5 oz)	30	10	0	7
Kretschmer					
Toasted Wheat Bran	⅓ cup	57	15	—	3
Mother's					
Oat Bran	½ cup	150	24	1	6
Quaker					
Oat Bran	½ cup (1.4 oz)	150	25	1	6
Unprocessed	2 tbsp	8	4	—	3
Roman Meal					
Oat	1 oz	94	13	0	5

FOOD	PORTION	CALS.	CARB.	SUG.	FIB.
Stone-Buhr					
Oat	⅓ cup (1 oz)	90	20	0	4

BREAD

(*see also* BAGEL, BISCUIT, BREADSTICK, CROISSANT, ENGLISH MUFFIN, MUFFIN, ROLL, SCONE)

CANNED

FOOD	PORTION	CALS.	CARB.	SUG.	FIB.
boston brown	1 slice (1.6 oz)	88	20	—	2
B&M					
Brown Bread	½ in slice (2 oz)	130	29	9	2
Brown Bread Raisins	½ in slice (2 oz)	130	29	11	2
FROZEN					
Kineret					
Challah	⅛ loaf (2 oz)	150	25	3	1
New York					
Garlic	1 slice (2 oz)	190	27	1	1
Garlic Reduced Fat	1 slice (2 oz)	160	29	1	1
Texas Garlic Toast	1 in slice (1.4 oz)	160	17	1	1
MIX					
cornbread	1 piece (2 oz)	189	29	—	1
Aunt Jemima					
Corn Bread Easy Mix	⅓ cup (1.3 oz)	150	26	6	1
Natural Ovens					
Cracked Wheat	2 slices (2.4 oz)	140	38	0	4
English Muffin Bread	2 slices (2.4 oz)	140	35	0	2
Executive Fitness Sunny Millet	2 slices (2.6 oz)	160	37	0	4
Garden Bread	1 oz	50	14	0	1
Glorious Cinnamon & Raisin Fat Free	2 slices (2.1 oz)	110	30	0	3
Honey 'N Flax	2 slices (2.5 oz)	140	30	0	4
Hunger Filler Bread	2 slices (2.1 oz)	110	28	0	5
Light Wheat	2 slices (2.2 oz)	84	30	0	5
Nutty Natural Wheat Bread	2 slices (2.5 oz)	140	32	0	6
Seven Grain Herb	2 slices (2.5 oz)	140	30	0	4
Soft Hearth Whole Wheat	2 slices (2 oz)	100	30	0	4
Soft Sandwich Very Low Fat	2 slices (2.3 oz)	110	26	0	2
Stay Slim	2 slices (2 oz)	100	20	0	4
READY-TO-EAT					
baguette whole wheat	2 oz	140	29	tr	1
cracked wheat	1 slice	65	12	—	1
italian	1 slice (1 oz)	81	15	—	1
oat bran	1 slice	71	12	—	1

FOOD	PORTION	CALS.	CARB.	SUG.	FIB.
oatmeal	1 slice	73	13	—	1
pita	1 reg (2 oz)	165	33	—	1
pita	1 sm (1 oz)	78	16	—	1
pita whole wheat	1 sm (1 oz)	76	16	—	2
pita whole wheat	1 reg (2 oz)	170	35	—	5
pumpernickel	1 slice	80	15	—	2
rye	1 slice	83	16	—	2
seven grain	1 slice	65	12	—	2
sourdough	1 slice (1 oz)	78	15	—	1
vienna	1 slice (1 oz)	78	15	—	1
wheat reduced calorie	1 slice	46	10	—	3
wheat berry	1 slice	65	12	—	1
wheat bran	1 slice	89	17	—	3
white	1 slice	67	12	—	1
white reduced calorie	1 slice	48	10	—	2
whole wheat	1 slice	70	13	—	2
Alvarado St. Bakery					
Barley	1 slice (1.2 oz)	70	15	3	2
California Style	1 slice (1.2 oz)	60	10	1	2
French	1 slice (1.2 oz)	80	15	2	2
Multi-Grain	1 slice (1.2 oz)	60	11	2	2
Multi-Grain No-Salt	1 slice (1.2 oz)	60	11	1	2
Oat Berry	1 slice (1.2 oz)	70	13	2	2
Raisin	1 slice (1.1 oz)	80	15	6	2
Rye Seed	1 slice (1.2 oz)	60	11	1	2
Sourdough	1 slice (1.2 oz)	80	15	2	2
Wheat	1 slice (1.3 oz)	90	18	3	3
Arnold					
12 Grain Natural	1 slice (0.8 oz)	60	10	—	1
Augusto Pan De Aqua	1 oz	80	14	—	1
Bran'nola Country Oat	1 slice (1.3 oz)	90	16	—	3
Bran'nola Dark Wheat	1 slice (1.3 oz)	90	15	—	3
Bran'nola Hearty Wheat	1 slice (1.3 oz)	100	15	—	3
Bran'nola Nutty Grains	1 slice (1.3 oz)	90	14	—	3
Bran'nola Original	1 slice (1.3 oz)	90	16	—	3
Cinnamon Chip	1 slice	80	13	—	tr
Cinnamon Raisin	1 slice (0.9 oz)	70	13	—	1
Country Bran Bakery Light	1 slice (0.8 oz)	40	7	—	3
Cranberry	1 slice (0.9 oz)	70	14	3	1
French Stick Savoni	1 oz	80	15	—	1
Italian Bakery Light	1 slice (0.7 oz)	40	7	—	2
Oatmeal Bakery	1 slice	60	12	—	2
Oatmeal Bakery Light	1 slice	40	8	—	2
Oatmeal Raisin	1 slice (0.9 oz)	60	12	—	2

FOOD	PORTION	CALS.	CARB.	SUG.	FIB.
Arnold (CONT.)					
Pumpernickel	1 slice (1.1 oz)	70	15	—	1
Rye Bakery Soft Light	1 slice (1.1 oz)	40	7	—	2
Rye Bakery Soft Seeded	1 slice (1.1 oz)	70	14	—	1
Rye Bakery Soft Unseeded	1 slice (1.1 oz)	70	14	—	1
Rye Dill	1 slice (1.1 oz)	60	10	—	1
Rye Real Jewish Dijon	1 slice	70	15	—	1
Rye Real Jewish Melba Thin	1 slice (0.7 oz)	40	9	—	1
Rye Real Jewish Unseeded	1 slice	80	16	—	1
Rye Real Jewish With Caraway	1 slice	70	13	—	1
Rye Real Jewish Without Seeds	1 slice (1.1 oz)	70	15	—	1
Sourdough Francisco	1 slice	90	19	—	1
Wheat Brick Oven	1 slice (0.8 oz)	60	9	—	2
Wheat Golden Light	1 slice (0.8 oz)	40	7	—	2
Wheat Natural	1 slice (1.3 oz)	80	15	—	2
Wheat Berry Honey	1 slice (1.1 oz)	80	13	—	2
White Brick Oven	1 slice (0.8 oz)	60	11	—	1
White Country	1 slice (1.3 oz)	100	18	—	1
White Extra Fiber Brick Oven	1 slice (0.9 oz)	50	10	—	2
White Light Brick Oven	1 slice (0.8 oz)	40	10	—	2
White Premium Light	1 slice	40	7	—	2
White Thin Sliced Brick Oven	1 slice	40	7	—	tr
Whole Wheat 100% Light Brick Oven	1 slice (0.8 oz)	40	6	—	3
Whole Wheat 100% Stoneground	1 slice (0.8 oz)	50	8	—	2
August Bros.					
Pumpernickel	1 slice	80	14	—	1
Rye Onion	1 slice	80	14	—	1
Rye Thin Unseeded	1 slice	40	8	—	1
Rye With Seeds	1 slice (1 lb loaf)	80	14	—	1
Rye Without Seeds	1 slice	80	14	—	1
Rye N' Pump	1 slice	90	18	—	1
Beefsteak					
Pumpernickel	1 slice (1 oz)	70	13	0	1
Rye Hearty	1 slice (1 oz)	70	13	tr	1
Rye Light	2 slices (1.6 oz)	70	17	2	5
Rye Mild	2 slices (1.4 oz)	90	18	1	2
Rye Soft	1 slice (1 oz)	70	13	0	1

FOOD	PORTION	CALS.	CARB.	SUG.	FIB.
Beefsteak (CONT.)					
Wheat Hearty	1 slice (1 oz)	70	13	tr	1
Wheat Soft	1 slice (1 oz)	70	13	tr	tr
White Robust	1 slice (1 oz)	70	13	tr	tr
Bread Du Jour					
Austrian Wheat	3 in slice (1 oz)	130	26	2	2
French	3 in slice (1 oz)	130	26	2	1
Brownberry					
Bran'nola Country Oat	1 slice	90	18	—	3
Bran'nola Hearty Wheat	1 slice	88	17	—	3
Bran'nola Nutty Grains	1 slice	85	17	—	3
Bran'nola Original	1 slice	85	18	—	3
Health Nut	1 slice	71	12	—	3
Oatmeal Natural	1 slice	63	13	—	1
Oatmeal Soft	1 slice	48	10	—	2
Raisin Bran	1 slice	61	12	—	2
Raisin Cinnamon	1 slice	66	12	—	1
Raisin Walnut	1 slice	68	11	—	2
Wheat Apple Honey	1 slice	69	11	—	2
Wheat Soft	1 slice	74	12	—	1
Cedar's					
Mountain Bread Six Grain	1 piece (2.4 oz)	200	35	3	4
Damascus Bakeries					
Mountain Shepard Lahvash	⅓ loaf (2 oz)	135	28	0	2
Dicarlo's					
Foccaccia	⅛ bread (2 oz)	130	25	1	1
French Parisian	2 slices (1 oz)	70	14	tr	tr
Freihofer's					
Country Potato	1 slice (1.3 oz)	100	19	2	1
Country White	1 slice (1.3 oz)	100	19	2	tr
Wheat Light	1 slice (1.6 oz)	80	17	2	4
White Light	2 slices (1.6 oz)	80	18	1	4
Whole Wheat 100%	1 slice (1.3 oz)	90	16	3	2
Home Pride					
Hearty Buttermilk & Biscuit White	1 slice (1.3 oz)	100	18	2	tr
Hearty Deli Rye	1 slice (2 oz)	140	26	1	3
Hearty Golden Honey Wheat	1 slice (1.3 oz)	90	18	2	2
Hearty Honey Oats & Cracked Wheat	1 slice (1.4 oz)	100	19	2	2
Hearty Seven Grain Multi Grain	1 slice (1.3 oz)	100	17	1	2
Honey Wheat	1 slice (1 oz)	70	13	1	1

FOOD	PORTION	CALS.	CARB.	SUG.	FIB.
Home Pride (CONT.)					
Seven Grain	1 slice (0.9 oz)	60	12	tr	1
Wheat	1 slice (0.9 oz)	70	13	tr	1
Wheat Light	3 slices (2.1 oz)	110	25	2	6
White	1 slice (0.9 oz)	70	13	2	0
White Grain	1 slice (1 oz)	60	13	—	2
White Light	3 slices (0.9 oz)	110	25	2	6
Whole Wheat Hearty 100% Stoneground	1 slice (1.4 oz)	90	18	2	3
Malsovit					
Bread	1 slice	66	12	—	4
Raisin	1 slice	77	12	—	3
Matthew's					
9 Grain & Nut	1 slice	80	9	—	2
Cinnamon	1 slice	70	13	—	2
Golden	1 slice	70	14	—	1
Oat Bran	1 slice	65	12	—	2
Pita Whole Wheat	1	210	45	—	7
Sodium Free	1 slice	70	12	—	2
Whole Wheat	1 slice	70	12	—	2
Meditarranean Magic					
Focaccia	⅕ loaf (1.8 oz)	140	27	2	tr
Monks' Bread					
Sunflower & Bran	1 slice	70	12	—	2
Pepperidge Farm					
7 Grain Hearty Slice	2 slices	180	36	—	2
Cinnamon	1 slice	90	15	—	2
Cracked Wheat	1 slice	70	13	—	1
Crunchy Oat 1½ lb Loaf	2 slices	190	34	—	3
Date Walnut	1 slice	90	14	—	2
French Fully Baked	2 oz	150	28	—	1
French Twin	1 oz	80	15	—	0
Honey Bran	1 slice	90	18	—	1
Italian Brown & Serve	1 oz	80	14	—	0
Oatmeal	1 slice	70	12	—	1
Oatmeal 1½ lb Loaf	1 slice	90	17	—	1
Oatmeal Light	1 slice	45	9	—	1
Pumpernickel Family	1 slice	80	15	—	2
Pumpernickel Party	4 slices	60	12	—	1
Rye Dijon	1 slice	50	9	—	1
Rye Dijon Thick Sliced	1 slice	70	15	—	2
Rye Family	1 slice (32 g)	80	16	—	2
Rye Party	4 slices	60	12	—	1
Rye Seedless Family	1 slice	80	16	—	2

FOOD	PORTION	CALS.	CARB.	SUG.	FIB.
Pepperidge Farm (CONT.)					
Sesame Wheat	2 slices	190	36	—	3
Sprouted Wheat	1 slice	70	11	—	2
Swirl Raisin Cinnamon	1 slice (1 oz)	80	14	6	1
Vienna Light	1 slice	45	10	—	1
Vienna Thick Sliced	1 slice	70	13	—	0
Wheat 1½ lb Loaf	1 slice	90	18	—	2
Wheat Family	1 slice	70	13	—	2
Wheat Light	1 slice	45	9	—	1
Wheat Very Thin Sliced	1 slice	35	7	—	0
White Country	2 slices	190	38	—	2
White Large Family Thin Slice	1 slice	70	13	—	0
White Sandwich	2 slices	130	24	—	0
White Thin Slice	1 slice	80	14	—	0
White Toasting	1 slice	90	17	—	1
White Very Thin Sliced	1 slice	40	8	—	0
Whole Wheat Thin Slice	1 slice	60	12	—	2
Roman Meal					
Brown & Serve Mini Loaf	½ loaf (2 oz)	136	24	4	1
Cracked Wheat	1 slice (1.4 oz)	92	15	2	2
Hearty Wheat Light	1 slice (0.8 oz)	42	7	1	2
Honey Nut Oat Bran	1 slice (1 oz)	72	11	2	1
Honey Oat Bran	1 slice (1 oz)	70	12	2	1
Oat	1 slice (1 oz)	69	12	1	1
Oat Bran	1 slice (1 oz)	68	12	2	1
Oat Bran Light	1 slice (0.8 oz)	42	7	1	2
Round Top	1 slice (1 oz)	67	12	2	1
Sandwich	1 slice (0.8 oz)	55	10	2	1
Seven Grain	1 slice (1 oz)	67	12	2	1
Seven Grain Light	1 slice (0.8 oz)	42	7	1	3
Sourdough Light	1 slice (0.8 oz)	41	7	1	3
Sourdough Whole Grain Light	1 slice (0.8 oz)	40	7	1	3
Sun Grain	1 slice (1 oz)	70	11	2	1
Twelve Grain	1 slice (1 oz)	70	11	1	1
Twelve Grain Light	1 slice (0.8 oz)	42	7	1	3
Wheat Light	1 slice (0.8 oz)	41	7	1	3
Wheatberry Honey	1 slice (1 oz)	67	12	2	1
Wheatberry Light	1 slice (0.8 oz)	42	7	1	2
White Light	1 slice (0.8 oz)	41	7	1	3
Whole Grain 100%	1 slice (1.4 oz)	91	16	3	2
Whole Grain Sourdough	1 slice (1 oz)	66	12	1	1
Whole Wheat 100%	1 slice (1 oz)	64	11	2	2

FOOD	PORTION	CALS.	CARB.	SUG.	FIB.
Roman Meal (CONT.)					
Whole Wheat 100% Light	1 slice (0.8 oz)	42	7	1	2
Sahara					
Pita Oat Bran	½ pocket (1 oz)	66	14	—	2
Sunmaid					
Raisin	1 slice	70	13	—	1
Tree Of Life					
100% Spelt	1 slice (1.8 oz)	130	22	1	3
Millet	1 slice (1.8 oz)	130	25	1	2
Rye Sour Dough	1 slice (1.8 oz)	110	24	2	5
Sprouted Seven Grain	1 slice (1.8 oz)	110	20	1	2
Valley Lahvosh					
Valley Wraps	1 (1 oz)	100	19	3	1
Wonder					
Calcium Enriched	1 slice (1 oz)	70	12	2	tr
Cinnamon Raisin	1 slice (1 oz)	70	14	1	tr
Cracked Wheat	1 slice (1 oz)	70	14	tr	1
French	1 slice (1 oz)	80	15	1	tr
French Light	2 slices (1.6 oz)	80	18	tr	5
Granola	1 slice (1.5 oz)	100	19	2	2
Honey Bran Light	2 slices (1.6 oz)	80	18	2	6
Italian	1 slice (1.1 oz)	80	15	1	tr
Italian Family	1 slice (1 oz)	70	13	tr	tr
Italian Light	2 slices (1.6 oz)	80	18	tr	5
Kid	1 slice (0.9 oz)	70	13	tr	tr
Light Calcium Enriched	2 slices (1.6 oz)	80	18	2	5
Nine Grain Light	2 slices (1.6 oz)	80	18	2	6
Oatmeal Light	2 slices (1.6 oz)	90	19	2	4
Rye	1 slice (1 oz)	70	13	tr	1
Rye Light	2 slices (1.6 oz)	70	17	2	5
Sourdough	1 slice (1.2 oz)	90	17	1	tr
Sourdough Light	2 slices (1.6 oz)	80	18	tr	5
Texas Toast	1 slice (1.4 oz)	100	19	1	1
Vienna	1 slice (1 oz)	70	13	tr	tr
Wheat Calcium Light	2 slices (1.6 oz)	80	18	2	6
Wheat Family	1 slice (0.9 oz)	70	13	tr	tr
Wheat Golden Country Style	2 slices (1.4 oz)	100	19	1	1
Wheat Light	2 slices (1.6 oz)	80	18	1	6
White	1 slice (0.9 oz)	70	13	tr	tr
White Calcium	2 slices (1.6 oz)	100	20	2	1
White Calcium Light	2 slices (1.6 oz)	80	18	2	5
White Light	2 slices (1.6 oz)	80	18	1	5
White With Buttermilk	1 slice (1 oz)	80	14	1	tr

FOOD	PORTION	CALS.	CARB.	SUG.	FIB.
Wonder (CONT.)					
Whole Wheat 100%	1 slice (1 oz)	70	12	1	2
Whole Wheat 100% Soft	2 slices (1.6 oz)	110	21	2	1
Whole Wheat 100% Stoneground	1 slice (1.2 oz)	80	14	1	2
ZA					
Pit-Za Hearty Multi-Grain	1/9 bread (2 oz)	130	25	2	2
Pit-Za Salt-Free Garlic Whole Wheat	1/9 bread (2 oz)	150	28	4	3
REFRIGERATED					
Roman Meal					
Loaf	1 slice (1 oz)	85	13	—	1
Stefano's					
Stuffed Bread Broccoli & Cheese	1/2 bread (6 oz)	450	54	5	7

BREAD COATING

FOOD	PORTION	CALS.	CARB.	SUG.	FIB.
Don's Chuck Wagon					
All Purpose Mix	1/4 cup (1 oz)	100	20	0	1
Fish & Chips Mix	1/4 cup (1 oz)	100	21	0	1
Fish Mix	1/4 cup (1 oz)	95	21	0	1
Frying Mix Chicken	1/4 cup (1 oz)	95	21	0	1
Frying Mix Seafood Seasoned	1/4 cup (1 oz)	95	21	0	1
Mushroom Mix	1/4 cup (1 oz)	95	21	0	1
Onion Ring Mix	1/4 cup (1 oz)	100	21	0	1
Ka-Me					
Tempura Batter Mix	1 oz	100	22	0	0
Oven Fry					
Extra Crispy For Chicken	1/8 pkg (0.5 oz)	60	10	2	0
Extra Crispy For Pork	1/8 pkg (0.5 oz)	60	11	1	0
Shake 'N Bake					
Buffalo Wings	1/10 pkg (0.4 oz)	40	8	3	0
Classic Italian Chicken or Pork	1/8 pkg (0.4 oz)	40	7	tr	0
Country Mild Recipe	1/8 pkg (0.3 oz)	35	5	0	0
Glazes Barbecue Chicken Or Pork	1/8 pkg (0.4 oz)	45	9	5	0
Glazes Honey Mustard Chicken Or Pork	1/8 pkg (0.4 oz)	45	9	6	0
Glazes Tangy Honey Chicken Or Pork	1/8 pkg (0.4 oz)	45	9	6	0
Home Style Flour Recipe For Chicken	1/8 pkg (0.4 oz)	40	7	0	0

FOOD	PORTION	CALS.	CARB.	SUG.	FIB.
Shake 'N Bake (CONT.)					
Hot & Spicy Chicken Or Pork	⅛ pkg (0.4 oz)	40	7	tr	0
Original For Chicken	⅛ pkg (0.4 oz)	40	7	tr	0
Original For Fish	¼ pkg (0.7 oz)	80	14	tr	tr
Original For Pork	⅛ pkg (0.4 oz)	45	8	tr	0
BREAD MACHINE MIX					
Dromedary					
Country White	½ in slice (2 oz)	140	28	3	1
Italian Herb	½ in slice (1.8 oz)	140	25	2	1
Stoneground Wheat	½ in slice (1.8 oz)	140	26	3	2
Pillsbury					
Cracked Wheat	¹⁄₁₂ pkg (1.3 oz)	130	25	3	2
Sassafras					
Apricot Oatmeal	1 slice (1.4 oz)	140	29	3	2
Wanda's					
Dried Tomato Cheddar	¼ cup mix per serv (1.2 oz)	140	22	4	3
European White	¼ cup mix per serv (1.2 oz)	130	26	2	1
Oatmeal	¼ cup mix per serv (1.2 oz)	120	24	7	1
Oatmeal Cinnamon	¼ cup mix per serv (1.2 oz)	120	19	7	1
Old World Rye	¼ cup mix per serv (1.9 oz)	90	27	9	3
Onion	¼ cup mix per serv (1.2 oz)	120	25	4	1
Orange Cinnamon	¼ cup mix per serv (1.3 oz)	130	28	7	1
Oregano Garlic	¼ cup mix per serv (1.2 oz)	130	25	2	2
Rosemary Basil	¼ cup mix per serv (1.2 oz)	130	26	3	1
Rye	¼ cup mix per serv (1.2 oz)	120	25	4	1
Rye Caraway	¼ cup mix per serv (1.2 oz)	120	25	4	1
Sourdough	¼ cup mix per serv (1.2 oz)	120	25	2	1
Sunflower Sesame Poppyseed	¼ cup mix per serv (1.2 oz)	120	25	4	2
Ten Grain	¼ cup mix per serv (1.4 oz)	140	27	3	3

FOOD	PORTION	CALS.	CARB.	SUG.	FIB.
Wanda's (CONT.)					
Wheat	¼ cup mix per serv (1.2 oz)	130	26	4	2
White	¼ cup mix per serv (1.2 oz)	130	26	3	1
Whole Wheat	¼ cup mix per serv (1.3 oz)	130	26	8	4

BREADCRUMBS

FOOD	PORTION	CALS.	CARB.	SUG.	FIB.
dry	1 cup	426	78	—	5
dry seasonsed	1 cup (4 oz)	441	85	—	5
fresh	⅔ cup	76	14	—	1
Arnold					
Italian	½ oz	50	8	—	tr
Plain	½ oz	50	8	—	tr
Contadina					
Plain	⅓ cup	100	19	1	1
Devonsheer					
Italian Style	1 oz	104	20	—	1
Plain	1 oz	108	21	—	1
Progresso					
Italian Style	¼ cup (1 oz)	110	20	1	1
Lemon Herb	¼ cup (0.9 oz)	100	20	2	2
Plain	¼ cup (1 oz)	100	19	1	1
Tomato Basil	¼ cup (1.1 oz)	120	22	3	2

BREADSTICKS

FOOD	PORTION	CALS.	CARB.	SUG.	FIB.
Angonoa					
Cheese	5 (1 oz)	120	20	tr	1
Cheese Mini	16 (1 oz)	120	20	tr	1
Garlic	6 (1 oz)	120	21	tr	1
Italian Style Plain	5 (1 oz)	120	20	tr	1
Low Sodium With Sesame Seed	6 (1 oz)	130	19	tr	2
Onion	6 (1 oz)	120	21	tr	2
Pizza Mini	26 (1 oz)	120	21	tr	1
Sesame Mini	16 (1 oz)	130	19	tr	2
Sesame Royale	6 (1 oz)	130	18	tr	2
Whole Wheat Mini	14 (1 oz)	130	19	tr	3
Bread Du Jour					
Italian	1 (1.9 oz)	130	25	tr	1
Sourdough	1 (1.9 oz)	130	25	tr	1
J.J. Cassone					
Garlic	1 (1.6 oz)	150	26	2	2

FOOD	PORTION	CALS.	CARB.	SUG.	FIB.
New York					
Garlic Soft	1 (1.5 oz)	140	23	1	1
Roman Meal					
Brown & Serve Soft	1 (2.7 oz)	181	32	5	3
Refrigerated	1 (1.4 oz)	117	18	—	1

BREAKFAST BAR

(*see also* BREAKFAST DRINKS, NUTRITIONAL SUPPLEMENTS)

FOOD	PORTION	CALS.	CARB.	SUG.	FIB.
Carnation					
Chewy Chocolate Chip	1 (1.26 oz)	150	22	10	tr
Chewy Peanut Butter Chocolate Chip	1 (1.26 oz)	140	21	9	tr
Nutri-Grain					
Apple Cinnamon	1 (1.3 oz)	140	27	12	1
Blueberry	1 (1.3 oz)	140	27	12	1
Peach	1 (1.3 oz)	140	27	12	1
Raspberry	1 (1.3 oz)	140	27	12	1
Strawberry	1 (1.3 oz)	140	27	13	1

BREAKFAST DRINKS

(*see also* BREAKFAST BAR, NUTRITIONAL SUPPLEMENTS)

FOOD	PORTION	CALS.	CARB.	SUG.	FIB.
orange drink powder	3 rounded tsp	93	24	—	—
orange drink powder as prep w/water	6 oz	86	22	—	—
Carnation					
Instant Breakfast Cafe Mocha	1 pkg	130	28	23	1
Instant Breakfast Cafe Mocha	1 pkg + skim milk (9 fl oz)	220	39	35	1
Instant Breakfast Cafe Mocha	1 can (10 fl oz)	220	35	33	0
Instant Breakfast Classic Chocolate Malt	1 pkg + skim milk (9 fl oz)	220	39	28	1
Instant Breakfast Classic Chocolate Malt	1 pkg	130	26	16	1
Instant Breakfast Creamy Milk Chocolate	1 pkg	130	28	22	1
Instant Breakfast Creamy Milk Chocolate	1 pkg + skim milk (9 fl oz)	220	39	34	1
Instant Breakfast Creamy Milk Chocolate	8 fl oz	220	36	35	1
Instant Breakfast Creamy Milk Chocolate	1 can (10 fl oz)	220	37	34	1
Instant Breakfast French Vanilla	1 pkg + skim milk	220	39	29	0

FOOD	PORTION	CALS.	CARB.	SUG.	FIB.
Carnation (CONT.)					
Instant Breakfast French Vanilla	1 pkg	130	27	17	0
Instant Breakfast No Sugar Added Classic Chocolate	1 pkg + skim milk (9 fl oz)	160	24	18	1
Instant Breakfast No Sugar Added Classic Chocolate	1 pkg	70	11	6	1
Instant Breakfast No Sugar Added Creamy Milk Chocolate	1 pkg + skim milk (9 fl oz)	160	24	18	1
Instant Breakfast No Sugar Added Creamy Milk Chocolate	1 pkg	70	12	6	1
Instant Breakfast No Sugar Added French Vanilla	1 pkg + skim milk (9 fl oz)	150	24	29	0
Instant Breakfast No Sugar Added French Vanilla	1 pkg	70	12	7	0
Instant Breakfast No Sugar Added Strawberry Creme	1 pkg + skim milk (9 fl oz)	150	24	19	0
Instant Breakfast No Sugar Added Strawberry Creme	1 pkg	70	12	7	0
Instant Breakfast Strawberry Creme	1 pkg	130	28	18	0
Instant Breakfast Strawberry Creme	1 pkg + skim milk	220	39	30	0
BROCCOFLOWER					
Dole					
Fresh	⅕ head	35	7	2	—
BROCCOLI					
FRESH					
chinese broccoli (gai lan) cooked	1 cup (3.1 oz)	19	3	—	2
chopped cooked	½ cup	22	4	—	2
raw chopped	½ cup	12	2	—	1
Dole					
Spear	1 med	40	4	—	5
FROZEN					
spears cooked	½ cup	25	5	—	3
spears cooked	10 oz pkg	69	13	—	4
Amy's Organic					
Pocket Sandwich Broccoli & Cheese	1 (4.5 oz)	270	37	4	3
Big Valley					
Chopped	¾ cup (3 oz)	25	4	1	2

FOOD	PORTION	CALS.	CARB.	SUG.	FIB.
Big Valley (CONT.)					
Cuts	¾ cup (3 oz)	25	4	1	2
Birds Eye					
Baby Broccoli Blend	1 cup (3.4 oz)	70	8	3	3
Baby Florets	1 cup (3 oz)	25	4	1	2
In Cheese Sauce	½ cup (3.9 oz)	110	7	3	2
Fresh Like					
Spear	3.5 oz	26	5	—	1
Green Giant					
Butter Sauce	4 oz	50	7	2	2
Cheese Sauce	⅔ cup (3.9 oz)	70	9	5	2
Chopped	¾ cup (2.8 oz)	25	4	1	2
Cuts	1 cup (2.9 oz)	25	4	1	2
Harvest Fresh Cut	⅔ cup (3.2 oz)	25	4	tr	2
Harvest Fresh Spears	3.5 oz	25	4	1	2
Select Florets	1⅓ cups (2.9 oz)	25	4	1	2
Select Spears	3 oz	25	4	2	2
Stouffer's					
Au Gratin	1 serv (4 oz)	100	10	3	2
Tree Of Life					
Broccoli	1 cup (3.1 oz)	25	4	1	2

BROWNIE
FROZEN
Weight Watchers

FOOD	PORTION	CALS.	CARB.	SUG.	FIB.
Brownie A La Mode	1 (3.14 oz)	190	34	23	2
Double Fudge Brownie Parfait	1 (5.3 oz)	190	39	20	2

HOME RECIPE

FOOD	PORTION	CALS.	CARB.	SUG.	FIB.
plain	1 (0.8 oz)	112	12	—	1
w/nuts	1 (0.8 oz)	95	11	—	—

MIX

FOOD	PORTION	CALS.	CARB.	SUG.	FIB.
plain	1 (1.2 oz)	139	20	—	1
plain low calorie	1 (0.8 oz)	84	16	—	1
Estee					
Lite	2	100	23	1	1
Jiffy					
Fudge as prep	1	160	28	18	tr

READY-TO-EAT

FOOD	PORTION	CALS.	CARB.	SUG.	FIB.
plain	1 lg (2 oz)	227	36	—	1
plain	1 sm (1 oz)	115	18	—	1
w/ nuts	1 (1 oz)	100	16	—	—
w/o nuts	1 (2 oz)	243	39	—	—
Greenfield					
Brownie HomeStyle	1 (1.4 oz)	120	29	21	1

FOOD	PORTION	CALS.	CARB.	SUG.	FIB.
Hostess					
Brownie Bites	5 (2 oz)	260	32	24	2
Brownie Bites Walnut	5 (2 oz)	270	31	24	2
Little Debbie					
Fudge	1 pkg (2.1 oz)	270	39	27	1
Fudge	1 pkg (3.6 oz)	450	65	45	2
Fudge	1 pkg (2.9 oz)	360	52	36	1
Fudge	1 pkg (2.5 oz)	310	44	31	1
Pepperidge Farm					
Charlotte Fudgey Brownie	1	220	28	—	2
Tahoe Milk Chocolate Pecan	1	210	30	—	1
Westport Fudgey Brownies w/ Walnuts	1	220	28	—	2
Sweet Rewards					
Double Fudge	1 (1.1 oz)	110	25	15	tr
Fat Free Brownie	1 bar (1 oz)	90	21	14	<1
Tastykake					
Brownie	1 (85 g)	340	53	—	5

BRUSSELS SPROUTS
FRESH

FOOD	PORTION	CALS.	CARB.	SUG.	FIB.
cooked	½ cup	30	7	—	3
raw	1 sprout	8	2	—	1
Dole					
Sprouts	½ cup	19	4	—	2
FROZEN					
Big Valley					
Whole	5-8 pieces (3 oz)	35	6	2	1
Birds Eye					
Brussels Sprouts	6 (3 oz)	35	7	2	3
Fresh Like					
Sprouts	3.5 oz	37	7	—	1
Green Giant					
Butter Sauce	⅔ cup (3.6 oz)	60	9	3	4

BUCKWHEAT

FOOD	PORTION	CALS.	CARB.	SUG.	FIB.
groats roasted cooked	1 cup (5.9 oz)	647	34	—	5
groats roasted uncooked	1 cup (5.7 oz)	567	123	—	17
Wolff's					
Kasha Coarse cooked	¼ cup (1.6 oz)	170	35	0	2
Kasha Fine cooked	¼ cup (1.6 oz)	170	35	0	2
Kasha Medium cooked	¼ cup (1.6 oz)	170	35	0	2
Kasha Whole cooked	¼ cup (1.6 oz)	170	35	0	2

FOOD	PORTION	CALS.	CARB.	SUG.	FIB.
BUFFALO					
water buffalo roasted	3 oz	111	0	0	0
BULGUR					
cooked	1 cup (6.3 oz)	151	34	—	8
uncooked	1 cup (4.9 oz)	479	106	—	26
Casbah					
Pilaf Mix as prep	1 cup	200	42	0	4
Salad Mix as prep	⅔ cup	90	20	0	1
Good Shepherd					
Bulgur	¼ cup (43 g)	150	33	—	1
Hodgson Mill					
Bulgur	¼ cup (1.4 oz)	120	24	0	1
BURBOT (FISH)					
fresh baked	3 oz	98	0	0	0
BUTTER					
(*see also* BUTTER BLENDS, BUTTER SUBSTITUTES, MARGARINE)					
clarified butter	3½ oz	876	0	0	0
stick	1 pat (5 g)	36	tr	—	—
stick	1 stick (4 oz)	813	tr	—	—
whipped	4 oz	542	tr	—	—
whipped	1 pat (4 g)	27	tr	—	—
Cabot					
Stick	1 tsp	35	0	0	0
Unsalted Stick	1 tsp	35	0	0	0
Crystal					
Salted Stick	1 tbsp (0.5 oz)	102	tr	0	0
Unsalted Stick	1 tbsp (0.5 oz)	102	tr	0	0
Hotel Bar					
Stick	1 tsp	35	0	0	0
Keller's					
Stick	1 tsp	35	0	0	0
Land O'Lakes					
Light Stick	1 tbsp	50	0	0	0
Light Unsalted Stick	1 tbsp	50	0	0	0
Stick	1 tbsp (0.5 oz)	100	0	0	0
Unsalted Stick	1 tbsp (0.5 oz)	100	0	0	0
Unsalted Tub	1 tbsp	60	0	0	0
Whipped	1 tbsp (0.3 oz)	70	0	0	0
BUTTER BEANS					
CANNED					
Allen					
Baby	½ cup (4.5 oz)	120	22	1	6

FOOD	PORTION	CALS.	CARB.	SUG.	FIB.
Allen (CONT.)					
Large	½ cup (4.5 oz)	120	20	tr	7
Green Giant					
Butter Beans	½ cup (4.5 oz)	90	16	1	4
Sunshine					
Butter Beans	½ cup (4.5 oz)	120	23	0	8
Trappey					
Baby White With Bacon	½ cup (4.5 oz)	130	21	2	6
Large White With Bacon	½ cup (4.5 oz)	110	21	tr	6
Van Camp's					
Butter Beans	½ cup	110	22	—	7
FROZEN					
Birds Eye					
Butter Beans	½ cup (2.7 oz)	100	20	1	4
Speckled	½ cup (2.7 oz)	100	20	1	4

BUTTER BLENDS

(*see also* BUTTER, BUTTER SUBSTITUTES, MARGARINE)

FOOD	PORTION	CALS.	CARB.	SUG.	FIB.
stick	1 stick	811	1	—	—
Blue Bonnet					
Better Blend Stick	1 tbsp	90	0	0	0
Better Blend Tub	1 tbsp	90	0	0	0
Better Blend Unsalted Stick	1 tbsp	90	0	0	0
Brummel & Brown					
Spread Make With Yogurt	1 tbsp (0.5 oz)	50	0	0	0
Country Morning					
Blend Light Stick	1 tbsp (0.5 oz)	50	0	0	0
Blend Light Tub	1 tbsp (0.5 oz)	50	0	0	0
Blend Stick	1 tbsp	100	0	0	0
Blend Tub	1 tbsp	100	0	0	0
Blend Unsalted Stick	1 tbsp	100	0	0	0

BUTTER SUBSTITUTES

(*see also* BUTTER BLENDS, MARGARINE)

FOOD	PORTION	CALS.	CARB.	SUG.	FIB.
Butter Buds					
Mix	1 tsp (2 g)	5	2	—	—
Sprinkles	1 tsp (2 g)	5	2	—	—
Molly McButter					
Cheese	1 tsp	5	1	—	—
Light Sodium	1 tsp	5	1	—	—
Natural Butter	1 tsp	5	1	—	—
Roasted Garlic	1 tsp	5	1	—	—
Morningstar Farms					
Roasted Soy Butter	2 tbsp (1.1 oz)	170	10	3	1

FOOD	PORTION	CALS.	CARB.	SUG.	FIB.
Mrs. Bateman's					
Butterlike Baking Butter	1 tbsp (0.5 oz)	36	8	0	0
Butterlike Saute Butter	1 tbsp (0.5 oz)	40	8	0	0
Natural Touch					
Roasted Soy Butter	2 tbsp (1.1 oz)	170	10	3	1
Watkins					
Butter Sprinkles	1 tsp (2 g)	5	1	0	0
Imitation Butter Flavored Mist	1 tbsp (0.5 oz)	120	0	0	0

BUTTERFISH

FOOD	PORTION	CALS.	CARB.	SUG.	FIB.
baked	3 oz	159	0	0	0
fillet baked	1 oz	47	0	0	0

BUTTERSCOTCH
(*see also* CANDY)

FOOD	PORTION	CALS.	CARB.	SUG.	FIB.
Nestle					
Morsels Butterscotch	1 tbsp	80	10	10	—

CABBAGE
(*see also* COLESLAW)

FRESH

FOOD	PORTION	CALS.	CARB.	SUG.	FIB.
danish raw	1 head (2 lbs)	228	49	—	18
danish raw shredded	½ cup (1.2 oz)	9	2	—	tr
danish shredded cooked	½ cup (2.6 oz)	17	3	—	1
green raw	1 head (2 lbs)	228	49	—	18
green raw shredded	½ cup (1.2 oz)	9	2	—	tr
green shredded cooked	½ cup (2.6 oz)	17	3	—	1
napa cooked	1 cup (3.8 oz)	13	2	—	0
red raw shredded	½ cup	10	2	—	1
red shredded cooked	½ cup	16	3	—	—
savoy shredded cooked	½ cup	18	4	—	—
Dole					
Cabbage	1/12 med head	18	3	—	2
Napa shredded	½ cup	6	1	—	tr

CAKE
(*see also* BROWNIE, COOKIE, DANISH PASTRY, DOUGHNUT, PIE)

FOOD	PORTION	CALS.	CARB.	SUG.	FIB.
angelfood	1 cake (11.9 oz)	876	197	—	5
angelfood home recipe	1/12 cake (1.9 oz)	142	32	—	1
bakewell tart	1 slice (3 oz)	410	39	—	2
battenburg cake	1 slice (2 oz)	204	28	—	1
boston cream pie frzn	1/6 cake (3.2 oz)	232	40	—	1
cheesecake	1/6 cake (2.8 oz)	256	20	—	2
coffeecake creme-filled chocolate frosting home recipe	1/6 cake (3.2 oz)	298	49	—	2

FOOD	PORTION	CALS.	CARB.	SUG.	FIB.
coffeecake crumb topped cinnamon home recipe	1/12 cake (2.1 oz)	240	30	—	2
crumpets toasted	2 (4 oz)	119	26	—	2
eccles cake	1 slice (2 oz)	285	36	—	1
eclair	1 (1.4 oz)	149	15	—	tr
madeira cake	1 slice (1 oz)	98	15	—	1
sour cream pound	1/10 cake (1 oz)	117	16	—	tr
tiramisu	1 cake (4.4 lbs)	5732	439	234	3
treacle tart	1 slice (2.5 oz)	258	42	—	1
vanilla slice	1 slice (2½ oz)	248	30	—	1
yellow w/ chocolate frosting	1/8 cake (2.2 oz)	242	36	—	1
Baby Watson					
Cheesecake	1 slice (3.8 oz)	390	23	20	2
Cheesecake Light	1/16 cake (3.9 oz)	280	24	18	3
Baker Maid					
Creole Royal Pineapple Apricot	3 slices (5 oz)	270	61	45	4
Creole Royal Pineapple Apricot	1 slice (1.7 oz)	90	20	15	1
Carousel					
New York Cheese Cake	1 cake (3 oz)	250	16	15	1
Drake's					
Mini Coffee Cakes	4 (1.83 oz)	220	33	20	1
Dutch Mill					
Dessert Shells Chocolate Covered	1 (0.5 oz)	80	8	6	0
Freihofer's					
Angel Food	1/5 cake (2 oz)	150	35	23	0
Cinnamon Swirl Buns	1 (2.8 oz)	290	47	24	1
Coffee Cake Cinnamon Pecan	1/8 cake (2 oz)	220	33	20	1
Crumb	1/8 cake (2 oz)	240	33	13	1
Homestyle Golden Loaf	1/8 cake (1.8 oz)	200	28	17	0
Pound	1/5 cake (2.8 oz)	330	41	24	0
Greenfield					
Blondie Apple Spice	1 (1.4 oz)	120	28	20	0
Blondie Chocolate Chip	1 (1.4 oz)	120	29	21	0
Hostess					
Angel Food Ring	1/6 cake (1.6 oz)	150	29	19	0
Apple Twist	1 (2.5 oz)	220	42	16	tr
Baseball Yellow Cakes	1 (1.6 oz)	160	32	19	0
Choco Licious	1 (1.5 oz)	170	28	17	1
Choco-Diles	1 (1.8 oz)	210	31	20	1
Cinnaminis Original	5 (2.4 oz)	300	37	19	2

FOOD	PORTION	CALS.	CARB.	SUG.	FIB.
Hostess (CONT.)					
Cinnamon Roll	1 (2.3 oz)	220	39	21	1
Crumb Cake	1 (1.9 oz)	210	33	16	1
Cup Cakes Chocolate	1 (1.6 oz)	170	28	16	tr
Cup Cakes Chocolate Light	1 (1.4 oz)	120	26	17	tr
Cup Cakes Orange	1 (1.5 oz)	160	28	18	0
Dessert Cups	1 (1 oz)	90	18	8	0
Ding Dongs	1 (1.3 oz)	160	21	15	tr
Fruit Cake Holiday	⅙ cake (5.3 oz)	490	93	39	3
Fruit Loaf	1 (3.8 oz)	350	67	28	2
Ho Ho's	1 (1 oz)	130	17	13	tr
Holiday Cakes	1 (1.6 oz)	160	32	19	0
Honey Bun Glazed	1 (2.7 oz)	320	35	21	2
Honey Bun Iced	1 (3.4 oz)	390	49	31	2
Hopper Cakes	1 (1.6 oz)	160	32	19	0
Lights Low Fat Cinnamon Crumb Cake	1 (1 oz)	90	19	16	0
Lil Angels	1 (1 oz)	90	17	11	0
Pecan Spinners	1 (1 oz)	110	15	8	tr
Pound Cake	⅕ cake (3.2 oz)	350	48	22	1
Sno Balls	1 (1.6 oz)	160	29	17	1
Suzy Q's	1 (2 oz)	220	35	21	2
Suzy Q's Banana	1 (2 oz)	220	32	18	tr
Swirls Caramel Pecan	1 (2 oz)	140	25	10	1
Tiger Tails	1 (1.5 oz)	160	26	14	tr
Twinkies	1 (1.4 oz)	140	25	13	0
Twinkies Banana	2 (2.7 oz)	300	42	24	tr
Twinkies Devil Food	2 (2.7 oz)	300	47	28	2
Twinkies Lights	1 (1.4 oz)	120	24	15	0
Twinkies Strawberry Fruit 'n Creme	1 (1.6 oz)	150	30	17	tr
Jell-O					
Cheesecake Snack Original	1 (3.3 oz)	160	23	19	0
Cheesecake Snack Strawberry	1 (3.3 oz)	150	26	23	0
Kellogg's					
Pop-Tarts Apple Cinnamon	1 (1.8 oz)	210	37	16	1
Pop-Tarts Blueberry	1 (1.8 oz)	210	36	16	1
Pop-Tarts Brown Sugar Cinnamon	1 (1.8 oz)	210	35	14	1
Pop-Tarts Cherry	1 (1.8 oz)	200	37	15	1
Pop-Tarts Chocolate Graham	1 (1.8 oz)	210	35	17	1
Pop-Tarts Frosted Apple Cinnamon	1 (1.8 oz)	190	39	19	1

FOOD	PORTION	CALS.	CARB.	SUG.	FIB.
Kellogg's (CONT.)					
Pop-Tarts Frosted Blueberry	1 (1.8 oz)	200	37	18	1
Pop-Tarts Frosted Brown Sugar Cinnamon	1 (1.8 oz)	210	34	17	1
Pop-Tarts Frosted Cherry	1 (1.8 oz)	200	38	19	1
Pop-Tarts Frosted Chocolate Vanilla Creme	1 (1.8 oz)	200	37	19	1
Pop-Tarts Frosted Chocolate Fudge	1 (1.8 oz)	200	37	19	1
Pop-Tarts Frosted Grape	1 (1.8 oz)	200	38	18	1
Pop-Tarts Frosted Raspberry	1 (1.8 oz)	210	37	18	1
Pop-Tarts Frosted S'mores	1 (1.8 oz)	200	36	18	1
Pop-Tarts Frosted Strawberry	1 (1.8 oz)	200	38	19	1
Pop-Tarts Frosted Wild Berry	1 (2 oz)	210	39	20	1
Pop-Tarts Frosted Wild Watermelon	1 (2 oz)	210	39	20	1
Pop-Tarts Low Fat Blueberry	1 (1.8 oz)	190	39	17	1
Pop-Tarts Low Fat Cherry	1 (1.8 oz)	190	39	17	1
Pop-Tarts Low Fat Frosted Brown Sugar Cinnamon	1 (1.8 oz)	190	39	20	1
Pop-Tarts Low Fat Frosted Chocolate Fudge	1 (1.8 oz)	190	39	18	2
Pop-Tarts Low Fat Frosted Strawberry	1 (1.8 oz)	190	39	20	1
Pop-Tarts Low Fat Strawberry	1 (1.8 oz)	190	39	17	1
Pop-Tarts Strawberry	1 (1.8 oz)	200	37	15	1
Little Debbie					
Apple Delights	1 pkg (1.2 oz)	140	24	13	1
Apple-Roos	1 pkg (1.5 oz)	150	32	23	1
Banana Nut Muffin Loaves	1 pkg (1.9 oz)	210	30	18	1
Banana Twins	1 pkg (2.2 oz)	250	40	29	0
Be My Valentine	1 pkg (2.2 oz)	280	39	32	1
Cherry Cordials	1 pkg (1.3 oz)	160	23	16	1
Choc-o-Jel	1 pkg (1.2 oz)	150	21	15	1
Choco-Cakes	1 pkg (2.1 oz)	250	35	27	1
Choco-Cakes	1 pkg (2.2 oz)	240	35	28	1
Chocolate	1 pkg (3 oz)	360	52	40	1
Chocolate Chip	1 pkg (2.4 oz)	290	42	34	1

FOOD	PORTION	CALS.	CARB.	SUG.	FIB.
Little Debbie (CONT.)					
Chocolate Twins	1 pkg (2.4 oz)	240	42	31	1
Christmas Tree Cakes	1 pkg (1.5 oz)	190	27	22	0
Coconut	1 pkg (2.1 oz)	270	38	30	1
Coconut	1 pkg (2.4 oz)	300	42	33	0
Coconut Rounds	1 pkg (1.2 oz)	140	22	14	1
Coffee Cake Apple	1 pkg (1.9 oz)	220	36	22	1
Coffee Cake Apple Streusel	1 pkg (2 oz)	220	37	23	1
Devil Cremes	1 pkg (1.6 oz)	190	28	20	0
Devil Cremes	1 pkg (3.2 oz)	380	57	41	1
Devil Squares	1 pkg (2.2 oz)	260	39	31	1
Easter Basket Cakes	1 pkg (2.5 oz)	310	44	35	1
Fancy Cakes	1 pkg (2.4 oz)	300	42	34	0
Fudge Crispy	1 pkg (1.1 oz)	170	20	13	1
Fudge Round	1 pkg (2.5 oz)	290	49	34	2
Fudge Round	1 pkg (3 oz)	350	59	41	2
Fudge Rounds	1 pkg (1.2 oz)	140	23	16	1
Golden Cremes	1 pkg (1.5 oz)	170	25	18	0
Golden Cremes	1 pkg (3 oz)	330	50	35	0
Holiday Cake Chocolate	1 pkg (2.4 oz)	290	43	33	1
Holiday Cake Vanilla	1 pkg (2.5 oz)	310	44	35	1
Honey Bun	1 pkg (4 oz)	510	53	23	5
Honey Bun	1 pkg (3 oz)	380	39	17	4
Jelly Rolls	1 pkg (2.1 oz)	230	41	34	0
Lemon Stix	1 pkg (1.5 oz)	210	30	18	1
Marshmallow Supremes	1 pkg (1.1 oz)	130	22	18	1
Mint Sprints	1 pkg (1.5 oz)	230	28	19	1
Nutty Bar	1 pkg (2 oz)	290	34	20	1
Pecan Twins	1 pkg (2 oz)	220	32	15	1
Pumpkin Delights	1 pkg (1.1 oz)	130	21	12	1
Smiley Faces Cherry	1 pkg (1.2 oz)	140	23	13	1
Smiley Faces Pumpkin	1 pkg (1 oz)	130	20	6	1
Snack Cake Chocolate	1 pkg (2.5 oz)	300	43	33	1
Snack Cake Vanilla	1 pkg (2.6 oz)	320	45	36	1
Spice	1 pkg (2.5 oz)	300	43	35	1
Star Crunch	1 pkg (1.1 oz)	140	21	15	1
Star Crunch	1 pkg (2.6 oz)	330	51	34	1
Swiss Rolls	1 pkg (2.1 oz)	250	38	26	1
Swiss Rolls	1 pkg (2.7 oz)	320	47	33	1
Swiss Rolls	1 pkg (3.2 oz)	380	57	45	1
Teddy Berries	1 pkg (1.2 oz)	130	23	12	1
Vanilla	1 pkg (3 oz)	370	53	42	0
Vanilla Cremes	1 pkg (1.4 oz)	170	25	18	0
Zebra Cakes	1 pkg (2.6 oz)	150	45	36	1

FOOD	PORTION	CALS.	CARB.	SUG.	FIB.
Nabisco					
Frosted Strawberry	1 (1.7 oz)	190	35	17	1
Nature's Choice					
Toaster Pastries Fat Free Apple Cinnamon	1 (1.9 oz)	180	41	21	4
Toaster Pastries Fat Free Blueberry	1 (1.9 oz)	180	41	21	4
Toaster Pastries Fat Free Raspberry	1 (1.9 oz)	180	41	20	3
Toaster Pastries Fat Free Strawberry	1 (1.9 oz)	180	41	20	3
Toaster Pastries Low Fat Cherry	1 (1.9 oz)	180	36	16	3
Toaster Pastries Low Fat Frosted Blueberry	1 (1.9 oz)	190	42	23	3
Toaster Pastries Low Fat Frosted Chocolate	1 (1.9 oz)	200	42	24	3
Toaster Pastries Low Fat Frosted Cinnamon	1 (1.9 oz)	190	42	23	3
Toaster Pastries Low Fat Frosted Strawberry	1 (1.9 oz)	190	42	23	3
Toaster Pastries Low Fat Peach Apricot	1 (1.9 oz)	180	36	16	3
Pepperidge Farm					
Berkshire Apple Crisp	1	250	43	—	1
Strawberry Shortcake Dessert Lights	1 piece (3 oz)	170	30	—	1
Perugina					
Pannettone Au Beurre	1/6 cake (2.9 oz)	310	47	21	2
Sara Lee					
Banana	1/6 cake (2.3 oz)	230	37	28	0
Banana Sundae	1/10 cake (2.8 oz)	270	32	24	tr
Carrot	1/6 cake (3.2 oz)	320	39	35	2
Cheesecake Cherry	1/4 cake (4.7 oz)	350	55	35	2
Cheesecake Chocolate Chip	1/4 cake (4.2 oz)	410	47	43	2
Cheesecake Chocolate Mousse	1/5 cake	400	37	27	2
Cheesecake French	1/6 cake	350	34	22	1
Cheesecake Singles Fudge Brownie Crumble	1 slice (4 oz)	400	43	36	2
Cheesecake Singles Strawberry Drizzle	1 slice (4 oz)	380	46	40	2
Cheesecake Strawberry	1/4 pie (4.7 oz)	330	49	36	2
Cheesecake Strawberry French	1/6 cake	320	43	26	1

FOOD	PORTION	CALS.	CARB.	SUG.	FIB.
Sara Lee (CONT.)					
Cheesecake Bars Chocolate Dipped Original	1 bar (2.7 oz)	190	14	12	0
Cheesecake Bites Chocolate Praline Pecan	5 pieces (4 oz)	480	44	33	3
Cheesecake Bites Chocolate Praline Pecan	1 piece (0.8 oz)	100	9	7	tr
Cheesecake Bites Chocolate Dipped Original	5 pieces (4 oz)	500	41	32	2
Cheesecake Bites Chocolate Dipped Original	1 piece (0.8 oz)	100	8	6	0
Cheesecake Bites Toasted Almond Crunch	5 pieces (4 oz)	470	43	24	2
Cheesecake Bites Toasted Almond Crunch	1 (0.8 oz)	90	9	5	0
Coffee Cake Butter Streusel	⅙ cake (1.9 oz)	220	25	11	tr
Coffee Cake Cheese	⅙ cake (1.9 oz)	180	28	11	0
Coffee Cake Crumb	⅛ cake (2 oz)	220	32	17	tr
Coffee Cake Pecan	⅙ cake (1.9 oz)	230	24	9	tr
Coffee Cake Raspberry	⅙ cake (1.9 oz)	200	27	13	tr
Harvest Pumpkin Spice	⅛ cake (2.9 oz)	270	33	25	1
Layer Cake Coconut	⅛ cake (2.8 oz)	280	34	25	2
Layer Cake Double Chocolate	⅛ cake (2.8 oz)	260	33	28	2
Layer Cake Fudge Golden	⅛ cake (2.8 oz)	270	36	30	1
Layer Cake German Chocolate	⅛ cake (2.9 oz)	280	34	30	2
Layer Cake Vanilla	⅛ cake (2.8 oz)	250	31	25	0
Original Cheesecake Reduced Fat	¼ cake (4.2 oz)	310	40	28	2
Pound Cake	¼ cake (2.7 oz)	320	38	21	1
Pound Cake Chocolate Swirl	1 slice (1 oz)	110	14	11	0
Pound Cake Family Size	⅙ cake (2.7 oz)	310	36	15	1
Pound Cake Free & Light	¼ cake (2.5 oz)	200	39	21	1
Pound Cake Golden	1 slice (1 oz)	120	15	11	0
Pound Cake Reduced Fat	1 slice (1 oz)	100	15	10	0
Pound Cake Strawberry	¼ cake (2.9 oz)	290	44	25	1
Red White & Blueberry	¹⁄₁₀ cake (3 oz)	210	31	21	1
Slice Chocolate	1 (3 oz)	320	42	16	tr
Strawberry Shortcake	⅛ cake (2.5 oz)	180	27	15	1
Sinbad					
Baklava	1 piece (2 oz)	337	44	29	2

FOOD	PORTION	CALS.	CARB.	SUG.	FIB.
Tastykake					
Butter Cream Cream Filled Cupcake	1 (32 g)	120	20	—	1
Chocolate Cream Filled Cupcake	1 (34 g)	130	21	—	1
Chocolate Cupcake	1 (30 g)	100	19	—	1
Honeybun Glazed	1 pkg (92 g)	360	42	—	4
Honeybun Iced	1 pkg (92 g)	350	50	—	1
Junior Chocolate	1 pkg (94 g)	340	57	—	4
Junior Coconut	1 pkg (94 g)	300	60	—	3
Junior Lemon	1 pkg (94 g)	310	75	—	1
Junior Orange	1 pkg (94 g)	340	61	—	1
Kandy Kake Chocolate	1 (19 g)	80	13	—	1
Kandy Kake Coconut	1 (19 g)	80	11	—	1
Kandy Kake Peanut Butter	1 (19 g)	90	11	—	1
Koffee Kake Cream Filled	1 (29 g)	110	18	—	0
Koffee Kake Junior	1 pkg (71 g)	260	44	—	1
Kreme Kup	1 (25 g)	90	15	—	1
Krimpet Butterscotch	1 (28 g)	100	19	—	0
Krimpet Jelly	1 (28 g)	90	19	—	1
Krimpet Strawberry	1 (28 g)	100	20	—	0
Pastry Pocket Cheese	1 (85 g)	330	38	—	1
Pastry Pocket Cherry	1 (85 g)	330	41	—	1
Royale Chocolate Cupcake	1 (46 g)	170	28	—	2
Tasty Too Chocolate Cream Filled Cupcake	1 (32 g)	100	21	—	1
Tasty Too Vanilla Cream Filled Cupcake	1 (32 g)	100	21	—	1
Thomas'					
Date Nut Loaf	1 oz	90	18	—	1
Toastettes					
Frosted Blueberry	1 (1.7 oz)	190	45	17	1
Frosted Brown Sugar Cinnamon	1 (1.7 oz)	190	35	18	1
Frosted Cherry	1 (1.7 oz)	190	35	17	1
Frosted Fudge	1 (1.7 oz)	190	34	15	3
Strawberry	1 (1.7 oz)	190	35	17	1
Tortuga					
Cayman Island Rum Cake	1 piece (2 oz)	194	27	8	0
Weight Watchers					
Chocolate Raspberry Royale	1 (3.5 oz)	190	39	22	2
Chocolate Chip Cookie Dough Sundae	1 (2.64 oz)	180	33	20	2

FOOD	PORTION	CALS.	CARB.	SUG.	FIB.
Weight Watchers (CONT.)					
Chocolate Eclair	1 (2.1 oz)	150	25	14	2
Coffee Cake Apple Cinnamon Danish	1 piece (1.9 oz)	160	30	13	1
Coffee Cake Cheese Danish	1 piece (1.9 oz)	160	29	11	1
Coffee Cake Raspberry Danish	1 piece (1.9 oz)	160	30	13	1
Double Fudge	1 piece (2.75 oz)	190	36	22	2
French Style Cheesecake	1 piece (3.9 oz)	180	28	9	2
New York Style Cheesecake	1 piece (2.5 oz)	150	21	17	0
Strawberry Parfait Royale	1 (5.24 oz)	180	35	22	0
Triple Chocolate Eclair	1 (2.14 oz)	160	25	13	1
Well-Bred Loaf					
Banana Bread	1 slice (3.5 oz)	330	52	33	tr
Banana Nut	1 slice (4.3 oz)	440	59	36	2
Blueberry	1 slice (4.3 oz)	440	69	42	1
Carrot	1 slice (4.3 oz)	480	64	38	2
Carrot Traditional	1 slice (4.3 oz)	440	71	46	2
Chocolate Chip	1 slice (4.3 oz)	490	74	46	2
Cinnamon Walnut	1 slice (4.3 oz)	480	72	44	1
Coconut Rum	1 slice (4.3 oz)	490	64	39	tr
Cranberry	1 slice (4.3 oz)	460	77	47	1
Marble	1 slice (4.3 oz)	530	83	49	1
Pound All Butter	1 slice (4.3 oz)	470	73	44	tr
Pound Mandarin Orange	1 slice (4 oz)	460	68	10	tr
Raisin	1 slice (4.3 oz)	460	76	49	2

CALABAZA

FOOD	PORTION	CALS.	CARB.	SUG.	FIB.
fresh	½ cup	32	8	—	—

CANADIAN BACON

FOOD	PORTION	CALS.	CARB.	SUG.	FIB.
grilled	1 pkg (6 oz)	257	2	—	0
Hormel					
Canadian Bacon	2 oz	70	0	0	0
Jones					
Slices	1	30	tr	—	—

CANDY

(*see also* MARSHMALLOW)

FOOD	PORTION	CALS.	CARB.	SUG.	FIB.
boiled sweets	¼ lb	327	87	—	0
crisped rice bar almond	1 bar (1 oz)	130	18	—	1
crisped rice bar chocolate chip	1 bar (1 oz)	115	21	9	1
marzipan	1 oz	128	15	—	2
milk chocolate w/ almonds	1 bar (1.45 oz)	215	22	20	—

FOOD	PORTION	CALS.	CARB.	SUG.	FIB.
100 Grand					
Bar	1 bar (1.5 oz)	200	30	27	tr
3 Musketeers					
Bar	2 fun size (1.2 oz)	140	25	22	0
Bar	1 (2.1 oz)	260	46	40	1
5th Avenue					
Bar	1 (2.1 oz)	290	39	—	—
After Eight					
Dark Chocolate Wafer Thin Mints	1	35	6	—	—
Almond Joy					
Bar	1 (1.76 oz)	250	28	—	—
Andes					
Chocolate Covered Mint Patties	1 (0.5 oz)	60	13	12	0
Baby Ruth					
Bar	1 (2.1 oz)	270	36	27	2
Fun Size	2 pieces	200	27	12	1
Bar None					
Candy	1 (1.5 oz)	240	23	—	—
Barricini					
Dark Chocolate Raspberry Creme Shells	1 piece (0.3 oz)	47	5	4	0
Bit-O-Honey					
Candy	1.7 oz	200	39	—	—
Bits O Brickle					
Candy	1 tbsp (0.5 oz)	80	9	9	0
Bonus					
Bar	1 bar (2.1 oz)	290	34	27	2
Breath Savers					
Sugar Free Mint Cinnamon	1 piece (2 g)	10	2	0	—
Sugar Free Peppermint	1 piece (2 g)	10	2	0	—
Sugar Free Spearmint	1 piece (2 g)	10	2	0	—
Sugar Free Wintergreen	1 piece (2 g)	10	2	0	—
Brock					
Butterscotch Discs	3 pieces (0.6 oz)	70	17	11	—
Candy Corn	21 pieces (1.4 oz)	150	37	29	—
Candy Rolls	2 rolls (0.5 oz)	50	12	12	—
Caramel Dots	3 pieces (1.3 oz)	140	25	14	tr
Cinnamon Discs	3 pieces (0.6 oz)	70	17	11	—
Circus Peanuts	11 pieces (2.5 oz)	260	65	60	—
Coconut Mountains	4 pieces (1.4 oz)	170	29	24	—
Fruit Basket	3 pieces (0.6 oz)	60	15	13	—
Fruit Kisses	3 pieces (0.6 oz)	70	17	11	—

FOOD	PORTION	CALS.	CARB.	SUG.	FIB.
Brock (CONT.)					
Glitters	2 pieces (0.5 oz)	50	13	8	—
Gummy Bears	5 pieces (1.4 oz)	130	30	25	—
Gummy Squirms	5 pieces (1.3 oz)	120	28	24	—
Jelly Beans	12 pieces (1.4 oz)	140	36	26	—
Lemon Drops	3 pieces (0.5 oz)	60	14	9	—
Orange Slices	4 pieces (1.5 oz)	140	36	27	—
Party Mints	9 pieces (0.5 oz)	60	15	15	—
Peanut Butter Crunch	3 pieces (0.6 oz)	80	15	10	—
Pops Assorted	2 (0.5 oz)	60	15	10	—
Sour Balls	3 pieces (0.6 oz)	70	17	11	—
Sour Sharks	23 pieces (2.5 oz)	30	60	45	—
Spearmint Starlights	3 pieces (0.6 oz)	60	16	10	—
Spice Drops	12 pieces (1.4 oz)	130	33	24	—
Starlight Mints	3 pieces (0.6 oz)	60	16	10	—
Toffee	6 pieces (1.5 oz)	170	31	27	—
Butterfinger					
BB's	1 pkg (1.7 oz)	230	34	32	1
Bar	1 (2.1 oz)	280	41	40	1
Fun Size	2 bars (1.6 oz)	200	30	29	1
Caramello					
Candy	1 (1.6 oz)	220	28	—	—
Cellas					
Chocolate Covered Cherries Milk Chocolate	2 pieces (1 oz)	110	18	17	2
Certs					
Breath Mints	1 piece (1.67 g)	6	2	—	—
Mini Sugar Free	1 piece (0.365 g)	1	tr	—	—
Sugar Free	1 piece (1.67 g)	7	2	—	—
Charms					
Blow Pop	1 (0.6 oz)	70	17	14	—
Lollipop Sour	1 (0.6 oz)	70	18	17	—
Lollipop Sweet	1 (0.6 oz)	70	18	17	—
Chuckles					
Candy	4 pieces (1.4 oz)	140	34	24	—
Chunky					
Bar	1 (1.4 oz)	200	22	20	2
Clorets					
Mints	1 piece (1.67 g)	6	2	—	—
Crunch					
Fun Size	4 bars (1.5 oz)	200	25	21	1
Dove					
Dark Chocolate	¼ bar (1.5 oz)	230	26	22	3
Dark Chocolate	1 bar (1.3 oz)	200	22	19	2

FOOD	PORTION	CALS.	CARB.	SUG.	FIB.
Dove (CONT.)					
Dark Chocolate Minatures	7 (1.5 oz)	220	26	21	2
Milk Chocolate	1 bar (1.3 oz)	200	22	21	1
Milk Chocolate	¼ bar (1.5 oz)	230	25	24	1
Milk Chocolate Miniatures	7 (1.5 oz)	230	25	24	1
Truffles	3 (1.2 oz)	200	19	18	1
Dream					
Caramel & Nougat In Milk Chocolate	1 bar (1 oz)	90	21	8	1
Estee					
Caramels Chocolate & Vanilla No Sugar Added	5 (1.3 oz)	150	26	3	0
Dark Chocolate	½ bar (1.4 oz)	200	23	15	0
Gum Drops Assorted Fruit Sugar Free	23 (1.4 oz)	140	36	30	0
Gum Drops Licorice	23 (1.4 oz)	140	36	0	—
Gummy Bears Sugar Free	16 (1.4 oz)	140	31	0	—
Hard Candies Assorted Fruit Sugar Free	5 (0.5 oz)	60	16	0	0
Hard Candies Assorted Mint Sugar Free	5 (0.5 oz)	60	16	0	0
Hard Candies Butterscotch Sugar Free	2 (0.4 oz)	50	12	0	—
Hard Candies Peppermint Swirls Sugar Free	3 (0.5 oz)	60	14	0	—
Hard Candies Tropical Fruit Sugar Free	5 (0.5 oz)	60	16	0	0
Lollipops Assorted Fruit Sugar Free	2 (0.5 oz)	60	16	0	—
Milk Chocolate	½ bar (1.4 oz)	230	17	15	0
Milk Chocolate With Almonds	½ bar (1.4 oz)	230	16	14	0
Milk Chocolate With Crisp Rice	1 bar (2.3 oz)	370	29	24	0
Milk Chocolate With Fruit & Nuts	½ bar (1.4 oz)	220	18	15	0
Mint Chocolate	½ bar (1.4 oz)	200	23	15	0
Peanut Brittle No Sugar Added	⅓ box (1.5 oz)	210	28	tr	1
Peanut Butter Cups	5 (1.3 oz)	200	19	13	1
Peanut Butter Cups	1 (0.3 oz)	40	3	3	0
Toffee Sugar Free	5 (0.5 oz)	60	16	0	—
Favorite Brands					
Candy Corn	24 pieces (1.4 oz)	150	37	34	—

FOOD	PORTION	CALS.	CARB.	SUG.	FIB.
Favorite Brands (CONT.)					
Cinnamon Imperials	52 (0.5 oz)	80	14	12	—
Circus Peanuts	5 pieces (1.6 oz)	160	39	33	—
Gummallo Apple Ring	5 pieces (1.4 oz)	120	27	20	—
Gummallo Peach Ring	5 pieces (1.4 oz)	120	27	20	—
Gummi Bears	18 pieces (1.4 oz)	130	30	19	—
Gummi Dinos	7 pieces (1.3 oz)	120	28	18	—
Gummi Worms	4 pieces (1.4 oz)	130	29	18	—
Jelly Beans	13 (1.4 oz)	150	37	28	—
Marshmallow Eggs	3 (1.3 oz)	140	34	32	—
Neon Worms	4 pieces (1.4 oz)	120	28	22	—
Sour Gummi Bears	16 pieces (1.4 oz)	110	26	20	—
Sour Gummi Worms	4 pieces (1.6 oz)	130	29	23	—
Ferrero Rocher					
Candy	2 pieces (0.9 oz)	150	11	11	0
Franklin					
Crunch 'N Munch Candied	1.25 oz	170	28	—	1
Crunch 'N Munch Caramel	1.25 oz	160	28	—	1
Crunch 'N Munch Maple Walnut	1.25 oz	160	28	—	1
Crunch 'N Munch Toffee	1.25 oz	160	28	—	1
Glenny's					
Brown Rice Treats Carob & Mint With Oat Bran	1 bar (1.75 oz)	180	37	—	2
Brown Rice Treats Cinnamon & Raisin	1 bar (1.75 oz)	170	38	—	—
Brown Rice Treats Peanut & Raisin	1 bar (2 oz)	210	39	—	—
Brown Rice Treats Plain & Fancy	1 bar (1.25 oz)	120	28	—	—
Brown Rice Treats Raisin Bran	1 bar (1.75 oz)	170	38	—	—
Brown Rice Treats Toasted Almond With Oat Bran	1 bar (1.75 oz)	200	34	—	2
Fruit Drops Black Cherry	1	6	1	—	—
Fruit Drops Gentle Mint	1	6	1	—	—
Fruit Drops Mandarin Orange	1	6	1	—	—
Fruit Drops Mixed Fruit	1	6	1	—	—
Fruit Drops Twist Of Lemon	1	6	1	—	—
Hard Candies Fruit	1	19	4	—	—
Hard Candies Peppermint	1	19	4	—	—
Lollipops C Pops	1	35	8	—	—
Lollipops Fruit	1	21	5	—	—

FOOD	PORTION	CALS.	CARB.	SUG.	FIB.
Glenny's (CONT.)					
Moist & Chewy Coconut Almondine Bar	1 bar (1.5 oz)	190	22	—	—
Moist & Chewy Oatmeal Raisin Bar	1 bar (1.5 oz)	160	30	—	—
Moist & Chewy Peanut Bar	1 bar (1.5 oz)	180	24	—	—
Moist & Chewy Sunflower Bar	1 bar (1.5 oz)	180	24	—	—
Snack Bar Fat-Free Apple-Cinnamon	1 (1.25 oz)	120	28	—	—
Snack Bar Fat-Free Caramel	1 (1.25 oz)	120	29	—	—
Snack Bar Fat-Free Chocolate	1 (1.25 oz)	120	28	—	—
Snack Bar Fat-Free Raspberry	1 (1.25 oz)	120	29	—	—
Godiva					
Almond Butter Dome	3 pieces (1.5 oz)	240	19	14	0
Bouchee Au Chocolat	1 piece (1.5 oz)	210	25	18	0
Bouchee Ivory Raspberry	1 pieces (1 oz)	160	17	11	0
Gold Ballotin	3 pieces (1.5 oz)	210	27	21	0
Truffle Amaretto Di Saronno	2 pieces (1.5 oz)	210	24	17	0
Truffle Deluxe Liqueur	2 pieces (1.5 oz)	210	23	16	0
Golden Almond					
Bar	½ bar	260	20	—	—
Golden III					
Bar	½ bar	250	26	—	—
Goldenberg's					
Peanut Chews	3 pieces (1.3 oz)	180	22	14	1
Goo Goo Supreme					
With Pecans	1 pkg (1.5 oz)	188	34	20	4
Goobers					
Peanuts	1 pkg (1.38 oz)	210	19	16	3
Good & Fruity					
Candy	1 box (1.8 oz)	140	35	12	2
Good & Plenty					
Snacksize	3 boxes (1.5 oz)	140	34	24	—
Haviland					
Chocolate Covered Thin Mints	6 (1.5 oz)	170	33	32	1
Heath					
Bar	1 (1.4 oz)	210	25	24	0
Hershey					
Amazin'Fruit Gummy Candy	2 snack pkg (1.4 oz)	130	30	19	—

FOOD	PORTION	CALS.	CARB.	SUG.	FIB.
Hershey (CONT.)					
Bar	1 (1.55 oz)	240	25	—	—
Bar With Almonds	1 (1.45 oz)	230	20	—	—
Kisses	9 pieces (1.46 oz)	220	23	—	—
Special Dark Sweet Chocolate Bar	1 (1.45)	220	25	—	—
Jolly Rancher					
Candies	3 pieces (0.6 oz)	60	14	9	—
Joyva					
Halvah	1.5 oz	240	16	7	2
Halvah Chocolate Covered	1 bar (2 oz)	380	20	19	3
Jells Raspberry	3 pieces (1.6 oz)	200	25	24	tr
Joys Raspberry	1 (1.6 oz)	200	25	24	tr
Marshmallow Twists Chocolate Covered	2 (1.5 oz)	190	21	23	0
Rings Orange & Raspberry	3 pieces (1.5 oz)	190	23	22	tr
Sesame Crunch	3 pieces (0.5)	80	7	7	0
Sticks Orange	3 pieces (1.6 oz)	200	25	24	tr
Twists Vanilla & Cherry	2 pieces (1.5 oz)	190	21	23	0
Juicefuls					
Candy	3 pieces (0.5 oz)	60	15	15	—
Junior Mints					
Snack Size	1 pkg (0.7 oz)	75	16	16	0
Just Born					
Hot Tamales	1 pkg (2.1 oz)	220	55	34	—
Mike and Ike Berry Fruits	1 pkg (2.1 oz)	220	55	34	—
Mike and Ike Cherry & Bubble Gum	1 pkg (2.1 oz)	220	55	34	—
Mike and Ike Chewy Grape	1 pkg (2.1 oz)	220	55	34	—
Mike and Ike Lemon Watermelon	1 pkg (2.1 oz)	220	55	34	—
Mike and Ike Original	1 pkg (1.2 oz)	220	55	34	—
Mike and Ike Strawberry & Banana	1 pkg (2.1 oz)	220	55	34	—
Mike and Ike Tropical Fruits	1 pkg (2.1 oz)	220	55	34	—
Super Hot Tamales	1 pkg (2.1 oz)	220	55	34	—
Teenee Beanee Assorted Fruits	36 pieces (1.4 oz)	150	36	23	—
Teenee Beanee Berry Berry	36 pieces (1.4 oz)	150	36	23	—
Teenee Beanee Tropical Mix	36 pieces (1.4 oz)	150	36	23	—
Kit Kat					
Bar	1 (1.625 oz)	250	29	—	—
Krackel					
Bar	1 (1.55 oz)	230	27	—	—

FOOD	PORTION	CALS.	CARB.	SUG.	FIB.
Laffy Taffy					
Apple Chews	1 oz	110	26	—	—
Banana Chews	1 oz	110	26	—	—
Grape Chews	1 oz	110	26	—	—
Passion Punch Chews	1 oz	110	26	—	—
Strawberry Chews	1 oz	110	26	—	—
Sweet & Sour Cherry Chews	1 oz	110	26	—	—
Watermelon Chews	1 oz	110	26	—	—
Lance					
Chocolaty Peanut Bar	1 (57 g)	320	29	—	—
Peanut Bar	1 pkg (50 g)	260	24	—	—
Popscotch	1 pkg (35 g)	160	24	—	—
Lifesavers					
Big Tablet Candy Cane	4 pieces (0.5 oz)	60	16	13	—
Cards 'N Candy	4 pieces (0.4 oz)	40	10	10	—
Christmas Tin	4 pieces (0.5 oz)	60	16	13	—
Egg-Sortment	1 roll (0.4 oz)	40	10	10	—
Fruit Juicers Lollipops	1	40	10	—	0
Gummi Bunnies	3 pkg (1.6 oz)	140	34	23	—
Gummi Savers Five Flavor	1 roll (1.5 oz)	130	32	22	—
Gummi Savers Five Flavor	1 pkg (1.8 oz)	160	38	26	—
Gummi Savers Mixed Berry	1 roll (1.5 oz)	130	32	22	—
Gummi Savers Mixed Berry	1 pkg (1.8 oz)	160	38	24	—
Gummi Savers Tangy Fruits	1 pkg (1.8 oz)	160	38	24	—
Gummi Savers Tangy Fruits	1 roll (1.5 oz)	130	32	22	—
Gummi Savers Variety	2 pkg (1.3 oz)	120	27	19	—
Gummi Savers Wacky Frootz	1 roll (1.5 oz)	130	32	22	—
Gummi Savers Wacky Frootz	1 pkg (1.8 oz)	160	38	24	—
Holes Five Flavor	20 pieces (5 g)	20	5	4	—
Holes Island Fruit	20 pieces (5 g)	20	5	4	—
Holes Sour 'N Sweet	16 pieces (5 g)	20	5	4	—
Holes Sunshine Fruits	20 pieces (0.2 oz)	20	5	4	—
Holes Super Tart	20 pieces (5 g)	20	5	5	—
Holes Tangerine	1 candy	2	1	—	0
Holes Wild Fruits	20 pieces (5 g)	20	5	4	—
Lollipops Candy Cane	1 (0.4 oz)	40	10	7	—
Lollipops Christmas	1 (0.4 oz)	40	10	10	—
Lollipops Easter	1 (0.4 oz)	40	10	7	—
Lollipops Fruit Flavors	1 (0.4 oz)	45	11	11	0
Lollipops Swirled Flavors	1 (0.4 oz)	40	10	7	—
Lollipops Valentine	1 (0.4 oz)	40	10	10	—

FOOD	PORTION	CALS.	CARB.	SUG.	FIB.
Lifesavers (CONT.)					
Roll Butter Rum	2 pieces (5 g)	20	5	4	—
Roll Candy Cane	4 pieces (0.4 oz)	40	10	8	—
Roll Cryst-O-Mint	2 pieces (5 g)	20	5	4	—
Roll Five Flavor	2 pieces (5 g)	20	5	4	—
Roll Fruits On Fire	2 pieces (5 g)	20	5	4	—
Roll Pep-O-Mint	3 pieces (5 g)	20	5	5	—
Roll Spear-O-Mint	3 pieces (5 g)	20	5	5	—
Roll Sunshine Fruits	2 pieces (5 g)	20	5	4	—
Roll Tangy Fruit Swirl	2 pieces (5 g)	20	5	4	—
Roll Tangy Fruit Watermelon	1 pieces (5 g)	20	5	4	—
Roll Tangy Fruits	2 pieces (5 g)	20	5	4	—
Roll Tropical Fruits	2 pieces (5 g)	20	5	4	—
Roll Wild Cherry	1 piece (5 g)	20	5	4	—
Roll Wild Flavors	2 pieces (5 g)	20	5	4	—
Roll Wild Sour Berries	2 pieces (5 g)	20	5	4	—
Roll Wint-O-Green	3 pieces (5 g)	20	5	5	—
Sack'it Butter Rum	4 pieces (0.5 oz)	60	15	13	—
Sack'it Five Flavor	4 pieces (0.5 oz)	60	16	13	—
Sack'it Holiday Tin	4 pieces (0.5 oz)	60	16	13	—
Sack'it Pep-O-Mint	4 pieces (0.5 oz)	60	16	15	—
Sack'it Tangy Fruits	4 pieces (0.5 oz)	60	16	13	—
Sack'it Wild Cherry	4 pieces (0.5 oz)	60	16	13	—
Sack'it Wint-O-Green	4 pieces (0.5 oz)	60	16	15	—
Sugar Free Iced Mint	1 piece (2 g)	10	2	0	—
Sugar Free Vanilla Mint	1 piece (2 g)	10	2	0	—
Valentine Book	2 pieces (5 g)	20	5	4	—
Lindt					
Truffles	3 pieces (1.3 oz)	220	14	12	0
M&M's					
Almond	1.5 oz	220	24	21	2
Almond	1 pkg (1.3 oz)	200	21	18	2
Mint	1 pkg (1.7 oz)	230	34	31	1
Mint	1.5 oz	200	30	27	1
Peanut	½ bag king size (1.6 oz)	240	28	23	2
Peanut	1 fun size (0.7 oz)	110	13	11	1
Peanut	1 pkg (1.7 oz)	250	30	25	2
Peanut	1.5 oz	220	25	21	2
Peanut Butter	1 fun size (0.7 oz)	110	12	10	1
Peanut Butter	1.5 oz	220	25	20	2
Peanut Butter	1 pkg (1.6 oz)	240	27	22	2
Plain	1 pkg fun size (0.7 oz)	100	15	13	0

FOOD	PORTION	CALS.	CARB.	SUG.	FIB.
M&M's (CONT.)					
Plain	½ pkg king size (1.6 oz)	220	32	29	1
Plain	1 pkg (1.7 oz)	230	34	31	1
Plain	1.5 oz	200	30	27	1
Mars					
Almond Bar	2 fun size (1.3 oz)	190	23	20	1
Almond Bar	1 bar (1.8 oz)	240	31	26	1
Mayfair					
Mints	5 pieces (1.3 oz)	180	26	24	tr
Milk Duds					
Pieces	1 box (1.8 oz)	230	38	19	0
Snack Size	4 boxes (1.3 oz)	160	26	19	0
Milkshake					
Bar	1 bar (1.8 oz)	220	38	25	0
Milky Way					
Bar	2 fun size (1.4 oz)	180	28	24	0
Bar	⅓ king size (1.2 oz)	160	24	21	0
Bar	1 (2.1 oz)	280	43	37	1
Dark	1 fun size (0.7 oz)	90	14	12	0
Dark	1 bar (1.8 oz)	220	36	30	1
Miniature	5 (1.5 oz)	190	30	26	0
Mounds					
Bar	1 (1.9 oz)	260	31	—	—
Mr. Goodbar					
Candy	1 (1.75 oz)	290	23	—	—
Nestle					
Areo Bar	1 bar (1.45 oz)	210	26	23	2
Buncha Crunch	1 pkg (1.4 oz)	90	26	20	tr
Crunch	1 bar (1.55 oz)	230	28	23	1
Milk Chocolate	1 bar (1.45 oz)	220	23	21	2
Turtles Pecan Caramel Candy	2 pieces (1.2 oz)	160	20	13	1
Newman's Own					
Organics Espresso Sweet Dark Chocolate	1 bar (1.2 oz)	190	19	15	0
Nips					
Butter Rum	2 pieces (0.5 oz)	60	12	12	—
Caramel	2 pieces (0.5 oz)	60	12	12	—
Chocolate Mint	2 pieces (0.5 oz)	60	11	11	—
Chocolate Parfait	2 pieces (0.5 oz)	60	11	10	—
Peanut Butter Parfait	2 pieces (0.5 oz)	60	11	11	—
Ocean Spray					
Fruit Waves Assorted	3 pieces (0.3 oz)	35	9	9	—

FOOD	PORTION	CALS.	CARB.	SUG.	FIB.
Oh Henry!					
Bar	1 (1.8 oz)	230	32	30	2
Palmer					
Milk Chocolate Lollipop	1 (0.9 oz)	130	16	15	2
PayDay					
Bar	1 (1.85 oz)	240	28	20	2
Pearson					
Licorice	2 pieces (0.5 oz)	60	12	12	—
Pez					
Candy	1 roll (0.3 oz)	30	8	0	—
Sugar Free	1 roll (0.3 oz)	30	8	0	0
Planters					
Original Peanut Bar	1 pkg (1.6 oz)	230	22	13	2
Raisinets					
Candy	1 pkg (1.58 oz)	200	31	28	2
Fun Size	3 pkg (1.7 oz)	210	33	30	1
Reese's					
Peanut Butter Cups	1 (1.8 oz)	280	26	—	—
Pieces	1.85 oz	260	32	—	—
Sticks	1 (0.7 oz)	120	11	8	—
Riesen					
Candy	5 pieces (1.4 oz)	180	29	20	3
Rolo					
Carmels In Milk Chocolate	8 pieces (1.93 oz)	270	37	—	—
Russell Stover					
Assorted Creams	3 pieces (1.4 oz)	180	29	25	0
Looney Tunes Peanut Butter Nougat w/ Peanuts in Milk Chocolate	1 snack size (0.7 oz)	90	14	7	tr
Pecan Roll	1 (2 oz)	300	26	21	3
Simply Lite					
Sugar Free Lil'l Bits Chocolately	36 pieces (1.4 oz)	130	28	0	1
Sugar Free Lil'l Bits Peanut Buttery	36 pieces (1.4 oz)	140	26	0	1
Sugar Free Patteez	5 pieces (1.3 oz)	110	29	0	1
Skittles					
Original	2 pkg fun size (1.6 oz)	180	41	35	0
Original	1 pkg (2.8 oz)	250	55	47	0
Original	½ king size (1.3 oz)	150	34	29	0
Original	1.5 oz	170	38	32	0
Tropical	1 bag (2.2 oz)	250	56	47	0

FOOD	PORTION	CALS.	CARB.	SUG.	FIB.
Skittles (CONT.)					
Tropical	1.5 oz	170	38	32	0
Tropical	2 bags fun size (1.4 oz)	160	36	31	0
Wild Berry	2 bags fun size (1.4 oz)	160	36	31	0
Wild Berry	1 bag (2.2 oz)	250	56	47	0
Wild Berry	1.5 oz	170	38	32	0
Skor					
Toffee Bar	1 (1.4 oz)	220	22	—	—
Smucker's					
Jelly Beans	1 pkg (0.7 oz)	70	18	14	0
Snickers					
Bar	1 bar (2.1 oz)	280	36	29	1
Bar	2 bars fun size (1.4 oz)	190	24	20	1
Bar	⅓ king size (1.2 oz)	170	21	17	1
Miniatures	4 (1.3 oz)	170	22	18	1
Munch Bar	1 (1.4 oz)	230	17	12	2
Peanut Butter	1 bar (2 oz)	310	28	23	1
Sno-Caps					
Candies	1 pkg (2.3 oz)	300	48	38	3
Solitaires					
Candies	½ bag	260	20	—	—
Sour Punch					
Candy Straws Sour Apple	6 pieces (1.4 oz)	130	31	20	—
Spice Stix					
And Drops	14 pieces (1.6 oz)	140	35	15	—
Starburst					
California Fruits	8 pieces (1.4 oz)	160	33	22	0
California Fruits	1 stick (2.1 oz)	240	48	32	0
Original Fruits	⅓ king size (1.2 oz)	140	28	19	0
Original Fruits	8 pieces (1.4 oz)	160	33	22	0
Orignal Fruits	1 stick (2.1 oz)	240	48	32	0
Strawberry Fruits	8 pieces (1.4 oz)	160	33	22	0
Strawberry Fruits	1 stick (2.1 oz)	240	48	32	0
Tropical Fruits	1 stick (2.1 oz)	240	48	32	0
Tropical Fruits	8 pieces (1.4 oz)	160	33	22	0
Swedish Fish					
Original	19 pieces (1.4 oz)	160	39	24	0
Sweet Escapes					
Triple Chocolate Wafer Bars	1 (0.7 oz)	80	14	12	—
Sweet'N Low					
Sugar Free Butter Toffee	4 pieces (0.5 oz)	30	15	—	—

FOOD	PORTION	CALS.	CARB.	SUG.	FIB.
Sweet'N Low (CONT.)					
Sugar Free Butterscotch	1 piece	7	4	—	—
Sugar Free Cinnamon	1 piece	7	4	—	—
Sugar Free Fancy Fruit	1 piece	7	4	—	—
Sugar Free Fruit Flavors	1 piece	7	4	—	—
Sugar Free Hard Candy Coffee	4 pieces (0.5 oz)	30	14	—	—
Sugar Free Peppermint	1 piece	7	4	—	—
Sugar Free Soft Candy Fruitie Flavors	1 piece	11	4	—	—
Sugar Free Soft Candy Tropical Flavors	1 piece	11	4	—	—
Sugar Free Watermelon	1 piece	7	4	—	—
Sugar Free Wild Cherry	1 piece	7	4	—	—
Switzer					
Cherry Bites	12 pieces (1.6 oz)	50	11	4	—
Licorice Bites	12 pieces (1.6 oz)	46	11	3	—
Symphony					
Almond Butterchips	1 (1.4 oz)	220	20	—	—
Milk Chocolate	1 (1.4 oz)	220	22	—	—
Terry's					
Orange Milk Chocolate	5 pieces (1.5 oz)	240	26	24	1
Twix					
Caramel	1 pkg (2 oz)	280	37	27	0
Caramel	1 (1 oz)	140	19	14	0
Caramel	1 fun size (0.5 oz)	80	10	8	0
Caramel	1 king size (0.8 oz)	120	15	11	1
Peanut Butter	1 (0.9 oz)	130	13	9	1
Twizzlers					
Candy	4 pieces (1.4 oz)	130	30	14	—
Pull-N-Peel Cherry	1 piece (1.1 oz)	110	23	13	—
Velamints					
Cocoamint	1 piece (1.7 g)	5	2	0	—
Peppermint	1 piece (1.7 g)	5	2	0	—
Spearmint	1 piece (1.7 g)	5	2	0	—
Wintergreen	1 piece (1.7 g)	5	2	0	—
Very Special					
Chocolate Bottles Liquor Filled	3 pieces (1 oz)	150	24	9	2
Whatchamacallit					
Bar	1 (1.8 oz)	260	30	—	—
Whitman's					
Assorted	3 pieces (1.4 oz)	190	27	22	0
Dark Chocolate	3 pieces (1.4 oz)	200	25	19	1

FOOD	PORTION	CALS.	CARB.	SUG.	FIB.
Whitman's (CONT.)					
Little Ambassadors	7 pieces (1.4 oz)	190	26	22	1
Pecan Delight	1 bar (2 oz)	310	27	17	2
Pecan Roll	1 bar (2 oz)	300	26	21	1
Sampler	3 pieces (1.4 oz)	200	25	19	1
Snoopy Treats Caramel Peanuts Milk Chocolate	1 snack size (1.4 oz)	80	24	18	tr
Whoppers					
Candy	1 pkg (1.8 oz)	230	36	28	1
Y&S					
Bites Cherry	1 oz	100	23	—	—
York					
Peppermint Patty	1 snack size (0.5 oz)	57	11	8	—
Peppermint Patty	1 (1.5 oz)	180	34	—	—
Zero					
Bar	2 pieces (1.4 oz)	170	28	21	0
CANTALOUPE					
fresh cubed	1 cup	57	13	—	1
fresh half	½	94	22	—	2
Big Valley					
Balls frzn	¾ cup (4.9 oz)	40	10	7	0
Dole					
Fresh	¼	50	11	—	0
CAPERS					
Progresso					
Capers	1 tsp (5 g)	0	0	0	0
CARIBOU					
roasted	3 oz	142	0	0	0
CARROT JUICE					
Hollywood					
Juice	6 fl oz	80	17	—	2
Odwalla					
Juice	8 fl oz	70	18	8	2
CARROTS					
CANNED					
slices	½ cup	17	4	—	1
slices low sodium	½ cup	17	4	—	1
Allen					
Sliced	½ cup (4.5 oz)	35	8	3	3
Crest Top					
Sliced	½ cup (4.5 oz)	35	8	3	3

FOOD	PORTION	CALS.	CARB.	SUG.	FIB.
Del Monte					
Cut	½ cup (4.3 oz)	35	8	5	3
Sliced	½ cup (4.3 oz)	35	8	5	3
Green Giant					
Sliced	½ cup (4.2 oz)	25	6	3	2
LeSueur					
Baby Whole	½ cup (4.2 oz)	35	8	5	3
S&W					
Diced Fancy	½ cup	30	7	—	—
Seneca					
Diced	½ cup	30	6	—	2
Sliced	½ cup	30	6	—	2
FRESH					
baby raw	1 (½ oz)	6	1	—	—
raw	1 (2.5 oz)	31	7	—	2
raw shredded	½ cup	24	6	—	2
Dole					
Medium	1	40	8	—	1
FROZEN					
Big Valley					
Carrots	½ cup (3 oz)	35	8	6	2
Birds Eye					
Baby Whole	⅔ cup (3 oz)	35	6	3	2
Fresh Like					
Carrots	3.5 oz	42	10	—	—
Green Giant					
Select Baby Cut	¾ cup (2.8 oz)	30	7	3	3
CASABA					
cubed	1 cup	45	11	—	—
CASHEWS					
Planters					
Fancy Oil Roasted	1 oz	170	8	tr	1
Fancy Oil Roasted	1 pkg (2 oz)	340	16	2	3
Halves Lightly Salted Oil Roasted	1 oz	160	9	0	2
Halves Oil Roasted	1 oz	170	8	tr	2
Honey Roasted	1 oz	150	11	5	1
Honey Roasted	1 pkg (2 oz)	310	23	9	3
Munch'N Go Honey Roasted	1 pkg (2 oz)	310	23	7	3
Munch'N Go Singles Oil Roasted	1 pkg (2 oz)	330	16	1	3
Oil Roasted	1 pkg (1 oz)	160	8	2	1

FOOD	PORTION	CALS.	CARB.	SUG.	FIB.
Planters (CONT.)					
Oil Roasted	1 pkg (1.5 oz)	250	12	0	2
CATFISH					
channel breaded & fried	3 oz	194	7	—	—
CATSUP					
(*see* KETCHUP)					
CAULIFLOWER					
FRESH					
cooked	½ cup (2.2 oz)	14	3	—	1
flowerets cooked	3 (2 oz)	12	2	—	1
flowerets raw	3 (2 oz)	14	3	—	1
green cooked	1½ cup (3.2 oz)	29	6	—	3
green raw	1 head 7 in diam (18 oz)	158	31	—	16
green raw	1 cup (2.2 oz)	20	4	—	2
green raw floweret	1 (0.9 oz)	8	2	—	1
raw	½ cup (1.8 oz)	13	3	—	1
Dole					
Cauliflower	⅙ med head	18	3	—	2
FROZEN					
Big Valley					
Florets	¾ cup (3 oz)	25	4	1	1
Birds Eye					
Frzn	⅔ cup	25	5	—	2
In Cheese Sauce	½ cup (4.1 oz)	80	7	3	1
Fresh Like					
Cauliflower	3.5 oz	26	5	—	1
Green Giant					
Cheese Sauce	½ cup (3.5 oz)	60	8	4	2
Florets	1 cup (2.8 oz)	25	4	1	2
CAVIAR					
black	1 tbsp	40	1	—	—
red	1 tbsp	40	1	—	—
CELERY					
FRESH					
raw	1 stalk (1.3 oz)	6	1	—	1
raw diced	½ cup	10	2	—	1
Dole					
Stalks	2 med	20	2	—	4
FROZEN					
Fresh Like					
Celery	3.5 oz	14	3	—	1

FOOD	PORTION	CALS.	CARB.	SUG.	FIB.

CEREAL

FOOD	PORTION	CALS.	CARB.	SUG.	FIB.
corn flakes low sodium	1 cup (0.9 oz)	100	22	—	tr
corn grits white regular & quick as prep w/ water & salt	¾ cup (6.4 oz)	109	24	—	tr
corn grits white regular or quick as prep	¾ cup (6.4 oz)	109	24	—	tr
corn grits yellow regular & quick as prep w/ water & salt	¾ cup (6.4 oz)	109	24	—	tr
corn grits yellow regular & quick not prep	1 cup (5.5 oz)	579	124	—	3
crispy rice	1 cup (1 oz)	111	25	—	tr
crispy rice low sodium	1 cup (0.9 oz)	105	23	—	tr
farina as prep w/ water	¾ cup (6.1 oz)	88	19	—	2
farina not prep	1 tbsp (0.4 oz)	40	9	—	tr
oatmeal instant w/ cinnamon & spice as prep w/ water	1 pkg (5.6 oz)	177	35	—	3
oatmeal instant w/ raisins & spice as prep w/ water	1 cup (5.5 oz)	161	32	—	2
oatmeal instant w/ bran & raisins as prep w/ water	1 pkg (6.8 oz)	158	30	—	6
oatmeal istant as prep w/ water	1 cup (8.2 oz)	138	24	—	4
oatmeal regular & quick as prep w/ water	¾ cup (6.1 oz)	149	19	—	3
oatmeal regular & quick not prep	⅓ cup (0.9 oz)	104	18	—	3
puffed rice	1 cup (0.5 oz)	56	13	—	tr
puffed wheat	1 cup (0.4 oz)	44	10	—	1
shredded mini wheats	1 cup (1.1 oz)	107	24	—	3
shredded wheat rectangular	1 biscuit (0.8 oz)	85	19	—	2
shredded wheat round	2 biscuits (1.3 oz)	136	31	—	4
whole wheat hot natural as prep w/ water	¾ cup (6.4 oz)	113	25	—	3
Albers					
Hominy Quick Grits uncooked	¼ cup	140	31	—	1
Arrowhead					
4 Grain + Flax	¼ cup (1.6 oz)	150	28	0	6
7 Grain	⅓ cup (1.4 oz)	140	25	0	5
Amaranth Flakes	1 cup (1.2 oz)	130	25	3	3

FOOD	PORTION	CALS.	CARB.	SUG.	FIB.
Arrowhead (CONT.)					
Apple Corns	1 cup (1.5 oz)	150	35	10	4
Bear Mush	¼ cup (1.6 oz)	160	33	0	2
Bran Flakes	1 cup (1 oz)	100	22	6	4
Kamut Flakes	1 cup (1.1 oz)	120	25	2	3
Maple Corns	1 cup (1.9 oz)	190	43	11	6
Multi Grain Flakes	1 cup (1.2 oz)	140	29	3	3
Nature O's	1 cup (1.1 oz)	130	24	1	3
Oat Bran Flakes	1 cup (1.2 oz)	110	22	8	4
Oat Flakes Rolled	⅓ cup (1.2 oz)	130	23	tr	4
Oat Groats	¼ cup (1.5 oz)	160	29	tr	4
Oatmeal Instant Original	1 oz	100	22	—	—
Puffed Corn	1 cup (0.8 oz)	80	16	0	1
Puffed Kamut	1 cup (0.6 oz)	50	11	0	2
Puffed Millet	1 cup (0.9 oz)	90	19	0	1
Puffed Rice	1 cup (0.8 oz)	90	19	0	1
Puffed Wheat	1 cup (0.9)	90	20	0	2
Rice & Shine	¼ cup (1.5 oz)	150	32	0	2
Spelt Flakes	1 cup (1.1 oz)	100	22	2	3
Wheat Flakes Rolled	⅓ cup (1.2 oz)	110	24	0	5
Aunt Jemima					
Enriched White Hominy Grits Regular	3 tbsp	101	22	—	1
Barbara's					
Apple Cinnamon Toasted O's	¾ cup	110	24	11	2
Bite Size Shredded Oats	1¼ cups (2 oz)	220	46	12	6
Breakfast O's	1 cup (1 oz)	120	22	2	3
Brown Rice Crisps	1 cup (1 oz)	120	25	2	1
Cocoa Crunch Stars	1 cup (1 oz)	110	26	8	1
Corn Flakes	1 cup (1 oz)	110	26	3	2
Frosted Corn Flakes	1 cup (1 oz)	110	27	8	4
Honey Crunch Stars	1 cup (1 oz)	110	26	8	2
Honey Nut Toasted O's	¾ cup	120	23	11	2
Organic Ultra Minis Frosted	¾ cup (1.9 oz)	190	46	12	7
Organic Ultra Minis Original	¾ cup (1.9 oz)	190	45	4	8
Organic Fruity Punch	1 cup (1 oz)	110	26	8	0
Puffins	¾ cup (0.9 oz)	90	23	5	5
Shredded Spoonfuls	¾ cup (1.1 oz)	120	23	5	4
Shredded Wheat	2 biscuits (1.4 oz)	140	31	0	5
Betty Crocker					
Dutch Apple	1 cup (1.9 oz)	220	47	18	1
Streusel	¾ cup (1 oz)	120	25	9	1

FOOD	PORTION	CALS.	CARB.	SUG.	FIB.
Cap'n Crunch					
Crunchberries	¾ cup	113	24	—	1
Original	¾ cup	113	24	—	1
Peanut Butter Crunch	¾ cup	119	22	—	1
Erewhon					
Aztec	1 oz	100	24	—	1
Barley Plus	1 oz	110	22	—	1
Crispy Brown Rice	1 oz	110	24	—	4
Fruit 'n Wheat	1 oz	100	21	—	3
Oat Bran With Toasted Wheat Germ	1 oz	115	18	—	3
Oatmeal Instant Dates & Walnuts	1.2 oz	130	24	—	3
Oatmeal Instant With Added Oat Bran	1.25 oz	125	23	—	4
Raisin Bran	1 oz	100	22	—	3
Super-O's	1 oz	110	24	—	4
Wheat Flakes	1 oz	100	22	—	4
Estee					
Corn Flakes	1 pkg (1 oz)	90	24	tr	4
Raisin Bran	1 pkg (1 oz)	90	21	6	3
General Mills					
Apple Cinnamon Cheerios	¾ cup (1 oz)	120	25	13	1
Basic 4	1 cup (1.9 oz)	200	43	14	3
Berry Berry Kix	¾ cup (1 oz)	120	26	9	0
Body Buddies Natural Fruit	1 cup (1 oz)	120	26	6	0
Booberry	1 cup (1 oz)	120	27	14	0
Cheerios	1 cup (1 oz)	110	22	1	3
Cinnamon Grahams	¾ cup (1 oz)	120	26	11	1
Cinnamon Toast Crunch	¾ cup (1 oz)	130	24	10	1
Cocoa Puffs	1 cup (1 oz)	120	27	14	0
Cookie Crisp	1 cup (1 oz)	120	25	12	0
Corn Chex	1 cup (1 oz)	110	26	3	0
Count Chocula	1 cup (1 oz)	120	26	14	0
Country Corn Flakes	1 cup (1 oz)	120	26	2	0
Crispy Wheaties 'n Raisins	1 cup (1.9 oz)	190	44	20	4
Fiber One	½ cup (1 oz)	60	24	0	13
Frankenberry	1 cup (1 oz)	120	27	14	0
French Toast Crunch	¾ cup (1 oz)	120	26	12	0
Frosted Cheerios	1 cup (1 oz)	120	25	13	1
Golden Grahams	¾ cup (1 oz)	120	25	11	1
Honey Frosted Wheaties	¾ cup (1 oz)	110	27	12	0
Honey Nut Cheerios	1 cup (1 oz)	120	24	11	2
Honey Nut Clusters	1 cup (1.9 oz)	210	46	16	3

FOOD	PORTION	CALS.	CARB.	SUG.	FIB.
General Mills (CONT.)					
Jurassic Park Crunch	1 cup (1 oz)	120	26	13	1
Kaboom	1¼ cup (1 oz)	120	24	6	1
Kix	1⅓ cup (1 oz)	120	26	3	1
Lucky Charms	1 cup (1 oz)	120	25	13	1
Multi-Bran Chex	1 cup (2 oz)	200	49	12	7
Multi-Grain Cheerios	1 cup (1 oz)	110	24	6	3
Oatmeal Crisp Almond	1 cup (1.9 oz)	220	42	15	4
Oatmeal Crisp Apple Cinnamon	1 cup (1.9 oz)	210	46	19	4
Oatmeal Crisp Raisin	1 cup (1.9 oz)	210	44	19	3
Raisin Nut Bran	¾ cup (1.9 oz)	200	41	16	5
Reese's Peanut Butter Puffs	¾ cup (1 oz)	130	24	13	0
Rice Chex	1¼ cup (1.1 oz)	120	27	2	0
S'Mores Grahams	¾ cup (1 oz)	120	26	13	0
Sun Crunchers	1 cup (1.9 oz)	220	45	16	2
Team Cheerios	1 cup (1 oz)	120	25	11	1
Total Corn Flakes	1⅓ cup (1 oz)	110	25	3	0
Total Raisin Bran	1 cup (1.9 oz)	180	43	19	5
Total Whole Grain	¾ cup (1 oz)	110	24	5	3
Trix	1 cup (1 oz)	120	26	13	1
Wheat Chex	1 cup (1.9 oz)	180	41	1	5
Wheat Hearts not prep	¼ cup (1.3 oz)	130	26	1	2
Wheaties	1 cup (1 oz)	110	24	4	3
Good Shepherd					
Millet Rice Flakes Wheat Free	1 oz	95	19	—	1
Spelt	1 oz	90	20	—	3
Spelt Flakes	1 oz	100	21	—	2
Grist Mill					
Apple Cinnamon Natural	½ cup (1.9 oz)	260	36	15	3
Bran	½ cup (1.9 oz)	250	37	8	11
Oat & Honey Natural	½ cup (1.9 oz)	270	34	11	4
Oat Honey & Raisin Natural	½ cup (1.9 oz)	260	35	14	4
H-O					
Farina Instant	1 pkg	110	22	—	3
Farina not prep	3 tbsp	120	26	—	3
Oatmeal Instant	½ cup	130	22	—	3
Oatmeal Instant	1 pkg	110	18	—	3
Oatmeal Instant Apple Cinnamon	1 pkg	130	26	—	3
Oatmeal Instant Maple Brown Sugar	1 pkg	160	32	—	3

FOOD	PORTION	CALS.	CARB.	SUG.	FIB.
H-O (CONT.)					
Oatmeal Instant Raisin & Spice	1 pkg	150	32	—	3
Oatmeal Instant Sweet 'n Mellow	1 pkg	150	30	—	3
Oats 'n Fiber	⅓ cup	100	15	—	3
Oats 'n Fiber	1 pkg	110	18	—	3
Oats 'n Fiber Apple & Bran	1 pkg	130	26	—	3
Oats 'n Fiber Raisin & Bran	1 pkg	150	32	—	3
Oats Gourmet	⅓ cup	100	18	—	3
Oats Quick	½ cup	130	22	—	3
Health Valley					
100% Natural Bran With Apples & Cinnamon	¼ cup (1 oz)	100	22	—	5
Amaranth Cereal With Bananas	½ cup (1 oz)	110	20	—	4
Amaranth Crunch With Raisins	¼ cup (1 oz)	110	20	—	3
Amaranth Flakes 100% Organic	½ cup (1 oz)	90	21	—	3
Blue Corn Flakes 100% Organic	½ cup (1 oz)	90	19	—	3
Bran Cereal With Dates 100% Organic	¼ cup (1 oz)	100	20	—	5
Bran Cereal With Raisins 100% Organic	¼ cup (1 oz)	100	20	—	5
Fiber 7 Flakes 100% Organic	½ cup (1 oz)	90	20	—	5
Fiber 7 Flakes With Raisins 100% Organic	½ cup (1 oz)	90	20	—	5
Fruit & Fitness	1 cup (2 oz)	220	37	—	11
Fruit Lites Corn	½ cup (0.5 oz)	45	10	—	tr
Fruit Lites Rice	½ cup (0.5 oz)	45	11	—	tr
Fruit Lites Wheat	½ cup (0.5 oz)	45	11	—	2
Healthy Crunch Almond Date	¼ cup (1 oz)	110	18	—	4
Healthy Crunch Apple Cinnamon	¼ cup (1 oz)	110	18	—	4
Healthy O's 100% Organic	¾ cup (1 oz)	90	18	—	3
Lites Puffed Corn	½ cup (1 oz)	50	11	—	tr
Lites Puffed Rice	½ cup (1 oz)	50	12	—	tr
Lites Puffed Wheat	½ cup (1 oz)	50	11	—	1
Oat Bran Flakes 100% Organic	½ cup (1 oz)	100	20	—	4

FOOD	PORTION	CALS.	CARB.	SUG.	FIB.
Health Valley (CONT.)					
Oat Bran Flakes Almonds/ Dates 100% Organic	½ cup (1 oz)	100	20	—	4
Oat Bran Flakes With Raisins 100% Organic	½ cup (1 oz)	100	20	—	4
Oat Bran Natural Apples & Cinnamon	¼ cup (1 oz)	100	19	—	4
Oat Bran Natural Raisins & Spice	¼ cup	100	19	—	4
Oat Bran O'S 100% Organic	½ cup (1 oz)	110	20	—	3
Oat Bran O'S Fruit & Nuts	½ cup (1 oz)	110	19	—	3
Orangeola Almonds & Dates	¼ cup	110	18	—	4
Orangeola Bananas & Hawaiian Fruit	¼ cup (1 oz)	120	20	—	4
Raisin Bran Flakes 100% Organic	½ cup (1 oz)	100	21	—	6
Real Oat Bran Almond Crunch	¼ cup (1 oz)	110	17	—	4
Real Oat Bran Hawaiian Fruit	¼ cup (1 oz)	130	22	—	5
Real Oat Bran Raisin Nut	¼ cup (1 oz)	130	21	—	5
Rice Bran O's	½ cup	110	22	—	2
Rice Bran With Almonds & Dates	½ cup (1 oz)	110	19	—	2
Sprouts 7 Bananas & Hawaiian Fruit	¼ cup (1 oz)	90	16	—	4
Sprouts 7 Raisin	¼ cup	90	16	—	5
Swiss Breakfast Raisin Nut	¼ cup (1 oz)	100	19	—	3
Swiss Breakfast Tropical Fruit	¼ cup (1 oz)	100	19	—	3
Healthy Choice					
Almond Crunch With Raisins	1 cup (2 oz)	210	46	16	5
Golden Multi- Grain Flakes	¾ cup (1.1 oz)	110	26	6	3
Toasted Brown Sugar Squares	1 cup (2 oz)	190	44	9	5
Heartland					
Coconut	1 oz	130	18	—	2
Plain	1 oz	130	18	—	2
Raisin	1 oz	130	18	—	2
Kashi					
5-Bran	2½ oz	281	47	—	16
Cereal	2 oz	177	38	—	5

FOOD	PORTION	CALS.	CARB.	SUG.	FIB.
Kashi (CONT.)					
Puffed	¾ oz	74	16	—	2
Kellogg's					
All-Bran	½ cup (1.1 oz)	80	24	6	10
All-Bran Bran Buds	⅓ cup (1 oz)	80	24	8	13
All-Bran Extra Fiber	½ cup (0.9 oz)	50	20	0	13
Apple Jacks	1 cup (1.2 oz)	120	30	16	1
Cocoa Frosted Flakes	¾ cup (1.1 oz)	120	28	13	0
Cocoa Krispies	¾ cup (1.1 oz)	120	27	13	0
Complete Oat Bran Flakes	¾ cup (1 oz)	110	23	6	4
Complete Wheat Bran Flakes	¾ cup (1 oz)	90	23	5	5
Corn Flakes	1 cup (1 oz)	100	24	2	1
Corn Pops	1 cup (1.1 oz)	120	28	14	0
Cracklin' Oat Bran	¾ cup (1.7 oz)	190	35	15	6
Crispix	1 cup (1 oz)	110	25	3	1
Froot Loops	1 cup (1.1 oz)	120	28	15	1
Frosted Flakes	¾ cup (1.1 oz)	120	28	13	1
Honey Crunch Corn Flakes	¾ cup (1.1 oz)	120	26	10	1
Just Right Crunchy Nuggets	1 cup (2 oz)	210	46	12	3
Just Right Fruit & Nut	1 cup (2.1 oz)	220	49	15	3
Mini-Wheat Frosted	1 cup (1.8 oz)	180	41	10	5
Mini-Wheat Strawberry Squares	¾ cup (1.8 oz)	170	40	9	5
Mini-Wheats Apple Cinnamon Squares	¾ cup (1.9 oz)	180	44	12	5
Mini-Wheats Blueberry Squares	¾ cup (1.9 oz)	180	43	11	5
Mini-Wheats Frosted Bite Size	24 pieces (2.1 oz)	200	48	12	6
Mini-Wheats Raisin Squares	¾ cup (1.9 oz)	180	42	12	5
Mueslix Apple & Almond Crunch	¾ cups (1.9 oz)	200	39	12	5
Mueslix Raisin & Almond	⅔ cup (1.9 oz)	200	41	17	4
Nutri-Grain Almond Raisin	1¼ cup (1.7 oz)	180	38	7	4
Nutri-Grain Golden Wheat	¾ cup (1 oz)	100	23	0	4
Product 19	1 cup (1 oz)	100	25	4	1
Raisin Bran	1 cup (2.1 oz)	200	47	18	8
Rice Krispies	1¼ cup (1.2 oz)	120	29	3	0
Rice Krispies Razzle Dazzle	¾ cup (1 oz)	110	25	10	0
Rice Krispies Treats	¾ cup (1 oz)	120	26	9	0
Smacks	¾ cup (1 oz)	100	24	15	1

FOOD	PORTION	CALS.	CARB.	SUG.	FIB.
Kellogg's (CONT.)					
Smart Start	1 cup (1.8 oz)	180	43	15	2
Special K	1 cup (1.1 oz)	110	21	4	1
Kolln					
Crispy Oats	1 cup (1.8 oz)	190	40	9	2
Oat Bran Crunch	⅔ cup (2.1 oz)	220	41	2	9
Oat Muesli Fruit	¾ cup (2 oz)	200	39	12	4
Kraft					
Morning Traditions Banana Nut Crunch	1 cup (2 oz)	250	43	12	4
Morning Traditions Blueberry Morning	1¼ cup (1.9 oz)	220	43	13	2
Morning Traditions Cranberry Almond Crunch	1 cup (1.9 oz)	220	44	15	3
Morning Traditions Great Grains Crunchy Pecan	⅔ cup (1.9 oz)	220	38	9	4
Morning Traditions Great Grains Raisins Dates & Pecans	⅔ cup (1.9 oz)	210	39	14	4
Little Crow					
Coco Wheat	3 tbsp (36 g)	130	28	—	4
Maltex					
Cereal	1 oz	105	21	—	3
Maypo					
30 Second	1 oz	100	19	—	2
Vermont Style	1 oz	105	20	—	2
With Oat Bran	1 oz	130	26	—	4
McCann's					
Irish Oatmeal	1 oz	110	20	0	3
Mother's					
Oatmeal Instant	½ cup (1.4 oz)	150	27	1	4
Whole Wheat Natural	½ cup (1.4 oz)	130	30	0	4
Mueslix					
Crispy Blend	⅔ cup (1.9 oz)	200	42	16	4
Nabisco					
100% Bran	⅓ cup (1 oz)	80	23	7	8
Cream Of Wheat Instant as prep	1 cup	120	25	0	1
Cream Of Wheat Quick as prep	1 cup	120	25	0	1
Cream Of Wheat Regular as prep	1 cup	120	25	0	1
Frosted Shredded Wheat Bite Size	1 cup (1.8 oz)	190	44	12	5

FOOD	PORTION	CALS.	CARB.	SUG.	FIB.
Nabisco (CONT.)					
Honey Nut Shredded Wheat Bite Size	1 cup (1.8 oz)	200	43	12	4
Mix'n Eat Cream Of Wheat Apple & Cinnamon	1 pkg (1¼ oz)	130	29	—	1
Mix'n Eat Cream Of Wheat Brown Sugar Cinnamon	1 pkg (1¼ oz)	130	29	—	1
Mix'n Eat Cream Of Wheat Maple Brown Sugar	1 pkg (1¼ oz)	130	29	—	1
Mix'n Eat Cream Of Wheat Our Original	1 pkg (1¼ oz)	100	21	—	1
Original Shredded Wheat	2 biscuits (1.6 oz)	160	38	0	5
Original Shredded Wheat 'N Bran	1¼ cup (2.1 oz)	200	47	tr	8
Original Shredded Wheat Spoon Size	1 cup (1.7 oz)	170	41	0	5
Nutri-Grain					
Almond Raisin	1¼ cup (2 oz)	200	43	8	4
Golden Wheat	¾ cup (1.1 oz)	100	24	0	4
Post					
Alpha-Bits	1 cup (1 oz)	130	27	13	1
Bran Flakes	¾ cup (1 oz)	100	24	6	5
Cocoa Pebbles	¾ cup (1 oz)	120	26	13	0
Fruit & Fibre Dates Raisins & Walnuts	1 cup (1.9 oz)	210	42	17	5
Fruit & Fibre Peaches Raisins & Almonds	1 cup (1.9 oz)	210	42	14	5
Fruity Pebbles	¾ cup (1 oz)	110	24	12	0
Golden Crisp	¾ cup (1 oz)	110	25	15	0
Grape-Nuts	¾ cup (1 oz)	100	24	5	3
Grape-Nuts	½ cup (2 oz)	200	47	7	5
Honey Bunches Of Oats	¾ cup (1 oz)	120	25	6	1
Honey Bunches Of Oats With Almonds	¾ cup (1.1 oz)	130	24	7	1
Honeycomb	1⅓ cups (1 oz)	110	26	11	tr
Marshmallow Alpha-Bits	1 cup (1 oz)	120	25	14	0
Post Toasties	1 cup (1 oz)	100	24	2	1
Raisin Bran	1 cup (2 oz)	190	47	20	8
Waffle Crisp	1 cup (1 oz)	130	24	11	0
Waffle Crisp	1 cup (1 oz)	130	24	11	0
Quaker					
100% Natural	¼ cup	127	18	—	2
100% Natural Apples & Cinnamon	¼ cup	126	19	—	2

FOOD	PORTION	CALS.	CARB.	SUG.	FIB.
Quaker (CONT.)					
100% Natural Raisin & Date	¼ cup	123	18	—	2
Crunchy Bran	⅔ cup	89	23	—	5
Crunchy Not Oh!s	1 cup	127	22	—	1
Enriched White Hominy Grits Quick	3 tbsp	101	22	—	1
Enriched Yellow Hominy Quick Grits	3 tbsp	101	22	—	1
Honey Graham Oh!s	1 cup	122	23	—	1
Instant Grits Original	1 pkg (1 oz)	100	22	—	1
Instant Grits With Imitation Bacon Bits	1 pkg	101	22	—	2
Instant Grits With Imitation Ham Bits	1 pkg	99	21	—	2
Instant Grits With Real Cheddar Cheese	1 pkg	104	22	—	1
King Vitaman	1½ cup	110	23	—	1
Life Cinnamon	⅔ cup	101	19	—	3
Life Original	⅔ cup	101	19	—	3
Multigrain	½ cup (1.4 oz)	130	29	1	5
Oat Squares	½ cup	105	21	—	2
Oatmeal Instant	1 pkg (1 oz)	100	19	0	3
Oatmeal Instant Apples & Cinnamon	1 pkg (1.2 oz)	130	27	11	3
Oatmeal Instant Bananas & Cream	1 pkg (1.2 oz)	130	26	11	2
Oatmeal Instant Blueberries & Cream	1 pkg (1.2 oz)	130	26	11	2
Oatmeal Instant Cinnamon & Spice	1 pkg (1.6 oz)	170	36	16	3
Oatmeal Instant Kid's Choice Chocolate Chip Cookie	1 pkg (1.5 oz)	160	32	12	3
Oatmeal Instant Kid's Choice Cookie'n Cream	1 pkg (1.5 oz)	160	31	12	2
Oatmeal Instant Kid's Choice Fruity Marshmallow	1 pkg (1.4 oz)	150	31	13	3
Oatmeal Instant Kid's Choice Oatmeal Raisin Cookie	1 pkg (1.5 oz)	160	32	14	2
Oatmeal Instant Kid's Choice Radical Raspberry	1 pkg (1.4 oz)	150	29	11	3

FOOD	PORTION	CALS.	CARB.	SUG.	FIB.
Quaker (CONT.)					
Oatmeal Instant Kid's Choice S'mores	1 pkg (1.5 oz)	160	32	14	2
Oatmeal Instant Kid's Choice Strawberries'n Stuff	1 pkg (1.4 oz)	150	30	13	3
Oatmeal Instant Kid's Choice Twisted Strawberry Banana	1 pkg (1.4 oz)	150	31	13	3
Oatmeal Instant Maple & Brown Sugar	1 pkg (1.5 oz)	160	33	13	3
Oatmeal Instant Peaches & Cream	1 pkg (1.2 oz)	140	27	12	2
Oatmeal Instant Raisin & Spice	1 pkg (1.5 oz)	150	33	16	3
Oatmeal Instant Raisin Date & Walnut	1 pkg (1.3 oz)	140	27	13	3
Oatmeal Instant Strawberries & Cream	1 pkg (1.2 oz)	140	27	11	2
Oatmeal Quick'n Hearty Microwave	1 pkg (1 oz)	110	19	1	2
Oatmeal Quick'n Hearty Microwave Apple Spice	1 pkg (1.6 oz)	170	35	15	3
Oatmeal Quick'n Hearty Microwave Brown Sugar Cinnamon	1 pkg (1.5 oz)	150	31	12	3
Oatmeal Quick'n Hearty Microwave Cinnamon Double Raisin	1 pkg (1.6 oz)	170	35	16	3
Oatmeal Quick'n Hearty Microwave Honey Bran	1 pkg (1.4 oz)	150	30	12	3
Oats Old Fashion	½ cup (1.4 oz)	150	27	1	4
Oats Quick	½ cup (1.4 oz)	150	27	1	4
Oats Steel Cut	½ cup (1.4 oz)	150	27	1	4
Popeye Sweet Crunch	1 cup	113	24	—	1
Puffed Rice	1 cup	54	13	—	tr
Puffed Wheat	1 cup	50	11	—	1
Shredded Wheat	2 biscuits	132	32	—	4
Whole Wheat Hot Natural	½ cup (1.4 oz)	130	30	0	4
Ralston					
Almond Delight	1 cup (1.8 oz)	210	41	12	4
Bran Flakes	¾ cup (1.1 oz)	110	24	5	5
Chex Multi-Bran	1¼ cup (2 oz)	220	46	11	7
Cocoa Crispy Rice	1 cup (1.8 oz)	200	45	18	tr

FOOD	PORTION	CALS.	CARB.	SUG.	FIB.
Ralston (CONT.)					
Cocoa Crunchies	¾ cup (1.1 oz)	120	26	13	0
Cookie Crisp	1 cup (1 oz)	120	25	12	0
Corn Flakes	1¼ cup (1.1 oz)	120	27	3	1
Crisp Crunch	¾ cup (1.1 oz)	120	26	14	tr
Crisp Rice	1¼ cup (1.2 oz)	130	28	2	0
Frosted Flakes	¾ cup (1.1 oz)	120	28	11	1
Fruit Rings	¾ cup (0.9 oz)	100	23	12	0
Magic Stair	¾ cup (1.1 oz)	120	26	11	tr
Muesli Blueberry	1 cup (1.9 oz)	200	41	14	4
Muesli Cranberry	¾ cup (1.9 oz)	200	40	14	4
Muesli Peach	¾ cup (1.9 oz)	200	39	12	4
Muesli Raspberry	¾ cup (2 oz)	220	44	14	4
Muesli Strawberry	1 cup (1.9 oz)	210	41	14	4
Multi Vitamin Whole Grain Flakes	1 cup (1.1 oz)	120	25	3	3
Nutty Nuggets	½ cup (1.7 oz)	180	38	4	5
Raisin Bran	¾ cup (1.9 oz)	190	41	16	6
Tasteeos	1¼ cup (1.1 oz)	130	22	2	3
Tasteeos Apple Cinnamon	1 cup (1.2 oz)	130	27	10	1
Tasteeos Honey Nut	1 cup (1.2 oz)	130	28	10	1
Roman Meal					
Apple Cinnamon	1.2 oz	105	18	4	6
Cream Of Rye	1.3 oz	111	20	0	5
Oats Wheat Dates Raisins Almonds	1.3 oz	129	24	7	3
Oats Wheat Honey Coconuts Almonds	1.3 oz	155	22	8	3
Original	1 oz	83	15	0	5
Original With Oats	1.2 oz	108	19	0	5
Stone-Buhr					
4 Grain	⅓ cup (1.6 oz)	140	31	0	5
7 Grain	⅓ cup (1.6 oz)	140	31	0	7
Bran Flakes	¼ cup (0.6 oz)	64	14	0	2
Cracked Wheat	¼ cup (2.4 oz)	210	48	2	6
Manna Golden	6 tsp (1.6 oz)	160	35	0	1
Rolled Oats Old Fashion	6 tsp (1.6 oz)	150	28	tr	5
Scotch Oats	¼ cup (1.6 oz)	150	28	tr	4
Sunbelt					
Muesli	1.9 oz	210	44	17	3
US Mills					
Poppets	1 oz	110	24	—	1
Uncle Sam	1 oz	110	20	—	7

FOOD	PORTION	CALS.	CARB.	SUG.	FIB.
Uncle Roy's					
Muesli Swiss Style	½ cup (1.6 oz)	170	32	8	3
Weetabix					
Cereal	2 (1.3 oz)	142	31	—	3
Wheatena					
Cereal	⅓ cup (1.4 oz)	150	32	0	5

CEREAL BARS
(*see also* GRANOLA BARS, NUTRITIONAL SUPPLEMENTS)

FOOD	PORTION	CALS.	CARB.	SUG.	FIB.
Cap'n Crunch					
Bar	1 (0.8 oz)	90	17	8	—
Golden Grahams Treats					
Chocolate Chunk	1 bar (0.8 oz)	90	17	—	tr
Honey Graham	1 bar (0.8 oz)	90	17	—	tr
Kellogg's					
Nutri-Grain Apple Cinnamon	1 (1.3 oz)	140	27	13	1
Nutri-Grain Blueberry	1 (1.3 oz)	140	27	13	1
Nutri-Grain Cherry	1 (1.3 oz)	140	27	13	1
Nutri-Grain Mixed Berry	1 (1.3 oz)	140	27	13	1
Nutri-Grain Peach	1 (1.3 oz)	140	27	13	1
Nutri-Grain Raspberry	1 (1.3 oz)	140	27	13	1
Nutri-Grain Strawberry	1 (1.3 oz)	140	27	13	1
Rice Krispies Treats	1 (0.8 oz)	90	18	8	0
Rice Krispies Treats Chocolate Chip Squares	1 (0.8 oz)	90	17	11	0
Nature's Choice					
Fat Free Apple	1 bar (1.3 oz)	110	27	14	2
Fat Free Blueberry	1 bar (1.3 oz)	110	27	14	2
Fat Free Cranberry	1 bar (1.3 oz)	110	27	13	2
Fat Free Peach	1 bar (1.3 oz)	110	27	14	2
Fat Free Raspberry	1 bar (1.3 oz)	110	27	13	2
Fat Free Strawberry	1 bar (1.3 oz)	110	27	13	2
Low Fat Triple Berry	1 bar (1.3 oz)	130	28	14	2
Low Fat Very Cherry	1 bar (1.3 oz)	130	28	14	2

CHAMPAGNE

FOOD	PORTION	CALS.	CARB.	SUG.	FIB.
sekt german champagne	3.5 fl oz	84	5	—	—
Andre					
Blush	1 fl oz	22	1	—	—
Brut	1 fl oz	21	1	—	—
Cold Duck	1 fl oz	25	2	—	—
Extra Dry	1 fl oz	23	1	—	—
Ballatore					
Spumante	1 fl oz	23	2	—	—

FOOD	PORTION	CALS.	CARB.	SUG.	FIB.
Eden Roc					
Brut	1 fl oz	21	1	—	—
Brut Rosé	1 fl oz	22	2	—	—
Extra Dry	1 fl oz	21	1	—	—
Tott's					
Blanc de Noir	1 fl oz	22	2	—	—
Brut	1 fl oz	20	tr	—	—
Extra Dry	1 fl oz	21	1	—	—

CHEESE

(*see also* CHEESE DISHES, CHEESE SUBSTITUTES, COTTAGE CHEESE, CREAM CHEESE)

FOOD	PORTION	CALS.	CARB.	SUG.	FIB.
cacio di roma sheep's milk cheese	1 oz	130	0	0	0
caerphilly	1.4 oz	150	0	0	0
chabichou	1 oz	95	tr	tr	0
chaource	1 oz	83	tr	tr	0
cheddar reduced fat	1.4 oz	104	0	0	0
cheshire reduced fat	1.4 oz	108	tr	—	0
comte	1 oz	114	tr	tr	0
coulommiers	1 oz	88	tr	tr	0
crottin	1 oz	105	tr	tr	0
derby	1.4 oz	161	0	0	0
edam reduced fat	1.4 oz	92	tr	—	0
fromage frais	1.6 oz	51	3	—	0
gloucester double	1.4 oz	162	0	0	0
goat fresh	1 oz	23	tr	tr	0
lancashire	1.4 oz	149	0	0	0
leicester	1.4 oz	160	0	0	0
lymeswold	1.4 oz	170	tr	—	0
maroilles	1 oz	97	tr	tr	0
stilton blue	1.4 oz	164	0	0	0
stilton white	1.4 oz	145	0	0	0
wensleydale	1.4 oz	151	0	0	0
whey cheese	3.5 oz	440	33	0	0
Alouette					
Brie Baby	1 oz	110	2	2	0
Brie Baby With Herbs	1 oz	110	2	2	0
French Onion	2 tbsp (0.8 oz)	70	1	1	0
Garlic	2 tbsp (0.8 oz)	70	1	1	0
Light Dill	2 tbsp (0.8 oz)	50	2	1	0
Light Garlic	2 tbsp (0.8 oz)	50	1	1	1
Light Herb	2 tbsp (0.8 oz)	50	2	1	0
Light Herbs & Garlic	2 tbsp (0.8 oz)	50	1	1	0

FOOD	PORTION	CALS.	CARB.	SUG.	FIB.
Alouette (CONT.)					
Light Spring Vegetable	2 tbsp (0.8 oz)	50	1	1	0
Salmon	2 tbsp (0.8 oz)	60	1	1	0
Scallions	2 tbsp (0.8 oz)	70	1	1	0
Spinach	2 tbsp (0.8 oz)	60	1	1	0
Alpine Lace					
American	1 slice (0.66 oz)	50	1	1	0
American Fat Free	1 piece (1 oz)	45	2	0	0
American Hot Pepper Less Fat Less Sodium	1 piece (1 oz)	80	2	0	0
American Less Fat Less Sodium	1 piece (1 oz)	80	2	0	0
Cheddar Fat Free	1 piece (1 oz)	45	2	0	0
Cheddar Reduced Fat	1 piece (1 oz)	80	1	0	0
Colby Reduced Fat	1 piece (1 oz)	80	1	0	0
Fat Free For Parmesan Lovers	2 tsp (5 g)	10	0	0	0
Fat Free Mexican Macho	2 tbsp (1 oz)	30	1	0	0
Fat Free Singles	1 slice (0.66 oz)	25	tr	0	0
Feta Reduced Fat	1 piece (1 oz)	60	1	0	0
Mozzarella Fat Free	1 piece (1 oz)	45	2	0	0
Mozzarella Reduced Sodium Part Skim	1 piece (1 oz)	70	1	0	0
Muenster Reduced Sodium	1 piece (1 oz)	100	1	0	0
Provolone Smoked Reduced Fat	1 piece (1 oz)	70	1	0	0
Swiss Reduced Fat	1 piece (1 oz)	90	1	0	0
BabyBel					
Mini Light	1 (0.7 oz)	45	0	0	0
Bongrain					
Chavrie	2 tbsp (0.8 oz)	40	1	0	0
Montrachet	1 oz	70	tr	0	0
Montrachet Chive	1 oz	70	tr	0	0
Montrachet Classic	1 oz	70	tr	0	0
Montrachet Classic Herb	1 oz	70	tr	0	0
Montrachet Herbs & Garlic	1 oz	70	tr	0	0
Montrachet In Oil drained	1 oz	70	tr	0	0
Montrachet With Ash	1 oz	70	tr	0	0
Breakstone's					
Ricotta	¼ cup (2.2 oz)	110	3	3	0
Bresse					
Brie	1 oz	110	2	2	0
Brie Light	1 oz	70	1	tr	tr
Brie With Herbs	1 oz	110	2	2	0

FOOD	PORTION	CALS.	CARB.	SUG.	FIB.
Bresse (CONT.)					
Creme De Brie	2 tbsp (1 oz)	90	tr	0	0
Creme De Brie Herb	2 tbsp (1 oz)	90	tr	0	0
Cabot					
Mediterranean Cheddar		110	1	0	0
Vermont Cheddar 50% Light	1 oz	70	1	0	0
Cheez Whiz					
Light	2 tbsp (1.2 oz)	80	6	3	0
Churney					
Feta	1 oz	80	tr	tr	0
Cracker Barrel					
Baby Swiss	1 oz	110	0	0	0
Cheddar Extra Sharp	1 oz	120	0	0	0
Cheddar Marbled Sharp	1 oz	110	tr	0	0
Cheddar New York Aged	1 oz	120	0	0	0
Cheddar Sharp	1 oz	120	0	0	0
Cheddar Vermont Sharp	1 oz	110	tr	0	0
Reduced Fat Cheddar Extra Sharp	1 oz	90	tr	0	0
Reduced Fat Cheddar Sharp	1 oz	90	tr	0	0
Reduced Fat Cheddar Vermont Sharp	1 oz	90	tr	0	0
Whipped Spreadable Cream Cheese & Extra Sharp Cheddar	2 tbsp (0.9 oz)	80	tr	0	0
Whipped Spreadable Cream Cheese & Sharp Cheddar	2 tbsp (0.9 oz)	80	tr	0	0
Whipped Spreadable Cream Cheese & Sharp Cheddar w/ Herbs	2 tbsp (0.9 oz)	80	tr	0	0
Delice De France					
Cheese	1 oz	110	2	2	0
With Herbs	1 oz	110	2	2	0
Delico					
Alouette Cajun	2 tbsp (0.8 oz)	70	1	1	0
Alouette French Onion	2 tbsp (0.8 oz)	70	1	1	0
Alouette Garden Vegetable	2 tbsp (0.8 oz)	60	1	1	0
Alouette Garlic	2 tbsp (0.8 oz)	70	1	1	0
Alouette Horseradish & Chive	2 tbsp (0.8 oz)	60	1	1	0
Alouette Spinach	2 tbsp (0.8 oz)	60	1	1	0

FOOD	PORTION	CALS.	CARB.	SUG.	FIB.
Di Giorno					
Parmesan Grated	2 tsp (5 g)	25	0	0	0
Parmesan Shredded	2 tsp (5 g)	20	0	0	0
Parmesan Shredded	2 tsp (5 g)	20	0	0	0
Romano Grated	2 tsp (5 g)	25	0	0	0
Romano Shredded	2 tsp (5 g)	20	0	0	0
Dorman					
Muenster	1 oz	110	0	0	0
Muenster Low Sodium	1 oz	110	0	0	0
Swiss	1 oz	100	0	0	0
Easy Cheese					
Spread American	2 tbsp (1.2 oz)	100	2	2	0
Spread Cheddar	2 tbsp (1.2 oz)	100	3	3	0
Spread Cheddar'n Bacon	2 tbsp (1.2 oz)	100	3	2	0
Spread Nacho	2 tbsp (1.2 oz)	100	3	3	0
Spread Sharp Cheddar	2 tbsp (1.2 oz)	100	3	2	0
Father Time					
Cheddar Extra-Sharp Premium	1 oz	110	1	0	0
Formagg					
Formaggio D'Oro	1 oz	70	1	0	0
Friendship					
Farmer	2 tbsp (1 oz)	50	0	0	0
Farmer No Salt Added	2 tbsp (1 oz)	50	0	0	0
Hoop	2 tbsp (1 oz)	20	0	0	0
Gerard					
Brie	1 oz	90	2	1	0
Handi-Snacks					
Cheez'n Breadsticks	1 pkg (1.1 oz)	120	12	3	0
Cheez'n Crackers	1 pkg (1.1 oz)	110	9	2	0
Cheez'n Pretzels	1 pkg (1 oz)	100	11	2	tr
Mozzarella String Cheese	1 piece (1 oz)	80	0	0	0
Nacho Stix'n Cheez	1 pkg (1.1 oz)	110	11	2	0
Heluva Good Cheese					
American	1 slice (0.7)	45	2	1	0
Cheddar Curds Snack	1 oz	113	1	0	0
Cheddar Extra-Sharp	1 oz	110	1	0	0
Cheddar Mild	1 oz	110	1	0	0
Cheddar Mild Reduced Fat	1 oz	80	1	0	0
Cheddar Mild White	1 oz	110	1	0	0
Cheddar Sharp	1 oz	110	1	0	0
Cheddar Sharp White	1 oz	110	1	0	0
Cheddar Shredded	¼ cup (1 oz)	110	1	0	0
Cheddar Very Low Sodium	1 oz	110	0	0	0

FOOD	PORTION	CALS.	CARB.	SUG.	FIB.
Heluva Good Cheese (CONT.)					
Cheddar White Extra-Sharp	1 oz	110	1	0	0
Cheddar White Very Low Sodium	1 oz	110	0	0	0
Cheddar White Shredded	¼ cup (1 oz)	110	1	0	0
Colby	1 oz	117	0	0	0
Colby-Jack	1 oz	110	0	0	0
Cold Pack Cheddar Sharp	2 tbsp (1 oz)	90	3	3	0
Cold Pack Cheddar Sharp With Bacon	2 tbsp (1 oz)	90	3	3	0
Cold Pack Cheddar Sharp With Horseradish	2 tbsp (1 oz)	90	3	3	0
Cold Pack Cheddar Sharp With Jalapenos	2 tbsp (1 oz)	90	3	3	0
Cold Pack Cheddar Sharp With Port Wine	2 tbsp (1 oz)	90	3	3	0
Monterey Jack	1 oz	100	0	0	0
Monterey Jack Shredded	¼ cup (1 oz)	100	1	0	0
Monterey Jack With Jalapenos	1 oz	100	0	0	0
Mozzarella Part Skim Low Moisture Shredded	¼ cup (1 oz)	80	1	0	0
Mozzarella Whole Milk	1 oz	80	tr	tr	0
Muenster	1 oz	100	0	0	0
Swiss	1 oz	112	0	0	0
Washed Curd Cheese	1 oz	110	1	0	0
Hoffman					
American Yellow	1 oz	110	1	0	0
Hot Pepper	1 oz	90	2	2	0
Super Sharp	1 oz	110	1	0	0
Keller's					
Chub	2 tbsp (1 oz)	100	1	1	0
Kraft					
Cheddar Extra Sharp	1 oz	120	0	0	0
Cheddar Medium	1 oz	110	tr	5	0
Cheddar Mild	1 oz	110	tr	0	0
Cheddar Sharp	1 oz	120	0	0	0
Cheddary Melts Medium Cheddar	1 oz	110	2	1	0
Cheddary Melts Mild Cheddar	1 oz	110	2	1	0
Cheddary Melts Shreds Medium Cheddar	¼ cup (1.1 oz)	120	2	1	0
Cheddary Melts Shreds Mild Cheddar	¼ cup (1.1 oz)	120	2	1	0

FOOD	PORTION	CALS.	CARB.	SUG.	FIB.
Kraft (CONT.)					
Cheese Food w/ Garlic	1 oz	90	2	2	0
Cheese Food w/ Jalapeno Peppers	1 oz	90	2	2	0
Colby	1 oz	110	tr	0	0
Colby Monterey Jack	1 oz	110	0	0	0
Deluxe American	1 oz	100	tr	0	0
Deluxe American White	1 oz	100	tr	0	0
Deluxe Singles American	1 (1 oz)	110	tr	0	0
Deluxe Singles American	1 (0.7 oz)	70	tr	0	0
Deluxe Singles Pimento	1 (1 oz)	100	tr	0	0
Deluxe Singles Swiss	1 (1 oz)	90	0	0	0
Deluxe Singles Swiss	1 slice (0.7 oz)	70	0	0	0
Free Grated	2 tsp (5 g)	15	3	tr	0
Free Shredded Cheddar	¼ cup (0.9 oz)	40	1	0	0
Free Shredded Mozzarella	¼ cup (1 oz)	45	2	0	tr
Grated Parm Plus! Garlic Herb	2 tsp (5 g)	15	2	0	0
Grated Parm Plus! Zesty Red Pepper	2 tsp (5 g)	15	2	0	0
Grated Parmesan	2 tsp (5 g)	20	0	0	0
Grated Romano	2 tsp (5 g)	20	0	0	0
Marbled Cheddar Mild	1 oz	110	tr	0	0
Marbled Cheddar & Monterey Jack	1 oz	110	tr	0	0
Marbled Cheddar & Whole Milk Mozzarella	1 oz	100	tr	0	0
Marbled Colby Monterey Jack	1 oz	110	0	0	0
Monterey Jack	1 oz	110	0	0	0
Monterey Jack w/ Jalapeno Peppers	1 oz	110	tr	0	0
Mozzarella Part Skim Low Moisture	1 oz	80	tr	0	0
Mozzarella String Cheese Low Moisture Part Skim	1 piece (1 oz)	80	0	0	0
Pizza Shredded Four Cheese	¼ cup (0.9 oz)	90	tr	0	0
Pizza Shredded Mozzarella & Cheddar	⅓ cup (1.1 oz)	120	1	0	0
Pizza Shredded Mozzarella & Provolone w/ Smoke Flavor	¼ cup (0.9 oz)	90	tr	0	0
Reduced Fat Cheddar Mild	1 oz	90	tr	0	0

FOOD	PORTION	CALS.	CARB.	SUG.	FIB.
Kraft (CONT.)					
Reduced Fat Cheddar Sharp	1 oz	90	tr	0	0
Reduced Fat Colby	1 oz	80	0	0	0
Reduced Fat Monterey Jack	1 oz	80	tr	0	0
Shredded Cheddar Medium	¼ cup (0.9 oz)	100	tr	0	0
Shredded Cheddar Mild	¼ cup (0.9 oz)	100	tr	0	0
Shredded Cheddar Sharp	1 oz (0.9 oz)	110	tr	0	0
Shredded Cheddar & Monterey Jack	¼ cup (0.9 oz)	100	tr	0	0
Shredded Colby & Monterey Jack	¼ cup (0.9 oz)	100	tr	0	0
Shredded Hearty Italian	⅓ cup (1.1 oz)	100	2	0	0
Shredded Italian Style Classic Garlic	⅓ cup (1.1 oz)	100	2	0	tr
Shredded Italian Style Mozzarelle & Parmesan	⅓ cup (1.1 oz)	100	1	0	0
Shredded Lower Fat Cheddar Mild	¼ cup (0.9 oz)	80	tr	0	0
Shredded Lower Fat Cheddar Sharp	¼ cup (0.9 oz)	80	tr	0	0
Shredded Lower Fat Colby & Monterey Jack	¼ cup (0.9 oz)	80	tr	0	0
Shredded Lower Fat Mozzarella	⅓ cup (1.1 oz)	80	tr	0	0
Shredded Lower Fat Pizza Cheese	⅓ cup (1.1 oz)	90	1	0	0
Shredded Mexican Style Cheddar & Monterey Jack	⅓ cup (1.1 oz)	120	tr	0	0
Shredded Mexican Style Cheddar & Monterey Jack w/ Jalapeno Peppers	⅓ cup (1.1 oz)	120	tr	0	0
Shredded Mexican Style Four Cheese	⅓ cup (1.1 oz)	120	tr	0	0
Shredded Mexican Style Taco Cheese	⅓ cup (1.1 oz)	120	1	0	0
Shredded Monterey Jack	¼ cup (0.9 oz)	100	tr	0	0
Shredded Parmesan	2 tsp (5 g)	20	0	0	0
Shredded Part Skim Mozzarella	¼ cup (1.1 oz)	90	tr	0	0
Shredded Swiss	¼ cup (0.9 oz)	100	tr	0	0
Shredded Whole Milk Mozzarella	¼ cup (1.1 oz)	100	1	0	0

FOOD	PORTION	CALS.	CARB.	SUG.	FIB.
Kraft (CONT.)					
Shredded Finely Cheddar Mild	¼ cup (1.1 oz)	120	tr	0	0
Shredded Finely Cheddar Sharp	¼ cup (1.1 oz)	120	tr	0	0
Shredded Finely Colby & Monterey Jack	¼ cup (1 oz)	110	tr	0	0
Shredded Finely Lower Fat Cheddar Milk	⅓ cup (1.1 oz)	100	1	0	0
Shredded Finely Lower Fat Cheddar Sharp	⅓ cup (1.1 oz)	100	1	0	0
Shredded Finely Part Skim Mozzarella	¼ cup (1.1 oz)	90	tr	0	0
Shredded Finely Swiss	¼ cup (0.9 oz)	110	tr	0	0
Singles American	1 (1.2 oz)	110	3	2	0
Singles American	1 (0.7 oz)	60	2	1	0
Singles American	1 (0.6 oz)	60	2	1	0
Singles Mild Mexican	1 (0.7 oz)	70	2	1	0
Singles Monterey	1 slice (0.7 oz)	70	2	1	0
Singles Pimento	1 (0.7 oz)	60	1	tr	0
Singles Reduced Fat American	1 (0.7 oz)	50	2	2	0
Singles Reduced Fat American White	1 (0.7 oz)	50	2	2	0
Singles Sharp	1 slice (0.7 oz)	70	tr	0	0
Singles Swiss	1 slice (0.7 oz)	70	1	1	0
Singles Nonfat American	1 (0.7 oz)	30	3	2	0
Singles Nonfat American White	1 (0.7 oz)	30	3	2	0
Singles Nonfat Sharp Cheddar	1 (0.7 oz)	35	3	2	0
Singles Nonfat Swiss	1 slice (0.7 oz)	30	3	2	0
Slices Cheddar Mild	1 (1 oz)	110	tr	0	0
Slices Colby	1 (1.6 oz)	180	tr	0	0
Slices Part Skim Mozzarella	1 (1.6 oz)	130	tr	0	0
Slices Part Skim Mozzarella	1 (1.5 oz)	120	tr	0	0
Slices Provolone Smoke Flavor	1 (1.5 oz)	150	tr	0	0
Slices Swiss	1 (1.5 oz)	170	tr	0	0
Slices Swiss	1 (1.6 oz)	180	tr	0	0
Slices Swiss	1 (1.3 oz)	150	tr	0	0
Slices Swiss	1 (0.8 oz)	90	0	0	0
Slices Swiss Aged	1 (1.5 oz)	170	tr	0	0
Slices Deli-Thin Part Skim Mozzarella	1 (1 oz)	80	tr	0	0

FOOD	PORTION	CALS.	CARB.	SUG.	FIB.
Kraft (CONT.)					
Slices Deli-Thin Swiss	1 (0.8 oz)	90	0	0	0
Slices Deli-Thin Swiss Aged	1 (0.8 oz)	90	0	0	0
Slices Reduced Fat Swiss	1 (1.3 oz)	130	tr	0	0
Spread Bacon	2 tbsp (1.1 oz)	90	tr	0	0
Spread Olive & Pimento	2 tbsp (1.1 oz)	70	3	2	0
Spread Pimento	2 tbsp (1.1 oz)	80	3	2	0
Spread Pineapple	2 tbsp (1.1 oz)	70	4	4	0
Spread Pineapple	2 tbsp (1.1 oz)	70	4	4	0
Spread Roka Brand Blue	2 tbsp (1.1 oz)	90	tr	0	0
Swiss	1 oz	110	0	0	0
Lactaid					
American	3.5 oz	328	7	—	0
Land O'Lakes					
American	1 slice (0.75 oz)	80	tr	0	0
American	2 slices (1 oz)	100	1	0	0
American	1 oz	110	tr	0	0
American Less Salt	1 oz	110	tr	0	0
American Light	1 oz	70	2	0	0
American Sharp	1 oz	110	tr	0	0
American & Swiss	1 oz	100	0	0	0
Baby Swiss	1 oz	110	0	0	0
Brick	1 oz	100	tr	0	0
Chedarella	1 oz	100	0	0	0
Cheddar Light	1 oz	70	tr	0	0
Jalapeno Light	1 oz	70	1	0	0
Monterey Jack	1 oz	110	tr	0	0
Mozzarella	1 oz	80	tr	0	0
Muenster	1 oz	100	0	0	0
Provolone	1 oz	100	tr	0	0
Swiss	1 oz	110	tr	0	0
Swiss Light	1 oz	80	tr	0	0
Laughing Cow					
Assorted Wedge	1 (1 oz)	70	1	1	0
Babybel	1 oz	90	0	0	0
Babybel Mini	1 (0.7 oz)	70	0	0	0
Bonbel	1 oz	100	0	0	0
Bonbel Mini	1 (0.7 oz)	70	0	0	0
Cheesebits	6 pieces (1 oz)	70	1	1	0
Gouda Mini	1 (0.7 oz)	80	0	0	0
Original Wedge	1 (1 oz)	70	1	1	0
Wedge Light	1 (1 oz)	50	1	1	0

FOOD	PORTION	CALS.	CARB.	SUG.	FIB.
Lifetime					
Cheddar Fat Free	1 oz	40	1	1	0
Cheddar Fat Free Lactose Free	1 oz	40	1	1	0
Garden Vegetable Fat Free	1 oz	40	1	1	0
Jalapeno Jack Fat Free	1 oz	40	1	1	0
Jalapeno Jack Fat Free Lactose Free	1 oz	40	1	1	0
Mild Mexican Fat Free	1 oz	40	1	1	0
Monterey Jack Fat Free	1 oz	40	1	1	0
Mozzarella Fat Free	1 oz	40	1	1	0
Mozzarella Fat Free Lactose Free	1 oz	40	1	1	0
Onions & Chives Fat Free	1 oz	40	1	1	0
Sharp Cheddar Fat Free	1 oz	40	1	1	0
Smoked Cheddar Fat Free	1 oz	40	1	1	0
Swiss Fat Free	1 oz	40	1	1	0
Light N'Lively					
Singles American	1 (0.7 oz)	45	2	1	0
MayBud					
Edam	1 oz	100	1	0	0
Gouda	1 oz	100	1	0	0
Gouda Round	1 oz	100	1	0	0
New Holland					
Cheese	1 oz	90	0	0	0
Garlic	1 oz	90	tr	0	0
Havarti Lower Fat Garden Vegetable	1 oz	80	0	0	0
Jalapeno	1 oz	80	tr	0	0
Natural Vegetable	1 oz	80	0	0	0
Old English					
American Sharp	1 slice (1 oz)	100	tr	0	0
Polly-O					
Mozzarella Free	1 oz	35	tr	—	—
String Lite	1 piece (1 oz)	60	tr	tr	0
President					
Feta Fat Free	1 oz	30	2	tr	0
Price's					
Cheese & Bacon Spread	2 tbsp (1.1 oz)	90	2	2	0
Jalapeno Nacho Dip Hot	2 tbsp (1.1 oz)	80	2	2	0
Jalapeno Nacho Dip Mild	2 tbsp (1.1 oz)	80	2	2	0
Pimento Cheese Spread	2 tbsp (1.1 oz)	80	2	2	0
Pimento Cheese Spread Light	2 tbsp (1.1 oz)	60	3	3	0

FOOD	PORTION	CALS.	CARB.	SUG.	FIB.
Price's (CONT.)					
Vegetable Garden	2 tbsp (1.1 oz)	70	3	3	0
Quaker					
Chub	2 tbsp (1 oz)	100	1	1	0
Rondele					
Light Soft Spreadable Garlic & Herb	2 tbsp (0.9 oz)	60	2	1	0
Soft Spreadable Garlic & Herbs	2 tbsp (1 oz)	100	1	tr	0
Sargento					
4 Cheese Mexican Recipe Blend Shredded	¼ cup (1 oz)	110	tr	0	0
6 Cheese Italian Recipe Blend Shredded	¼ cup (1 oz)	90	0	0	0
Blue Crumbled	¼ cup (1 oz)	100	1	0	0
Cheddar	1 slice (1 oz)	110	1	1	0
Cheddar Mild Shredded Classic Supreme	¼ cup (1 oz)	110	1	tr	0
Cheddar Mild Shredded Fancy Supreme	¼ cup (1 oz)	110	1	tr	0
Cheddar Mild Shredded Preferred Light	¼ cup (1 oz)	70	tr	0	0
Cheddar Mild White Shredded Classic Supreme	¼ cup (1 oz)	110	1	tr	0
Cheddar New York Sharp Shredded Classic Supreme	¼ cup (1 oz)	110	1	tr	0
Cheddar Sharp Shredded Classic Supreme	¼ cup (1 oz)	110	1	tr	0
Cheddar Sharp Shredded Fancy Supreme	¼ cup (1 oz)	110	1	tr	0
Cheese For Nachos & Tacos Shredded	¼ cup (1 oz)	110	1	0	0
Cheese For Pizza Shredded	¼ cup (1 oz)	90	0	0	0
Cheese For Tacos Shredded	¼ cup (1 oz)	110	1	0	0
Cheese For Tacos Shredded Preferred Light	¼ cup (1 oz)	70	tr	0	0
Colby	1 slice (1 oz)	110	0	0	0
Colby-Jack Shredded Fancy Supreme	¼ cup (1 oz)	110	tr	0	0
Gourmet Parm	1 tbsp	20	tr	—	—
Jarlsberg	1 slice (1.2 oz)	120	1	0	0
Monterey Jack	1 slice (1 oz)	100	0	0	0

FOOD	PORTION	CALS.	CARB.	SUG.	FIB.
Sargento (CONT.)					
MooTown Snackers Cheddar	1 piece (0.8 oz)	100	1	tr	0
MooTown Snackers Cheddar Mild Light	1 piece (0.8 oz)	60	tr	0	0
MooTown Snackers Cheese & Pretzels	1 pkg (1 oz)	90	12	1	0
MooTown Snackers Cheese & Sticks	1 pkg (1 oz)	100	13	3	0
MooTown Snackers Colby-Jack	1 piece (0.8 oz)	90	tr	tr	0
MooTown Snackers Pizza Cheese & Sticks	1 pkg (1 oz)	100	13	3	0
MooTown Snackers String	1 piece (0.8 oz)	70	tr	0	0
MooTown Snackers String Light	1 piece (0.8 oz)	60	tr	0	0
Mozzarella	1 slice (1.5 oz)	130	2	0	0
Mozzarella Preferred Light	1 slice (1.5 oz)	100	0	0	0
Mozzarella Shredded Classic Supreme	¼ cup (1 oz)	80	1	0	0
Mozzarella Shredded Fancy Supreme	¼ cup (1 oz)	80	1	0	0
Mozzarella Shredded Preferred Light	¼ cup (1 oz)	70	tr	0	0
Muenster	1 slice (1 oz)	100	tr	0	0
Parmesan Fresh	1 oz	111	1	—	—
Parmesan Shredded	¼ cup (1 oz)	110	1	0	0
Parmesan & Romano Shredded	¼ cup (1 oz)	110	1	0	0
Pizza Double Cheese Shredded	¼ cup (1 oz)	90	1	0	0
Provolone	1 slice (1 oz)	100	0	0	0
Ricotta Light	¼ cup (2.2 oz)	60	3	3	0
Ricotta Old Fashioned	¼ cup (2.2 oz)	90	3	3	0
Ricotta Part Skim	¼ cup (2.2 oz)	80	2	3	0
Swiss	1 slice (0.7 oz)	80	0	0	0
Swiss Preferred Light	1 slice (1 oz)	80	tr	0	0
Swiss Shredded Fancy Supreme	¼ cup (1 oz)	110	0	0	0
Swiss Wafer Thin	2 slices (1 oz)	110	0	0	0
Smart Beat					
American Fat Free	1 slice (0.6 oz)	25	3	—	—
Lactose Free Fat Free	1 slice (0.6 oz)	25	3	—	—
Mellow Cheddar Fat Free	1 slice (0.6 oz)	25	3	—	—

FOOD	PORTION	CALS.	CARB.	SUG.	FIB.
Smart Beat (CONT.)					
Sharp Cheddar Fat Free	1 slice (0.6 oz)	25	3	—	—
Treasure Cave					
Blue Crumbled	1 oz	110	tr	0	0
Feta Crumbled	1 oz	80	tr	0	0
Velveeta					
Light	1 oz	60	3	2	0
Shredded	¼ cup (1.3 oz)	130	3	3	0
Shredded Mild Mexican w/ Jalapeno Pepper	¼ cup (1.3 oz)	120	3	2	0
Spread	1 oz	90	3	2	0
Spread Hot Mexican	1 oz	90	3	2	0
Spread Mild Mexican	1 oz	90	3	2	0
Weight Watchers					
Cheddar Mild Yellow	1 oz	80	1	0	0
Cheddar Sharp Yellow	1 oz	80	1	0	0
Fat Free Grated Italian Topping	1 tbsp	20	2	1	0
Fat Free Reduced Sodium American Yellow	2 slices (0.75 oz)	30	3	2	0
Fat Free Sharp Cheddar	2 slices (0.75 oz)	30	3	2	0
Fat Free Swiss	2 slices (0.75 oz)	30	2	2	0
Fat Free White	2 slices (0.75 oz)	30	3	2	0
Fat Free Yellow	2 slices (0.75 oz)	30	3	2	0
WisPride					
Chunk	1 oz	110	4	4	0
Garlic & Herb Cup	2 tbsp (1.1 oz)	100	4	4	0
Hickory Smoked Cup	2 tbsp (1.1 oz)	100	4	4	0
Port Wine Ball	2 tbsp (1.1 oz)	100	4	4	0
Port Wine Cup	2 tbsp (1.1 oz)	100	4	4	0
Port Wine Light Cup	2 tbsp (1.1 oz)	80	5	5	0
Sharp Ball	2 tbsp (1.1 oz)	100	4	4	0
Sharp Cheddar Ball	2 tbsp (1.1 oz)	100	4	4	0
Sharp Cup	2 tbsp (1.1 oz)	100	4	4	0
Sharp Light Cup	2 tbsp (1.1 oz)	80	5	5	0
Swiss Ball	2 tbsp (1.1 oz)	110	5	5	0

CHEESE DISHES
FROZEN

Stouffer's

Welsh Rarebit	½ cup (2.5 oz)	120	5	2	0

HOME RECIPE

welsh rarebit as prep w/ 1 white toast	1 slice	228	14	—	1

FOOD	PORTION	CALS.	CARB.	SUG.	FIB.

CHEESE SUBSTITUTES

Formagg

FOOD	PORTION	CALS.	CARB.	SUG.	FIB.
American White	1 slice (0.66 oz)	60	tr	tr	0
American Yellow	1 slice (0.66 oz)	60	tr	tr	0
Caesar's Italian Garden American	1 oz	60	1	0	0
Cheddar	1 slice (0.66 oz)	60	tr	tr	0
Cheddar Shredded	1 oz	60	1	0	0
Classic American	1 oz	60	1	0	0
Macaroni And Cheese Sauce	⅔ cup (5 oz)	190	35	2	0
Mozzarella Shredded	1 oz	60	1	0	0
Old World Mozzarella	1 oz	60	1	0	0
Parmesan Grated	2 tsp (5 g)	15	tr	0	tr
Swiss	1 oz	60	1	0	0
Swiss White	1 slice (0.66 oz)	60	tr	tr	0
Vintage Provolone	1 oz	60	1	0	0
Zesty Jalapeno American	1 oz	60	1	0	0

Georgio's

FOOD	PORTION	CALS.	CARB.	SUG.	FIB.
Imitation Cheddar Shredded	¼ cup (1 oz)	90	1	0	0
Imitation Mozzarella Shredded	¼ cup (1 oz)	90	1	0	0

Sargento

FOOD	PORTION	CALS.	CARB.	SUG.	FIB.
Classic Supreme Cheddar Shredded	¼ cup (1 oz)	90	2	0	0
Classic Supreme Mozzarella Shredded	¼ cup (1 oz)	80	tr	0	0
Fancy Supreme Cheddar Shredded	¼ cup (1 oz)	90	2	0	0

CHERRIES

CANNED

Del Monte

FOOD	PORTION	CALS.	CARB.	SUG.	FIB.
Dark Pitted In Heavy Syrup	½ cup (4.2 oz)	120	24	24	tr
Sweet Dark Whole Unpitted In Heavy Syrup	½ cup (4.2 oz)	120	24	23	tr

DRIED

Sonoma

FOOD	PORTION	CALS.	CARB.	SUG.	FIB.
Pitted	¼ cup (1.4 oz)	140	34	25	2

FRESH

Dole

FOOD	PORTION	CALS.	CARB.	SUG.	FIB.
Cherries	1 cup	90	19	—	3

FOOD	PORTION	CALS.	CARB.	SUG.	FIB.
FROZEN					
Big Valley					
Dark Sweet	¾ cup (4.9 oz)	90	20	14	3
CHERRY JUICE					
After The Fall					
Black Cherry	1 can (12 oz)	170	42	37	0
Capri Sun					
Wild Cherry Drink	1 pkg (7 oz)	100	30	30	0
Hi-C					
Box	8.45 fl oz	140	35	34	—
Drink	8 fl oz	130	33	33	—
Kool-Aid					
Black Cherry Drink as prep w/ sugar	1 serv (8 oz)	100	25	25	0
Bursts Cherry Drink	1 (7 oz)	100	25	25	0
Drink as prep w/ sugar	1 serv (8 oz)	100	25	25	0
Splash Drink	1 serv (8 oz)	110	29	29	0
Sugar Free Drink Mix as prep	1 serv (8 oz)	5	0	0	0
Tree Of Life					
Concentrate	8 tsp (1.4 oz)	110	28	28	—
Veryfine					
Juice-Ups	8 fl oz	130	33	33	0
CHESTNUTS					
creme de marrons	1 oz	73	18	10	1
CHEWING GUM					
Bazooka					
Fruit Chunk	1 piece (6 g)	25	5	5	—
Fruit Soft	1 piece (6 g)	25	5	5	—
Gum	1 piece (4 g)	15	4	3	—
Gum	1 piece (6 g)	25	5	5	—
Beech-Nut					
Peppermint	1 stick (3 g)	10	2	2	0
Spearmint	1 stick (3 g)	10	2	2	0
Brock					
Bubble Gum	1 piece (0.2 oz)	20	4	3	—
Bubble Yum					
Bananaberry Split	1 piece (0.3 oz)	25	6	6	—
Cotton Candy	1 piece (0.3 oz)	25	6	6	—
Grape	1 piece (0.3 oz)	25	6	6	—
Luscious Lime	1 piece (0.3 oz)	25	6	6	—
Regular	1 piece (0.3 oz)	25	6	6	0

FOOD	PORTION	CALS.	CARB.	SUG.	FIB.
Bubble Yum (CONT.)					
Sour Apple	1 piece (0.3 oz)	25	6	5	1
Sour Cherry	1 piece (0.3 oz)	25	6	5	0
Sugarless	1 piece (0.2 oz)	15	3	0	—
Sugarless Grape	1 piece (0.2 oz)	15	3	0	—
Sugarless Peppermint	1 piece (0.2 oz)	15	3	0	—
Sugarless Strawberry	1 piece (0.2 oz)	15	3	0	—
Sugarless Variety	1 piece (0.2 oz)	15	3	0	—
Variety Pack	1 piece (0.3 oz)	25	6	5	0
Watermelon	1 piece (0.3 oz)	25	6	6	0
Wild Strawberry	1 piece (0.3 oz)	25	6	6	0
Care*Free					
Sugarless Bubble Gum	1 stick (3 g)	10	2	0	—
Sugarless Cinnamon	1 piece (3 g)	5	2	0	—
Sugarless Peppermint	1 piece (3 g)	5	2	0	—
Sugarless Spearmint	1 piece (3 g)	5	2	0	—
Sugarless Wild Cherry	1 stick (3 g)	10	2	0	—
Fruit Stripe					
Bubble Gum Jumbo Pack	1 stick (3 g)	10	2	2	0
Variety Pack Chewing & Bubble Gum	1 stick (3 g)	10	2	2	0
Rain-Blo					
Bubble Gum Balls	1 piece (2 g)	5	2	0	—
Stick*Free					
Sugarless Peppermint	1 stick (3 g)	10	2	0	—
Sugarless Spearmint	1 stick (3 g)	10	2	0	—
Swell					
Bubble Gum	1 piece (3 g)	10	2	2	—
Winterfresh					
Stick	1 stick (3 g)	10	2	2	—

CHICKEN

(*see also* CHICKEN DISHES, CHICKEN SUBSTITUTES, DINNER, HOT DOGS)

FOOD	PORTION	CALS.	CARB.	SUG.	FIB.
CANNED					
w/ broth	½ can (2.5 oz)	117	0	0	0
w/ broth	1 can (5 oz)	234	0	0	0
Swanson					
White	2½ oz	100	0	0	0
White & Dark	2½ oz	100	0	0	0
FRESH					
broiler/fryer back w/ skin roasted	1 oz	96	0	0	0
broiler/fryer back w/ skin stewed	½ back (2.1 oz)	158	0	0	0

FOOD	PORTION	CALS.	CARB.	SUG.	FIB.
broiler/fryer breast w/ skin roasted	2 oz	115	0	0	0
broiler/fryer breast w/ skin roasted	½ breast (3.4 oz)	193	0	0	0
broiler/fryer breast w/ skin stewed	½ breast (3.9 oz)	202	0	0	0
broiler/fryer breast w/o skin roasted	½ breast (3 oz)	142	0	0	0
broiler/fryer breast w/o skin stewed	2 oz	86	0	0	0
broiler/fryer dark meat w/ skin roasted	3.5 oz	256	0	0	0
broiler/fryer dark meat w/ skin stewed	3.9 oz	256	0	0	0
broiler/fryer dark meat w/o skin roasted	1 cup (5 oz)	286	0	0	0
broiler/fryer dark meat w/o skin stewed	1 cup (5 oz)	269	0	0	0
broiler/fryer dark meat w/o skin stewed	3 oz	165	0	0	0
broiler/fryer drumstick w/ skin stewed	1 (2 oz)	116	0	0	0
broiler/fryer drumstick w/o skin fried	1 (1.5 oz)	82	0	0	0
broiler/fryer drumstick w/o skin roasted	1 (1.5 oz)	76	0	0	0
broiler/fryer drumstick w/o skin stewed	1 (1.6 oz)	78	0	0	0
broiler/fryer leg w/ skin roasted	1 (4 oz)	265	0	0	0
broiler/fryer leg w/ skin stewed	1 (4.4 oz)	275	0	0	0
broiler/fryer leg w/o skin roasted	1 (3.3 oz)	182	0	0	0
broiler/fryer leg w/o skin stewed	1 (3.5 oz)	187	0	0	0
broiler/fryer light meat w/ skin roasted	2.8 oz	175	0	0	0
broiler/fryer light meat w/ skin stewed	3.2 oz	181	0	0	0
broiler/fryer light meat w/o skin roasted	1 cup (5 oz)	242	0	0	0
broiler/fryer light meat w/o skin stewed	1 cup (5 oz)	223	0	0	0

FOOD	PORTION	CALS.	CARB.	SUG.	FIB.
broiler/fryer neck w/ skin stewed	1 (1.3 oz)	94	0	0	0
broiler/fryer neck w/o skin stewed	1 (.6 oz)	32	0	0	0
broiler/fryer skin roasted	from ½ chicken (2 oz)	254	0	0	0
broiler/fryer skin stewed	from ½ chicken (2.5 oz)	261	0	0	0
broiler/fryer thigh w/ skin roasted	1 (2.2 oz)	153	0	0	0
broiler/fryer thigh w/ skin stewed	1 (2.4 oz)	158	0	0	0
broiler/fryer thigh w/o skin roasted	1 (1.8 oz)	109	0	0	0
broiler/fryer thigh w/o skin stewed	1 (1.9 oz)	107	0	0	0
broiler/fryer w/ skin roasted	½ chicken (10.5 oz)	715	0	0	0
broiler/fryer w/ skin stewed	½ chicken (11.7 oz)	730	0	0	0
broiler/fryer w/o skin roasted	1 cup (5 oz)	266	0	0	0
broiler/fryer w/o skin stewed	1 oz	54	0	0	0
broiler/fryer w/o skin stewed	1 cup (5 oz)	248	0	0	0
broiler/fryer wing w/ skin roasted	1 (1.2 oz)	99	0	0	0
broiler/fryer wing w/ skin stewed	1 (1.4 oz)	100	0	0	0
cornish hen w/ skin roasted	1 hen (8 oz)	595	0	0	0
cornish hen w/o skin & bone roasted	1 hen (3.8 oz)	144	0	0	0
cornish hen w/o skin & bone roasted	½ hen (2 oz)	72	0	0	0
cornish hen w/skin roasted	½ hen (4 oz)	296	0	0	0
roaster dark meat w/o skin roasted	1 cup (5 oz)	250	0	0	0
roaster light meat w/o skin roasted	1 cup (5 oz)	214	0	0	0
roaster w/ skin roasted	½ chicken (1.1 lbs)	1071	0	0	0
roaster w/o skin roasted	1 cup (5 oz)	469	0	0	0
stewing dark meat w/o skin stewed	1 cup (5 oz)	361	0	0	0
stewing w/ skin stewed	½ chicken (9.2 oz)	744	0	0	0
stewing w/ skin stewed	6.2 oz	507	0	0	0
Perdue					
Boneless Breasts Cooked	3 oz	120	0	0	0
Boneless Breast Tenderloins Cooked	3 oz	100	0	0	0

FOOD	PORTION	CALS.	CARB.	SUG.	FIB.
Perdue (CONT.)					
Boneless Thighs Roasted	2 (3.5 oz)	200	0	0	0
Breast Quarters Cooked	3 oz	180	0	0	0
Burger Cooked	1 (3 oz)	170	0	0	0
Chicken Breast Seasoned Barbecue Cooked	3 oz	110	5	4	—
Chicken Breast Seasoned Italian Cooked	3 oz	100	2	1	—
Chicken Breast Seasoned Oriental Cooked	3 oz	100	3	2	—
Cornish Hen Split Dark Meat Roasted	1 half (6.5 oz)	210	0	0	0
Cornish Hen White Meat Cooked	3 oz	170	0	0	0
Drumsticks Roasted	1 (2 oz)	110	0	0	0
Drumsticks Skinless Roasted	2 (3.5 oz)	150	0	0	0
Ground Cooked	3 oz	180	0	0	0
Jumbo Drumsticks Roasted	1 (2 oz)	110	0	0	0
Jumbo Split Breast Roasted	1 (7 oz)	370	0	0	0
Jumbo Thighs Roasted	1 (3 oz)	240	0	0	0
Jumbo Whole Leg Roasted	2 (5.5 oz)	360	0	0	0
Jumbo Wings Roasted	2 (3 oz)	210	0	0	0
Leg Quarters Cooked	3 oz	210	0	0	0
Oven Stuffer Boneless Breast Cooked	3 oz	120	0	0	0
Oven Stuffer Boneless Breast Thin Sliced Cooked	1 slice (2 oz)	80	0	0	0
Oven Stuffer Boneless Thighs Roasted	1 (3.5 oz)	170	0	0	0
Oven Stuffer Dark Meat Roasted	3 oz	200	0	0	0
Oven Stuffer Drumstick Roasted	1 (3.5 oz)	190	0	0	0
Oven Stuffer White Meat Roasted	3 oz	160	0	0	0
Oven Stuffer Whole Breast Cooked	3 oz	150	0	0	0
Oven Stuffer Wing Drummettes Roasted	2 (2.5 oz)	170	0	0	0
Split Breast Skinless Roasted	1 (6 oz)	250	0	0	0

FOOD	PORTION	CALS.	CARB.	SUG.	FIB.
Perdue (CONT.)					
Split Breasts Roasted	1 (7 oz)	370	0	0	0
Thighs Roasted	1 (3 oz)	240	0	0	0
Thighs Skinless Roasted	1 (2.5 oz)	160	0	0	0
Whole White Meat Cooked	3 oz	160	0	0	0
Whole Leg Roasted	1 (5.5 oz)	360	0	0	0
Wingettes Roasted	3 (3 oz)	200	0	0	0
Wings Roasted	2 (3 oz)	210	0	0	0
Tyson					
Breast	3 oz	116	0	0	0
Drumstick	3 oz	131	0	0	0
Thigh	3 oz	152	0	0	0
Whole	3 oz	134	0	0	0
Wing	3 oz	147	0	0	0
Wampler Longacre					
Ground raw	1 oz	50	0	0	0
FROZEN					
Banquet					
Country Fried	1 serv (3 oz)	270	13	1	1
Drum Snackers	2.25 oz	190	12	—	1
Fried Breast	1 piece (4.45 oz)	240	18	2	4
Fried Hot & Spicy	1 serv (3 oz)	260	13	1	1
Fried Original	1 serv (3 oz)	270	13	1	1
Fried Thigh & Drumsticks	1 serv (3 oz)	260	10	1	2
Hot & Spicy Nuggets	2.5 oz	230	11	—	1
Hot Popcorn Chicken	1 pkg (3 oz)	290	18	0	2
Nuggets	3 oz	240	12	2	1
Nuggets Chicken & Cheddar	2.7 oz	280	13	2	1
Nuggets Chicken & Mozzarella	6 (2.8 oz)	210	20	3	2
Nuggets Southern Fried	6 (4.5 oz)	340	22	0	2
Nuggets Sweet & Sour	6 (4.5 oz)	320	25	0	2
Patties	1 (2.5 oz)	180	10	2	tr
Patties Southern Fried	1 (2.5 oz)	190	12	—	tr
Skinless Fried	1 serv (3 oz)	210	7	1	2
Skinless Fried Honey BBQ	1 serv (3 oz)	210	7	1	2
Southern Fried	1 serv (3 oz)	270	13	1	1
Tenders	3 pieces (3 oz)	260	16	1	2
Tenders Southern Fried	3 pieces (3 oz)	260	16	tr	1
Wings Hot & Spicy	4 pieces (5 oz)	230	5	0	1
Country Skillet					
Chicken Chunks	5 (3.1 oz)	270	18	2	1
Chicken Nuggets	10 (3.3 oz)	280	16	2	1

FOOD	PORTION	CALS.	CARB.	SUG.	FIB.
Country Skillet (CONT.)					
Chicken Patties	2.5 oz	190	12	3	1
Southern Fried Chicken Chunks	5 (3.1 oz)	250	16	4	1
Southern Fried Chicken Patties	1 (2.5 oz)	190	12	3	1
Empire					
Nuggets	5 (3 oz)	180	12	1	1
Stix	4 (3.1 oz)	180	6	0	2
Ozark Valley					
Nuggets	4 (2.9 oz)	210	16	0	2
Patties	1 (3 oz)	210	14	0	1
Sensible Chef					
Fried Breast	1 (3 oz)	200	8	0	2
Tyson					
Boneless Skinless Breast	3.5 oz	130	0	0	0
Boneless Skinless Thighs	3.5 oz	200	0	0	0
Drums & Thighs	3.5 oz	270	0	0	0
Skinless Breast Tenders	3.5 oz	120	0	0	0
READY-TO-EAT					
poultry salad sandwich spread	1 tbsp (13 g)	109	1	—	—
Carl Buddig					
Chicken	1 oz	50	1	—	0
Chicken By George					
Cajun	1 breast (4 oz)	130	3	0	0
Caribbean Grill	1 breast (4 oz)	150	8	6	0
Garlic & Herb	1 breast (4 oz)	120	3	1	0
Italian Bleu Cheese	1 breast (4 oz)	130	2	0	0
Lemon Herb	1 breast (4 oz)	120	3	2	0
Lemon Oregano	1 breast (4 oz)	130	3	1	0
Mesquite Barbecue	1 breast (4 oz)	130	5	3	0
Mustard Dill	1 breast (4 oz)	140	2	1	0
Roasted	1 breast (4 oz)	110	1	0	0
Teriyaki	1 breast (4 oz)	130	6	4	0
Tomato Herb With Basil	1 breast (4 oz)	140	5	4	0
Empire					
Barbacue Whole	5 oz	280	1	4	0
Battered & Breaded Cutlets	1 (3.3 oz)	200	11	4	2
Battered & Breaded Fried Breasts	3 oz	170	3	0	tr
Battered & Breaded Nuggets	5 (3 oz)	200	9	0	1
Bologna	3 slices (1.8 oz)	200	2	0	0

FOOD	PORTION	CALS.	CARB.	SUG.	FIB.
Empire (CONT.)					
Fried Drum & Thigh	3 oz	240	7	0	2
Healthy Choice					
Deli-Thin Oven Roasted Breast	6 slices (2 oz)	45	0	0	0
Deli-Thin Smoked Breast	6 slices (2 oz)	60	1	0	0
Fresh-Trak Oven Roasted Breast	1 slice (1 oz)	30	0	0	0
Oven Roasted Breast	1 slice (1 oz)	25	0	0	0
Smoked Breast	1 slice (1 oz)	35	0	0	0
Louis Rich					
Carving Board Classic Baked	2 slices (1.6 oz)	45	2	0	0
Carving Board Grilled	2 slices (1.6 oz)	45	2	0	0
Deli-Thin Oven Roasted Breast	4 slices (1.8 oz)	50	1	tr	0
Oven Roasted Deluxe Breast	1 slice (1 oz)	30	1	0	0
Oscar Mayer					
Free Oven Roasted Breast	4 slices (1.8 oz)	45	1	tr	0
Lunchables Chicken/ Monterey Jack	1 pkg (4.5 oz)	350	20	5	1
Lunchables Deluxe Chicken/Turkey	1 pkg (5.1 oz)	380	24	7	1
Lunchables Dessert Chocolate Pudding/ Chicken/ Jack	1 pkg (6.2 oz)	370	33	16	0
Perdue					
Cafe Meal Kit Stir Fry	1 serv (8.2 oz)	360	65	17	3
Cornish Hen Dark Meat Cooked	3 oz	200	0	0	0
Cornish Hen Split White Meat Roasted	½ hen (6.5 oz)	200	0	0	0
Nuggets Chicken & Cheese	5 (3 oz)	220	11	1	2
Nuggets Chik-Tac-Toe Cooked	5 (3 oz)	200	15	2	2
Nuggets Football Basketball Baseball	4 (3 oz)	230	14	2	—
Nuggets Original	5 (3 oz)	200	15	2	2
Nuggets Star & Drumstick	4 (3 oz)	200	15	2	2
Original Tenderloins Cooked	3 oz	160	7	2	2
Original Cutlets Cooked	1 (3.5 oz)	230	18	2	2
Oven Roasted Breast	1 (5 oz)	190	0	1	0

FOOD	PORTION	CALS.	CARB.	SUG.	FIB.
Perdue (CONT.)					
Oven Roasted Drumsticks	2 (2.5 oz)	100	0	1	0
Oven Roasted Half Dark Meat	3 oz	170	0	1	0
Oven Roasted Half White Meat	3 oz	140	0	1	0
Oven Roasted Thighs	1 (3 oz)	170	0	1	0
Oven Roasted Whole Chicken Dark Meat	3 oz	170	0	1	0
Oven Roasted Whole Chicken White Meat	3 oz	140	0	1	0
Short Cuts Italian	3 oz	110	1	1	0
Short Cuts Mesquite	3 oz	110	2	1	0
Short Cuts Oven Roasted	3 oz	110	2	1	0
Wings Barbecued	3 oz	200	3	3	1
Wings Hot & Spicy	3 oz	190	2	2	1
Tyson					
Roasted Drumsticks w/ Skin	2 (3.8 oz)	220	1	1	—
Wings Barbecue	6-7 (3.5 oz)	218	0	0	0
Wings Hot & Spicy	6-7 (3.5 oz)	218	0	0	0
Wings Roasted	6-7 (3.5 oz)	218	0	0	0
Wings Teriyaki	6-7 (3.5 oz)	218	0	0	0

CHICKEN DISHES
CANNED
Dinty Moore					
Noodles & Chicken	1 can (7.5 oz)	180	19	2	1
Stew	1 cup (8.5 oz)	220	16	3	2

FROZEN
Croissant Pocket					
Stuffed Sandwich Chicken Broccoli & Cheddar	1 piece (4.5 oz)	300	37	5	5
Hot Pocket					
Stuffed Sandwich Chicken & Cheddar With Broccoli	1 (4.5 oz)	300	37	6	tr
Jimmy Dean					
Grilled Breast Sandwich	1 (5.5 oz)	330	27	4	1
Lean Pockets					
Stuffed Sandwich Chicken Fajita	1 (4.5 oz)	260	36	4	3
Stuffed Sandwich Chicken Parmesan	1 (4.5 oz)	260	34	5	1

FOOD	PORTION	CALS.	CARB.	SUG.	FIB.
Lean Pockets (CONT.)					
Stuffed Sandwich Glazed Chicken Supreme	1 (4.5 oz)	240	34	6	1
Luigino's					
Chicken A La King With Noodles	1 pkg (8 oz)	240	28	0	2
Noodles With Chicken Peas & Carrots	1 cup (6.3 oz)	260	33	1	2
Noodles With Chicken Peas & Carrots	1 pkg (8 oz)	300	38	1	2
Sweet & Sour Chicken With Rice	1 pkg (8 oz)	300	50	14	2
Mrs. Paterson's					
Aussie Pie Chicken	1 (5.5 oz)	460	45	3	2
Aussie Pie Chicken Low Fat	1 (5.5 oz)	380	44	3	1
White Castle					
Grilled Chicken Sandwich	2 (4 oz)	250	24	2	5
Grilled Chicken Sandwich w/ Sauce	2 (4.8 oz)	290	33	2	5
MIX					
Chicken Skillet Helper					
Stir-Fried Chicken as prep	1 cup	270	30	1	1
Hamburger Helper					
Cheddar Spirals Reduced Sodium Chicken Recipe as prep	1 cup	240	27	5	1
Italian Herb Reduced Sodium Chicken Recipe as prep	1 cup	200	29	6	2
Southwestern Beef Reduced Sodium Chicken Recipe as prep	1 cup	220	32	6	2
SHELF-STABLE					
Dinty Moore					
Microwave Cup Chicken & Dumpling	1 pkg (7.5 oz)	200	21	1	1
Microwave Cup Stew	1 pkg (7.5 oz)	180	18	2	2

CHICKEN SUBSTITUTES

FOOD	PORTION	CALS.	CARB.	SUG.	FIB.
Harvest Direct					
TVP Poultry Chunks	3.5 oz	280	32	—	18
TVP Poultry Ground	3.5 oz	280	32	—	18
Knox Mountain Farm					
Chick'N Wheat Mix	1 serv (⅙ pkg)	110	3	—	2

FOOD	PORTION	CALS.	CARB.	SUG.	FIB.
Loma Linda					
Chicken Supreme Mix not prep	⅓ cup (0.9 oz)	90	6	0	4
Chik Nuggets	5 pieces (3 oz)	240	13	tr	5
Fried Chik'n w/ Gravy	2 pieces (2.8 oz)	210	3	tr	2
Morningstar Farms					
Chik Nuggets	4 pieces (3 oz)	160	17	2	5
Chik Patties	1 (2.5 oz)	150	15	1	2
Soy Is Us					
Chicken Not!	½ cup (1.75 oz)	140	15	4	9
White Wave					
Meatless Sandwich Slices	2 slices (1.6 oz)	80	8	3	0
Worthington					
Chic-Ketts	2 slices (1.9 oz)	120	2	0	2
Chicken Sliced	2 slices (2 oz)	80	1	0	tr
ChikStiks	1 (1.6 oz)	110	3	tr	2
CrispyChik Patties	1 (2.5 oz)	170	15	1	4
Cutlets	1 slice (2.1 oz)	70	3	0	2
Diced Chik	¼ cup (1.9 oz)	40	1	0	1
FriChik	2 pieces (3.2 oz)	120	1	0	1
FriChik Low Fat	2 pieces (3 oz)	80	2	0	1
Golden Croquettes	4 pieces (3 oz)	210	14	1	6
Sliced Chik	3 slices (3.2 oz)	70	2	0	2

CHICKPEAS
CANNED

FOOD	PORTION	CALS.	CARB.	SUG.	FIB.
Allen					
Garbanzo	½ cup (4.4 oz)	120	19	0	8
East Texas Fair					
Garbanzo	½ cup (4.4 oz)	120	19	0	8
Eden					
Organic	½ cup (4.6 oz)	120	19	—	5
Goya					
Spanish Style	7.5 oz	150	32	—	9
Green Giant					
Garbanzo	½ cup (4.4 oz)	110	18	tr	5
Old El Paso					
Garbanzo	½ cup (4.6 oz)	120	20	0	7
Progresso					
Chick Peas	½ cup (4.6 oz)	120	20	0	7

CHILI
CANNED

FOOD	PORTION	CALS.	CARB.	SUG.	FIB.
Allen					
Mexican Chili Beans	½ cup (4.5 oz)	120	22	1	8

FOOD	PORTION	CALS.	CARB.	SUG.	FIB.
Brown Beauty					
Mexican Chili Beans	½ cup (4.5 oz)	120	22	1	8
Del Monte					
Sauce	1 tbsp (0.6 oz)	20	0	4	0
Eden					
Organic Chili Beans w/ Jalapeno & Red Peppers	½ cup (4.6 oz)	130	21	1	7
Gebhardt					
Hot With Beans	1 cup	470	47	—	6
Plain	1 cup	530	20	—	1
With Beans	1 cup	495	47	—	6
Health Valley					
Mild Vegetarian With Beans	5 oz	160	21	—	12
Mild Vegetarian With Beans No Salt Added	5 oz	160	21	—	12
Mild Vegetarian With Lentils	5 oz	140	15	—	7
Mild Vegetarian With Lentils No Salt Added	5 oz	140	15	—	7
Spicy Vegetarian With Beans	5 oz	160	21	—	12
Hormel					
Chunky With Beans	1 cup (8.7 oz)	270	34	5	7
Hot No Beans	1 cup (8.3 oz)	210	17	3	3
Hot With Beans	1 cup (8.7 oz)	270	33	5	7
No Beans	1 cup (8.3 oz)	210	17	3	3
Turkey No Beans	1 cup (8.3 oz)	190	17	4	3
Turkey With Beans	1 cup (8.7 oz)	210	30	6	5
Vegetarian	1 cup (8.7 oz)	200	38	6	7
With Beans	1 cup (8.7 oz)	270	33	5	7
With Beans	1 cup (8.7 oz)	270	33	5	7
Hunt's					
Chili Beans	½ cup (4.5 oz)	87	17	8	6
Just Rite					
Hot With Beans	4 oz	195	16	—	1
With Beans	4 oz	200	16	—	1
Without Beans	4 oz	180	9	—	tr
Natural Touch					
Vegetarian	1 cup (8.1 oz)	170	21	2	11
Old El Paso					
Chili With Beans	1 cup (8 oz)	200	15	0	6
Van Camp's					
Chilee Beanee Weenee	1 can (8 oz)	240	27	—	9
Chili With Beans	1 cup (8.9 oz)	350	28	—	7

FOOD	PORTION	CALS.	CARB.	SUG.	FIB.
Worthington					
Chili	1 cup (8.1 oz)	290	21	2	9
Low Fat	1 cup (8.1 oz)	170	21	2	11
DRIED					
Gebhardt					
Chili Powder	1 tsp	15	3	—	tr
Chili Quik Seasoning	1 tsp	10	2	—	tr
Hurst					
HamBeens Chili Beans	1 serv	130	22	1	10
Nile Spice					
Chili'n Beans Original	1 pkg	150	25	5	6
Chili'n Beans Spicy	1 pkg	150	25	5	6
Old El Paso					
Chili Seasoning Mix	1 tbsp (0.3 oz)	25	4	0	1
Watkins					
Chili Seasoning	1¼ tsp (4 g)	15	2	0	0
Powder	¼ tsp (0.5 g)	0	0	0	0
FROZEN					
Amy's Organic					
Whole Meals Chili & Cornbread	1 pkg (10.5 oz)	320	59	14	8
Lean Cuisine					
Three Bean w/ Rice	1 pkg (10 oz)	250	38	9	9
Luigino's					
Chili-Mac	1 pkg (8 oz)	230	29	0	3
Stouffer's					
With Beans	1 pkg (8.75 oz)	270	29	7	8
Tabatchnick					
Vegetarian	7.5 oz	210	28	6	10
SHELF-STABLE					
Hormel					
Microcup Meals Chili Mac	1 cup (7.5 oz)	200	17	3	2
Microcup Meals Hot With Beans	1 cup (7.3 oz)	220	27	4	6
Microcup Meals No Beans	1 cup (7.3 oz)	190	15	3	2
Microcup Meals With Beans	1 cup (7.3 oz)	220	27	4	6

CHINESE CABBAGE
(*see* CABBAGE)

CHINESE FOOD
(*see* ASIAN FOOD)

CHIPS
(*see also* POPCORN, PRETZELS, SNACKS)
CORN
barbecue	1 oz	148	16	—	1

FOOD	PORTION	CALS.	CARB.	SUG.	FIB.
barbecue	1 bag (7 oz)	1036	111	—	10
plain	1 bag (7 oz)	1067	113	—	9
plain	1 oz	153	16	—	1
puffs cheese	1 bag (8 oz)	1256	122	—	2
puffs cheese	1 oz	157	15	—	tr
twists cheese	1 bag (8 oz)	1256	122	—	2
twists cheese	1 oz	157	15	—	tr
Energy Food Factory					
Corn Pops Fat Free	½ oz	50	11	0	1
Corn Pops Nacho	½ oz	50	12	1	1
Corn Pops Original	½ oz	50	11	0	1
Fritos					
Chili Cheese	34 pieces (1 oz)	160	15	—	1
Crisp 'N Thin	18 pieces (1 oz)	160	16	—	1
Dip Size	13 pieces (1 oz)	150	16	—	1
Non-Stop Nacho Cheese	34 pieces (1 oz)	150	16	—	1
Rowdy Rustlers Bar-B-Q	34 pieces (1 oz)	150	17	—	1
Wild 'N Mild	32 pieces (1 oz)	160	16	—	1
Health Valley					
Chips	1 oz	160	13	—	1
No Salt Added	1 oz	160	13	—	1
With Cheddar Cheese	1 oz	160	15	—	1
Planters					
Corn Chips	34 chips (1 oz)	170	17	1	2
King Size	17 chips (1 oz)	160	16	tr	2
Snacks To Go	1 pkg (1.5 oz)	240	23	1	3
Snyder's					
BBQ	1 oz	160	14	—	2
Chips	1 oz	160	14	—	2
Wise					
Dipsy Doodles	1 pkg (1.5 oz)	240	24	0	1
MULTIGRAIN					
Barbara's					
Pinta Chips	13 (1 oz)	130	19	0	2
Pinta Chips Salsa	12 (1 oz)	130	19	0	2
POTATO					
sticks	1 oz	148	15	—	1
sticks	½ cup (0.6 oz)	94	10	—	1
Barbara's					
No Salt Added	1¼ cups (1 oz)	150	15	0	0
Regular	1¼ cups (1 oz)	150	15	0	0
Ripple	1¼ cups (1 oz)	150	15	0	1
Yogurt & Green Onion	1¼ cups (1 oz)	150	15	tr	1

FOOD	PORTION	CALS.	CARB.	SUG.	FIB.
Barrel O' Fun					
Barbeque	1 oz	145	16	0	0
Chips	1 oz	150	15	0	0
Sour Cream & Onion	1 oz	150	15	0	0
Butterfield					
Sticks	1 pkg (1.7 oz)	250	26	0	3
Sticks	⅔ cup (1 oz)	150	16	0	2
Cape Cod					
Chips	19 chips (1 oz)	150	17	tr	1
Energy Food Factory					
Potato Pops Au Gratin	½ oz	60	12	1	1
Potato Pops Fat Free	½ oz	50	13	0	1
Potato Pops Herb & Garlic	½ oz	50	11	0	1
Potato Pops Mesquite	½ oz	50	12	2	1
Potato Pops Original	½ oz	50	11	0	1
Potato Pops Salt N' Vinegar	½ oz	50	11	0	1
Health Valley					
Country Ripple	1 oz	160	15	—	1
Country Ripple No Salt Added	1 oz	160	15	—	1
Dip Chips	1 oz	160	15	—	1
Dip Chips No Salt Added	1 oz	160	15	—	1
Natural	1 oz	160	15	—	1
Natural No Salt Added	1 oz	160	15	—	1
Herr's					
Potato	1 oz	140	16	—	1
Kelly's					
Bar-B-Q	1 oz	150	15	—	1
Chips	1 oz	150	14	—	2
Crunchy	1 oz	150	17	—	2
Rippled	1 oz	150	14	—	2
Sour Cream n' Onion	1 oz	150	15	—	1
Lay's					
Baked KC Masterpiece	11 pieces (1 oz)	110	23	3	2
Baked Original	12 chips (1 oz)	110	23	1	2
Baked Sour Cream & Onion	12 chips (1 oz)	110	23	3	2
Bar-B-Q	17 pieces (1 oz)	150	15	—	1
Cheddar Cheese	17 pieces (1 oz)	150	14	—	1
Crunch Tators	16 pieces (1 oz)	150	17	—	1
Crunch Tators Amazin' Cajun	16 pieces (1 oz)	150	17	—	—
Crunch Tators Hoppin' Jalapeno	16 pieces (1 oz)	140	18	—	1
Flamin' Hot	17 pieces (1 oz)	150	15	—	1

FOOD	PORTION	CALS.	CARB.	SUG.	FIB.
Lay's (CONT.)					
Reduced Fat Original	21 chips (1 oz)	150	18	0	1
Salt & Vinegar	17 pieces (1 oz)	150	14	—	1
Tangy Ranch	17 pieces (1 oz)	160	15	—	1
Unsalted	17 pieces (1 oz)	150	15	—	1
Wow Original	25 chips (1 oz)	80	19	—	1
Wow Original	1 pkg (0.75 oz)	55	13	0	1
Louise's					
"1g" Mesquite BBQ	1 oz	110	24	1	2
"1g" Original	1 oz	110	24	0	2
70% Less Fat Mesquite BBQ	1 oz	110	21	1	2
70% Less Fat Original	1 oz	110	21	0	2
Fat-Free Maui Onion	1 oz	110	23	0	2
Fat-Free Mesquite BBQ	1 oz	110	23	1	2
Fat-Free No Salt	1 oz	110	24	0	2
Fat-Free Original	1 oz	110	23	0	2
Fat-Free Vinegar & Salt	1 oz	110	23	0	2
Mr. Phipps					
Tater Crisps Bar-B-Que	21 (1 oz)	130	21	3	1
Tater Crisps Original	23 (1 oz)	120	20	2	1
Tater Crisps Sour Cream 'n Onion	22 (1 oz)	130	21	2	1
Pringles					
Fat Free	15 chips (1 oz)	75	17	tr	2
Ruffles					
Cheddar Cheese & Sour Cream	18 chips (1 oz)	160	15	—	1
Chips	18 chips (1 oz)	150	15	—	1
Mesquite Grille B-B-Q	18 chips (1 oz)	160	15	—	1
Monterey Jack Cheese Attack	18 chips (1 oz)	160	15	—	1
Ranch	18 chips (1 oz)	160	15	—	1
Reduced Fat	16 chips (1 oz)	140	18	0	1
Sour Cream & Onion	18 chips (1 oz)	160	15	—	1
Snyder's					
BBQ	1 oz	150	13	—	1
Cheddar Bacon	1 oz	150	13	—	1
Chips	1 oz	150	13	—	1
Coney Island	1 oz	150	13	—	1
Grilled Steak & Onion	1 oz	150	13	—	1
Hot Buffalo Wings	1 oz	150	13	—	1
Kosher Dill	1 oz	150	13	—	1
No Salt	1 oz	150	13	—	1

FOOD	PORTION	CALS.	CARB.	SUG.	FIB.
Snyder's (CONT.)					
Salt & Vinegar	1 oz	150	13	—	1
Sausage Pizza	1 oz	150	13	—	1
Sour Cream & Onion	1 oz	150	13	—	1
Sour Cream & Onion Unsalted	1 oz	150	13	—	1
State Line					
Chips	1 pkg (0.5 oz)	80	7	0	tr
Utz					
Wavy	20 chips (1 oz)	150	14	0	1
TORTILLA					
nacho	1 bag (8 oz)	1131	142	—	12
plain	1 bag (7.5 oz)	1067	134	—	14
plain	1 oz	142	18	—	2
Barbara's					
Blue Corn	15 (1 oz)	140	16	tr	1
Blue Corn No Salt Added	15 (1 oz)	140	16	tr	1
Barrel O' Fun					
Nacho	1 oz	140	19	0	1
Tostada Yellow	1 oz	140	19	0	0
White	1 oz	140	20	0	0
Doritos					
Reduced Fat Cooler Ranch	13 chips (1 oz)	130	20	2	1
Reduced Fat Nacho Cheeiser	13 chips (1 oz)	130	19	2	1
Wow Nacho Cheese	11 chips (1 oz)	97	21	—	1
Wow Nacho Cheesier	1 pkg (0.75 oz)	70	13	tr	1
Frito Lay					
Salsa 'N Cheese	16 (1 oz)	150	17	—	2
Guiltless Gourmet					
Baked	22-26 chips (1 oz)	110	21	—	1
Herr's					
Restaurant Style White Corn	10 chips (1 oz)	140	18	1	2
Louise's					
95% Fat-Free	1 oz	120	23	0	1
Mr. Phipps					
Nacho	28 (1 oz)	130	20	3	3
Original	28 (1 oz)	130	21	3	3
Old El Paso					
NACHIPS	9 chips (1 oz)	150	17	0	2
White Corn	11 chips (1 oz)	140	18	0	1
Santitas					
Cantina Style	1 oz	140	19	—	2

FOOD	PORTION	CALS.	CARB.	SUG.	FIB.
Santitas (CONT.)					
Cantina Style Fajita	1 oz	140	19	—	2
Chips	1 oz	140	19	—	2
Strips	1 oz	140	19	—	2
Snyder's					
Chips	1 oz	140	18	—	2
Enchilada	1 oz	140	18	—	2
Nacho Cheese	1 oz	140	18	—	2
No Salt	1 oz	140	18	—	2
Ranch	1 oz	140	18	—	2
Tostitos					
Baked Cool Ranch	11 chips (1 oz)	120	21	0	1
Baked Original	9 chips (1 oz)	110	24	0	2
Baked Unsalted	13 chips (1 oz)	110	24	0	2
Bite Size	16 pieces (1 oz)	150	18	—	2
Chips	11 pieces (1 oz)	140	18	—	2
Restaurant Style Lime 'N Chili	7 pieces (1 oz)	150	18	—	2
Restaurant Style White Corn	7 pieces (1 oz)	150	20	—	2
VEGETABLE					
Eden					
Vegetable Chips	50 (1 oz)	130	24	2	0
Wasabi Chip Hot & Spicy	50 (1 oz)	130	24	2	0
Hain					
Carrot Chips	1 oz	150	16	—	0
Carrot Chips Barbecue	1 oz	140	16	—	0
Carrot Chips No Salt Added	1 oz	150	16	—	0
Health Valley					
Carrot Lites	0.5 oz	75	9	—	tr
Robert's American Gourmet					
Spirulina Spirals	1 oz	120	22	4	3
Terra Chips					
Sweet Potato	1 oz	140	18	2	1
Sweet Potato Spiced	1 oz	140	16	6	3
Taro Spiced	1 oz	130	20	2	2
Vegetable	1 oz	140	18	1	3

CHITTERLINGS

pork cooked	3 oz	258	0	0	0

CHIVES

fresh chopped	1 tsp	0	tr	—	—

FOOD	PORTION	CALS.	CARB.	SUG.	FIB.
CHOCOLATE					
(see also CANDY, CAROB, COCOA, ICE CREAM TOPPINGS, MILK DRINKS)					
BAKING					
grated unsweetened	1 cup (4.6 oz)	690	37	—	18
squares unsweetened	1 square (1 oz)	148	8	—	4
Baker's					
Bittersweet	½ square (0.5 oz)	70	7	5	1
German's Sweet	2 squares (0.5 oz)	60	8	8	tr
Semi-Sweet	½ square (0.5 oz)	70	8	7	1
Unsweetened	½ square (0.5 oz)	70	4	0	2
White	½ square (0.5 oz)	80	8	8	0
Nestle					
Choco Bake	½ oz	80	5	0	3
Premier White	½ oz	80	8	8	—
Semi-Sweet	½ oz	70	9	7	2
Unsweetened	½ oz	80	5	—	3
CHIPS					
Baker's					
Chips	1 oz	143	18	17	—
Real Milk Chocolate	½ oz	70	9	8	0
Real Semi-Sweet	½ oz	60	9	8	1
Semi-Sweet	½ oz	70	10	9	0
M&M's					
Baking Bits Milk Chocolate	0.5 oz	70	10	9	0
Baking Bits Semi-Sweet	0.5 oz	70	9	7	1
Nestle					
Morsels Milk Chocolate	1 tbsp	70	10	9	—
Morsels Mint Chocolate	1 tbsp	70	9	7	2
Morsels Rainbow	1 tbsp	70	10	9	1
Morsels Mini Semi-Sweet	1 tbsp	70	9	7	2
Semi-Sweet Morsels	1 tbsp	40	9	7	2
MIX					
Quik					
Chocolate Powder	2 tbsp (0.8 oz)	90	19	18	1
Chocolate Powder No Sugar Added	2 tbsp (0.4 oz)	40	7	1	2
CHOCOLATE MILK					
(see CHOCOLATE, COCOA, MILK DRINKS, MILKSHAKE)					
CHOCOLATE SYRUP					
Estee					
Choco-Syp	2 tbsp (1.2 oz)	50	11	9	—
Marzetti					
Syrup	2 tbsp	40	21	20	0

FOOD	PORTION	CALS.	CARB.	SUG.	FIB.
Quik					
Chocolate	2 tbsp (1.3 oz)	100	23	17	tr
Red Wing					
Syrup	2 tbsp (1.4 oz)	110	25	19	0
Tollhouse					
Mint-Chocolate	2 tbsp (1.5 oz)	130	25	22	1
Semi-Sweet	2 tbsp (1.5 oz)	130	24	22	1
CHUTNEY					
apple	1.2 oz	68	18	—	1
coconut	¼ cup	74	4	—	2
tomato	1.2 oz	54	14	—	1
Sonoma					
Dried Tomato	1 tbsp (0.7 g)	35	9	8	0
CILANTRO					
fresh	1 tsp (2 g)	tr	tr	—	tr
fresh	1 cup (1.6 oz)	11	2	—	1
Watkins					
Dried	¼ tsp (0.5 oz)	0	0	0	0
CINNAMON					
sticks	0.5 oz	39	8	0	3
Watkins					
Ground	¼ tsp (0.5 g)	0	0	0	0
CISCO					
raw	3 oz	84	0	0	0
smoked	1 oz	50	0	0	0
CLAMS					
CANNED					
Progresso					
Creamy Clam	½ cup (4.2 oz)	100	8	0	0
Minced	¼ cup (2 oz)	25	2	0	0
Red Clam	½ cup (4.4 oz)	80	8	5	1
White Clam Sauce	½ cup (4.4 oz)	120	1	0	0
COCOA					
(*see also* CHOCOLATE)					
powder unsweetened	1 tbsp (5 g)	11	3	—	2
powder unsweetened	1 cup (3 oz)	197	47	—	29
Nestle					
Cocoa	1 tbsp	15	3	0	2
Swiss Miss					
Cocoa Diet	6 oz	20	3	—	0
Hot Cocoa Bavarian Chocolate	6 oz	110	20	—	0

FOOD	PORTION	CALS.	CARB.	SUG.	FIB.
Swiss Miss (CONT.)					
Hot Cocoa Double Rich	6 oz	110	22	—	0
Hot Cocoa Milk Chocolate	6 oz	110	24	—	0
Hot Cocoa Milk Chocolate	1 serv	110	24	17	1
Hot Cocoa Mini-Marshmallow	1 serv	109	24	18	1
Hot Cocoa Rich Chocolate	1 serv	110	24	19	1
Hot Cocoa Sugar Free	1 serv	67	13	10	1
Hot Cocoa Sugar Free Milk Chocolate	1 serv	49	10	7	1
Hot Cocoa Sugar Free Mini-Marshmallow	1 serv	51	11	7	1
Hot Cocoa White Chocolate	1 serv	109	21	21	tr
Hot Cocoa With Mini Marshmallows	6 oz	110	23	—	0
Hot Cocoa Lite	1 serv	74	17	16	2
Lite as prep	6 oz	70	17	—	0
Sugar Free With Sugar Free Marshmallows as prep	6 oz	50	9	—	0
Sugar Free as prep	6 oz	60	10	—	0
Ultra Slim-Fast					
Hot Cocoa as prep w/ water	8 oz	190	35	—	5
Weight Watchers					
Hot Cocoa Mix as prep	1 pkg	70	7	6	1

COCONUT

FOOD	PORTION	CALS.	CARB.	SUG.	FIB.
fresh	1 piece (1.5 oz)	159	7	—	4
fresh shredded	1 cup	283	12	—	7
Baker's					
Angel Flake	1 tbsp (0.5 oz)	70	6	5	1
Angel Flake (canned)	2 tbsp (0.5 oz)	70	6	5	1
Premium Shred	2 tbsp (0.5 oz)	70	6	5	1

COD
CANNED

FOOD	PORTION	CALS.	CARB.	SUG.	FIB.
atlantic	3 oz	89	0	0	0
atlantic	1 can (11 oz)	327	0	0	0
DRIED					
atlantic	3 oz	246	0	0	0
FRESH					
atlantic cooked	1 fillet (6.3 oz)	189	0	0	0
atlantic cooked	3 oz	89	0	0	0
pacific baked	3 oz	95	0	0	0
tarama	3.5 oz	547	6	tr	—

FOOD	PORTION	CALS.	CARB.	SUG.	FIB.
FROZEN					
Van De Kamp's					
Lightly Breaded Fillets	1 (4 oz)	220	19	3	0
COFFEE					
(*see also* COFFEE BEVERAGES, COFFEE SUBSTITUTES)					
REGULAR					
brewed	6 oz	4	1	—	—
COFFEE BEVERAGES					
(*see also* COFFEE SUBSTITUTES)					
General Foods					
Cappuccino Coolers French Vanilla as prep w/ 2% milk	1 serv	180	27	—	0
International Coffee Sugar Free Cafe Vienna as prep	1 serv (8 oz)	30	3	0	0
International Coffee Sugar Free Fat Free Suisse Mocha as prep	1 serv (8 oz)	25	5	0	tr
International Coffees Cafe Francais as prep	1 serv (8 oz)	60	7	4	0
International Coffees Cafe Vienna as prep	1 serv (8 oz)	70	11	9	tr
International Coffees Decaffeinated French Vanilla Cafe as prep	1 serv (8 oz)	60	10	7	0
International Coffees Decaffeinated Suisse Mocha as prep	1 serv (8 oz)	60	9	7	0
International Coffees French Vanilla Cafe as prep	1 serv (8 oz)	60	10	7	0
International Coffees Hazelnut Belgian Cafe as prep	1 serv (8 oz)	70	12	9	0
International Coffees Irish Creme Cafe as prep	1 serv (8 oz)	60	10	8	0
International Coffees Italian Cappuccino as prep	1 serv (8 oz)	60	10	8	0
International Coffees Kahlua Cafe as prep	1 serv (8 oz)	60	10	7	0
International Coffees Orange Cappuccino as prep	1 serv (8 oz)	70	11	9	tr

FOOD	PORTION	CALS.	CARB.	SUG.	FIB.
General Foods (CONT.)					
International Coffees Suisse Mocha as prep	1 serv (8 oz)	60	8	7	0
International Coffees Viennese Chocolate Cafe as prep	1 serv (8 oz)	50	10	9	0
International Coffees Sugar Free Fat Free Decaffeinated French Vanilla	1 serv (8 oz)	25	5	0	0
International Coffees Sugar Free Fat Free Decaffeinated Suisse Mocha	1 serv (8 oz)	25	5	0	tr
International Coffees Sugar Free Fat Free French Vanilla Cafe as prep	1 serv (8 oz)	25	5	0	0
Maxwell House					
Cafe Cappuccino Amaretto as prep	1 serv (8 oz)	90	19	18	0
Cafe Cappuccino Decaffeinated Mocha as prep	1 serv (8 oz)	100	17	16	0
Cafe Cappuccino Decaffeinated Vanilla as prep	1 serv (8 oz)	90	19	18	0
Cafe Cappuccino Irish Cream as prep	1 serv (8 oz)	90	19	18	0
Cafe Cappuccino Mocha as prep	1 serv (8 oz)	100	17	16	0
Cafe Cappuccino Sugar Free Mocha as prep	1 serv (8 oz)	60	7	0	tr
Cafe Cappuccino Sugar Free Vanilla as prep	1 serv (8 oz)	60	7	0	0
Cafe Cappuccino Vanilla as prep	1 serv (8 oz)	90	19	18	0
Iced Cappuccino as prep w/ 2% milk	1 serv (8 oz)	180	27	27	tr
Starbucks					
Frappuccino	1 bottle (9.5 fl oz)	190	39	30	0

COFFEE SUBSTITUTES

Natural Touch

Kaffree Roma	1 tsp (2 g)	10	2	0	0

FOOD	PORTION	CALS.	CARB.	SUG.	FIB.
Natural Touch (CONT.)					
Roma Cappuccino	3 tbsp (0.4 oz)	50	5	4	0
Postum					
Instant Coffee Flavor as prep	1 serv (8 oz)	10	3	0	0
Instant as prep	1 serv (8 oz)	10	3	0	0

COFFEE WHITENERS
(*see also* MILK SUBSTITUTES)

FOOD	PORTION	CALS.	CARB.	SUG.	FIB.
Hood					
Non Dairy	1 tbsp (0.5 oz)	20	2	tr	0
International Delight					
Amaretto	1 tbsp (0.6 fl oz)	45	7	5	0
Cinnamon Hazelnut	1 tbsp (0.6 fl oz)	45	7	5	0
Irish Creme	1 tbsp (0.6 fl oz)	45	7	5	0
No Fat Amaretto	1 tbsp (0.5 fl oz)	30	7	5	0
No Fat French Vanilla Royale	1 tbsp (0.5 fl oz)	30	7	5	0
No Fat Hawaiian Macadamia	1 tbsp (0.5 fl oz)	30	7	5	0
No Fat Irish Creme	1 tbsp (0.5 fl oz)	30	7	5	0
Suisse Chocolate Mocha	1 tbsp (0.6 fl oz)	45	7	5	0
Mocha Mix					
Fat-Free	1 tbsp (0.5 fl oz)	10	1	0	0
Lite	1 tbsp (0.5 fl oz)	10	tr	0	0
Lite	4 fl oz	80	3	—	0
Original	1 tbsp (0.5 fl oz)	20	1	1	0
Signature Flavors French Vanilla	1 tbsp (0.5 fl oz)	35	8	7	—
Signature Flavors Irish Creme	1 tbsp (0.5 fl oz)	35	8	7	—
Signature Flavors Kahlua	1 tbsp (0.5 fl oz)	35	8	7	—
Signature Flavors Mauna Loa Macadamia Nut	1 tbsp (0.5 fl oz)	35	8	7	—
N-Rich Creamer					
Whitener	1 tsp	10	1	—	0

COLESLAW

FOOD	PORTION	CALS.	CARB.	SUG.	FIB.
Fresh Express					
Cole Slaw	1½ cups (3 oz)	25	6	3	2

COLLARDS
CANNED

FOOD	PORTION	CALS.	CARB.	SUG.	FIB.
Allen					
Collards	½ cup (4.1 oz)	30	5	1	3

FOOD	PORTION	CALS.	CARB.	SUG.	FIB.
Sunshine					
Collards	½ cup (4.1 oz)	30	5	1	3

COOKIES
(*see also* BROWNIE, CAKE, DOUGHNUT, PIE)
MIX
Estee

Chocolate Chip	3	130	17	10	0

READY-TO-EAT

butter	1 (5 g)	23	3	—	tr
chocolate chip	1 (0.4 oz)	48	7	—	tr
chocolate chip soft-type	1 (0.5 oz)	69	9	—	tr
chocolate w/ creme filling	1 (0.35 oz)	47	7	—	tr
digestive biscuits plain	2	141	21	—	1
fig bars	1 (0.56 oz)	56	11	—	1
fortune	1 (0.28 oz)	30	7	—	tr
fudge	1 (0.73 oz)	73	17	—	tr
graham honey	1 (0.24 oz)	30	5	—	tr
oatmeal	1 (0.6 oz)	81	12	—	1
oatmeal	1 (0.52 oz)	71	9	—	tr
oatmeal soft-type	1 (0.5 oz)	61	10	—	tr
oatmeal raisin	1 (0.6 oz)	81	12	—	1
oatmeal raisin soft-type	1 (0.5 oz)	61	10	—	tr
peanut butter soft-type	1 (0.5 oz)	69	9	—	tr
shortbread pecan	1 (0.49 oz)	79	8	—	tr
vanilla sandwich	1 (0.35 oz)	48	7	—	tr
Archway					
Almond Crescents	2 (0.8 oz)	100	17	6	tr
Apple N'Raisin	1 (1.1 oz)	130	20	11	1
Apricot Filled	1 (1 oz)	110	18	9	tr
Bells And Stars	3 (1 oz)	150	19	7	tr
Blueberry Filled	1 (1 oz)	110	19	14	tr
Carrot Cake	1 (1 oz)	120	18	14	0
Cherry Filled	1 (1 oz)	110	19	14	tr
Cherry Nougat	3 (1 oz)	150	18	12	0
Chocolate Chip	1 (1 oz)	130	19	8	0
Chocolate Chip & Toffee	1 (1 oz)	140	19	9	tr
Chocolate Chip Bag	3 (0.9 oz)	130	17	9	0
Chocolate Chip Drop	1 (1 oz)	140	11	9	0
Chocolate Chip Ice Box	1 (1 oz)	140	19	9	0
Chocolate Chip Mini	12 (1.1 oz)	150	20	9	0
Cinnamon Snaps	12 (1.1 oz)	150	19	9	0
Coconut Macaroon	1 (0.8 oz)	90	14	9	2
Cookie Jar Hermits	1 (1 oz)	110	19	9	tr

FOOD	PORTION	CALS.	CARB.	SUG.	FIB.
Archway (CONT.)					
Dark Chocolate	1 (1 oz)	110	20	7	tr
Dutch Chocolate	1 (1 oz)	120	19	13	0
Fig Bars Low Fat	2 (1.1 oz)	100	23	12	1
Frosty Lemon	1 (1 oz)	120	19	15	0
Frosty Orange	1 (1 oz)	120	19	8	1
Fruit And Honey Bar	1 (1 oz)	110	18	14	tr
Fruit Bar No Fat	1 (1 oz)	90	21	11	0
Fruit Cake	1 (1.1 oz)	140	20	12	2
Fudge Nut Bar	1 (1 oz)	110	17	8	tr
Fun Chip Mini	12 (1.1 oz)	140	21	9	0
Gingersnaps	5 (1.1 oz)	130	22	12	0
Granola No Fat	1 (0.5 oz)	50	11	7	tr
Holiday Pak	3 (1.1 oz)	150	19	9	tr
Iced Gingerbread	3 (1.1 oz)	140	23	10	0
Iced Molasses	1 (1 oz)	110	19	8	tr
Iced Oatmeal	1 (1 oz)	120	19	15	1
Lemon Snaps	12 (1.1 oz)	150	19	9	0
New Orleans Cake	1 (1 oz)	110	18	8	tr
Nutty Nougat	3 (1.1 oz)	160	18	7	0
Oatmeal	1 (0.9 oz)	110	19	10	tr
Oatmeal Apple Filled	1 (1 oz)	110	18	14	0
Oatmeal Date Filled	1 (1 oz)	110	18	15	tr
Oatmeal Mini	12 (1.1 oz)	150	19	7	1
Oatmeal Pecan	1 (1 oz)	120	18	9	1
Oatmeal Raisin	1 (1 oz)	110	19	13	tr
Oatmeal Raisin Bran	1 (1 oz)	110	19	9	tr
Old Fashioned Molasses	1 (1 oz)	120	20	10	0
Old Fashioned Windmill	1 (0.7 oz)	100	15	9	0
Party Treats	3 (1.1 oz)	140	20	9	0
Peanut Butter	1 (1 oz)	140	16	8	tr
Peanut Butter & Chip	3 (0.9 oz)	130	16	8	0
Peanut Butter N' Chips	1 (1 oz)	140	16	9	tr
Peanut Butter Nougat	3 (1.1 oz)	160	18	8	1
Pecan Crunch	6 (1.1 oz)	150	18	8	0
Pecan Ice Box	1 (1 oz)	140	18	9	0
Pecan Malted Nougat	3 (1.1 oz)	160	17	11	2
Pfeffernusse	2 (1.3 oz)	140	32	22	tr
Pineapple Filled	1 (0.9 oz)	100	16	8	1
Raisin Oatmeal	1 (1 oz)	130	19	9	1
Raisin Oatmeal Bag	3 (1 oz)	130	19	10	1
Raspberry Filled	1 (1 oz)	110	18	9	tr
Rocky Road	1 (1 oz)	130	18	9	tr
Ruth's Golden Oatmeal	1 (1 oz)	120	19	11	tr

FOOD	PORTION	CALS.	CARB.	SUG.	FIB.
Archway (CONT.)					
Select Assortment	3 (0.9 oz)	130	18	9	0
Soft Molasses Drop	1 (1 oz)	110	18	6	1
Soft Sugar	1 (1 oz)	110	18	11	0
Strawberry Filled	1 (1 oz)	110	18	9	tr
Sugar	1 (1 oz)	120	20	11	0
Vanilla Wafer	5 (1.1 oz)	130	22	15	0
Wedding Cakes	3 (1.1 oz)	160	20	9	0
Bakery Wagon					
Apple Walnut Raisin	1	100	16	8	1
Cobbler Apple Cranberry Fat Free	1	70	16	10	1
Cobbler Apple Fat Free	1	70	17	9	1
Cobbler Mixed Fruit Fat Free	1	70	16	21	1
Cobbler Raspberry Fat Free	1	70	17	7	1
Ginger Snaps	5	160	22	10	1
Honey Fruit Bars	1	100	17	8	1
Iced Molasses	1	100	18	9	1
Iced Molasses Mini	3	130	18	12	1
Oatmeal Apple Filled	1	90	14	7	1
Oatmeal Chocolate Chunk	1	100	16	4	1
Oatmeal Date Filled	1	90	17	5	1
Oatmeal Raspberry Filled	1	100	16	7	1
Oatmeal Soft	1	100	16	10	1
Oatmeal Walnut Raisin	1	100	17	4	1
Vanilla Wafers Cholesterol Free	6	130	22	14	1
Baking On The Lite Side					
Oatmeal Crunchy	2 (0.6 oz)	60	13	2	0
Raspberry Linzer	1 (0.6 oz)	55	12	2	0
Barbara's					
Animal Cookies Vanilla	8 (1 oz)	130	20	4	1
Chocolate Chip	1 (0.6 oz)	80	10	5	1
Double Dutch Chocolate	1 (0.6 oz)	80	10	5	1
Fat Free Homestyle Chewy Chocolate	2 (0.9 oz)	80	20	11	2
Fat Free Homestyle Chocolate Mint	2 (0.9 oz)	80	20	12	2
Fat Free Homestyle Nutt'n Crispies	2 (0.9 oz)	80	20	11	2
Fat Free Homestyle Oatmeal Raisin	2 (0.9 oz)	80	20	12	2
Fat Free Mini Carmel Apple	6 (1 oz)	110	24	12	1

FOOD	PORTION	CALS.	CARB.	SUG.	FIB.
Barbara's (CONT.)					
Fat Free Mini Cocoa Mocha	6 (1 oz)	100	23	11	1
Fat Free Mini Double Chocolate	6 (1 oz)	100	23	12	1
Fat Free Mini Oatmeal Raisin	6 (1 oz)	110	24	12	2
Fig Bars Fat Free	1 (0.7 oz)	60	15	11	1
Fig Bars Fat Free Raspberry	1 (0.7 oz)	60	15	11	1
Fig Bars Fat Free Whole Wheat	1 (0.7 oz)	60	15	11	2
Fig Bars Fat Free Whole Wheat Apple Cinnamon	1 (0.7 oz)	60	14	10	2
Fig Bars Low Fat	1 (0.7 oz)	60	14	9	1
Fig Bars Low Fat Blueberry	1 (0.7 oz)	60	14	9	1
Old Fashioned Oatmeal	1 (0.6 oz)	70	11	5	1
Snackimals Chocolate Chip	8 (1 oz)	120	18	8	1
Snackimals Oatmeal Wheat Free	8 (1 oz)	120	19	8	2
Snackimals Vanilla	8 (1 oz)	120	19	7	1
Traditional Shortbread	1 (0.6 oz)	80	10	3	1
Barnum's					
Animal Crackers	12 (1.1 oz)	140	23	8	1
Animal Crackers Chocolate	10 (1 oz)	130	23	8	1
Biscos					
Sugar Wafers	8 (1 oz)	140	21	13	tr
Waffle Cremes	4 (1.2 oz)	180	24	17	tr
Cadbury					
Fingers	3	85	11	6	tr
Chip-A-Roos					
Cookies	3 (1.3 oz)	190	23	10	1
Chips Ahoy!					
Bit Size Chocolate Chip	14 (1.1 oz)	170	21	10	tr
Chewy Chocolate Chip	3 (1.3 oz)	170	23	14	tr
Chunky Chocolate Chip	1 (0.5 oz)	80	11	7	tr
Real Chocolate Chip	3 (1.1 oz)	160	21	10	1
Reduced Fat	3 (1.1 oz)	150	23	10	1
Sprinkled Real Chocolate Chip	3 (1.3 oz)	170	24	12	tr
Striped Chocolate Chip	1 (0.5 oz)	80	10	6	tr
Chortles					
Cookies	½ pkg. (1 oz)	125	23	11	1
Cookie Lover's					
Blue Ribbon Brownies	1 (0.8 oz)	90	14	7	0
Classic Shortbread	1 (0.8 oz)	110	12	4	0

FOOD	PORTION	CALS.	CARB.	SUG.	FIB.
Cookie Lover's (CONT.)					
Dutch Chocolate Chip	1 (0.8 oz)	90	12	4	0
Fancy Peanut Butter	1 (0.8 oz)	100	10	4	0
Grahams Cinnamon Honey	2 (1 oz)	110	24	6	1
Grahams Honey	2 (1 oz)	100	22	5	1
Old-Time Raisin	1 (0.8 oz)	90	14	6	0
Delacre					
Cookie Assortment	4 (1.1 oz)	130	18	10	1
Dutch Mill					
Chocolate Chip	3 (1.1 oz)	160	18	10	1
Coconut Macaroons	3 (1 oz)	120	14	12	0
Oatmeal Raisin	3 (1 oz)	130	18	10	1
Estee					
Chocolate Chip	4 (1.1 oz)	150	21	5	tr
Coconut	4 (1 oz)	140	19	5	tr
Creme Wafers Chocolate	7 (1.1 oz)	160	21	9	tr
Creme Wafers Lemon	5 (1.2 oz)	170	23	10	0
Creme Wafers Peanut Butter	5 (1.2 oz)	170	21	7	0
Creme Wafers Triple Decker Banana Split	3 (0.9 oz)	140	18	8	0
Creme Wafers Triple Decker Chocolate Caramel & Peanut Butter	3 (0.9 oz)	140	17	7	0
Creme Wafers Vanilla	7 (1.1 oz)	160	22	9	0
Creme Wafers Vanilla & Strawberry	5 (1.2 oz)	170	23	10	0
Fig Bars Apple Low Fat	2 (1 oz)	100	22	14	3
Fig Bars Cranberry Low Fat	2 (1 oz)	100	22	14	3
Fig Bars Low Fat	2 (1 oz)	100	23	13	3
Fudge	4 (1 oz)	150	19	5	1
Lemon	4 (1 oz)	140	19	5	tr
Oatmeal Raisin	4 (1 oz)	130	19	6	1
Sandwich Chocolate	3 (1.2 oz)	160	24	9	1
Sandwich Original	3 (1.2 oz)	160	24	10	1
Sandwich Peanut Butter	3 (1.2 oz)	160	22	7	1
Sandwich Vanilla	3 (1.2 oz)	160	25	7	tr
Shortbread Reduced Fat	4 (1 oz)	130	22	5	tr
Vanilla	4 (1 oz)	140	19	5	tr
Freihofer's					
Chocolate Chip	2 (0.9 oz)	120	16	10	1
Girl Scout					
Chalet Cremes Sugar Free	4 (1 oz)	150	22	0	1
Do-si-dos	3 (1.2 oz)	170	22	11	1

FOOD	PORTION	CALS.	CARB.	SUG.	FIB.
Girl Scout (CONT.)					
Samoas	2 (1 oz)	160	17	12	2
Snaps	7 (1.1 oz)	130	26	10	1
Striped Chocolate Chip	3 (1.2 oz)	180	20	11	1
Tagalongs	2 (0.9 oz)	150	13	8	2
Thin Mints	4 (1 oz)	140	18	10	1
Trefoils	5 (1.1 oz)	160	20	7	1
Golden Fruit					
Apple	1 (0.7 oz)	80	15	6	tr
Cranberry	1 (0.7 oz)	70	15	7	tr
Cranberry Low Fat	1 (0.7 oz)	70	15	7	tr
Raisin	1 (0.7 oz)	80	15	7	tr
Handi-Snack					
Cookie Jammers Cookies & Fruit Spread	1 pkg (1.3 oz)	130	26	14	tr
Health Valley					
Amaranth Cookies	1	70	12	—	2
Fancy Fruit Chunks Apricot Almond	2	90	12	—	2
Fancy Fruit Chunks Date Pecan	2	90	13	—	2
Fancy Fruit Chunks Raisin Oat Bran	2	70	13	—	2
Fancy Fruit Chunks Tropical Fruit	2	90	15	—	2
Fancy Peanut Chunks	2	90	12	—	2
Fat Free Apple Spice	3	75	17	—	3
Fat Free Apricot Delight	3	75	16	—	3
Fat Free Date Delight	3	75	17	—	3
Fat Free Hawaiian Fruit	3	75	16	—	3
Fat Free Jumbos Apple Raisin	1	70	16	—	3
Fat Free Jumbos Raisin	1	70	16	—	3
Fat Free Jumbos Raspberry	1	70	16	—	3
Fat Free Raisin Oatmeal	3	75	17	—	3
Fiber Jumbos Blueberry Nut	1	100	14	—	3
Fiber Jumbos Chunky Pecan	1	100	14	—	3
Fiber Jumbos Raisin Nut	1	100	14	—	3
Fruit & Fitness	5	200	34	—	6
Fruit Jumbos Almond Date	1	70	10	—	1
Fruit Jumbos Oat Bran	1	70	12	—	2
Fruit Jumbos Raisin Nut	1	70	10	—	1

FOOD	PORTION	CALS.	CARB.	SUG.	FIB.
Health Valley (CONT.)					
Fruit Jumbos Tropical Fruit	1	70	10	—	2
Graham Amaranth	7	110	25	—	3
Graham Honey	7	100	18	—	2
Graham Oat Bran	7	120	20	—	5
Honey Jumbos Crisp Cinnamon	1	70	9	—	1
Honey Jumbos Crisp Peanut Butter	1	70	11	—	1
Honey Jumbos Fancy Oat Bran	2	130	20	—	4
Oat Bran Animal Cookies	7	110	17	—	3
Oat Bran Fruit & Nut	2	110	17	—	3
The Great Tofu	2	90	14	—	4
The Great Wheat Free	2	80	14	—	3
Heyday					
Caramel & Peanut	1 (0.8 oz)	110	13	11	tr
Fudge	1 (0.8 oz)	110	13	11	tr
Honey Maid					
Cinnamon Grahams	10 (1.1 oz)	140	26	11	1
Honey Grahams	8 (1 oz)	120	22	7	1
Hydrox					
Original	3	150	21	11	1
Reduced Fat	3 (1.1 oz)	130	24	12	1
LU					
Chocolatiers	4 (1.1 oz)	170	20	10	2
Chocolatiers Dipped	3 (1 oz)	170	17	—	1
Le Petit Ecolier Dark Chocolate	2 (0.9 oz)	130	17	9	1
Little Schoolboy Milk Chocolate	2 (0.9 oz)	130	15	8	0
Marie Lu	3 (1.2 oz)	170	25	6	1
Truffle Lu	4 (1.2 oz)	180	18	15	1
La Choy					
Fortune	1	15	4	—	tr
Little Debbie					
Animal	1 pkg (1.5 oz)	190	33	8	0
Apple Flips	1 (1.2 oz)	150	24	13	tr
Caramel Cookie Bars	1 pkg (1.2 oz)	160	23	17	1
Chocolate Chip Chewy	1 pkg (2 oz)	370	47	25	1
Chocolate Chip Crisp	1 pkg (1.5 oz)	210	26	10	1
Cookie Wreaths	1 pkg (0.6 oz)	90	11	6	0
Creme Filled Chocolate	1 pkg (1.2 oz)	180	24	13	1
Creme Filled Chocolate	1 pkg (1.8 oz)	260	36	16	1

FOOD	PORTION	CALS.	CARB.	SUG.	FIB.
Little Debbie (CONT.)					
Easter Puffs	1 pkg (1.2 oz)	140	25	22	0
Figaroos	1 pkg (1.5 oz)	160	31	22	3
Figaroos	1 pkg (2 oz)	200	40	30	2
Fudge Macaroons	1 pkg (1 oz)	140	18	13	1
Ginger	1 pkg (0.7 oz)	90	14	7	1
Oatmeal Crisp	1 pkg (1.5 oz)	210	27	14	1
Oatmeal Lights	1 pkg (1.3 oz)	140	28	15	1
Oatmeal Raisin	1 pkg (2.7 oz)	320	50	29	2
Peanut Butter	1 pkg (1.5 oz)	210	27	15	1
Peanut Butter & Jelly Sandwich	1 pkg (1.1 oz)	130	22	14	1
Peanut Butter Bars	1 pkg (1.9 oz)	270	33	20	1
Peanut Clusters	1 pkg (1.4 oz)	190	23	17	1
Pecan Spinwheels	1 pkg (1 oz)	110	16	7	1
Pecan Shortbread	1 pkg (1.5 oz)	220	26	13	0
Lorna Doone					
Cookies	4 (1 oz)	140	19	6	tr
Mallomars					
Cookies	2 (0.9 oz)	120	17	13	1
Mallopuffs					
Cookies	1 (0.6 oz)	70	12	6	tr
Manischewitz					
Macaroons Chocolate	2 (0.9 oz)	90	15	6	4
Mother's					
Almond Shortbread	3	180	19	6	1
Butter	5	140	21	—	—
Checkerboard Wafers	8	150	20	10	1
Chocolate Chip	2	160	20	11	0
Chocolate Chip Angel	3	180	21	8	1
Chocolate Chip Bag	4	140	23	9	1
Chocolate Chip Parade	4	130	19	8	1
Circus Animals	6	140	20	12	0
Cocadas	5	150	20	6	2
Cookie Parade	4	140	18	9	2
Dinosaur Grrrahams	2	130	24	—	—
Double Fudge	3	170	22	11	2
Duplex Creme	3	170	23	12	1
English Tea	2	180	26	12	1
Fig Bar	2	130	24	11	0
Fig Bar Fat Free	1	70	16	9	1
Fig Bar Whole Wheat	2	130	20	12	3
Fig Bar Whole Wheat Fat Free	1	70	17	12	1

FOOD	PORTION	CALS.	CARB.	SUG.	FIB.
Mother's (CONT.)					
Flaky Flix Fudge	2	140	17	12	2
Flaky Flix Vanilla	2	140	17	14	1
Frosted Holiday	4	130	19	11	0
Fudge Bowl Crowns	2	140	21	12	1
Fudge Bowl Nuggets	2	140	21	12	1
Gaucho Peanut Butter	2	190	22	7	2
Gingerbread Man	6	140	21	7	1
Iced Oatmeal	2	120	20	10	1
Iced Oatmeal Bag	4	120	20	10	1
Iced Raisin	2	180	24	12	1
MLB Double Header Duplex	3	170	23	12	1
Macaroon	2	150	18	8	2
Marias	3	170	28	9	1
North Poles	2	140	17	15	0
Oatmeal	2	110	17	14	1
Oatmeal Chocolate Chip	2	120	19	9	1
Oatmeal Raisin	5	150	20	9	2
Oatmeal Walnut Chocolate Chip	2	130	17	9	1
Pecan Goldens	2	170	17	9	5
Rainbow Wafers	8	150	20	10	1
Striped Shortbread	3	170	22	8	1
Sugar	2	140	19	8	1
Taffy	2	180	25	11	2
Triplet Assortment	2	140	18	11	1
Vanilla Wafers	6	150	24	14	1
Walnut Fudge	2	130	16	7	1
Zoo Pals	14	140	23	6	1
Mystic Mint					
Cookies	1 (0.5 oz)	90	11	8	0
Nabisco					
Brown Edge Wafers	5 (1 oz)	140	21	10	tr
Bugs Bunny Chocolate Graham	13 (1.1 oz)	140	22	9	1
Bugs Bunny Cinnamon Graham	13 (1.1 oz)	140	23	8	tr
Bugs Bunny Graham	13 (1.1 oz)	140	23	7	1
Cameo	2 (1 oz)	130	21	10	tr
Chocolate Grahams	3 (1.1 oz)	160	21	12	1
Chocolate Chip Snaps	7 (1.1 oz)	150	24	10	tr
Chocolate Snaps	7 (1.1 oz)	140	23	9	1
Cookie Break	3 (1.1 oz)	160	23	11	tr
Danish Imported	5 (1.1 oz)	170	22	8	1

FOOD	PORTION	CALS.	CARB.	SUG.	FIB.
Nabisco (CONT.)					
Family Favorites Fudge Covered Grahams	3 (1 oz)	140	19	10	1
Family Favorites Fudge Striped Shortbread	3 (1.1 oz)	160	22	11	1
Family Favorites Oatmeal	1 (0.5 oz)	80	12	5	tr
Family Favorites Vanilla Sandwich	3 (1.2 oz)	170	25	12	0
Famous Chocolate Wafers	5 (1.1 oz)	140	24	11	1
Ginger Snaps Old Fashioned	4 (1 oz)	120	22	10	tr
Grahams	8 (1 oz)	120	22	7	1
Marshmallow Puffs	1 (0.75 oz)	90	14	11	0
Marshmallow Twirls	1 (1 oz)	130	20	15	tr
Nilla Wafers	8 (1.1 oz)	140	24	12	0
Pecan Passion	1 (0.5 oz)	90	9	3	0
Pinwheels	1 (1 oz)	130	21	16	tr
National					
Arrowroot	1 (5 g)	20	3	1	tr
Newman's Own					
Fig Newman's Organic	2 (1.3 oz)	120	28	15	1
Newtons					
Apple Fat Free	2 (1 oz)	100	24	14	1
Cranberry Fat Free	2 (1 oz)	100	23	15	1
Fig	2 (1.1 oz)	110	20	13	1
Fig Fat Free	1 (1 oz)	100	22	15	2
Raspberry Fat Free	2 (1 oz)	100	23	14	tr
Strawberry Fat Free	2 (1 oz)	100	23	16	tr
Nutra/Balance					
Chocolate Chip	1 (2 oz)	260	34	—	8
Oatmeal Raisin	1 (2 oz)	240	36	—	8
Nutter Butter					
Bites Peanut Butter Sandwich	10 (1.1 oz)	150	20	10	1
Peanut Butter Sandwich	2 (1 oz)	130	19	8	1
Peanut Creme Patties	5 (1.1 oz)	160	17	8	1
Oreo					
Cookies	3 (1.2 oz)	160	23	13	1
Double Stuf	2 (1 oz)	140	19	12	tr
Fudge Covered	1 (0.75 oz)	110	14	10	tr
Halloween Treats	2 (1 oz)	140	19	13	1
Reduced Fat	3 (1.2 oz)	140	24	13	1
White Fudge Covered	1 (0.75 oz)	110	14	10	tr

FOOD	PORTION	CALS.	CARB.	SUG.	FIB.
Pally					
Butter	4 (0.88 oz)	100	17	5	—
Pepperidge Farm					
Beacon Hill Chocolate Chocolate Walnut	1	120	14	—	1
Blondie Chocolate Chip Fat Free	1 (1.4 oz)	120	29	21	tr
Bordeaux	2	70	11	—	0
Brussels	2	110	13	—	0
Cheasapeake Chocolate Chunk Pecan	1	120	14	—	1
Cheyenne Peanut Butter Milk Chocolate Chunk	1	110	13	—	1
Chocolate Chip	2	100	12	—	0
Dakota Milk Chocolate Oatmeal	1	110	15	—	1
Nantucket Chocolate Chunk	1	120	15	—	1
Old Fashioned Chocolate Chip	2	100	12	—	0
Ripple Milk Chocolate Fat Free	1 (0.6 oz)	60	13	7	tr
Sante Fe Oatmeal Raisin	1	100	16	—	1
Sausalito Milk Chocolate Macadamia	1	120	14	—	0
Ritz					
Chocolate Covered	3 (1 oz)	150	17	9	1
Sargento					
MooTown Snackers Cookies & Creme Honey Graham Sticks & Vanilla Creme w/Sprinkle	1 pkg (1.1 oz)	140	19	11	0
MooTown Snackers Cookies & Creme Vanilla Sticks & Chocolate Fudge Creme	1 pkg (1.1 oz)	140	20	12	0
SnackWell's					
Fat Free Double Fudge	1 (0.5 oz)	50	12	6	tr
Golden Devil's Food	1 (0.5 oz)	50	12	8	0
Reduced Fat Chocolate Chip	13 (1 oz)	130	22	10	1
Reduced Fat Chocolate Sandwich With Chocolate Creme	2 (0.9 oz)	100	20	11	1
Reduced Fat Oatmeal Raisin	2 (1 oz)	110	20	10	1

FOOD	PORTION	CALS.	CARB.	SUG.	FIB.
SnackWell's (CONT.)					
Reduced Fat Vanilla Sandwich	2 (0.9 oz)	110	21	10	1
Social Tea					
Cookies	6 (1 oz)	120	20	7	tr
Stella D'Oro					
Egg Jumbo	1	u0	9	—	—
Indulgente Cashew Biscottini	1 (1.1 oz)	150	19	8	tr
Sunshine					
Almond Crescents	4 (1.1 oz)	150	22	10	tr
Animal Crackers	1 box (2 oz)	260	43	13	1
Animal Crackers	14 (1.1 oz)	140	24	7	tr
Classics Chocolate Chip With Pecans	1 (0.7 oz)	110	11	5	tr
Classics Chocolate Chip With Walnuts	1 (0.7 oz)	100	11	6	1
Classics Premier Chocolate Chip	1 (0.7 oz)	100	13	7	tr
Dixie Vanilla	2 (0.9 oz)	120	19	6	tr
Fig Bars	2 (1 oz)	110	20	11	1
Fudge Family Bears Vanilla	2 (1 oz)	140	20	10	tr
Fudge Mint Patties	2 (0.8 oz)	130	16	10	tr
Fudge Striped Shortbread	3 (1.1 oz)	160	20	9	1
Ginger Snaps	7 (1 oz)	130	22	9	tr
Grahams Cinnamon	2 (1.1 oz)	140	22	8	tr
Grahams Fudge Dipped	4 (1.2 oz)	170	21	11	1
Grahams Honey	2 (1 oz)	120	20	6	1
Grahamy Bears	1 pkg (2 oz)	260	41	11	2
Grahamy Bears	10 (1.1 oz)	140	22	6	1
Iced Gingerbread	5 (1 oz)	130	19	6	tr
Iced Oatmeal	2 (0.9 oz)	120	18	9	tr
Jingles	6 (1.1 oz)	150	22	9	tr
Lemon Coolers	5 (1 oz)	140	21	10	tr
Mini Chocolate Chip Cookies	5 (1.1 oz)	160	20	8	tr
Mini Fudge Royals	15 (1.1 oz)	160	20	8	1
Oatmeal Chocolate Chip	3 (1.3 oz)	170	23	11	2
Oatmeal Country Style	3 (1.2 oz)	170	24	10	1
School House Cookies	20 (1.1 oz)	140	23	7	tr
Sugar Wafers Chocolate	3 (0.9 oz)	130	17	11	tr
Sugar Wafers Peanut Butter	4 (1.1 oz)	170	19	10	1
Sugar Wafers Vanilla	3 (0.9 oz)	130	18	13	tr
Tru Blu Chocolate	1 (0.6 oz)	80	11	4	tr

FOOD	PORTION	CALS.	CARB.	SUG.	FIB.
Sunshine (CONT.)					
Tru Blu Lemon	1 (0.6 oz)	80	11	4	tr
Tru Blu Vanilla	1 (0.5 oz)	80	11	4	tr
Vanilla Wafers	7 (1.1 oz)	150	20	10	tr
Vienna Fingers	2 (1 oz)	140	21	8	tr
Tastykake					
Chocolate Chip Bar	1 (43 g)	190	28	—	1
Chocolate Chunk Macadamia Nut	1 pkg (56 g)	310	42	—	2
Fudge Bar	1 (50 g)	200	35	—	1
Oatmeal Raisin Bar	1 (50 g)	210	32	—	1
Soft'N Chewy Chocolate Chip	1 (39 g)	170	25	—	1
Soft'n Chewy Chocolate Chocolate Chip	1 (32 g)	170	26	—	1
Soft'n Chewy Oatmeal Raisin	1 (39 g)	160	27	—	1
Vanilla Sugar Wafer	1 (6 g)	36	4	—	0
Teddy Grahams					
Chocolate	24 (1 oz)	140	22	9	1
Cinnamon	24 (1 oz)	140	23	8	1
Honey	24 (1 oz)	140	22	8	1
Tree Of Life					
Creme Supremes	2 (0.9 oz)	120	18	10	1
Creme Supremes Mint	2 (0.9 oz)	120	18	10	1
Fat Free Classic Carrot Cake	1 (0.8 oz)	60	14	6	1
Fat Free Devil's Food Chocolate	1 (0.8 oz)	70	15	7	1
Fat Free Golden Oatmeal Raisin	1 (0.8 oz)	70	16	7	1
Fat Free Harvest Fruit & Nut	1 (0.8 oz)	70	16	7	1
Fat Free Toasted Almond Butter	1 (0.8 oz)	70	16	7	1
Fruit Bars Apple Spice	2 (1.3 oz)	120	22	9	2
Fruit Bars Fat Free Fig	1 (0.8 oz)	70	16	11	2
Fruit Bars Fat Free Peach Apricot	1 (0.8 oz)	70	17	9	1
Fruit Bars Fat Free Wildberry	1 (0.8 oz)	70	16	7	2
Fruit Bars Fig	2 (1.3 oz)	120	21	10	3
Fruit Bars Peach Apricot	2 (1.3 oz)	120	22	11	2
Honey-Sweet Colossal Carrot Cake	1 (0.8 oz)	110	16	5	1
Honey-Sweet Lemon Burst	1 (0.8 oz)	110	15	5	1

FOOD	PORTION	CALS.	CARB.	SUG.	FIB.
Tree Of Life (CONT.)					
Honey-Sweet Oh-So-Oatmeal	1 (0.8 oz)	110	14	4	1
Honey-Sweet Pecans-A-Plenty	1 (0.8 oz)	125	14	4	1
Monster Fat Free Carrot Cake	¼ cookie (0.9 oz)	60	15	10	1
Monster Fat Free Devil's Food Chocolate	¼ cookie (0.9 oz)	80	20	12	2
Monster Fat Free Gingerbread	¼ cookie (0.9 oz)	80	19	9	2
Monster Fat Free Maple Pecan	¼ cookie (0.9 oz)	90	20	10	2
Royal Vanilla	2 (0.9 oz)	120	17	10	0
Small World Animal Grahams	7 (1 oz)	120	21	6	3
Small World Chocolate Chip	7 (1 oz)	120	20	6	3
Soft-Bake Chocolate Chip	1 (0.8 oz)	125	15	5	1
Soft-Bake Double Fudge	1 (0.8 oz)	110	16	5	2
Soft-Bake Maui Macaroon	1 (0.8 oz)	135	12	4	2
Soft-Bake Oatmeal	1 (0.8 oz)	115	16	5	2
Soft-Bake Peanut Butter	1 (0.8 oz)	125	13	4	1
Wheat-Free American Oatmeal	1 (0.8 oz)	90	11	3	1
Wheat-Free California Carob	1 (0.8 oz)	105	14	4	6
Wheat-Free Georgia Peanut Butter	1 (0.8 oz)	95	8	3	1
Wheat-Free Mountain Maple Walnut	1 (0.8 oz)	100	9	4	6
Vienna Fingers					
Low Fat	2 (1 oz)	130	23	10	tr
Walkers					
Shortbread Triangles	2 (0.7 oz)	100	12	4	0
Weight Watchers					
Apple Raisin Bar	1 (0.75 oz)	70	14	4	2
Chocolate Chip	2 (1.06 oz)	140	22	15	1
Chocolate Sandwich	2 (1.06)	140	23	16	1
Fruit Filled Fig	1 (0.7 oz)	70	16	9	0
Fruit Filled Raspberry	1 (0.7 oz)	70	16	7	0
Oatmeal Raisin	2 (1.06 oz)	120	22	13	1

FOOD	PORTION	CALS.	CARB.	SUG.	FIB.
Weight Watchers (CONT.)					
Vanilla Sandwich	2 (1.06 oz)	140	25	10	1

CORN

(*see also* BRAN, CEREAL, CORNMEAL)

CANNED

FOOD	PORTION	CALS.	CARB.	SUG.	FIB.
yellow	½ cup	66	15	—	1
Del Monte					
Cream Style Golden	½ cup (4.4 oz)	90	20	5	2
Cream Style Golden 50% Less Salt	½ cup (4.4 oz)	90	20	5	2
Cream Style Golden No Salt Added	½ cup (4.4 oz)	90	20	5	2
Cream Style Supersweet Golden	½ cup (4.4 oz)	60	14	7	2
Cream Style White	½ cup (4.4 oz)	100	21	6	2
Whole Kernel Golden	½ cup (4.4 oz)	90	18	6	3
Whole Kernel Golden Supersweet 50% Less Salt	½ cup (4.4 oz)	60	11	6	3
Whole Kernel Golden Supersweet No Salt Added	½ cup (4.4 oz)	60	11	7	3
Whole Kernel Golden Supersweet No Sugar	½ cup (4.4 oz)	60	11	7	3
Whole Kernel Golden Supersweet Vacuum Packed	½ cup (3.7 oz)	70	13	4	3
Whole Kernel Golden Supersweet Vacuum Packed No Salt Added	½ cup (3.7 oz)	70	13	4	3
Whole Kernel White Sweet	½ cup (4.4 oz)	80	17	7	2
Green Giant					
Cream Style	½ cup (4.5 oz)	100	22	11	1
Mexicorn	⅓ cup (2.7 oz)	60	14	4	2
Niblets	⅓ cup (2.7 oz)	70	15	4	2
Niblets 50% Less Sodium	⅓ cup (2.7 oz)	60	14	3	1
Niblets Extra Sweet	⅓ cup (2.6 oz)	50	10	4	2
Niblets No Added Sugar or Salt	⅓ cup (2.7 oz)	60	13	3	2
White Shoepeg	⅓ cup	80	16	3	1
Whole Sweet	½ cup (4.3 oz)	80	18	6	2
Whole Sweet 50% Less Sodium	½ cup (4.2 oz)	80	17	4	2

FOOD	PORTION	CALS.	CARB.	SUG.	FIB.
Ka-Me					
Baby	½ cup (4.5 oz)	20	3	3	2
Stir Fry	½ cup (4.5 oz)	20	3	3	2
Seneca					
Cream Style	½ cup	80	18	—	1
Whole Kernel	½ cup	90	21	—	2
Whole Kernel Natural Pack	½ cup	80	18	—	2
DRIED					
Goya					
Giant White	⅓ cup (1.6 oz)	160	35	1	4
FROZEN					
Birds Eye					
Baby Corn Blend	⅔ cup (2.9 oz)	60	11	2	2
Baby Gold & White	⅔ cup (3.3 oz)	80	15	6	2
In Butter Sauce	½ cup (4.6 oz)	110	23	5	2
Fresh Like					
Cob Corn	1 ear (3 in)	96	24	—	1
Cob Corn	1 ear (5 in)	96	23	—	1
Cut	3.5 oz	85	21	—	1
Green Giant					
Butter Sauce Niblets	⅔ cup (4.3 oz)	130	23	5	3
Butter Sauce Shoepeg White	¾ cup (4 oz)	120	21	5	3
Cream Corn	½ cup (4.1 oz)	110	23	6	2
Extra Sweet Niblets	⅔ cup (3.1 oz)	70	13	6	2
Harvest Fresh Niblets	⅔ cup (3.4 oz)	80	17	3	3
Harvest Fresh Shoepeg White	½ cup (2.6 oz)	70	14	3	2
Niblets	⅔ cup (2.9 oz)	80	17	3	2
On The Cob Extra Sweet	1 ear (4.4 oz)	120	22	13	3
On The Cob Nibblers	1 ear (2.1 oz)	70	14	2	1
On The Cob Niblets	1 ear (5 oz)	160	32	6	3
Select Extra Sweet White	⅔ cup (2.9 oz)	50	10	3	3
Select Shoepeg White	¾ cup (3.2 oz)	100	20	2	3
Ore Ida					
Cob Corn	1 ear (6.1 oz)	180	33	5	4
Cob Corn Mini-Gold	1 ear (3.1 oz)	90	16	2	2
Stouffer's					
Souffle	½ cup (6 oz)	170	21	7	1
Tree Of Life					
Corn	⅔ cup (3.2 oz)	80	19	5	1
SHELF-STABLE					
Pantry Express					
Golden Whole Kernel	½ cup	60	18	—	1

FOOD	PORTION	CALS.	CARB.	SUG.	FIB.
CORN CHIPS					
(*see* CHIPS)					
CORNISH HENS					
(*see* CHICKEN)					
CORNMEAL					
white	1 cup (4.8 oz)	505	107	—	10
whole grain	1 cup (4.3 oz)	442	94	—	9
yellow	1 cup (4.8 oz)	505	107	—	10
yellow self-rising	1 cup (4.3 oz)	407	86	—	8
Albers					
White	3 tbsp	110	34	—	tr
Yellow	3 tbsp	110	34	—	tr
Arrowhead					
Yellow	¼ cup (1.2 oz)	120	27	0	3
Aunt Jemima					
White	3 tbsp	102	22	—	1
Yellow	3 tbsp	102	22	—	1
Quaker					
White	3 tbsp	102	22	—	1
Yellow	3 tbsp	102	22	—	1
MIX					
Arrowhead					
Corn Bread	¼ cup (1.2 oz)	120	24	3	4
Aunt Jemima					
Self Rising White Mix	3 tbsp	98	21	—	1
Hodgson Mill					
Yellow	¼ cup (1 oz)	100	22	0	3
Yellow Self Rising	¼ cup (1 oz)	90	21	0	3
Kentucky Kernal					
White Corn Meal Mix	¼ cup (1 oz)	100	22	0	2
Miracle Maize					
Complete as prep	1 piece (1.5 oz)	193	34	—	2
Country Style as prep	1 piece 2 in x 2 in (1.8 oz)	230	38	—	2
Sweet as prep	1 piece 2 in x 2 in (1.8 oz)	236	41	—	1
Stone-Buhr					
Yellow Corn Meal	¼ cup (1 oz)	100	23	0	1
READY-TO-EAT					
Aurora					
Polenta	½ cup (5 oz)	110	24	2	1
CORNSTARCH					
cornstarch	1 cup (4.5 oz)	488	117	—	1

FOOD	PORTION	CALS.	CARB.	SUG.	FIB.

COTTAGE CHEESE

Axelrod

Nonfat	½ cup (4.4 oz)	90	7	5	0

Breakstone's

2% Fat Large Curd	½ cup (4.2 oz)	90	4	3	0
2% Fat Small Curd	½ cup (4.2 oz)	90	4	3	0
4% Fat Large Curd	½ cup (4.2 oz)	120	5	4	0
4% Fat Small Curd	½ cup (4.2 oz)	120	5	4	0
Dry Curd	¼ cup (1.9 oz)	45	3	3	0
Free	½ cup (4.4 oz)	80	6	5	0
Snack 2% Fat Small Curd	1 pkg (4 oz)	90	4	3	0
Snack 4% Fat Small Curd	1 pkg (4 oz)	110	4	4	0
Snack Free	1 pkg (4 oz)	70	6	4	0

Friendship

California Style	½ cup (4 oz)	115	4	4	0
Lowfat No Salt Added	½ cup (4 oz)	90	4	4	0
Lowfat Pineapple	½ cup (4 oz)	120	17	15	0
Lowfat 1%	½ cup (4 oz)	90	4	4	0
Nonfat	½ cup (4 oz)	80	5	5	0
Nonfat Plus Peach	½ cup (4 oz)	110	15	14	0
Pot Style	½ cup (4 oz)	90	3	3	0
With Pineapple	½ cup (4 oz)	140	15	14	0

Hood

1% Fat	½ cup (4 oz)	90	6	5	0
1% Fat Chive & Onion	½ cup (4 oz)	90	6	5	0
1% Fat No Salt Added	½ cup (4 oz)	90	6	5	0
1% Fat Pepper & Herb	½ cup (4 oz)	90	6	5	0
1% Fat Pineapple Cherry	½ cup (4 oz)	110	15	12	0
4% Fat	½ cup (4 oz)	120	5	4	0
4% Fat Chive	½ cup (4 oz)	130	5	4	0
4% Fat Pineapple	½ cup (4 oz)	130	15	13	0
Nonfat	½ cup (4 oz)	80	6	5	0
Nonfat Pineapple	½ cup (4 oz)	110	16	13	0

Knudsen

1.5% Fat Small Curd Pineapple	½ cup (4.6 oz)	120	14	12	0
2% Fat Small Curd	½ cup (4.2 oz)	100	5	4	0
4% Fat Large Curd	½ cup (4.5 oz)	130	4	3	0
4% Fat Small Curd	½ cup (4.3 oz)	120	4	3	0
Free	½ cup (4.2 oz)	80	4	3	0
On The Go! 1.5% Fat Peach	1 pkg (4 oz)	110	13	12	0
On The Go! 1.5% Fat Pineapple	1 pkg (4 oz)	110	13	11	0

FOOD	PORTION	CALS.	CARB.	SUG.	FIB.
Knudsen (CONT.)					
On The Go! 1.5% Fat Strawberry	1 pkg (4 oz)	110	13	11	0
On The Go! 1.5% Fat Tropical Fruit	1 pkg (4 oz)	110	13	11	0
On The Go! 2% Fat	1 pkg (4 oz)	90	5	3	0
On The Go! Free	1 pkg (4 oz)	70	4	3	0
Light N'Lively					
1% Fat	½ cup (4 oz)	80	5	4	0
1% Fat Garden Salad	½ cup (4.2 oz)	80	5	5	0
1% Fat Peach & Pineapple	½ cup (4.3 oz)	110	15	14	0
Fat Free	½ cup (4.4 oz)	80	6	4	0
Weight Watchers					
1%	½ cup	90	4	4	0
2%	½ cup	90	4	4	0

COUGH DROPS
Lifesavers

Menthol	2 (0.5 oz)	60	14	14	—

COUSCOUS

cooked	1 cup (5.5 oz)	176	36	—	2
dry	1 cup (6.1 oz)	650	134	—	9
Casbah					
Almond Chicken Vegetarian	1 pkg (1.5 oz)	160	29	0	tr
Asparagus Au Gratin Organic	1 pkg (1.5 oz)	150	28	0	1
Cheddar Broccoli	1 pkg (1.3 oz)	130	23	0	tr
Hearty Harvest Zestful Organic as prep	1 pkg (10 fl oz)	180	36	—	2
Moroccan Stew	1 pkg (2 oz)	180	36	6	1
Pilaf as prep	1 cup	200	40	0	tr
Tomato Parmesan	1 pkg (1.8 oz)	170	34	5	2
Kitchen Del Sol					
Aegean Citrus as prep	½ cup (1.1 oz)	110	20	1	1
Moroccan Ginger as prep	½ cup (1.1 oz)	120	21	2	1
Spicy Vegetable as prep	½ cup (1.1 oz)	120	20	1	1
Tomato & Olive	½ cup (1 oz)	120	19	1	1
Tomato & Olive	½ cup (1.1 oz)	120	19	1	1
Melting Pot					
Calypso Cranberry	1 cup	200	42	6	1
Lentil Curry	1 cup	170	35	3	1
Lucky Seven	1 cup	190	38	5	1
Mango Salsa	1 cup	190	40	6	1
Roasted Garlic	1 cup	170	34	3	1

FOOD	PORTION	CALS.	CARB.	SUG.	FIB.
Melting Pot (CONT.)					
Sesame Ginger	1 cup	180	36	5	0
Sun-Dried Tomatoes	1 cup	190	36	3	1
Wild Mushroom	1 cup	190	38	3	1
Near East					
As Prep	1¼ cup	260	46	1	2

CRAB
CANNED

blue	1 cup	133	0	0	0
blue	3 oz	84	0	0	0
FRESH					
alaska king cooked	3 oz	82	0	0	0
alaska king cooked	1 leg (4.7 oz)	129	0	0	0
blue cooked	3 oz	87	0	0	0
blue cooked	1 cup	138	0	0	0
queen steamed	3 oz	98	0	0	0

CRACKER CRUMBS

graham cracker crumbs	½ cup (4.4 oz)	540	97	—	3
Honey Maid					
Graham Cracker	0.5 oz	70	13	4	tr
Kellogg's					
Corn Flake Crumbs	2 tbsp (0.4 oz)	40	9	1	0
Nabisco					
Nilla Cookie Crumbs	2 tbsp (0.5 oz)	70	13	7	tr
Oreo					
Cookie Crumbs	2 tbsp (0.5 oz)	80	13	5	1
Premium					
Fat Free Cracker Crumbs	¼ cup (1 oz)	100	23	tr	1
Ritz					
Cracker Crumbs	⅓ cup (1 oz)	140	17	2	1
Sunshine					
Graham	3 tbsp (0.6 oz)	80	13	2	tr

CRACKERS
(*see also* CRACKER CRUMBS)

cheese w/ peanut butter filling	1 (0.24 oz)	34	4	—	tr
crispbread	3	61	9	—	1
crispbread rye	1 (0.35 oz)	37	8	—	2
crispbread rye	3	77	17	—	3
melba toast plain	1 (5 g)	19	4	—	tr
melba toast pumpernickel	1 (5 g)	19	4	—	tr
melba toast rye	1 (5 g)	19	4	—	tr
melba toast wheat	1 (5 g)	19	4	—	tr

FOOD	PORTION	CALS.	CARB.	SUG.	FIB.
oyster cracker	1 (1 g)	4	1	—	tr
saltines	1 (3 g)	13	2	—	tr
saltines low salt	1 (3 g)	13	2	—	tr
snack cracker	1 (3 g)	15	2	—	tr
snack cracker low salt	1 (3 g)	15	2	—	tr
soup cracker	1 (1 g)	4	1	—	tr
water biscuits	3	92	16	—	1
wheat thins	7 (0.5 oz)	67	9	—	1
wheat thins low salt	7 (0.5 oz)	67	9	—	1
zwieback	3½ oz	374	73	—	4
Adrienne's					
Gourmet Flatbread Ten Grain	2	20	3	—	1
Ak-mak					
100% Whole Wheat	5 (1 oz)	116	19	2	4
Armenian Cracker Bread	1 sheet (1 oz)	100	19	2	2
Armenian Cracker Bread Whole Wheat	1 sheet (1 oz)	116	19	2	4
Round Cracker Bread No Seeds	1 (1 oz)	100	20	2	1
Round Cracker Bread Seeded	1 (1 oz)	100	19	2	2
Round Cracker Bread Whole Wheat	1 (1 oz)	116	19	2	4
American Heritage					
Sesame	9 (1.1 oz)	160	17	1	1
Wheat & Bran	9 (1 oz)	140	17	2	2
Barbara's					
Cheese Bites	26 (1 oz)	120	24	0	1
French Onion	3	60	12	tr	tr
Rite Lite Rounds	5 (0.5 oz)	55	12	1	0
Roasted Garlic & Herb	3	60	12	tr	tr
Sundried Tomato & Basil	3	60	12	tr	tr
Toasted Sesame	3	60	11	tr	tr
Wheatines All Flavors	1 lg sq (0.5 oz)	50	10	tr	1
Better Cheddars					
Crackers	22 (1 oz)	70	17	tr	tr
Low Sodium	22 (1 oz)	150	18	0	tr
Reduced Fat	24 (1 oz)	140	19	tr	tr
Burns & Ricker					
Bagel Crisps Garlic	5 (1 oz)	100	22	1	1
Cheez-It					
Crackers	27 (1 oz)	160	16	tr	tr
Crackers	1 pkg (1.5 oz)	220	23	tr	1

FOOD	PORTION	CALS.	CARB.	SUG.	FIB.
Cheez-It (CONT.)					
Crackers	1 pkg (2 oz)	290	31	tr	2
Hot & Spicy	26 (1 oz)	160	17	tr	1
Hot & Spicy	1 pkg (1.5 oz)	220	25	1	1
Low Sodium	27 (1 oz)	160	16	tr	tr
Party Mix	½ cup (1 oz)	140	19	1	1
Reduced Fat	30 (1 oz)	130	19	tr	tr
White Cheddar	1 pkg (1.5 oz)	220	24	1	tr
White Cheddar	26 (1 oz)	160	17	tr	tr
Crown Pilot					
Crackers	1 (0.5 oz)	70	13	0	tr
Devonsheer					
Melba Rounds Garlic	½ oz	56	9	—	1
Melba Rounds Honey Bran	½ oz	52	9	—	1
Melba Rounds Onion	½ oz	51	10	—	1
Melba Rounds Plain	½ oz	53	10	—	1
Melba Rounds Plain Unsalted	½ oz	52	10	—	1
Melba Rounds Rye	½ oz	53	10	—	1
Melba Rounds Sesame	½ oz	57	8	—	1
Eden					
Brown Rice	5 (1 oz)	120	22	tr	2
Estee					
Unsalted	1 (0.5 oz)	70	10	0	0
Harvest Crisps					
5 Grain	13 (1.1 oz)	130	23	4	1
Oat	13 (1.1 oz)	140	22	3	1
Health Valley					
Herb Stoned Wheat	13	55	9	—	2
Herb Stoned Wheat No Salt	13	55	9	—	2
Rice Bran	7	130	19	—	2
Sesame Stoned Wheat	13	55	9	—	2
Sesame Stoned Wheat No Salt Added	13	55	9	—	2
Seven Grain Vegetable Stoned Wheat	13	55	9	—	2
Seven Grain Vegetable Stoned Wheat No Salt Added	13	55	9	—	2
Stoned Wheat	13	55	9	—	2
Stoned Wheat No Salt Added	13	55	9	—	2
Healthy Choice					
Bread Crisps Garlic Herb	11 (1 oz)	110	22	3	2

FOOD	PORTION	CALS.	CARB.	SUG.	FIB.
Hi Ho					
Butter Flavored	9 (1.1 oz)	160	19	2	tr
Cracked Pepper	9 (1.1 oz)	160	18	2	tr
Crackers	9	160	18	2	tr
Low Salt	9 (1.1 oz)	160	18	2	tr
Multi Grain	9 (1.1 oz)	160	18	2	1
Reduced Fat	10 (1.1 oz)	140	21	3	tr
Whole Wheat	9 (1.1 oz)	150	18	2	2
J.J. Flats					
Breadflats Caraway	1	52	10	—	1
Breadflats Caraway And Salt	1	51	9	—	1
Breadflats Cinnamon	1	53	10	—	1
Breadflats Flavorall	1	52	10	—	1
Breadflats Garlic	1	52	10	—	1
Breadflats Oat Bran	1	49	8	—	2
Breadflats Onion	1	53	10	—	1
Breadflats Plain	1	53	10	—	1
Breadflats Poppy	1	53	9	—	1
Breadflats Sesame	1	55	9	—	1
Kavli					
Crackers	1 piece	40	10	—	2
Krispy					
Cracked Pepper	5 (0.5 oz)	60	10	tr	tr
Fat Free	5 (0.5 oz)	60	12	0	tr
Mild Cheddar	5 (0.5 oz)	60	10	0	tr
Original	5 (0.5 oz)	60	10	tr	tr
Soup & Oyster Crackers	17 (0.5 oz)	60	11	tr	tr
Unsalted Tops	5 (0.5 oz)	60	10	tr	tr
Whole Wheat	5 (0.5 oz)	60	10	tr	tr
Little Debbie					
Cheese Crackers With Peanut Butter	1 pkg (1.4 oz)	210	23	5	1
Cheese Crackers With Peanut Butter	1 pkg (0.9 oz)	140	16	4	1
Toasty Crackers With Peanut Butter	1 pkg (0.9 oz)	140	16	3	1
Toasty Crackers With Peanut Butter	1 pkg (1.4 oz)	200	20	3	1
Wheat Crackers With Cheddar Cheese	1 pkg (0.9 oz)	140	16	2	0
NABS					
Cheese Peanut Butter Sandwich	6 (1.4 oz)	190	24	3	1

FOOD	PORTION	CALS.	CARB.	SUG.	FIB.
NABS (CONT.)					
Peanut Butter Toast Sandwich	6 (1.4 oz)	190	24	4	1
Nabisco					
Bacon Flavored	15 (1.1 oz)	160	19	2	tr
Chicken In A Biskit	14 (1 oz)	160	17	2	tr
Garden Crisps	15 (1 oz)	130	22	4	1
Oat Thins	18 (1 oz)	140	20	2	2
Royal Lunch	1 (0.4 oz)	50	8	tr	0
Swiss	15 (1 oz)	140	18	2	tr
Tid-Bit Cheese	32 (1 oz)	150	17	tr	tr
Vegetable Thins	14 (1.1 oz)	160	19	2	1
Wheat Thins Original	16 (1 oz)	140	19	2	2
Wheat Thins Reduced Fat	18 (1 oz)	120	21	3	2
Zings!	1 pkg (1.8 oz)	240	34	2	2
Nips					
Cheese	29 (1 oz)	150	18	0	tr
Old London					
Melba Toast Pumpernickel	½ oz	54	10	—	1
Melba Toast Sesame	½ oz	55	8	—	1
Melba Toast Sesame Unsalted	½ oz	55	8	—	1
Melba Toast Wheat	½ oz	51	10	—	1
Melba Toast White	½ oz	51	10	—	1
Melba Toast White Unsalted	½ oz	51	10	—	1
Melba Toast Whole Grain	½ oz	52	9	—	1
Melba Toast Whole Grain Unsalted	½ oz	53	10	—	1
Rounds Bacon	½ oz	53	9	—	1
Rounds Garlic	½ oz	56	9	—	1
Rounds Onion	½ oz	52	10	—	1
Rounds Sesame	½ oz	56	8	—	1
Rounds White	½ oz	48	9	—	1
Rounds Whole Grain	½ oz	54	9	—	1
Oysterettes					
Crackers	19 (0.5 oz)	60	10	0	tr
Partners					
Walla Walla Sweet Onion Perservative Free	0.5 oz	65	8	2	tr
Pepperidge Farm					
Butter Thins	4	70	10	—	0
Cracked Wheat	3	100	14	—	1
English Water Biscuits	4	70	13	—	0
Goldfish Cheddar Cheese	1 pkg (1½ oz)	190	28	—	1

FOOD	PORTION	CALS.	CARB.	SUG.	FIB.
Pepperidge Farm (CONT.)					
Goldfish Cheddar Cheese	1 oz	120	19	—	1
Goldfish Original	1 oz	130	18	—	1
Goldfish Parmesan Cheese	1 oz	120	19	—	1
Goldfish Pizza Flavored	1 oz	130	19	—	1
Goldfish Pretzel	1 oz	110	20	—	1
Hearty Wheat	4	100	13	—	1
Sesame	4	80	12	—	2
Snack Mix Classic	1 oz	140	14	—	1
Snack Mix Lightly Smoked	1 oz	150	13	—	1
Snack Sticks Cheese	8	130	19	—	1
Snack Sticks Pretzel	8	120	23	—	1
Snack Sticks Pumpernickel	8	140	20	—	1
Snack Sticks Sesame	8	140	19	—	1
Spicy Lightly Smoked	1 oz	140	14	—	1
Toasted Wheat With Onion	4	80	12	—	0
Planters					
Cheese Peanut Butter Sandwiches	1 pkg (1.4 oz)	190	24	3	1
Toast Peanut Butter Sandwiches	1 pkg (1.4 oz)	190	24	4	1
Premium					
Saltine Bits	34 (1 oz)	150	19	0	tr
Saltine Fat Free	5 (0.5 oz)	50	11	0	0
Saltine Low Sodium	5 (0.5 oz)	60	10	0	tr
Saltine Original	5 (0.5 oz)	60	10	0	tr
Saltine Unsalted Tops	5 (0.5 oz)	60	10	0	tr
Soup & Oyster	23 (0.5 oz)	60	11	0	tr
Ralston					
Oat Bran Krisp	2	60	6	—	3
Ritz					
Bits	48 (1 oz)	160	18	3	1
Bits Sandwiches With Peanut Butter	13 (1 oz)	150	17	3	1
Bits Sandwiches With Real Cheese	14 (1.1 oz)	160	17	4	1
Crackers	5 (0.5 oz)	80	10	1	tr
Low Sodium	5 (0.5 oz)	80	10	1	tr
Sandwiches With Real Cheese	1 pkg (1.4 oz)	210	21	4	1
Rykrisp					
Natural	2	40	7	—	4
Seasoned	2	45	8	—	3
Seasoned Twindividuals	2	45	8	—	3

FOOD	PORTION	CALS.	CARB.	SUG.	FIB.
Rykrisp (CONT.)					
Sesame	2	50	7	—	3
Savory Thins					
Toasted Onion & Garlic	15 (1 oz)	110	23	2	2
Sesmark					
Brown Rice	15 (1 oz)	120	25	0	tr
Cheese Thins	15 (1 oz)	130	26	0	tr
Rice Thins Original	15 (1 oz)	130	24	0	tr
Rice Thins Teriyaki Flavored	13 (1 oz)	130	24	0	tr
Savory Thins Original	15 (1 oz)	125	25	tr	1
Sesame Thins Cheddar	9 (1 oz)	150	15	tr	3
Sesame Thins Garlic	9 (1 oz)	150	16	tr	3
Sesame Thins Original	9 (1 oz)	150	16	1	2
Sesame Thins Unsalted	11 (1 oz)	150	17	tr	3
SnackWell's					
Cracked Pepper	7 (0.5 oz)	60	13	1	tr
Fat Free Wheat	5 (0.5 oz)	60	12	2	1
Reduced Fat Cheese	38 (1 oz)	130	23	0	1
Reduced Fat Classic Golden	6 (0.5 oz)	60	11	2	0
Salsa Cheddar	32 (1 oz)	120	23	2	1
Snorkles					
Cheddar	56 (1 oz)	140	19	0	1
Sociables					
Crackers	7 (0.5 oz)	80	9	tr	tr
Sunshine					
Saltines Cracked Pepper	5 (0.5 oz)	60	10	tr	tr
Tree Of Life					
Bite Size Fat Free Corn & Salsa	12	60	12	0	0
Bite Size Fat Free Cracked Pepper	12	55	12	1	0
Bite Size Fat Free Garden Vegetable	12	55	12	1	0
Bite Size Fat Free Garlic & Herb	12	55	12	1	0
Bite Size Fat Free Soya Nut	12	60	12	0	0
Bite Size Fat Free Toasted Onion	12	60	12	1	0
Bite Size Fat Free Whole Wheat	12	60	12	1	2
Fat Free Oyster	40 (0.5 oz)	60	13	0	0
Saltine Cracked Pepper Fat Free	4 (0.5 oz)	60	13	0	1
Saltine Fat Free	4 (0.5 oz)	50	11	0	0

FOOD	PORTION	CALS.	CARB.	SUG.	FIB.
Triscuit					
Crackers	7 (1.1 oz)	140	21	0	4
Deli-Style Rye	7 (1.1 oz)	140	22	0	4
Garden Herb	6 (1 oz)	130	20	tr	3
Low Sodium	7 (1.1 oz)	150	21	0	3
Reduced Fat	8 (1.1 oz)	130	24	0	4
Wheat 'n Bran	7 (1.1 oz)	140	22	0	4
Twigs					
Sesame & Cheese Sticks	15 (1 oz)	150	17	1	tr
Uneeda Biscuit					
Unsalted Tops	2 (0.5 oz)	60	11	0	tr
Venus					
Armenian Thin Bread	2 (0.9 oz)	100	19	—	—
Bran Wafers Salt Free	5 (0.5 oz)	60	11	—	2
Corn Crackers Salt Free	5 (0.5 oz)	60	10	—	2
Oat Bran Wafers	5 (0.5 oz)	60	11	—	2
Oat Bran Wafers Salt Free	5 (0.5 oz)	60	11	—	1
Old Brussels Jalapeno Waferettes	5 (0.5 oz)	80	7	—	1
Wheat Wafers Low Salt	5 (0.5 oz)	60	10	—	1
Wasa					
Crisp	3 (0.5 oz)	50	11	0	2
Crisp'N Light Sourdough Rye	3 (0.6 oz)	60	12	1	1
Crisp'N Light Wheat	2 (0.5 oz)	50	10	1	1
Crispbread Cinnamon Toast	1 (0.6 oz)	60	11	2	1
Crispbread Fiber Rye	1 (0.4 oz)	30	4	0	2
Crispbread Gluten & Wheat Free Corn	1 (0.4 oz)	40	7	0	0
Crispbread Hearty Rye	1 (0.5 oz)	45	9	0	2
Crispbread Light Rye	1 (0.3 oz)	25	5	0	1
Crispbread Multi Grain	1 (0.5 oz)	45	8	0	2
Crispbread Organic Rye	1 (0.3 oz)	25	7	0	1
Crispbread Sodium Free Rye	1 (0.3 oz)	30	7	0	2
Crispbread Sourdough Rye	1 (0.4 oz)	35	7	0	1
Crispbread Toasted Wheat	1 (0.5 oz)	50	8	0	1
Crispbread Whole Wheat	1 (0.5 oz)	50	11	—	1
Waverly					
Crackers	5 (0.5 oz)	70	10	0	0
Wheat Thins					
Low Salt	16 (1 oz)	140	20	2	2
Multi-Grain	17 (1 oz)	130	21	4	2

FOOD	PORTION	CALS.	CARB.	SUG.	FIB.
Wheatworth					
Stone Ground	5 (0.5 oz)	80	10	1	1
Zwieback					
Crackers	1 (8 g)	35	5	1	tr

CRANBERRIES
CANNED
Ocean Spray

CranOrange	¼ cup	120	30	29	1
Cranberry Sauce Jellied	¼ cup	110	27	26	tr
Whole Berry Sauce	¼ cup	110	28	27	1

DRIED
Ocean Spray

Craisins	⅓ cup (1.4 oz)	130	33	31	2

CRANBERRY JUICE
After The Fall

Cape Cod Cranberry	1 bottle (10 oz)	130	30	26	—
Cranberry Ginger Ale	1 can (12 oz)	140	35	35	0
Crystal Light					
Cranberry Breeze Drink	1 serv (8 oz)	5	0	0	0
Cranberry Breeze Drink Mix as prep	1 serv (8 oz)	5	0	0	0
Everfresh					
Cranberry Cocktail	1 can (8 oz)	140	36	36	0
Ocean Spray					
Cocktail	8 fl oz	140	34	34	0
Lightstyle Low Calorie Cranberry Juice Cocktail	8 fl oz	40	10	10	0
Reduced Calorie Cocktail	8 fl oz	50	13	13	0
Seneca					
Cocktail frzn as prep	8 fl oz	140	36	—	0
Tree Of Life					
Concentrate	8 tsp (1.4 oz)	110	28	15	—
Tropicana					
Twister Ruby Red	8 fl oz	120	30	28	—
Twister Ruby Red	1 bottle (10 fl oz)	150	37	34	—
Veryfine					
Cocktail	1 bottle (10 oz)	180	45	44	0

CRAYFISH
(see also LOBSTER)

cooked	3 oz	97	0	0	0
raw	8	24	0	0	0

FOOD	PORTION	CALS.	CARB.	SUG.	FIB.

CREAM
(*see also* SOUR CREAM, SOUR CREAM SUBSTITUTES, WHIPPED TOPPINGS)
LIQUID
Farmland

FOOD	PORTION	CALS.	CARB.	SUG.	FIB.
Half & Half	2 tbsp	40	2	1	0
Light Cream	2 tbsp	30	1	1	0
Hood					
Half & Half	2 tbsp (1 oz)	40	1	1	0
Heavy	1 tbsp (0.5 oz)	50	0	0	0
Light	1 tbsp (0.5 oz)	30	tr	tr	0
Whipping Cream	1 tbsp (0.5 oz)	45	tr	tr	0
Parmalat					
Half & Half	2 tbsp (1 oz)	40	2	1	0

CREAM CHEESE
Alpine Lace

FOOD	PORTION	CALS.	CARB.	SUG.	FIB.
Fat Free Garden Vegetable	2 tbsp (1 oz)	30	1	0	0
Fat Free Garlic & Herbs	2 tbsp (1 oz)	30	1	0	0
Breakstone's					
Temp-Tee Whipped	2 tbsp (0.8 oz)	80	tr	tr	0
Fleur De Lait					
Bermuda Onion & Chives	2 tbsp (0.9 oz)	90	2	2	0
Cinnamon Raisin	2 tbsp (0.9 oz)	90	6	5	0
Date Nut Rum	2 tbsp (0.9 oz)	90	4	4	0
Fresh Cut Garden Vegetable	2 tbsp (0.9 oz)	80	1	tr	0
Garden Vegetable	2 tbsp (0.9 oz)	80	1	tr	0
Garlic & Spice	2 tbsp (0.9 oz)	90	1	tr	0
Herb & Spice	2 tbsp (0.9 oz)	90	2	1	0
Irish Creme	2 tbsp (0.9 oz)	100	2	2	0
Lemon	2 tbsp (0.9 oz)	90	5	5	0
Lox	2 tbsp (0.9 oz)	90	1	1	0
Mandarin Orange	2 tbsp (0.9 oz)	90	3	3	0
Peach	2 tbsp (0.9 oz)	90	3	3	0
Pineapple	2 tbsp (0.9 oz)	90	3	3	0
Plain	2 tbsp (1 oz)	100	1	1	0
Strawberry	2 tbsp (0.9 oz)	90	3	3	0
Toasted Onion	2 tbsp (0.9 oz)	90	2	1	0
Wildberry	2 tbsp (0.9 oz)	90	4	3	0
Fresh Cut					
Bac'n & Horseradish	2 tbsp (0.9 oz)	90	1	tr	0
Bermuda Onion & Chives	2 tbsp (0.9 oz)	90	2	2	0
Date Nut & Rum	2 tbsp (0.9 oz)	90	4	4	0
Garlic & Spice	2 tbsp (0.9 oz)	90	1	tr	0
Herb & Spice	2 tbsp (0.9 oz)	90	2	1	0

FOOD	PORTION	CALS.	CARB.	SUG.	FIB.
Fresh Cut (CONT.)					
Lox	2 tbsp (0.9 oz)	90	1	tr	0
Peaches & Cream	2 tbsp (0.9 oz)	90	3	3	0
Strawberry	2 tbsp (0.9 oz)	90	3	3	0
Friendship					
NY Style Reduced Fat	2 tbsp (1 oz)	50	0	0	0
Heluva Good Cheese					
Cream Cheese	1 tbsp (1 oz)	100	1	1	0
Philadelphia					
Free	1 oz	30	2	1	0
Regular	1 oz	100	tr	tr	0
Soft	2 tbsp (1 oz)	100	1	1	0
Soft Apple Cinnamon	2 tbsp (1.1 oz)	100	5	5	0
Soft Cheesecake	2 tbsp (1 oz)	110	4	4	0
Soft Chives & Onions	2 tbsp (1.1 oz)	110	2	2	0
Soft Garden Vegetable	2 tbsp (1.1 oz)	110	1	tr	0
Soft Honey Nut	2 tbsp (1.1 oz)	110	4	3	0
Soft Pineapple	2 tbsp (1.1 oz)	100	4	4	0
Soft Salmon	3 tbsp (1.1 oz)	100	2	1	0
Soft Strawberry	2 tbsp (1.1 oz)	100	5	5	0
Soft Free	2 tbsp (1.2 oz)	30	2	1	0
Soft Free Garden Vegetable	2 tbsp (1.2 oz)	30	2	1	0
Soft Free Strawberries	2 tbsp (1.2 oz)	45	6	5	0
Soft Light	2 tbsp (1.1 oz)	70	2	2	0
Soft Light Jalapeno	2 tbsp (1.1 oz)	60	2	2	0
Soft Light Raspberry	2 tbsp (1.1 oz)	70	6	5	0
Soft Light Roasted Garlic	2 tbsp (1.1 oz)	70	2	2	0
Whipped	2 tbsp (0.7 oz)	70	tr	tr	0
Whipped Chives	2 tbsp (0.7 oz)	70	tr	tr	0
Whipped Smoked Salmon	2 tbsp (0.7 oz)	70	1	tr	0
With Chives	1 oz	90	tr	tr	0
Ultra Delight					
Cheddar Cream Cheese	2 tbsp (0.9 oz)	60	2	1	1
Chive	2 tbsp (0.9 oz)	60	2	1	1
Garlic	2 tbsp (0.9 oz)	60	2	1	1
Mixed Berry	2 tbsp (0.9 oz)	70	5	4	1
Nacho	2 tbsp (0.9 oz)	60	2	1	1
Salsa	2 tbsp (0.9 oz)	60	2	1	1
Shrimp	2 tbsp (0.9 oz)	60	2	1	1
Strawberry	2 tbsp (0.9 oz)	60	4	3	1
Vegetable	2 tbsp (0.9 oz)	50	2	1	1

FOOD	PORTION	CALS.	CARB.	SUG.	FIB.
Weight Watchers					
Light	2 tbsp	40	1	1	0
CRESS					
(*see also* WATERCRESS)					
CROISSANT					
apple	1 (2 oz)	145	21	—	1
cheese	1 (2 oz)	236	27	—	2
plain	1 (2 oz)	232	26	—	2
plain	1 mini (1 oz)	115	13	—	1
Pepperidge Farm					
Croissant Sandwich Quartet	1	170	22	—	tr
Rudy's Farm					
Ham & Swiss Sandwich	1 (3.4 oz)	310	27	0	1
CROUTONS					
plain	1 cup (1 oz)	122	22	—	2
seasoned	1 cup (1.4 oz)	186	25	—	2
Arnold					
Crispy Cheddar Romano	½ oz	64	8	—	tr
Crispy Cheese Garlic	½ oz	60	9	—	tr
Crispy Fine Herbs	½ oz	50	10	—	1
Crispy Italian	½ oz	60	8	—	tr
Brownberry					
Ceasar Salad	½ oz	62	8	—	1
Cheddar Cheese	½ oz	63	8	—	tr
Onion & Garlic	½ oz	60	9	—	tr
Seasoned	½ oz	59	8	—	1
Toasted	½ oz	56	10	—	tr
CUCUMBER					
FRESH					
raw	1 (11 oz)	38	8	—	3
raw sliced	½ cup (1.8 oz)	7	1	—	1
CUSK					
fillet baked	3 oz	106	0	0	0
CUSTARD					
MIX					
Jell-O					
Americana Custard Dessert as prep w/ 2% milk	½ cup (5 oz)	140	25	23	0

FOOD	PORTION	CALS.	CARB.	SUG.	FIB.
Jell-O (CONT.)					
Flan as prep w/ 2% milk	½ cup (5.1 oz)	140	26	25	0
READY-TO-EAT					
Kozy Shack					
Flan	1 pkg (4 oz)	150	25	23	0

DANISH PASTRY
FROZEN
Morton

Honey Buns	1 (2.28 oz)	250	35	16	2
Honey Buns Mini	1 (1.23 oz)	160	19	6	tr
READY-TO-EAT					
Hostess					
Apple	1 (3.8 oz)	400	47	22	2
Apple Fruit Roll	1 (2 oz)	180	33	13	1
Coffee Cake Raspberry	1 (1.2 oz)	110	21	10	tr

DATES
DRIED
Sonoma

Dried	5-6 (1.4 oz)	110	30	21	5

DEER
(*see* VENISON)

DELI MEATS/COLD CUTS
(*see also* CHICKEN, HAM, MEAT SUBSTITUTES, TURKEY)

corned beef loaf	1 oz	43	0	0	0
Carl Buddig					
Beef	1 oz	40	1	—	0
Corned Beef	1 oz	40	1	—	0
Pastrami	1 oz	40	1	—	0
Healthy Choice					
Bologna	1 slice (1 oz)	30	1	1	0
Bologna Beef	1 slice (1 oz)	35	3	1	0
Deli-Thin Bologna	4 slices (1.8 oz)	60	3	1	0
Well-Pack Bologna	1 slice (1 oz)	30	1	1	0
Hillshire					
Pepperoni	1 oz	110	0	0	0
Salami Hard	1 oz	100	0	0	0
Hormel					
Liverwurst Spread	4 tbsp (2 oz)	130	2	1	0
Pepperoni Chunk	1 oz	140	0	0	0
Pepperoni Sliced	15 slices (1 oz)	140	0	0	0
Pepperoni Twin	1 oz	140	0	0	0
Pillow Pack Genoa Salami	2 oz	160	0	0	0

FOOD	PORTION	CALS.	CARB.	SUG.	FIB.
Hormel (CONT.)					
Pillow Pack Pepperoni	16 slices (1 oz)	140	0	0	0
Jordan's					
Healthy Trim 95% Fat Free Macaroni & Cheese Loaf	2 slices (1.6 oz)	50	3	3	0
Healthy Trim 95% Fat Free Olive Loaf	2 slices (1.6 oz)	50	2	2	0
Healthy Trim 95% Fat Free Pickle & Pepper Loaf	2 slices (1.6 oz)	50	2	2	0
Healthy Trim 97% Fat Free Corned Beef	2 slices (1.6 oz)	45	0	0	0
Healthy Trim Low Fat Cooked Salami	3 slices (2 oz)	70	2	2	0
Healthy Trim Low Fat German Brand Bologna	3 slices (2 oz)	70	3	3	0
Oscar Mayer					
Bologna	1 slice (1 oz)	90	1	tr	0
Bologna Beef	1 slice (1 oz)	90	1	tr	0
Bologna Garlic	1 slice (1.4 oz)	110	1	tr	0
Bologna Wisconsin Made Ring	2 oz	180	2	1	0
Braunschweiger Spread	2 oz	190	2	tr	0
Brunschweiger	1 slice (1 oz)	100	1	0	0
Free Bologna	1 slice (1 oz)	20	2	tr	0
Head Cheese	1 slice (1 oz)	50	0	0	0
Light Bologna	1 slice (1 oz)	60	2	tr	0
Light Bologna Beef	1 slice (1 oz)	60	2	tr	0
Liver Cheese	1 slice (1.3 oz)	120	1	0	0
Lunchables Bologna/ American	1 pkg (4.5 oz)	450	19	3	0
Lunchables Deluxe Turkey/ Ham	1 pkg (5.1 oz)	360	23	6	1
Lunchables Dessert Jello/ Honey Turkey/Cheddar	1 pkg (5.7 oz)	320	27	16	tr
Lunchables Fun Pack Bologna/Wild Cherry	1 pkg (11.2 oz)	530	58	45	tr
Lunchables Fun Pack Ham/ Fruit Punch	1 pkg (11.2 oz)	450	53	39	tr
Lunchables Ham/Swiss	1 pkg (4.5 oz)	320	19	4	0
Lunchables Pepperoni/ American	1 pkg (4.5 oz)	480	19	3	0
Lunchables Salami/ American	1 pkg (4.5 oz)	430	18	3	0
Luncheon Loaf Spiced	1 slice (1 oz)	70	2	1	0

FOOD	PORTION	CALS.	CARB.	SUG.	FIB.
Oscar Mayer (CONT.)					
New England Brand Sausage	2 slices (1.6 oz)	60	1	tr	0
Old Fashioned Loaf	1 slice (1 oz)	70	2	1	0
Olive Loaf	1 slice (1 oz)	70	2	tr	0
Pepperoni	15 slices (1 oz)	140	0	0	0
Pickle And Pimiento Loaf	1 slice (1 oz)	80	3	2	0
Salami Cotto	1 slice (1 oz)	70	1	0	0
Salami Cotto Beef	1 slice (1 oz)	60	1	tr	0
Salami For Beer	1 slices (1.6 oz)	110	1	tr	0
Salami Genoa	3 slices (1 oz)	100	0	0	0
Salami Hard	3 slices (1 oz)	100	0	0	0
Salami Machaich Brand Beef	2 slices (1.6 oz)	120	1	tr	0
Sandwich Spread	2 oz	130	8	4	0
Summer Sausage	2 slices (1.6 oz)	140	0	0	0
Summer Sausage Beef	2 slices (1.6 oz)	140	1	tr	0
Russer					
Bologna	2 oz	180	3	3	—
Bologna Jalapeno Pepper	2 oz	170	3	2	—
Bologna Wunderbar German Brand	2 oz	190	5	4	—
Bologna Beef	2 oz	180	3	2	—
Bologna Garlic	2 oz	180	3	2	—
Bologna Italian Brand Sweet Red Pepper	2 oz	180	3	2	—
Braunschweiger	2 oz	170	3	2	—
Cooked Salami	2 oz	120	3	2	—
Dutch Brand	2 oz	130	6	4	—
Hot Cooked Salami	2 oz	110	3	2	—
Italian Brand Loaf	2 oz	130	5	3	—
Jalapeno Loaf With Monterey Jack Cheese	2 oz	160	4	3	—
Kielbasa Loaf	2 oz	120	5	3	—
Light Bologna	2 oz	120	3	2	—
Light Bologna Beef	2 oz	120	3	2	—
Light Braunschweiger	2 oz	120	3	2	—
Light Old Fashioned Loaf	2 oz	90	4	3	—
Light P&P Loaf	2 oz	100	4	3	—
Light Salami Cooked	2 oz	90	4	2	—
Olive Loaf	2 oz	160	4	3	—
P&P Loaf	2 oz	160	4	3	—
Pepper Loaf	2 oz	90	6	4	—
Polish Loaf	2 oz	140	7	4	—

FOOD	PORTION	CALS.	CARB.	SUG.	FIB.
Sara Lee					
Pastrami Beef	2 oz	100	1	—	1
Shofar					
Salami Beef	2 oz	160	0	0	0
Spam					
Less Salt	2 oz	170	0	0	0
Lite	2 oz	110	0	0	0
Original	2 oz	170	0	0	0
Smoked	2 oz	170	0	0	0

DIETING AIDS
(*see* NUTRITIONAL SUPPLEMENTS)

DILL
Watkins					
Liquid Spice	1 tbsp (0.5 oz)	120	0	0	0

DINNER
(*see also* ASIAN FOOD, PASTA DISHES, POT PIES, SPANISH FOOD)
FROZEN

FOOD	PORTION	CALS.	CARB.	SUG.	FIB.
Amy's Organic					
Whole Meals Country Dinner	1 pkg (11 oz)	380	60	14	9
Armour					
Classics Chicken Parmigiana	1 meal (10.75 oz)	360	25	8	7
Classics Chicken & Noodles	1 meal (11 oz)	280	30	—	6
Classics Chicken Mesquite	1 meal (9.5 oz)	280	39	16	5
Classics Chicken w/ Wine & Mushroom	1 meal (10 oz)	260	20	4	4
Classics Glazed Chicken	1 meal (10.75 oz)	280	20	7	4
Classics Meatloaf	1 meal (11.25 oz)	300	33	4	7
Classics Salisbury Steak	1 meal (11.25 oz)	330	20	6	4
Classics Swedish Meatballs	1 meal (10 oz)	300	20	2	4
Classics Turkey and Dressing	1 meal (11.25 oz)	270	34	1	5
Classics Veal Parmigiana	1 meal (11.25 oz)	400	35	8	5
Classics Lite Beef Pepper	1 meal (11 oz)	210	29	5	5
Classics Lite Chicken Burgundy	1 meal (10 oz)	210	20	2	4
Classics Lite Salisbury Steak	1 meal (11.5 oz)	260	26	6	6
Classics Lite Shrimp Creole	1 meal (10 oz)	220	49	6	16
Classics Lite Sweet & Sour Chicken	1 meal (11 oz)	220	38	0	4

FOOD	PORTION	CALS.	CARB.	SUG.	FIB.
Banquet					
BBQ Style Chicken	1 meal (9 oz)	320	36	15	3
Beef	1 meal (9 oz)	240	19	12	12
Chicken Parmigiana	1 pkg (9.5 oz)	290	27	3	3
Chicken & Dumplings	1 meal (10 oz)	260	35	16	16
Chicken Fried Steak	1 pkg (10 oz)	400	39	9	4
Chicken Nuggets	1 pkg (6.75 oz)	410	38	11	11
Extra Helping All White Chicken	1 meal (18 oz)	820	72	13	8
Extra Helping Chicken Parmigiana	1 meal (19 oz)	650	64	9	9
Extra Helping Chicken Fried Steak	1 meal (18.5 oz)	800	73	14	6
Extra Helping Fried Chicken	1 meal (18 oz)	790	72	14	8
Extra Helping Meatloaf	1 meal (19 oz)	650	49	13	10
Extra Helping Mexican Style	1 meal (22 oz)	820	100	35	20
Extra Helping Salisbury Steak	1 meal (19 oz)	740	52	3	11
Extra Helping Southern Fried Chicken	1 meal (17.5 oz)	750	67	14	9
Extra Helping Turkey Dinner	1 meal (18.8 oz)	560	63	26	7
Family Entree Beef Stew	1 serv (8.13 oz)	160	17	3	4
Family Entree Chicken Parmigiana	1 serv (4.67 oz)	240	18	4	2
Family Entree Chicken & Dumplings	1 serv (7.47 oz)	290	30	2	2
Family Entree Gravy & Sliced Turkey	1 serv (4.8 oz)	100	5	0	tr
Family Entree Gravy w/ Charbroiled Beef	1 serv (4.67 oz)	180	7	0	2
Family Entree Onion Gravy w/ Beef	1 serv (4.67 oz)	180	7	5	2
Family Entree Salisbury Steak	1 serv (4.67 oz)	200	7	0	2
Family Entree Veal Parmigiana	1 serv (4.67 oz)	230	19	2	2
Family Entrees Gravy & Sliced Beef	1 serv (5.6 oz)	100	7	2	tr
Fried Chicken	1 meal (9 oz)	470	35	1	6
Gravy w/ Beef Patty	1 pkg (9.5 oz)	300	21	2	2
Hot Sandwich Toppers Chicken Ala King	1 pkg (4.5 oz)	100	7	3	1

FOOD	PORTION	CALS.	CARB.	SUG.	FIB.
Banquet (CONT.)					
Hot Sandwich Toppers Creamed Chipped Beef	1 pkg (4 oz)	100	8	1	0
Hot Sandwich Toppers Gravy & Sliced Beef	1 pkg (4 oz)	70	5	tr	tr
Hot Sandwich Toppers Gravy & Sliced Turkey	1 pkg (5 oz)	90	7	1	tr
Hot Sandwich Toppers Salisbury Steak	1 pkg (5 oz)	220	8	1	2
Hot Sandwich Toppers Sloppy Joe	1 meal (4 oz)	140	12	1	1
Meatloaf	1 meal (9.5 oz)	280	23	2	2
Mexican Style Combo Meal	1 pkg (11 oz)	380	55	7	9
Mexican Style Meal	1 pkg (11 oz)	340	56	7	10
Oriental Style Chicken	1 pkg (9 oz)	260	34	16	4
Salisbury Steak	1 meal (9.5 oz)	310	28	2	2
Southern Fried Chicken Meal	1 pkg (8.75 oz)	260	44	6	4
Turkey	1 meal (9.25 oz)	270	31	2	3
Veal Parmagiana	1 pkg (9 oz)	530	35	14	7
Western Style Meal	1 meal (9.5 oz)	210	28	4	5
White Meat Chicken Meal	1 pkg (8.75 oz)	470	33	2	2
Birds Eye					
Easy Recipe Meal Starter Cacciatore as prep	1 serv	280	30	10	2
Easy Recipe Meal Starter Orange Glaze Chicken as prep	1 serv	280	30	17	2
Easy Recipe Meal Starter Southwestern	1 serv	280	30	6	2
Easy Recipe Meal Starter Sweet & Sour as prep	1 serv	280	30	28	2
Green Giant					
Create A Meal Broccoli Stir Fry as prep	1⅓ cups (9.9 oz)	290	16	7	4
Create A Meal Cheese & Herb Primavera as prep	1¼ cups (10 oz)	330	27	3	4
Create A Meal Garlic Herb as prep	1¼ cups (10 oz)	340	30	4	4
Create A Meal Hearty Vegetable Stew as prep	1¼ cups (10 oz)	280	25	5	3
Create A Meal Lemon Herb as prep	1½ cups (10 oz)	360	37	12	3
Create A Meal Mushroom & Wine as prep	1¼ cups (10 oz)	390	31	5	4

FOOD	PORTION	CALS.	CARB.	SUG.	FIB.
Green Giant (CONT.)					
Create A Meal Vegetable Almond Stir Fry as prep	1⅓ cups (10 oz)	320	22	9	6
Healthy Choice					
Beef & Peppers Cantonese	1 meal (11.5 oz)	270	40	18	5
Beef Pepper Steak Oriental	1 meal (9.5 oz)	250	34	0	3
Beef Tips Francais	1 meal (9.5 oz)	280	40	1	4
Beef Tips With Sauce	1 meal (11 oz)	290	40	31	5
Chicken Cantonese	1 meal (11.25)	210	31	15	5
Chicken Parmigiana	1 meal (11.5 oz)	300	47	3	6
Chicken & Vegetables Marsala	1 meal (11.5 oz)	220	32	1	3
Chicken Bangkok	1 meal (9.5 oz)	270	35	3	5
Chicken Dijon	1 meal (11 oz)	280	41	21	9
Chicken Imperial	1 meal (9 oz)	230	31	2	3
Chicken Picante	1 meal (11.25 oz)	220	30	25	6
Chicken Teriyaki	1 meal (12.25 oz)	270	42	24	5
Classics Beef Broccoli Beijing	1 meal (12 oz)	330	55	2	5
Classics Cacciatore Chicken	1 meal (12.5 oz)	260	36	5	6
Classics Chicken Fransesca	1 meal (12.5 oz)	360	51	4	5
Classics Country Inn Roast Turkey	1 meal (10 oz)	250	29	3	6
Classics Ginger Chicken Hunan	1 meal (12.6 oz)	350	59	11	5
Classics Mesquite Beef Barbecue	1 meal (11 oz)	310	45	5	6
Classics Salisbury Steak	1 meal (11 oz)	260	32	3	5
Classics Sesame Chicken Shanghai	1 meal (12 oz)	310	42	2	5
Classics Shrimp & Vegetables Maria	1 meal (12.5 oz)	260	46	tr	5
Country Glazed Chicken	1 meal (8.5 oz)	200	30	tr	3
Country Herb Chicken	1 meal (11.5 oz)	270	40	29	6
Country Roast Turkey With Mushroom	1 meal (8.5 oz)	220	28	0	3
Country Turkey & Pasta	1 meal (12.6 oz)	300	42	18	6
Homestyle Turkey With Vegetables	1 meal (9.5 oz)	260	34	1	3
Honey Mustard Chicken	1 meal (9.5 oz)	260	40	4	4
Lemon Pepper Fish	1 meal (10.7 oz)	290	47	20	7
Mandarin Chicken	1 meal (10 oz)	280	44	9	4
Mesquite Chicken Barbecue	1 meal (10.5 oz)	320	55	38	6

FOOD	PORTION	CALS.	CARB.	SUG.	FIB.
Healthy Choice (CONT.)					
Shrimp Marinara	1 meal (10.5 oz)	220	44	27	5
Smoky Chicken Barbecue	1 meal (12.75 oz)	380	57	37	7
Southwestern Glazed Chicken	1 meal (12.5 oz)	300	48	24	6
Sweet & Sour Chicken	1 meal (11.5 oz)	310	42	15	5
Traditional Breast Of Turkey	1 meal (10.5 oz)	280	40	14	7
Traditional Meat Loaf	1 meal (12 oz)	320	46	24	7
Traditional Beef Tips	1 meal (11.25 oz)	260	32	5	6
Tradtional Salisbury Steak	1 meal (11.5 oz)	320	48	5	7
Yankee Pot Roast	1 meal (11 oz)	280	38	2	5
Kid Cuisine					
Chicken Sandwiche	1 pkg (9.43 oz)	480	71	20	4
Chicken Nuggets	1 pkg (9.1 oz)	440	54	12	5
Fish Sticks	1 pkg (8.25 oz)	370	55	21	4
Fried Chicken	1 pkg (10.1 oz)	440	49	12	5
Macaroni & Beef	1 pkg (9.6 oz)	370	58	23	5
Lean Cuisine					
American Favorite Baked Chicken	1 pkg (8.6 oz)	230	31	4	5
American Favorite Baked Fish	1 pkg (9 oz)	270	36	6	3
American Favorite Beef Pot Roast	1 pkg (9 oz)	210	25	4	6
American Favorite Beef Tips Barbecue	1 pkg (8.75 oz)	290	47	12	7
American Favorite Chicken Medallions w/ Creamy Cheese	1 pkg (9.37 oz)	260	31	6	4
American Favorite Country Vegetables & Beef	1 pkg (9 oz)	210	33	9	3
American Favorite Honey Roasted Chicken	1 pkg (8.5 oz)	290	46	9	5
American Favorite Meatloaf & Whipped Potatoes	1 pkg (9.4 oz)	250	30	4	4
American Favorite Oven Roasted Beef	1 pkg (9.25 oz)	260	28	7	4
American Favorite Roasted Turkey Breast	1 pkg (9.75 oz)	270	49	25	5
American Favorite Salisbury Steak	1 pkg (9.5 oz)	280	29	2	4
American Favorite Scalloped Potatoes w/ Turkey Ham	1 pkg (10 oz)	250	38	7	6

FOOD	PORTION	CALS.	CARB.	SUG.	FIB.
Lean Cuisine (CONT.)					
Cafe Classics Chicken Carbonara	1 pkg (9 oz)	280	33	7	2
Cafe Classics Chicken Mediterranean	1 pkg (10.5 oz)	270	40	5	2
Cafe Classics Chicken Breast In Wine Sauce	1 pkg (8.1 oz)	210	23	7	2
Cafe Classics Chicken Parmesan	1 meal (10.9 oz)	220	27	10	4
Cafe Classics Chicken Piccata	1 pkg (9 oz)	270	41	7	2
Cafe Classics Chicken w/ Basil Cream Sauce	1 pkg (8.5 oz)	270	35	4	3
Cafe Classics Glazed Turkey	1 pkg (9 oz)	240	37	19	5
Cafe Classics Grilled Chicken Salsa	1 pkg (8.9 oz)	270	36	6	4
Cafe Classics Herb Roasted Chicken	1 pkg (8 oz)	210	27	5	3
Cafe Classics Honey Mustard Chicken	1 pkg (8 oz)	250	39	12	3
Cafe Classics Mesquite Beef w/ Rice	1 pkg (9 oz)	290	42	10	5
Cafe Classics Sirlion Beef Peppercorn	1 pkg (8.75 oz)	220	23	6	2
Chicken & Vegetables	1 pkg (10.5 oz)	250	31	3	4
Chicken A L'Orange	1 pkg (9 oz)	250	40	11	3
Chicken In Peanut Sauce	1 pkg (9 oz)	290	35	8	4
Fiesta Chicken w/ Rice & Vegetables	1 pkg (8.5 oz)	250	34	5	3
Glazed Chicken w/ Vegetable Rice	1 pkg (8.5 oz)	240	25	7	0
Homestyle Turkey	1 pkg (9.4 oz)	230	30	8	3
Mandarin Chicken	1 pkg (9 oz)	250	38	9	3
Oriental Beef	1 pkg (9.25 oz)	220	33	8	2
Stuffed Cabbage w/ Whipped Potatoes	1 pkg (9.5 oz)	170	24	5	5
Swedish Meatballs w/ Pasta	1 pkg (9.1 oz)	280	33	2	3
Life Choice					
Garden Potato Casserole	1 meal (13.4 oz)	160	37	11	9
Morton					
Breaded Chicken Pattie	1 meal (6.75 oz)	280	24	12	4
Chicken Nugget	1 meal (7 oz)	320	30	12	3
Fried Chicken	1 meal (9 oz)	420	30	4	4

FOOD	PORTION	CALS.	CARB.	SUG.	FIB.
Morton (CONT.)					
Meatloaf	1 meal (9 oz)	250	24	17	5
Mexican	1 meal (10 oz)	260	40	3	8
Salisbury Steak	1 meal (9 oz)	210	23	7	3
Turkey	1 meal (9 oz)	230	27	5	5
Veal Parmagiana	1 meal (8.75 oz)	280	30	8	4
Western	1 meal (9 oz)	290	26	3	6
Patio					
Chili	1 cup (8 oz)	260	13	5	4
Ranchera	1 pkg (13 oz)	410	14	11	14
Stouffer's					
Baked Chicken Breast w/ Mashed Potatoes	1 serv (12.2 oz)	330	25	2	3
Beef Stroganoff	1 pkg (9.75 oz)	390	30	2	2
Chicken A La King	1 pkg (9.5 oz)	350	41	5	2
Creamed Chicken	1 pkg (6.5 oz)	260	8	5	0
Creamed Chipped Beef	½ cup (5.5 oz)	160	6	5	1
Creamy Chicken & Broccoli	1 pkg (8.9 oz)	320	26	7	2
Escalloped Chicken & Noodles	1 pkg (10 oz)	430	30	4	3
Fish w/ Macaroni & Cheese	1 serv (9.5 oz)	460	47	8	2
Glazed Chicken w/ Rice	1 serv (11.8 oz)	290	39	9	2
Green Pepper Steak	1 pkg (10.5 oz)	330	45	4	3
Homestyle Baked Chicken & Gravy & Whipped Potatoes	1 pkg (8.9 oz)	270	19	1	2
Homestyle Beef Pot Roast & Browned Potatoes	1 pkg (8.9 oz)	250	29	3	4
Homestyle Fish Filet w/ Macaroni & Cheese	1 pkg (9 oz)	430	37	7	2
Homestyle Fried Chicken & Whipped Potatoes	1 pkg (7.5 oz)	310	33	1	5
Homestyle Meatloaf & Whipped Potatoes	1 pkg (9.9 oz)	330	26	4	3
Homestyle Roast Turkey w/ Gravy Stuffing & Whipped Potatoes	1 pkg (9.6 oz)	320	31	4	3
Homestyle Salisbury Steak & Gravy & Macaroni & Cheese	1 pkg (9.6 oz)	350	27	2	2
Meatloaf	1 serv (5.5 oz)	210	9	1	1
Meatloaf w/ Whipped Potatoes	1 serv (11.5 oz)	380	33	3	4

FOOD	PORTION	CALS.	CARB.	SUG.	FIB.
Stouffer's (CONT.)					
Stuffed Pepper	1 pkg (10 oz)	200	27	8	3
Swedish Meatballs	1 pkg (10.25 oz)	480	43	2	3
Ultra Slim-Fast					
Beef Pepper Steak	12 oz	270	36	—	0
Chicken Fettucini	12 oz	380	38	—	1
Chicken & Vegetable	12 oz	290	45	—	4
Country Style Vegetable & Beef Tips	12 oz	230	26	—	4
Mesquite Chicken	12 oz	360	61	—	5
Roasted Chicken In Mushroom Sauce	12 oz	280	30	—	0
Shrimp Creole	12 oz	240	45	—	5
Shrimp Marinara	12 oz	290	53	—	0
Sweet & Sour Chicken	12 oz	330	57	—	0
Turkey Medallions In Herb Sauce	12 oz	280	33	—	0
Weight Watchers					
Smart Ones Fiesta Chicken	1 pkg (8.5 oz)	220	38	9	5
Smart Ones Grilled Salisbury Steak	1 pkg (8.5 oz)	260	24	3	3
Smart Ones Honey Mustard Chicken	1 pkg (8.5 oz)	200	37	10	3
Smart Ones Lemon Herb Chicken Piccata	1 pkg (8.5 oz)	200	34	8	3
Smart Ones Pepper Steak	1 pkg (10 oz)	240	33	6	4
Smart Ones Risotto w/ Cheese & Mushrooms	1 pkg (10 oz)	290	44	5	4
Smart Ones Roast Turkey Medallions & Mushrooms	1 pkg (8.5 oz)	190	32	3	2
Smart Ones Shrimp Marinara	1 pkg (9 oz)	190	35	6	4
Smart Ones Stuffed Turkey Breast	1 pkg (10 oz)	260	37	10	5
Smart Ones Swedish Meatballs	1 pkg (9 oz)	300	33	3	2
SHELF-STABLE					
My Own Meal					
Beef Stew	1 pkg (10 oz)	260	22	3	4
Chicken Mediterranean	1 pkg (10 oz)	270	28	4	4
Chicken Noodles	1 pkg (10 oz)	270	29	4	3
Chicken & Black Beans	1 pkg (10 oz)	240	30	3	6

FOOD	PORTION	CALS.	CARB.	SUG.	FIB.
My Own Meal (CONT.)					
Old World Stew	1 pkg (10 oz)	310	31	3	3
DIP					
Breakstone's					
Bacon & Onion	2 tbsp (1.1 oz)	60	2	1	0
Chesapeake Clam	2 tbsp (1.1 oz)	50	1	tr	0
Free Creamy Salsa	2 tbsp (1.1 oz)	20	3	2	0
Free French Onion	2 tbsp (1.1 oz)	25	4	2	0
Free Ranch	2 tbsp (1.1 oz)	25	4	2	0
French Onion	2 tbsp (1.1 oz)	50	2	1	0
Toasted Onion	2 tbsp (1.1 oz)	50	2	1	0
Cheez Whiz					
Medium Cheese & Salsa	2 tbsp (1.2 oz)	100	3	2	0
Mild Cheese & Salsa	2 tbsp (1.2 oz)	100	3	2	0
Chi-Chi's					
Fiesta Bean	2 tbsp (0.9 oz)	35	4	0	1
Fiesta Cheese	2 tbsp (0.9 oz)	40	3	1	0
Durkee					
Sour Cream as prep	2 tbsp	25	4	1	0
Guiltless Gourmet					
Black Bean Mild	1 oz	25	5	—	1
Black Bean Spicy	1 oz	25	5	—	1
Pinto Bean	1 oz	25	5	—	1
Heluva Good Cheese					
Bacon Horseradish	2 tbsp (1.1 oz)	60	2	2	0
Clam	2 tbsp (1.1 oz)	50	2	1	0
French Onion	2 tbsp (1.1 oz)	50	2	1	0
Homestyle Onion	2 tbsp (1.1 oz)	60	3	2	0
Light French Onion	2 tbsp (1.1 oz)	35	3	2	0
Light Jalapeno Cheddar	2 tbsp (1.1 oz)	40	3	2	0
Ranch	2 tbsp (1.1 oz)	60	2	1	0
Knudsen					
Free Creamy Salsa	2 tbsp (1.1 oz)	20	3	2	0
Free French Onion	2 tbsp (1.1 oz)	25	4	2	0
Free Ranch	2 tbsp (1.1 oz)	25	4	2	0
Kraft					
Avocado	2 tbsp (1.1 oz)	60	4	tr	0
Bacon & Horseradish	2 tbsp (1.1 oz)	60	3	tr	0
Clam	2 tbsp (1.1 oz)	60	3	tr	0
Free French Onion	2 tbsp (1.1 oz)	25	4	2	0
Free Ranch	2 tbsp (1.1 oz)	25	4	2	0
Free Salsa	2 tbsp (1.1 oz)	20	3	2	0
French Onion	2 tbsp (1.1 oz)	60	4	tr	0

FOOD	PORTION	CALS.	CARB.	SUG.	FIB.
Kraft (CONT.)					
Green Onion	2 tbsp (1.1 oz)	60	4	tr	0
Jalapeno Cheese	2 tbsp (1.1 oz)	60	3	tr	0
Premium Sour Cream	2 tbsp (1.1 oz)	50	1	1	0
Premium Sour Cream Bacon & Horseradish	2 tbsp (1.1 oz)	60	2	1	0
Premium Sour Cream Bacon & Onion	2 tbsp (1.1 oz)	60	2	1	0
Premium Sour Cream Creamy Onion	2 tbsp (1.1 oz)	45	2	1	0
Premium Sour Cream French Onion	2 tbsp (1.1 oz)	45	2	1	0
Premium Sour Cream Ranch	2 tbsp (1.1 oz)	50	2	1	0
Ranch	2 tbsp (1.1 oz)	60	3	tr	0
Lay's					
Low Fat Sour Cream & Onion	2 tbsp (1 oz)	40	6	tr	tr
Louise's					
Fat Free Honey Mustard	1 oz	40	9	7	0
Fat Free Sour Cream & Onion	1 oz	25	4	1	0
Fat Free White Cheese Peppercorn	1 oz	25	4	1	0
Marzetti					
Blue Cheese Veggie	2 tbsp	200	1	0	0
Lemon Dill Veggie	2 tbsp	140	2	1	0
Light Ranch Veggie	2 tbsp	60	5	3	1
Ranch Veggie	2 tbsp	140	1	1	0
Sour Cream & Onion	2 tbsp	130	2	1	0
Southwestern Veggie	2 tbsp	130	1	1	0
Spinach Veggie	2 tbsp	130	1	1	0
Old El Paso					
Black Bean	2 tbsp (1 oz)	20	4	0	1
Cheese 'n Salsa Medium	2 tbsp (1 oz)	40	3	0	0
Cheese 'n Salsa Mild	2 tbsp (1 oz)	40	3	0	0
Chunky Salsa Medium	2 tbsp (1 oz)	15	3	2	1
Chunky Salsa Mild	2 tbsp (1 oz)	15	3	2	1
Jalapeno	2 tbsp (1 oz)	30	4	0	2
Ruffles					
Low Fat French Onion	1 tbsp (1 oz)	40	6	tr	tr
Snyder's					
Mustard Pretzel	2 tbsp (1.2 oz)	90	13	12	1

FOOD	PORTION	CALS.	CARB.	SUG.	FIB.
Taco Bell					
Fat Free Black Bean	2 tbsp (1.2 oz)	30	6	tr	2
Salsa Con Queso Medium	2 tbsp (1.2 oz)	45	5	tr	tr
Salsa Con Queso Mild	2 tbsp (1.2 oz)	45	5	tr	tr
Tostitos					
Low Fat Con Queso	2 tbsp (1 oz)	40	5	tr	tr
DOGFISH					
raw	3½ oz	193	0	0	0
DOLPHINFISH					
fresh baked	3 oz	93	0	0	0
fresh fillet baked	5.6 oz	174	0	0	0
DOUGHNUTS					
cake type unsugared	1 (1.6 oz)	198	23	—	1
chocolate glazed	1 (1.5 oz)	175	24	—	1
chocolate sugared	1 (1.5 oz)	175	24	—	1
chocolate coated	1 (1.5 oz)	204	21	—	1
frosted	1 (1.5 oz)	204	21	—	1
honey bun	1 (2.1 oz)	242	27	—	1
old fashioned	1 (1.6 oz)	198	23	—	1
sugared	1 (1.6 oz)	192	23	—	1
yeast glazed	1 (2.1 oz)	242	27	—	1
Dutch Mill					
Cider	1 (2.1 oz)	240	35	23	1
Cinnamon	1 (1.8 oz)	210	26	12	1
Donut Holes Double-Dipped Chocolate	3 (1.4 oz)	220	19	5	0
Donut Holes Shootin' Stars	3 (1.4 oz)	190	23	12	0
Double-Dipped Chocolate	1 (2.1 oz)	280	31	9	1
Glazed	1 (2.1 oz)	250	34	23	1
Glazed Chocolate	1 (2.4 oz)	270	40	10	1
Plain	1 (1.8 oz)	210	25	9	1
Sugared	1 (1.8 oz)	220	27	12	1
Freihofer's					
Assorted	1 (2 oz)	270	26	15	0
Hostess					
Assorted Regular	1 (1.6 oz)	200	23	14	tr
Cinnamon Family Pack	1 (1 oz)	110	15	8	tr
Cinnamon Swirl	1 (1.6 oz)	180	28	10	tr
Crumb Regular	1 (1 oz)	130	14	8	tr
Frosted Regular	1 (1.4 oz)	180	20	12	1
Gem Donettes Cinnamon	6 (3 oz)	320	53	28	1
Gem Donettes Frosted	6 (3 oz)	390	42	21	2

FOOD	PORTION	CALS.	CARB.	SUG.	FIB.
Hostess (CONT.)					
Gem Donettes Frosted Strawberry Filled	3 (3 oz)	240	29	15	1
Gem Donettes Powdered	6 (3 oz)	350	47	23	1
Gem Donettes Powdered Strawberry Filled	3 (3 oz)	210	31	15	tr
Glazed Party	1 (2.3 oz)	260	39	14	1
Jumbo Frosted	1 (2 oz)	260	28	14	1
Jumbo Plain	1 (1.1 oz)	140	16	8	tr
Jumbo Powdered	1 (1.3 oz)	160	19	11	tr
Mini Chocolate	5 (2 oz)	220	33	20	1
O's Raspberry Filled Powdered	1 (2.2 oz)	230	35	17	tr
Old Fashioned Glazed	1 (2.1 oz)	250	33	15	tr
Old Fashioned Glazed Honey Wheat	1 (2.1 oz)	250	33	15	1
Old Fashioned Plain	1 (1.5 oz)	170	21	9	tr
Plain Regular	1 (1 oz)	120	13	8	tr
Powdered Family Pack	1 (1 oz)	110	15	8	1
Little Debbie					
Donut Sticks	1 pkg (1.6 oz)	210	25	14	1
Donut Sticks	1 pkg (2.5 oz)	320	37	21	1
Donut Sticks	1 pkg (3 oz)	390	45	26	1
Donut Sticks	1 pkg (2 oz)	250	30	17	1
Tastykake					
Cinnamon	1 (47 g)	180	26	—	1
Frosted Rich	1 (57 g)	260	28	—	3
Frosted Rich Mini	1 (14 g)	44	8	—	1
Honey Wheat	1 (57 g)	210	32	—	1
Honey Wheat Mini	1 (12 g)	40	7	—	0
Orange Glazed	1 (57 g)	210	32	—	1
Plain	1 (47 g)	190	22	—	1
Powdered Sugar	1 (46 g)	180	24	—	1
Powdered Sugar Mini	1 (12 g)	40	7	—	0

DRESSING

(*see* STUFFING/DRESSING)

DRINK MIXERS

(*see also* SODA, MINERAL/BOTTLED WATER)

FOOD	PORTION	CALS.	CARB.	SUG.	FIB.
Bacardi					
Margarita Mix w/o liquor	8 fl oz	100	25	23	—
Pina Colada	8 fl oz	140	34	32	—
Rum Runner	8 fl oz	140	35	33	—
Strawberry Daiquiri w/o liquor	8 fl oz	140	35	33	—

FOOD	PORTION	CALS.	CARB.	SUG.	FIB.
Canada Dry					
Collins Mixer	8 fl oz	120	25	25	0
Sour Mixer	8 fl oz	90	22	22	0
Schweppes					
Collins Mixer	8 fl oz	100	24	24	0
Tabasco					
Bloody Mary Mix	1 serv (8.4 oz)	56	11	8	1
Bloody Mary Mix Extra Spicy	1 serv (8.4 oz)	58	11	10	2

DRUM

FOOD	PORTION	CALS.	CARB.	SUG.	FIB.
freshwater fillet baked	5.4 oz	236	0	0	0
freshwater baked	3 oz	130	0	0	0

DUCK

FOOD	PORTION	CALS.	CARB.	SUG.	FIB.
w/ skin roasted	1 cup (4.9 oz)	472	0	0	0
w/ skin w/ bone leg roasted	3 oz	184	0	0	0
w/ skin w/o bone breast roasted	3 oz	172	0	0	0
w/o skin roasted	1 cup (4.9 oz)	281	0	0	0
w/o skin w/ bone leg braised	1 cup (6.1 oz)	310	0	0	0
w/o skin w/o bone breast broiled	1 cup (6.1 oz)	244	0	0	0

EEL

FOOD	PORTION	CALS.	CARB.	SUG.	FIB.
fresh cooked	1 fillet (5.6 oz)	375	0	0	0
smoked	3.5 oz	330	0	0	0

EGG

(*see also* EGG DISHES, EGG SUBSTITUTES)

CHICKEN

FOOD	PORTION	CALS.	CARB.	SUG.	FIB.
hard cooked	1	77	1	—	—
poached	1	74	1	—	—
scrambled plain	2	200	2	—	—
EggsPlus					
Fresh	1 (1.8 oz)	70	0	0	0

OTHER POULTRY

FOOD	PORTION	CALS.	CARB.	SUG.	FIB.
duck raw	1 (2.5 oz)	130	1	—	0

EGG DISHES

FROZEN

Weight Watchers

FOOD	PORTION	CALS.	CARB.	SUG.	FIB.
Handy Ham & Cheese Omelet	1 (4 oz)	220	30	7	2

EGG ROLLS

(*see also* ASIAN FOOD)

Chun King

FOOD	PORTION	CALS.	CARB.	SUG.	FIB.
Chicken	8 (4.4 oz)	270	40	2	4

FOOD	PORTION	CALS.	CARB.	SUG.	FIB.
Chun King (CONT.)					
Pork & Shrimp	8 (4.4 oz)	290	39	2	4
Shrimp	8 (4.4 oz)	260	39	2	4
Empire					
Large	1 (3 oz)	190	28	4	2
Miniature	6 (4.8 oz)	280	43	6	4
La Choy					
Almond Chicken Restaurant Style	1 (3 oz)	170	23	6	3
Chicken Mini	14 (7.25 oz)	430	67	11	6
Chicken Restaurant Style	1 (3 oz)	170	25	4	4
Lobster Mini	14 (7.25 oz)	410	65	6	9
Meat & Shrimp Mini	15 (3.75 oz)	240	31	2	3
Mu Sho Pork Restaurant Style	1 (3 oz)	190	25	8	2
Pork Restaurant Style	1 (3 oz)	150	20	—	—
Pork & Shrimp Mini	14 (7.25 oz)	430	65	10	7
Shrimp Mini	14 (7.25 oz)	410	68	10	7
Shrimp Restaurant Style	1 (3 oz)	150	24	6	3
Sweet & Sour Restaurant Style	1 (3 oz)	180	29	10	3
Lean Cuisine					
Vegetable	1 pkg (9 oz)	340	64	19	3
Lo-An					
White Meat Chicken	1 (2.7 oz)	140	20	3	1
Luigino's					
Chicken	1 pkg (6 oz)	360	48	1	2
Pork & Shrimp	1 pkg (6 oz)	340	51	0	3
Shrimp	1 pkg (6 oz)	350	39	2	4
Sweet & Sour Chicken	1 pkg (6 oz)	400	59	9	4
Sweet & Sour Pork	1 pkg (6 oz)	360	56	10	4
Szechwan Vegetable	1 pkg (6 oz)	350	38	4	3
Worthington					
Vegetarian Egg Rolls	1 (3 oz)	180	20	tr	2

EGG SUBSTITUTES

FOOD	PORTION	CALS.	CARB.	SUG.	FIB.
Egg Beaters					
Eggs Substitute	¼ cup	25	1	—	0
Healthy Choice					
Cholesterol Free	¼ cup (2 oz)	25	tr	tr	0
Morningstar Farms					
Better'n Eggs	¼ cup (2 oz)	20	0	0	0
Breakfast Sandwich Bagel Scramblers Pattie Cheese	1 (5.9 oz)	320	40	6	4

FOOD	PORTION	CALS.	CARB.	SUG.	FIB.
Morningstar Farms (CONT.)					
Breakfast Sandwich English Muffin Scramblers Pattie	1 (5.1 oz)	240	32	3	5
Breakfast Sandwich English Muffin Scramblers Pattie Cheese	1 (6 oz)	280	35	5	5
Scramblers	¼ cup (2 oz)	35	2	2	0
Simply Eggs					
Egg Substitute	1.75 fl oz	35	1	—	1

EGGNOG
Hood

Fat Free	4 fl oz	100	21	18	0
Golden	4 fl oz	180	22	20	0
Light	4 fl oz	120	23	21	0
Select	4 fl oz	210	22	21	0

EGGPLANT
CANNED
Progresso

Appetizer	2 tbsp (1 oz)	30	2	2	2

ELK

roasted	3 oz	124	0	0	0

ENDIVE

raw chopped	½ cup	4	1	—	—

ENERGY BARS
(*see* BREAKFAST BARS, CEREAL BARS, GRANOLA BARS, NUTRITIONAL SUPPLEMENTS)

ENGLISH MUFFIN
FROZEN
Weight Watchers

Sandwich	1 (4 oz)	210	28	1	2
READY-TO-EAT					
whole wheat	1	134	27	—	4
Arnold					
Extra Crisp	1	130	26	—	1
Sourdough	1	130	25	—	1
Matthew's					
9 Grain & Nut	1	140	26	—	5
Cinnamon Raisin	1	160	33	—	4
Golden White	1	140	23	—	1
Whole Wheat	1	150	31	—	4

FOOD	PORTION	CALS.	CARB.	SUG.	FIB.
Roman Meal					
English Muffin	1 (2.2 oz)	135	25	4	3
Thomas'					
Oat Bran	1	116	26	—	3
Sandwich Size	1 (92 g)	210	42	2	2
Wonder					
English Muffin	1 (2 oz)	120	25	4	1
Raisin Rounds	1 (2.1 oz)	150	30	5	2
Sourdough	1 (2 oz)	120	25	4	1
REFRIGERATED					
Roman Meal					
English Muffin	½ muffin (1.1 oz)	66	14	—	1
Honey Nut Oat Bran	½ muffin (1.1 oz)	81	16	—	1
EPAZOTE					
fresh	1 tbsp (1 g)	tr	tr	—	tr
fresh sprig	1 (2 g)	1	tr	—	tr
FALAFEL					
Casbah					
as prep	5	130	20	0	2
Near East					
As Prep	2½ patties	230	18	3	5
FAST FOODS					
(*see individual foods in Part Two*)					
FAT					
(*see also* BUTTER, BUTTER BLENDS, BUTTER SUBSTITUTES, MARGARINE, OIL)					
beef cooked	1 oz	193	0	0	0
beef suet	1 oz	242	0	0	0
beef tallow	1 tbsp (13 g)	115	0	0	0
chicken	1 cup	1846	0	0	0
chicken	1 tbsp	115	0	0	0
cocoa butter	1 tbsp	120	0	0	0
duck	1 tbsp (13 g)	115	0	0	0
goose	1 tbsp	115	0	0	0
goose	3.5 oz	900	0	0	0
lamb new zealand raw	1 oz	182	0	0	0
lard	1 cup (205 g)	1849	0	0	0
lard	1 tbsp (13 g)	115	0	0	0
nutmeg butter	1 tbsp	120	0	0	0
pork backfat	1 oz	230	0	0	0
pork cooked	1 oz	178	0	0	0
salt pork	1 oz	212	0	0	0

FOOD	PORTION	CALS.	CARB.	SUG.	FIB.
shortening	1 tbsp	113	0	0	0
shortening	1 cup	1812	0	0	0
turkey	1 tbsp	115	0	0	0
ucuhuba butter	1 tbsp	120	0	0	0
Crisco					
Butter Flavor	1 tbsp	110	0	0	0
Shortening	1 tbsp	110	0	0	0
Shortening	1 tbsp (0.4 oz)	110	0	0	0
Sticks	1 tbsp (0.4 oz)	110	0	0	0
Sticks Butter Flavor	1 tbsp (0.4 oz)	110	0	0	0
Empire					
Chicken Fat Rendered	1 tbsp (0.5 oz)	120	tr	0	0
Wesson					
Shortening	1 tbsp	100	0	0	0

FAT SUBSTITUTES
Soy Is Us

Fat Not! Organic	3 tbsp	66	7	2	4

FAVA BEANS
Progresso

Fava Beans	½ cup (4.6 oz)	110	20	0	5

FENNEL

leaves	3.5 oz	24	3	—	4

FIBER
Delta

Natural Fiber	½ cup (1 oz)	20	2	—	20

FIGS
DRIED

California	½ cup (3.5 oz)	200	58	—	17
whole	10	477	122	—	17
Sonoma					
White Misson	3-4 (1.4 oz)	110	26	20	5

FIREWEED

leaves chopped	1 cup (0.8 oz)	24	4	—	2

FISH
(*see also individual names,* FISH SUBSTITUTES, SUSHI)
CANNED
Holmes

Finest Kippered Snacks drained	1 can (3.2 oz)	135	0	0	0
Port Clyde					
Fish Steaks In Louisiana Hot Sauce	1 can (3.75 oz)	150	2	0	0

FOOD	PORTION	CALS.	CARB.	SUG.	FIB.
Port Clyde (CONT.)					
Fish Steaks In Mustard Sauce	1 can (3.75 oz)	140	1	0	0
Fish Steaks In Soybean Oil With Hot Chilies drained	1 can (3.3 oz)	155	0	0	0
Fish Steaks In Soybean Oil drained	1 can (3.3 oz)	220	0	0	0
FROZEN					
Gorton's					
Grilled Fillets Cajun Blackened	1 piece (3.8 oz)	120	1	1	—
Kineret					
Fish Sticks	5 pieces (4 oz)	280	27	2	1
Van De Kamp's					
Battered Fish Fillets	1 (2.6 oz)	180	12	3	0
Battered Fish Nuggets	8 (4 oz)	280	20	6	0
Battered Fish Portions	2 pieces (5 oz)	350	26	5	0
Battered Fish Sticks	6 (4 oz)	260	18	4	0
Breaded Fillets	2 (3.5 oz)	280	17	2	0
Breaded Fish Portions	3 pieces (4.5 oz)	330	23	3	0
Breaded Fish Sticks	6 (4 oz)	290	23	3	0
Breaded Mini Fish Sticks	13 (3.3 oz)	250	19	2	0
Crisp & Healthy Breaded Fillets	2 (3.5 oz)	150	20	5	0
Crisp & Healthy Fish Sticks	6 (4 oz)	180	26	6	0
Fish 'n Fries	1 pkg (6.6 oz)	380	41	3	2
FISH PASTE					
fish paste	2 tsp	15	tr	—	0
FISH SUBSTITUTES					
Loma Linda					
Ocean Platter not prep	⅓ cup (0.9 oz)	90	8	0	4
Worthington					
Fillets	2 (3 oz)	180	8	tr	4
Tuno	½ cup (1.9 oz)	80	2	0	1
FLAXSEED					
Arrowhead					
Flaxseed	3 tbsp (1 oz)	140	11	0	6
Stone-Buhr					
Flaxseed	1 tsp (1 oz)	150	11	0	5
FLOUNDER					
FRESH					
cooked	1 fillet (4.5 oz)	148	0	0	0

FOOD	PORTION	CALS.	CARB.	SUG.	FIB.
FROZEN					
Van De Kamp's					
Lightly Breaded Fillets	1 (4 oz)	230	19	3	0
Natural Fillets	1 (4 oz)	110	0	0	0
FLOUR					
buckwheat whole groat	1 cup (4.2 oz)	402	85	—	12
corn masa	1 cup (4 oz)	416	87	—	11
rice brown	1 cup (5.5 oz)	574	121	—	7
rice white	1 cup (5.5 oz)	578	127	—	4
rye dark	1 cup (4.5 oz)	415	88	—	29
rye light	1 cup (3.6 oz)	374	82	—	15
rye medium	1 cup (3.6 oz)	361	79	—	15
triticale whole grain	1 cup (4.6 oz)	439	95	—	19
white all-purpose	1 cup (4.4 oz)	455	95	—	2
white bread	1 cup (4.8 oz)	495	99	—	3
white cake unsifted	1 cup (4.8 oz)	496	107	—	2
white self-rising	1 cup (4.4 oz)	443	93	—	3
white unbleached	1 cup (4.4 oz)	455	95	—	3
whole wheat	1 cup (4.2 oz)	407	87	—	15
Arrowhead					
Kamut	¼ cup (1.2 oz)	110	25	0	4
Pastry	⅓ cup (1.1 oz)	100	22	0	3
Rye Whole Grain	¼ cup (1.6 oz)	160	34	0	6
Spelt	¼ cup (1.2 oz)	100	24	0	5
Teff	¼ cup (1.4 oz)	140	29	0	5
Unbleached White	⅓ cup (1.6 oz)	160	33	0	0
Whole Grain Wheat	¼ cup (1.6 oz)	160	34	0	7
Whole Wheat	¼ cup (1.2 oz)	130	25	0	4
Aunt Jemima					
Self-Rising	3 tbsp	90	20	0	1
Gold Medal					
Whole Wheat	1 cup	350	78	—	10
Whole Wheat Blend	1 cup	380	84	—	8
Hodgson Mill					
50/50 Flour	¼ cup (1 oz)	100	21	0	2
Best For Bread	¼ cup (1 oz)	100	22	0	1
Buckwheat	⅓ cup (1.6 oz)	160	33	0	2
Oat Bran Blend	¼ cup (1 oz)	110	24	0	3
Oat Bran Flour	¼ cup (1 oz)	110	23	0	3
Rye	¼ cup (1 oz)	90	22	0	5
Seasoned Flour	¼ cup (1 oz)	90	20	0	0
White	¼ cup (1 oz)	100	23	0	3
Whole Wheat	¼ cup (1 oz)	100	22	0	3

FOOD	PORTION	CALS.	CARB.	SUG.	FIB.
King Arthur					
All Purpose Unbleached	¼ cup (1 oz)	100	22	1	tr
Robin Hood					
Rye Stone Ground	1 cup	360	86	—	13
Stone Ground Mills					
White Unbleached Organic	¼ cup (1.4 oz)	130	25	0	1
Whole Wheat 100% Stone Ground	3 tbsp (1 oz)	90	20	0	3

FRANKFURTER
(*see* HOT DOG)

FRENCH FRIES
(*see* POTATOES)

FRENCH TOAST
FROZEN

french toast	1 slice (2 oz)	126	19	—	2
Aunt Jemima					
Cinnamon Swirl	2 pieces (4.1 oz)	240	37	—	2
Slices	2 pieces (4.1 oz)	240	38	—	1

FROSTING
(*see* CAKE ICING)

FRUCTOSE
Estee

Fructose	1 tsp (4 g)	15	4	4	—
Packet	1 pkg (3 g)	10	3	3	—

FRUIT DRINKS
(*see also individual names,* LEMONADE)
FROZEN
Dole

100% Juice Blend Country Raspberry as prep	8 fl oz	140	34	28	0
100% Juice Blend Orchard Peach as prep	8 fl oz	140	34	28	0
Mountain Cherry 100% Juice Blend as prep	8 fl oz	120	30	28	0
Pineapple Grapefruit as prep	8 fl oz	130	29	25	0
Pineapple Orange as prep	8 fl oz	120	29	24	0
Pineapple Orange Banana as prep	8 fl oz	130	31	22	0
Pineapple Orange Guava as prep	8 fl oz	120	30	26	0

FOOD	PORTION	CALS.	CARB.	SUG.	FIB.
Dole (CONT.)					
Pineapple Passion Banana as prep	8 fl oz	120	30	24	0
Tropical Fruit as prep	8 fl oz	140	34	27	0
Five Alive					
Berry Citrus	8 fl oz	120	30	28	—
Citrus	8 fl oz	120	30	28	—
Tropical Citrus	8 fl oz	120	29	27	—
Minute Maid					
Berry Punch	8 fl oz	130	31	30	—
Citrus Punch	8 fl oz	120	31	30	—
Fruit Punch	8 fl oz	120	31	30	—
Limeade	8 fl oz	100	26	24	—
Pineapple Orange	8 fl oz	120	31	29	—
Tropical Punch	8 fl oz	120	31	30	—
Seneca					
Cranberry-Apple Juice Cocktail frzn as prep	8 fl oz	140	33	—	0
Raspberry- Cranberry Juice Cocktail frzn as prep	8 fl oz	140	36	—	0
MIX					
Crystal Light					
Fruit Punch as prep	1 serv (8 oz)	5	0	0	0
Lemon-Lime Drink as prep	1 serv (8 oz)	5	0	0	0
Passion Fruit Pineapple Drink as prep	1 serv (8 oz)	5	tr	0	0
Pineapple Orange Drink as prep	1 serv (8 oz)	5	0	0	0
Strawberry Orange Banana as prep	1 serv (8 oz)	5	0	0	0
Strawberry Kiwi as prep	1 serv (8 oz)	5	0	0	0
Watermelon Strawberry as prep	1 serv (8 oz)	5	0	0	0
Kool-Aid					
Cherry as prep	1 serv (8 oz)	60	16	16	0
Grape Berry Splash Drink as prep	1 serv (8 oz)	70	17	17	0
Grape Berry Splash Drink as prep w/ sugar	1 serv (8 oz)	100	25	25	0
Kickin' Kiwi Lime Drink as prep	1 serv (8 oz)	60	16	16	0
Kickin' Kiwi Lime Drink as prep w/ sugar	1 serv (8 oz)	100	25	25	0
Lemon-Lime Drink as prep w/ sugar	1 serv (8 oz)	100	25	25	0

FOOD	PORTION	CALS.	CARB.	SUG.	FIB.
Kool-Aid (CONT.)					
Man-O-Mango Berry Drink as prep	1 serv (8 oz)	60	16	16	0
Man-O-Mango Berry Drink as prep w/ sugar	1 serv (8 oz)	100	25	25	0
Oh Yeah Orange Pinapple Drink as prep w/ sugar	1 serv (8 oz)	100	25	25	0
Oh Yeah Orange Pineapple Drink as prep	1 serv (8 oz)	60	16	16	0
Pina-Pineapple Drink as prep	1 serv (8 oz)	60	17	17	0
Pina-Pineapple Drink as prep w/ sugar	1 serv (8 oz)	100	25	25	0
Rainbow Punch	8 oz	98	25	25	—
Roarin' Raspberry Cranberry Drink as prep	1 serv (8 oz)	70	17	17	0
Roarin' Raspberry Cranberry Drink as prep w/ sugar	1 serv (8 oz)	100	25	25	0
Slammin' Strawberry Kiwi Drink as prep	1 serv (8 oz)	70	17	17	0
Slammin' Strawberry Kiwi Drink as prep w/ sugar	1 serv (8 oz)	100	25	25	0
Strawberry Raspberry Drink as prep	1 serv (8 oz)	60	16	16	0
Strawberry Raspberry Drink as prep w/ sugar	1 serv (8 oz)	100	25	25	0
Sugar Free Tropical Punch as prep	1 serv (8 oz)	5	0	0	0
Tropical Punch as prep	1 serv (8 oz)	60	16	16	0
Tropical Punch as prep w/ sugar	1 serv (8 oz)	100	25	25	0
Watermelon Cherry Drink as prep	1 serv (8 oz)	60	16	16	0
Watermelon Cherry Drink as prep w/ sugar	1 serv (8 oz)	100	25	25	0
Tang					
Orange Pineapple as prep	1 serv (8 oz)	100	24	24	0
READY-TO-DRINK					
After The Fall					
Amaretto Almond	1 can (12 oz)	170	42	41	0
American Pie Cherry	1 can (12 oz)	190	35	34	0
Apple Apricot	1 cup (8 oz)	100	26	22	0
Apple Raspberry	1 bottle (10 oz)	110	29	24	—

FOOD	PORTION	CALS.	CARB.	SUG.	FIB.
After The Fall (CONT.)					
Apple Strawberry	1 bottle (10 oz)	120	30	24	—
Banana Casablanca	1 bottle (10 oz)	120	24	23	—
Berrymeister	1 can (12 oz)	160	40	35	0
Cranberry Meets Raspberry	1 bottle (10 oz)	120	29	24	—
Georgia Peach Blend	1 bottle (10 oz)	130	33	31	—
Mango Montage	1 bottle (10 oz)	140	33	29	—
Maui Grove	1 bottle (10 oz)	120	29	28	—
Nantucket Ginger Ale	1 can (12 oz)	140	35	33	0
Orange Icicle Cream	1 can (12 oz)	170	42	41	0
Oregon Berry	1 bottle (10 oz)	130	31	28	—
Passion Of The Islands	1 bottle (10 oz)	125	32	31	—
Peach Vanilla	1 can (12 oz)	170	42	35	0
Strawberry Vanilla	1 can (12 oz)	160	42	41	0
Twist O' Strawberry	1 can (12 oz)	190	37	34	0
Vanilla Bean Cream	1 can (12 oz)	170	42	41	0
Capri Sun					
Fruit Punch	1 pkg (7 oz)	100	26	26	0
Maui Punch	1 pkg (7 oz)	100	27	27	0
Mountain Cooler	1 pkg (7 oz)	90	24	24	0
Pacific Cooler	1 pkg (7 oz)	100	26	26	0
Red Berry	1 pkg (7 oz)	100	26	26	0
Safari Punch	1 pkg (7 oz)	100	25	25	0
Strawberry Kiwi Drink	1 pkg (7 oz)	100	26	26	0
Surfer Cooler Drink	1 pkg (7 oz)	100	27	27	0
Coco Lopez					
Mango Kiwi	8 fl oz	130	33	33	—
Crystal Geyser					
Juice Squeeze Citrus Grape	1 bottle (12 fl oz)	145	35	31	—
Juice Squeeze Orange & Passion Fruit	1 bottle (12 fl oz)	130	31	30	—
Juice Squeeze Passion Fruit & Mango	1 bottle (12 fl oz)	125	31	27	—
Juice Squeeze Wild Berry	1 bottle (12 fl oz)	130	31	30	—
Crystal Light					
Fruit Punch	1 serv (8 oz)	5	0	0	0
Kiwi Strawberry	1 serv (8 oz)	5	0	0	0
Orange Strawberry Banana Drink	1 serv (8 oz)	5	0	0	0
Everfresh					
Cranberry-Apple Drink	1 can (8 oz)	120	31	31	0
Grape-Strawberry	1 can (8 oz)	120	31	31	0
Kiwi-Strawberry	1 can (8 oz)	120	30	30	0
Mandarin Orange Mango Drink	1 can (8 oz)	120	29	29	0

FOOD	PORTION	CALS.	CARB.	SUG.	FIB.
Everfresh (CONT.)					
Orange Banana Strawberry Drink	1 can (8 oz)	120	30	30	0
Tropical Fruit Punch	1 can (8 oz)	120	30	30	0
Wild Blackberry Lime Drink	1 can (8 oz)	120	29	29	0
Five Alive					
Citrus	1 bottle (16 fl oz)	120	31	29	—
Citrus	1 can (11.5 fl oz)	170	43	41	—
Citrus Chilled	8 fl oz	120	30	28	—
Fresh Samantha					
Banana Strawberry	1 cup (8 oz)	148	36	—	2
Beta Yet	1 cup (8 oz)	98	24	—	2
Carrot Orange	1 cup (8 oz)	107	24	—	1
Colossal C	1 cup (8 oz)	116	30	—	2
Desperately Seeking C	1 cup (8 oz)	129	30	—	3
Protein Blast	1 cup (8 oz)	156	30	—	2
Spirulina Fruit Blend	1 cup (8 oz)	129	30	—	2
Strawberry Orange	1 cup (8 oz)	120	27	—	1
The Big Bang	1 cup (8 oz)	97	24	—	2
Fruitopia					
Fruit Integration	8 fl oz	110	29	29	—
Hi-C					
Boppin Berry Box	8.45 fl oz	140	33	33	—
Boppin' Berry	8 fl oz	130	32	31	—
Double Fruit Box	8.45 fl oz	130	32	32	—
Double Fruit Cooler	8 fl oz	130	31	30	—
Ecto Cooler	8 fl oz	130	32	31	—
Ecto Cooler	1 can (11.5 fl oz)	180	45	44	—
Ecto Cooler Box	8.45 fl oz	130	32	32	—
Fruit Punch	8 fl oz	130	32	31	—
Fruit Punch	1 can (11.5 fl oz)	190	46	45	—
Fruit Punch Box	8.45 fl oz	140	32	32	—
Fruity Bubble Gum	8 fl oz	120	30	30	—
Fruity Bubble Gum Box	8.45 fl oz	130	32	31	—
Hula Punch	8 fl oz	120	29	28	—
Hula Punch	1 can (11.5 fl oz)	170	42	41	—
Hula Punch Box	8.45 fl oz	120	30	29	—
Jammin' Apple Box	8.45 fl oz	130	33	32	—
Stompin' Banana Berry	8 fl oz	130	31	30	—
Stompin' Banana Berry Box	8.45 fl oz	130	32	31	—
Wild Berry	8 fl oz	120	30	30	—
Wild Berry Box	8.45 fl oz	130	32	31	—
Hood					
Natural Blenders Apple Cranberry Raspberry	1 cup (8 oz)	130	32	32	—

FOOD	PORTION	CALS.	CARB.	SUG.	FIB.
Hood (CONT.)					
Natural Blenders Apple Grape Cherry	1 cup (8 oz)	130	32	32	—
Natural Blenders Apple Peach Pear	1 cup (8 oz)	120	30	30	—
Natural Blenders Apple Wild Blueberry Strawberry	1 cup (8 oz)	120	30	30	—
Natural Blenders Pineapple Orange Kiwi	1 cup (8 oz)	120	30	30	—
Kool-Aid					
Bursts Great Bluedini	1 (7 oz)	100	24	24	0
Bursts Kickin' Kiwi Lime	1 (7 oz)	100	24	24	0
Bursts Oh Yeah Orange Pineapple	1 (7 oz)	100	24	24	0
Bursts Slammin' Strawberry Kiwi	1 (7 oz)	100	24	24	0
Bursts Tropical Punch	1 (7 oz)	100	24	24	0
Splash Grape Berry Punch	1 serv (8 oz)	120	31	31	0
Splash Kiwi Strawberry Drink	1 serv (8 oz)	110	29	29	0
Splash Tropical Punch	1 serv (8 oz)	120	31	31	0
Mauna La'i					
Island Guava Hawaiian Guava Fruit Juice Drink	8 fl oz	130	32	32	0
Mango & Hawaiian Guava Fruit Juice Drink	8 fl oz	130	33	33	0
Paradise Guava Hawaiian Guava & Passion Fruit Juice Drink	8 fl oz	130	32	32	0
Minute Maid					
Berry Punch Box	8.45 fl oz	130	31	30	—
Berry Punch Chilled	8 fl oz	130	31	30	—
Citrus Punch Chilled	8 fl oz	130	31	30	—
Fruit Punch Box	8.45 fl oz	120	31	30	—
Fruit Punch Chilled	8 fl oz	120	31	30	—
Juices To Go Citrus Punch	1 can (11.5 fl oz)	180	45	43	—
Juices To Go Citrus Punch	1 bottle (10 fl oz)	160	39	38	—
Juices To Go Concord Punch	1 can (11.5 fl oz)	180	46	45	—
Juices To Go Concord Punch	1 bottle (10 fl oz)	160	40	39	—
Juices To Go Concord Punch	1 bottle (16 fl oz)	130	32	31	—

FOOD	PORTION	CALS.	CARB.	SUG.	FIB.
Minute Maid (CONT.)					
Juices To Go Fruit Punch	1 can (11.5 fl oz)	180	44	43	—
Juices To Go Fruit Punch	1 bottle (10 fl oz)	160	39	37	—
Juices To Go Fruit Punch	1 bottle (16 fl oz)	120	31	30	—
Juices To Go Orange Blend	1 bottle (10 fl oz)	150	37	35	—
Juices To Go Orange Blend	1 can (11.5 fl oz)	170	43	40	—
Naturals Apple Cranberry	8 fl oz	170	42	40	—
Naturals Concord Medley	8 fl oz	130	32	31	—
Naturals Fruit Medley	8 fl oz	120	31	30	—
Naturals Orange Grape Medley	8 fl oz	120	30	27	—
Naturals Tropical Medley	8 fl oz	120	31	30	—
Tropical Punch Box	8.45 fl oz	130	32	31	—
Tropical Punch Chilled	8 fl oz	120	31	30	—
Mott's					
Apple Cranberry Blend	10 fl oz	180	44	34	0
Apple Cranberry From Concentrate as prep	8 fl oz	120	30	24	0
Apple Grape From Concentrate as prep	8 fl oz	120	30	24	0
Apple Raspberry Blend	10 fl oz	140	33	26	0
Apple Raspberry From Concentrate	8.45 fl oz	120	30	24	0
Fruit Basket Apple Raspberry Juice Cocktail as prep	8 fl oz	130	30	29	0
Fruit Basket Tropical Blend Juice Cocktail as prep	8 fl oz	120	30	29	0
Fruit Punch From Concentrate	8.45 fl oz	120	29	26	0
Fruit Punch From Concentrate	10 fl oz	170	42	33	0
Grape Apple	10 fl oz	170	41	32	0
Pineapple Orange	10 fl oz	170	42	34	0
Nantucket Nectars					
Orange Mango	8 fl oz	130	32	29	0
Ocean Spray					
Cran*Grape	8 fl oz	170	41	41	0
Cran*Raspberry	8 fl oz	140	36	36	0
Cran*Strawberry	8 fl oz	140	36	35	tr
Cranapple	8 fl oz	160	41	40	tr
Cranapple Reduced Calorie	8 fl oz	50	13	13	0
Fruit Punch	8 fl oz	130	32	32	0

FOOD	PORTION	CALS.	CARB.	SUG.	FIB.
Ocean Spray (CONT.)					
Kiwi Strawberry Cooler	8 fl oz	120	31	31	0
Ruby Red & Tangerine Grapefruit Juice Drink	8 fl oz	130	32	32	0
Odwalla					
Boyzenberry Mango	8 fl oz	140	34	29	2
C Monster	16 fl oz	300	72	68	4
Fruitshake Blackberry	8 fl oz	160	39	34	3
Guanaba Dabba Doo!	8 fl oz	130	29	23	0
Lotta Colada	8 fl oz	160	33	31	2
Mango Tango	8 fl oz	150	37	29	6
Mo Beta	16 fl oz	280	69	58	3
Raspberry Smoothie	8 fl oz	140	35	27	2
Strawberry Banana Smoothie	8 fl oz	100	26	23	2
Strawberry Go Man Go	8 fl oz	100	26	21	2
Super Protein	16 fl oz	400	40	19	5
Pek					
Mango Guava Ecstasy	1 bottle (20 fl oz)	110	27	25	0
Passionate Peach Grapefruit	8 fl oz	110	27	25	0
Shasta Plus					
Apple-Strawberry	1 can (11.5 oz)	160	41	41	0
Fruit Punch	1 can (11.5 oz)	160	39	39	0
Pineapple-Cherry	1 can (11.5 oz)	160	40	40	0
Smucker's					
Apple Cranberry	8 oz	120	32	—	—
Tropicana					
Berry Punch	8 fl oz	120	29	28	—
Citrus Punch	8 fl oz	140	36	33	—
Citrus Punch	1 bottle (10 fl oz)	180	45	41	—
Cranberry Punch	8 fl oz	140	34	33	—
Cranberry Punch	1 bottle (10 fl oz)	170	43	42	—
Cranberry Punch	1 can (11.5 fl oz)	200	49	48	—
Fruit Punch	1 container (10 fl oz)	160	39	38	—
Fruit Punch	8 fl oz	130	31	32	—
Fruit Punch	1 bottle (10 fl oz)	150	39	38	—
Fruit Punch	1 can (11.5 fl oz)	170	42	41	—
Orange Pineapple	8 fl oz	110	27	24	—
Orange Pineapple	1 bottle (10 fl oz)	130	32	30	—
Pineapple Punch	1 bottle (10 fl oz)	160	39	38	—

FOOD	PORTION	CALS.	CARB.	SUG.	FIB.
Tropicana (CONT.)					
Pineapple Punch	8 fl oz	120	31	30	—
Season's Best Cranberry Medley	8 fl oz	120	29	26	—
Tropics Apple Cranberry Kiwi	8 fl oz	120	30	28	—
Tropics Orange Strawberry Banana	8 fl oz	110	27	23	—
Tropics Orange Kiwi Passion	8 fl oz	100	26	23	—
Tropics Orange Peach Mango	8 fl oz	110	28	24	—
Tropics Orange Pineapple	8 fl oz	110	27	24	—
Tropics Pineapple Passion	8 fl oz	120	30	28	—
Twister Apple Raspberry Blackberry	1 can (11.5 fl oz)	180	44	40	—
Twister Apple Raspberry Blackberry	8 fl oz	120	31	28	—
Twister Apple Raspberry Blackberry	1 bottle (10 fl oz)	150	38	34	—
Twister Cranberry Raspberry Strawberry	8 fl oz	120	31	28	—
Twister Cranberry Raspberry Strawberry	1 bottle (10 fl oz)	160	39	34	—
Twister Light Cranberry Raspberry Strawberry	8 fl oz	45	11	9	—
Twister Light Cranberry Raspberry Strawberry	1 container (10 fl oz)	50	13	11	—
Twister Light Orange Cranberry	8 fl oz	30	7	4	—
Twister Light Orange Cranberry	1 container (10 fl oz)	35	9	6	—
Twister Light Orange Cranberry	1 container (10 fl oz)	35	9	6	—
Twister Light Orange Raspberry	8 fl oz	35	9	7	—
Twister Light Orange Raspberry	1 container (10 fl oz)	45	11	9	—
Twister Light Orange Strawberry Banana	1 container (10 fl oz)	45	11	8	—
Twister Orange Cranberry	8 fl oz	120	29	27	—
Twister Orange Cranberry	1 bottle (10 fl oz)	140	36	34	—
Twister Orange Peach	8 fl oz	120	29	26	—

FOOD	PORTION	CALS.	CARB.	SUG.	FIB.
Tropicana (CONT.)					
Twister Orange Peach	1 bottle (10 fl oz)	140	36	33	—
Twister Orange Peach	1 can (11.5 fl oz)	160	41	38	—
Twister Orange Raspberry	1 bottle (10 fl oz)	140	36	34	—
Twister Orange Raspberry	8 fl oz	120	29	27	—
Twister Orange Strawberry Banana	1 container (10 fl oz)	140	35	32	—
Twister Strawberry Banana	1 bottle (10 fl oz)	140	35	32	—
Twister Strawberry Banana	1 can (11.5 fl oz)	160	41	37	—
Twister Strawberry Banana	8 fl oz	120	29	26	—
Twister Strawberry Guava	8 fl oz	110	28	25	—
Twister Strawberry Guava	1 bottle (10 fl oz)	140	35	31	—
Veryfine					
Apple Cherryberry	8 fl oz	130	33	—	—
Apple Cranberry	1 bottle (10 oz)	190	48	48	0
Apple Quenchers Black Cherry White Grape	8 fl oz	120	30	30	0
Apple Quenchers Cranberry Tangerine	8 fl oz	120	31	31	0
Apple Quenchers Peach Kiwi	8 fl oz	130	33	31	0
Apple Quenchers Peach Plum	8 fl oz	130	32	31	0
Apple Quenchers Pear Passionfruit	8 fl oz	120	31	29	0
Apple Quenchers Raspberry Cherry	8 fl oz	120	31	30	0
Apple Quenchers Raspberry Lime	8 fl oz	120	30	30	0
Apple Quenchers Strawberry Banana	8 fl oz	120	30	29	0
Chillers Artic Mango Tangerine	8 fl oz	110	27	24	tr
Chillers Freezing Fruit Punch	8 fl oz	130	33	33	0
Chillers Lemon Lime Blizzard	8 fl oz	120	29	29	0
Chillers Shivering Strawberry Melon	1 can (11.5 oz)	160	41	40	0
Chillers Tropical Freeze	8 fl oz	120	30	29	0
Cranberry Raspberry	8 fl oz	160	41	41	0
Fruit Punch	1 bottle (10 oz)	170	42	41	0

FOOD	PORTION	CALS.	CARB.	SUG.	FIB.
Veryfine (CONT.)					
Juice-Ups Berry	8 fl oz	140	34	34	0
Juice-Ups Fruit Punch	8 fl oz	140	34	34	0
Juice-Ups Orange Punch	8 fl oz	140	35	35	0
Orange Strawberry	8 fl oz	120	31	31	0
Papaya Punch	1 bottle (10 oz)	160	39	38	0
Pineapple Orange	1 bottle (10 oz)	160	39	38	0
Strawberry Banana	1 can (1l.5 oz)	160	40	40	0
Strawberry Banana Punch	1 can (11.5 oz)	190	48	47	0
White House					
Apple Cherry	6 fl oz	90	22	—	0

FRUIT MIXED
(*see also individual names*)

CANNED

FOOD	PORTION	CALS.	CARB.	SUG.	FIB.
Del Monte					
Fruit Cocktail Fruit Naturals	½ cup (4.4 oz)	60	15	14	1
Fruit Cocktail In Heavy Syrup	½ cup (4.5 oz)	100	24	23	1
Fruit Cocktail Lite	½ cup (4.4 oz)	60	15	14	1
Lite Mixed Fruits Chunky	½ cup (4.4 oz)	60	15	14	1
Mixed Fruits Chunky Fruit Naturals	½ cup (4.4 oz)	60	15	14	1
Mixed Fruits Chunky In Heavy Syrup	½ cup (4.5 oz)	100	24	23	1
Snack Cups Mixed Fruit Fruit Naturals	1 serv (4.5 oz)	60	16	15	1
Snack Cups Mixed Fruit Fruit Naturals EZ-Open Lid	1 serv (4.5 oz)	60	15	14	1
Snack Cups Mixed Fruit In Heavy Syrup	1 serv (4.5 oz)	100	24	23	1
Snack Cups Mixed Fruit In Heavy Syrup EZ-Open Lid	1 serv (4.2 oz)	90	23	22	1
Snack Cups Mixed Fruit Lite	1 serv (4.5 oz)	60	16	15	1
Snack Cups Mixed Fruit Lite EZ-Open Lid	1 serv (4.5 oz)	60	15	14	1
Hunt's					
Fruit Cocktail	½ cup (4.5 oz)	90	23	22	1
Libby					
Chunky Mixed Lite	½ cup (4.3 oz)	60	14	12	1
Fruit Cocktail Lite	½ cup (4.3 oz)	60	15	11	1

FOOD	PORTION	CALS.	CARB.	SUG.	FIB.
Mott's					
Fruitsations Mixed Berry	1 pkg (4 oz)	90	22	20	1
DRIED					
Del Monte					
Mixed	⅓ cup (1.4 oz)	110	30	17	5
Planters					
Fruit'n Nut Mix	1 oz	140	13	8	2
Sonoma					
Diced	⅓ cup (1.4 oz)	120	31	8	3
Mixed Fruit	5-8 pieces (1.4 oz)	120	30	9	3
FROZEN					
Big Valley					
Burst O' Berries	⅔ cup (4.9 oz)	70	16	6	3
California Tropics	⅔ cup (4.9 oz)	60	15	8	2
Cup A Fruit	1 pkg (4 oz)	50	7	10	2
Mixed	4.9 oz	60	14	8	2
Birds Eye					
Mixed Fruit	½ cup (4.4 oz)	90	23	21	—
FRUIT SNACKS					
Betty Crocker					
Fruit Roll-Ups Peel 'N Build	2 rolls (1 oz)	110	24	10	—
Brock					
Beauty & The Beast	1 pkg (0.9 oz)	90	21	14	—
Cinderella	1 pkg (0.9 oz)	90	21	14	—
Dinosaurs	1 pkg (0.9 oz)	90	21	14	—
Ninja Trolls	1 pkg (0.9 oz)	90	21	14	—
Sharks	1 pkg (0.9 oz)	90	21	14	—
Del Monte					
Sierra Trail Mix	¼ cup (1.2 oz)	150	20	17	3
Sierra Trail Mix	1 pkg (1 oz)	120	16	13	2
Sierra Trail Mix	1 pkg (0.9 oz)	110	15	13	2
Favorite Brands					
Cherry Fruit Snack	1 pkg (0.9 oz)	80	19	14	—
Creepy Crawler Fruit Snacks	1 pkg (0.9 oz)	80	19	14	—
Dinosaur Fruit Snack	1 pkg (0.9 oz)	80	19	14	—
Grape Fruit Snack	1 pkg (0.9 oz)	80	19	13	—
Space Alien Fruit Snack	1 pkg (0.9 oz)	80	19	14	—
Sports Fruit Snacks	1 pkg (0.9 oz)	80	19	14	—
Strawberry Fruit Snack	1 pkg (0.9 oz)	80	19	14	—
Teenage Mutant Ninja Turtle Fruit Snacks	1 pkg (0.9 oz)	80	19	14	—
The Mega Roll Strawberry	1 pkg (1 oz)	110	22	14	2

FOOD	PORTION	CALS.	CARB.	SUG.	FIB.
Favorite Brands (CONT.)					
The Roll Cherry	1 pkg (0.75 oz)	80	16	10	1
The Roll Strawberry	1 pkg (0.75 oz)	80	16	10	1
Troll Fruit Snacks	1 pkg (0.9 oz)	80	19	14	0
Zoo Animal Fruit Snacks	1 pkg (0.9 oz)	80	19	14	—
Health Valley					
Bakes Apple	1 bar	100	16	—	3
Bakes Date	1 bar	100	16	—	3
Bakes Raisin	1 bar	100	16	—	3
Fat Free Fruit Bars 100% Organic Apple	1 bar	140	33	—	4
Fat Free Fruit Bars 100% Organic Apricot	1 bar	140	33	—	4
Fat Free Fruit Bars 100% Organic Date	1 bar	140	33	—	4
Fat Free Fruit Bars 100% Organic Raisin	1 bar	140	33	—	4
Fruit & Fitness Bars	2 bars	200	35	—	5
Oat Bran Bakes Apricot	1 bar	100	16	—	2
Oat Bran Bakes Fig & Nut	1 bar	110	16	—	2
Oat Bran Jumbo Fruit Bar Almond & Date	1 bar	170	28	—	7
Oat Bran Jumbo Fruit Bars Raisin & Cinnamon	1 bar	160	32	—	6
Rice Bran Jumbo Fruit Bars Almond & Date	1 bar	160	27	—	4
Seneca					
Apple Chips	12 chips (1 oz)	140	20	11	2
Sensible Foods					
Crackin' Fruit Cherry Berry	1 pkg (0.6 oz)	51	13	14	1
Crackin' Fruit Tropical Fruit	1 pkg (0.6 oz)	65	16	14	1
Sonoma					
Trail Mix	¼ cup (1.4 oz)	160	24	19	2
Sovex					
Fruit Bites Jungle Pals	1 pkg (0.9 oz)	90	21	—	—
Stretch Island					
Fruit Leather Chunky Cherry	2 pieces (1 oz)	90	24	22	2
Fruit Leather Great Grape	2 pieces (1 oz)	90	24	21	2
Fruit Leather Organic Apple	2 pieces (1 oz)	90	24	26	2
Fruit Leather Organic Grape	2 pieces (1 oz)	90	24	22	2
Fruit Leather Organic Raspberry	2 pieces (1 oz)	90	25	24	2
Fruit Leather Rare Raspberry	2 pieces (1 oz)	90	24	23	2

FOOD	PORTION	CALS.	CARB.	SUG.	FIB.
Stretch Island (CONT.)					
Fruit Leather Snappy Apple	2 pieces (1 oz)	90	25	18	3
Fruit Leather Tangy Apricot	2 pieces (1 oz)	90	23	14	2
Fruit Leather Truly Tropical	2 pieces (1 oz)	90	22	19	1
Sunbelt					
Fruit Boosters Apple	1 (1.3 oz)	130	27	20	0
Fruit Boosters Blueberry	1 (1.3 oz)	130	27	19	1
Fruit Boosters Strawberry	1 (1.3 oz)	130	27	19	0
Fruit Jammers	1 (1 oz)	100	23	19	0
Weight Watchers					
Apple & Cinnamon	1 pkg (0.5 oz)	50	13	9	2
Apple Chips	1 pkg (0.75 oz)	70	18	13	3
Peach & Strawberry	1 pkg (0.5 oz)	50	13	11	2

GARBANZO
(*see* CHICKPEAS)

GARLIC

FOOD	PORTION	CALS.	CARB.	SUG.	FIB.
powder	1 tsp	9	2	—	—
Watkins					
Garlic & Chive Seasoning	1 tbsp (7 g)	25	2	0	0
Garlic Lover's Herb Blend	¼ tsp (0.5 oz)	0	0	0	0
Liquid Spice	1 tbsp (0.5 oz)	120	0	0	0

GELATIN
MIX

FOOD	PORTION	CALS.	CARB.	SUG.	FIB.
low calorie	½ cup	8	0	—	0
mix artificially sweetened as prep	½ cup (4.1 oz)	8	1	tr	—
mix artificially sweetened as prep	1 pkg 4 serv (16.5 oz)	33	3	tr	—
mix as prep	½ cup (4.7 oz)	80	19	11	—
mix as prep	1 pkg 4 serv (19 oz)	319	76	43	—
Emes					
Kosher-Jel Plain	1 tbsp (7 g)	21	5	—	1
Jell-O					
1-2-3-Brand Strawberry as prep	⅔ cup (5.2 oz)	130	26	22	0
Apricot as prep	½ cup (5 oz)	80	19	19	0
Berry Black as prep	½ cup (5 oz)	80	19	19	0
Berry Blue as prep	½ cup (5 oz)	80	19	19	0
Black Cherry as prep	½ cup (5 oz)	80	19	19	0
Cherry as prep	½ cup (5 oz)	80	19	19	0
Cranberry Raspberry as prep	½ cup (5 oz)	80	19	19	0

FOOD	PORTION	CALS.	CARB.	SUG.	FIB.
Jell-O (CONT.)					
Cranberry Strawberry as prep	½ cup (5 oz)	80	19	19	0
Cranberry as prep	½ cup (5 oz)	80	19	19	0
Grape as prep	½ cup (5 oz)	80	19	19	0
Lemon as prep	½ cup (5 oz)	80	19	19	0
Lime as prep	½ cup (5 oz)	80	19	19	0
Mango as prep	½ cup (5 oz)	80	19	19	0
Mixed Fruit as prep	½ cup (5 oz)	80	19	19	tr
Orange as prep	½ cup (5 oz)	80	19	19	0
Peach as prep	½ cup (5 oz)	80	19	19	0
Peach Passion Fruit as prep	½ cup (5 oz)	80	19	19	0
Pineapple as prep	½ cup (5 oz)	80	19	19	0
Raspberry as prep	½ cup (5 oz)	80	19	19	0
Sparkling White Grape as prep	½ cup (5 oz)	80	19	19	0
Strawberry Banana as prep	½ cup (5 oz)	80	19	19	0
Strawberry Kiwi as prep	½ cup (5 oz)	80	19	19	0
Strawberry as prep	½ cup (5 oz)	80	19	19	0
Sugar Free Cherry as prep	½ cup (4.2 oz)	10	0	0	0
Sugar Free Cranberry as prep	½ cup (4.2 oz)	10	0	0	0
Sugar Free Lemon	½ cup (4.2 oz)	10	0	0	0
Sugar Free Lime as prep	½ cup (4.2 oz)	10	0	0	0
Sugar Free Mixed Fruit as prep	½ cup (4.2 oz)	10	0	0	0
Sugar Free Orange as prep	½ cup (4.2 oz)	10	0	0	0
Sugar Free Raspberry as prep	½ cup (4.2 oz)	10	0	0	0
Sugar Free Strawberry Banana as prep	½ cup (4.2 oz)	10	0	0	0
Sugar Free Strawberry as prep	½ cup (4.2 oz)	10	0	0	0
Sugar Free Strawberry Kiwi as prep	½ cup (4.2 oz)	10	0	0	0
Sugar Free Watermelon as prep	½ cup (4.2 oz)	10	0	0	0
Watermelon as prep	½ cup (5 oz)	80	19	19	0
Wild Strawberry as prep	½ cup (5 oz)	80	19	19	0
Kojel					
Diet	1 serv	10	4	—	—
READY-TO-EAT					
Del Monte					
Gel Snack Cups Blue Berry	1 serv (3.5 oz)	70	19	19	tr

FOOD	PORTION	CALS.	CARB.	SUG.	FIB.
Del Monte (CONT.)					
Gel Snack Cups Cherry	1 serv (3.5 oz)	70	19	19	tr
Gel Snack Cups Orange	1 serv (3.5 oz)	70	19	19	tr
Gel Snack Cups Strawberry	1 serv (3.5 oz)	70	19	19	tr
Handi-Snacks					
Gels Blue Raspberry	1 serv (4 oz)	80	20	20	0
Gels Cherry	1 serv (4 oz)	80	20	20	0
Gels Orange	1 serv (3.5 oz)	80	20	20	0
Gels Strawberry	1 serv (3.5 oz)	80	20	20	0
Hunt's					
Snack Pack Juicy Gels Cherry	1 (4 oz)	100	25	24	0
Snack Pack Juicy Gels Lemon Lime	1 (4 oz)	100	25	24	0
Snack Pack Juicy Gels Mixed Fruit	1 (4 oz)	100	25	24	0
Snack Pack Juicy Gels Orange	1 (4 oz)	100	25	24	0
Snack Pack Juicy Gels Strawberry	1 (4 oz)	100	25	24	0
Jell-O					
Berry Black	1 serv (3.5 oz)	70	17	17	0
Berry Blue	1 serv (3.5 oz)	70	17	17	0
Cherry	1 serv (3.5 oz)	70	17	17	0
Orange	1 serv (3.5 oz)	70	17	17	0
Orange Strawberry Banana	1 serv (3.5 oz)	70	17	17	0
Raspberry	1 serv (3.5 oz)	70	17	17	0
Rhymin' Lymon	1 serv (3.5 oz)	70	17	17	0
Strawberry	1 serv (3.5 oz)	70	17	17	0
Strawberry Kiwi	1 serv (3.5 oz)	10	0	0	0
Sugar Free Orange	1 serv (3.2 oz)	10	0	0	0
Sugar Free Raspberry	1 serv (3.2 oz)	10	0	0	0
Sugar Free Strawberry	1 serv (3.2 oz)	10	0	0	0
Tropical Berry	1 serv (3.5 oz)	10	0	0	0
Tropical Fruit Punch	1 serv (3.5 oz)	70	17	17	0
Wild Watermelon	1 serv (3.5 oz)	70	17	17	0
Kozy Shack					
Gel Treat Cherry	1 pkg (4 oz)	100	25	23	1
Gel Treat Lemon Lime	1 pkg (4 oz)	100	25	23	1
Gel Treat Orange	1 pkg (4 oz)	100	25	23	1
Gel Treat Strawberry	1 pkg (4 oz)	100	25	23	1
Gel Treat Sugar Free Orange	1 pkg (4 oz)	10	2	1	1
Gel Treat Sugar Free Strawberry	1 pkg (4 oz)	10	2	1	1

FOOD	PORTION	CALS.	CARB.	SUG.	FIB.
GIBLETS					
capon simmered	1 cup (5 oz)	238	0	0	0
GINGER					
ground	1 tsp (1.8 g)	6	1	—	—
root fresh	5 slices	8	2	—	—
Ka-Me					
Crystallized Slices	5 pieces (1 oz)	100	25	24	1
Sliced	20 pieces (0.5 oz)	0	0	1	0
GOAT					
roasted	3 oz	122	0	0	0
GOOSE					
w/ skin roasted	½ goose (1.7 lbs)	2362	0	0	0
w/ skin roasted	6.6 oz	574	0	0	0
w/o skin roasted	5 oz	340	0	0	0
w/o skin roasted	½ goose (1.3 lbs)	1406	0	0	0
GRANOLA					
BARS					
(*see also* CEREAL BARS, NUTRITIONAL SUPPLEMENTS)					
almond	1 (1 oz)	140	18	1	—
almond	1 (0.8 oz)	117	15	1	—
chewy chocolate coated chocolate chip	1 (1 oz)	132	18	—	1
chewy chocolate coated chocolate chip	1 (1.25 oz)	165	23	—	1
chewy raisin	1 (1 oz)	127	19	—	1
chewy raisin	1 (1.5 oz)	191	28	—	2
chocolate chip	1 (0.8 oz)	103	17	7	1
chocolate chip	1 (1 oz)	124	20	8	1
chocolate chip chewy	1 (1 oz)	119	10	13	1
chocolate chip chewy	1 (1.5 oz)	178	29	20	2
chocolate chip graham & marshmallow chewy	1 (1 oz)	121	20	—	1
nut & raisin chewy	1 (1 oz)	129	18	—	2
peanut	1 (1 oz)	136	18	8	—
peanut	1 (0.8 oz)	113	15	6	1
peanut butter	1 (0.8 oz)	114	15	5	—
peanut butter	1 (1 oz)	137	18	6	—
peanut butter chewy	1 (1 oz)	121	18	10	1
peanut butter & chocolate chip chewy	1 (1 oz)	122	18	—	1
plain	1 (1 oz)	134	18	7	2
plain	(0.9 oz)	115	19	6	1
plain chewy	1 (1 oz)	126	19	—	1

FOOD	PORTION	CALS.	CARB.	SUG.	FIB.
Carnation					
Chocolate Chunk	1 (1.26 oz)	140	23	10	1
Honey & Oats	1 (1.26 oz)	130	23	9	1
Fi-Bar					
Coconut	1	120	20	—	6
Peanut Butter	1	130	20	—	6
General Mills					
Nature Valley Cinnnamon	1	120	17	6	1
Nature Valley Oat Bran Honey Graham	1	110	16	6	1
Nature Valley Oats N'Honey	1	120	17	6	1
Nature Valley Peanut Butter	1	120	15	6	1
Nature Valley Rice Bran Cinnamon Graham	1	90	13	6	1
Grist Mill					
Chewy Apple Cinnamon	1 (1 oz)	120	21	9	1
Chewy Chocolate Chip	1 (1 oz)	130	21	10	1
Chewy Chunky Nut & Raisin	1 (1 oz)	130	18	9	1
Chewy Peanut Butter	1 (1 oz)	130	20	10	1
Chewy Peanut Butter Chocolate	1 (1 oz)	130	20	10	2
Chocolate Snack Chocolate Chip	1 (1.2 oz)	180	21	14	1
Chocolate Snack Nutty Fudge	1 (1.3 oz)	190	19	13	2
Crunchy Cinnamon	1 (0.8 oz)	110	16	7	1
Crunchy Oats 'N Honey	1 (0.8 oz)	110	15	7	1
Kudos					
Chocolate Chunk	1 (0.7 oz)	90	13	5	1
Chocolate Coated Chocolate Chip	1 (1 oz)	120	18	11	1
Chocolate Coated Milk & Cookies	1 (1 oz)	130	18	13	1
Chocolate Coated Nutty Fudge	1 (1 oz)	130	18	13	1
Chocolate Coated Peanut Butter	1 (1 oz)	130	18	11	1
Low Fat Blueberry	1 (0.7 oz)	90	15	7	1
Low Fat Strawberry	1 (0.7 oz)	80	15	7	1
Nature Valley					
Low Fat Chewy Chocolate Chip	1 bar (1 oz)	110	21	—	2
Nature's Choice					
Carob Chip	1 bar (0.7 oz)	80	16	8	2

FOOD	PORTION	CALS.	CARB.	SUG.	FIB.
Nature's Choice (CONT.)					
Cinnamon & Raisin	1 bar (0.7 oz)	80	16	7	3
Oats 'n Honey	1 bar (0.7 oz)	80	15	7	2
Peanut Butter	1 bar (0.7 oz)	80	14	7	2
Quaker					
Chewy Chocolate Chip	1	128	19	—	1
Chewy Chunky Nut & Raisin	1	131	17	—	2
Chewy Cinnamon Raisin	1	128	19	—	1
Chewy Honey & Oats	1	125	19	—	1
Chewy Peanut Butter	1	128	18	—	1
Chewy Peanut Butter Chocolate Chip	1	131	17	—	1
Dipps Caramel Nut	1	148	21	—	1
Dipps Chocolate Chip	1	139	19	—	1
Dipps Peanut Butter	1	170	9	—	1
Sunbelt					
Chewy Chocolate Chip	1 (1.25 oz)	160	23	15	2
Chewy Chocolate Chip	1 (1.8 oz)	220	32	21	2
Chewy Oats & Honey	1 (1 oz)	130	19	11	1
Chewy Oats & Honey	1 (1.7 oz)	210	32	19	2
Chewy With Almonds	1 (1 oz)	130	17	10	2
Chewy With Almonds	1 (1.5 oz)	190	25	15	2
Chewy With Raisins	1 (1.2 oz)	150	25	16	2
Fudge Dipped Chewy Chocolate Chip	1 (1.5 oz)	190	28	18	2
Fudge Dipped Chewy Macaroo	1 bar (2 oz)	280	32	21	3
Fudge Dipped Chewy Macaroo	1 (1.4 oz)	200	22	14	2
Fudge Dipped Chewy With Peanuts	1 bar (1.5 oz)	210	24	15	2
Fudge Dipped Chewy With Peanuts	1 (2 oz)	270	32	22	2
CEREAL					
granola	½ cup (2.1 oz)	285	32	—	6
Erewhon					
With Bran	1 oz	130	17	—	4
Good Shepherd					
Crunchy	1 oz	130	19	—	2
Honey Almond	1 oz	120	20	—	2
Organic 5 Grain Muesli	1 oz	160	27	—	3
Organic Brown Rice	1 oz	130	16	—	4
Organic Wheat Free	1 oz	90	39	—	2

FOOD	PORTION	CALS.	CARB.	SUG.	FIB.
Good Shepherd (CONT.)					
Organic Wheat Free Apple Cinnamon	1 oz	125	20	—	3
Organic Wheat Free Blueberry Amaranth	1 oz	110	22	—	2
Organic Wheat Free Strawberry Amaranth	1 oz	110	22	—	2
Grist Mill					
Low-Fat With Raisins	⅔ cup (1.9 oz)	220	42	14	3
Kellogg's					
Low Fat	½ cup (1.7 oz)	190	39	14	3
Low Fat With Raisins	⅔ cup (2.1 oz)	220	47	16	3
Nature Valley					
100% Natural Oat Cinnamon & Raisin	¾ cup (1.9 oz)	240	38	14	3
100% Natural Oat Fruit & Nut	⅔ cup (1.9 oz)	250	34	13	3
Low Fat Fruit	⅔ cup (1.9 oz)	210	44	19	3
Stone-Buhr					
Hot Apple	⅓ cup (1.6 oz)	153	31	3	5
Sun Country					
100% Natural With Almonds	¼ cup	130	19	—	1
100% Natural With Raisins & Dates	¼ cup	123	20	—	2
With Raisins	¼ cup	125	19	—	2
Sunbelt					
Banana Nut	1.9 oz	250	37	13	4
Fruit & Nut	1.9 oz	230	38	18	4
Low Fat	1.9 oz	200	42	20	4
Uncle Roy's					
Cashew Raisin	½ cup (1.6 oz)	180	32	6	3
Fat Free Apple Cinnamon	½ cup (1.6 oz)	175	38	11	3
Fat Free Wild Cherry	½ cup (1.6 oz)	175	38	11	3
Fruit & Nut	½ cup (1.6 oz)	175	30	8	3
Low Fat Berries Jubilee	½ cup (1.6 oz)	175	34	10	3
Low Fat Crispy	½ cup (1.4 oz)	160	31	9	3
Low Fat Luscious Raspberry	½ cup (1.6 oz)	175	34	10	3
Low Fat True Blueberry	½ cup (1.6 oz)	175	34	10	3
Maple Date Nut	½ cup (1.6 oz)	180	29	5	3
Nut Butter & Almonds	½ cup (1.6 oz)	195	29	5	3
Organic Golden Honey	½ cup (1.6 oz)	190	30	8	3
Organic Maple Nut'N Rice	½ cup (1.4 oz)	170	27	6	3

FOOD	PORTION	CALS.	CARB.	SUG.	FIB.
Uncle Roy's (CONT.)					
Organic Maple Raisin	½ cup (1.6 oz)	190	30	6	3
GRAPE JUICE					
Bright & Early					
Frozen	8 fl oz	140	34	33	—
Capri Sun					
Drink	1 pkg (7 oz)	100	25	25	0
Everfresh					
Juice	1 can (8 oz)	150	38	38	0
Hi-C					
Box	8.45 fl oz	130	33	33	—
Drink	8 fl oz	130	32	31	—
Drink	1 can (11.5 fl oz)	180	46	45	—
Kool-Aid					
Bursts Grape Drink	1 (7 oz)	100	25	25	0
Drink as prep w/ sugar	1 serv (8 oz)	100	25	25	0
Drink Mix as prep	1 serv (8 oz)	60	16	16	0
Sugar Free Drink Mix as prep	1 serv (8 oz)	5	0	0	0
Minute Maid					
Chilled	8 fl oz	130	33	32	—
Grape Punch frzn	8 fl oz	130	32	31	—
Punch Chilled	8 fl oz	130	32	31	—
Mott's					
Drink	10 fl oz	170	42	36	0
Fruit Basket Cocktail as prep	8 fl oz	130	32	31	0
Seneca					
Blush Grape Juice frzn as prep	8 fl oz	170	39	—	0
Fortified With Vitamin C frzn as prep	8 fl oz	170	39	—	0
Sweetened frzn as prep	8 fl oz	140	39	—	0
White Grape Juice frzn as prep	8 fl oz	140	33	—	0
Shasta Plus					
Grape Drink	1 can (11.5 oz)	160	39	39	0
Tropicana					
Season's Best	8 fl oz	160	39	36	—
Veryfine					
100% Juice	1 bottle (10 oz)	200	47	43	0
Chillers Glacial Grape	1 can (11.5 oz)	160	41	41	0

FOOD	PORTION	CALS.	CARB.	SUG.	FIB.
Veryfine (CONT.)					
Grape Drink	1 bottle (10 oz)	160	41	37	0
Juice-Ups	8 fl oz	130	32	32	0

GRAPE LEAVES

FOOD	PORTION	CALS.	CARB.	SUG.	FIB.
canned	1 (4 g)	3	tr	—	0
fresh raw	1 (3 g)	3	1	—	tr
Cedar's					
Grape Leaves Stuffed With Rice	6 pieces (4.9 oz)	180	22	—	8

GRAPEFRUIT

FOOD	PORTION	CALS.	CARB.	SUG.	FIB.
pink	½	37	9	—	1
pink sections	1 cup	69	18	—	1
white	½	39	10	—	1
white sections	1 cup	76	19	—	1
Dole					
Fresh	½	50	14	—	6

GRAPEFRUIT JUICE

FOOD	PORTION	CALS.	CARB.	SUG.	FIB.
After The Fall					
Pink	1 bottle (10 oz)	100	23	19	—
Apple & Eve					
Made In The Shade Ruby Red	8 fl oz	130	32	32	—
Crystal Geyser					
Juice Squeeze	1 bottle (12 fl oz)	150	36	31	—
Del Monte					
Juice	8 fl oz	100	24	20	1
Everfresh					
Juice	1 can (8 oz)	90	22	22	0
Ruby Red Cocktail	1 can (8 oz)	130	32	32	0
Fresh Samantha					
Juice	1 cup (8 oz)	101	24	—	tr
Hood					
Select	1 cup (8 oz)	100	23	23	—
Minute Maid					
Frozen	8 fl oz	100	23	19	—
Juices To Go	1 can (11.5 oz)	140	33	28	—
Juices To Go	1 bottle (10 fl oz)	120	29	24	—
Juices To Go	1 bottle (16 fl oz)	100	23	19	—
Juices To Go Pink Cocktail	1 bottle (10 fl oz)	140	34	31	—
Juices To Go Pink Cocktail	1 bottle (16 fl oz)	110	27	25	—
Juices to Go Pink Cocktail	8 fl oz	160	39	36	—

FOOD	PORTION	CALS.	CARB.	SUG.	FIB.
Mott's					
From Concentrate as prep	8 fl oz	120	27	20	0
Ocean Spray					
100% Juice	8 oz	100	24	23	tr
Pink Juice Cocktail	8 oz	110	28	28	0
Ruby Red Drink	8 oz	130	33	33	0
Odwalla					
Juice	8 fl oz	90	20	16	—
Tree Of Life					
Juice	8 fl oz	100	26	16	0
Tropicana					
Juice	8 fl oz	90	23	18	—
Juice	1 container (6 fl oz)	80	19	15	—
Ruby Red	8 fl oz	100	25	20	—
Ruby Red	1 container (10 fl oz)	120	30	25	—
Season's Best	1 bottle (10 fl oz)	110	27	23	—
Season's Best	1 bottle (7 fl oz)	80	19	16	—
Season's Best	8 fl oz	90	22	18	—
Season's Best	1 can (11.5 fl oz)	120	31	27	—
Twister Light Pink	8 fl oz	40	10	8	—
Twister Light Pink	1 container (10 fl oz)	50	12	10	—
Twister Pink	1 can (11.5 fl oz)	160	40	35	—
Twister Pink	8 fl oz	110	28	25	—
Twister Pink	1 container (10 fl oz)	140	35	31	—
Veryfine					
100% Juice	1 bottle (10 oz)	110	25	21	0
Pink	1 bottle (10 oz)	150	38	34	0
Ruby Red	8 fl oz	120	29	27	0
GRAPES					
FRESH					
grapes	10	36	9	—	tr
Dole					
Grapes	1½ cup	85	24	—	2
GRAVY					
(see also SAUCE)					
CANNED					
Rudy's Farm					
Sausage Gravy	¼ cup (2 oz)	50	7	0	0
MIX					
Bovril					
Extract	1 heaping tsp	9	tr	—	0

FOOD	PORTION	CALS.	CARB.	SUG.	FIB.
Durkee					
Au Jus as prep	¼ cup	5	1	0	0
Brown as prep	¼ cup	10	3	0	0
Brown Herb as prep	¼ cup	15	3	0	0
Brown Mushroom as prep	¼ cup	15	3	0	0
Brown Onion as prep	¼ cup	15	4	0	0
Chicken as prep	¼ cup	20	4	0	0
Country as prep	¼ cup	35	5	1	0
Homestyle as prep	¼ cup	15	3	0	0
Mushroom as prep	¼ cup	15	3	0	0
Onion as prep	¼ cup	10	3	0	0
Pork as prep	¼ cup	10	3	0	0
Sausage as prep	¼ cup	35	5	1	0
Swiss Steak as prep	¼ cup	15	4	0	0
Turkey as prep	¼ cup	20	4	1	0
French's					
Au Jus as prep	¼ cup	5	1	0	0
Brown as prep	¼ cup	10	3	0	0
Chicken as prep	¼ cup	25	4	0	0
Country as prep	¼ cup	35	5	1	0
Herb Brown as prep	¼ cup	15	3	0	0
Homestyle as prep	¼ cup	10	3	0	0
Mushroom as prep	¼ cup	10	3	0	0
Onion	¼ cup	15	4	0	0
Pork as prep	¼ cup	10	3	0	0
Sausage as prep	¼ cup	35	5	1	0
Turkey as prep	¼ cup	20	4	1	0
Loma Linda					
Gravy Quik Brown	1 tbsp (5 g)	20	4	0	0
Gravy Quik Chicken	1 tbsp (5 g)	20	3	0	0
Quik Gravy Country	1 tbsp (5 g)	25	4	0	0
Quik Gravy Mushroom	1 tbsp (5 g)	15	3	0	tr
Quik Gravy Onion	1 tbsp (5 g)	20	3	0	tr

GREAT NORTHERN BEANS
CANNED

FOOD	PORTION	CALS.	CARB.	SUG.	FIB.
great northern	1 cup	300	55	—	14
Allen					
Great Northern	½ cup (4.5 oz)	100	19	1	7
Green Giant					
Great Northern	½ cup (4.4 oz)	100	18	0	6
Trappey					
With Sausage	½ cup (4.5 oz)	100	18	3	7

DRIED

FOOD	PORTION	CALS.	CARB.	SUG.	FIB.
Hurst					
HamBeens w/ Ham	3 tbsp (1.2 oz)	120	22	1	11

FOOD	PORTION	CALS.	CARB.	SUG.	FIB.

GREEN BEANS
CANNED

FOOD	PORTION	CALS.	CARB.	SUG.	FIB.
green beans	½ cup	13	3	—	1
italian	½ cup	13	3	—	1
italian low sodium	½ cup	13	3	—	1
low sodium	½ cup	13	3	—	1
Allen					
Cut	½ cup (4.2 oz)	30	6	3	3
Cut No Added Salt	½ cup (4.2 oz)	15	3	1	2
French Style	½ cup (4.2 oz)	25	4	1	2
Italian	½ cup (4.2 oz)	35	7	2	3
Shell Outs	½ cup (4.5 oz)	30	6	2	2
Alma					
Cut	½ cup (4.2 oz)	30	6	3	3
Crest Top					
Cut	½ cup (4.2 oz)	30	6	3	3
Del Monte					
Cut	½ cup (4.3 oz)	20	4	2	2
Cut 50% Less Salt	½ cup (4.3 oz)	20	4	2	2
Cut Italian	½ cup (4.3 oz)	30	6	2	3
Cut No Salt Added	½ cup (4.3 oz)	20	4	2	2
French Style	½ cup (4.3 oz)	20	4	2	2
French Style 50% Less Salt	½ cup (4.3 oz)	20	4	2	2
French Style No Salt Added	½ cup (4.3 oz)	20	4	2	2
French Style Seasoned	½ cup (4.3 oz)	20	4	2	2
Whole	½ cup (4.3 oz)	20	4	2	2
GaBelle					
Cut	½ cup (4.2 oz)	30	6	3	3
Green Giant					
Cut	½ cup (4.2 oz)	20	4	2	1
Cut 50% Less Sodium	½ cup (4.2 oz)	20	4	2	1
French Style	½ cup (4.1 oz)	20	4	2	1
Kitchen Sliced	½ cup (4.2 oz)	20	4	2	1
Whole	½ cup (4.1 oz)	25	5	2	2
Seneca					
Cut	½ cup	20	6	—	2
Cuts Natural Pack	½ cup	25	6	—	2
French	½ cup	20	6	—	2
French Natural Pack	½ cup	25	6	—	2
Whole	½ cup	20	6	—	2
Sunshine					
Cut	½ cup (4.2 oz)	30	6	3	3
Italian	½ cup (4.2 oz)	35	7	2	3

FOOD	PORTION	CALS.	CARB.	SUG.	FIB.
FRESH					
raw	½ cup	17	4	—	1
FROZEN					
Birds Eye					
French w/ Toasted Almonds	¾ cup (4.1 oz)	80	7	3	3
Fresh Like					
Cut	3.5 oz	29	7	—	1
French	3.5 oz	29	7	—	1
Italian	3.5 oz	35	8	—	1
Whole	3.5 oz	29	6	—	1
Green Giant					
Cut	¾ cup (2.8 oz)	25	5	2	2
Harvest Fresh & Almonds	⅔ cup (2.8 oz)	60	5	2	2
Harvest Fresh Cut	⅔ cup (2.9 oz)	25	5	2	2
Stouffer's					
Green Bean Mushroom Casserole	1 serv (4 oz)	130	12	5	2
Tree Of Life					
Green Beans	⅔ cup (2.8 oz)	25	4	2	2
SHELF-STABLE					
Pantry Express					
Cut	½ cup	12	3	—	1
GREENS					
CANNED					
Allen					
Mixed	½ cup (4.2 oz)	30	8	tr	4
Sunshine					
Mixed	½ cup (4.2 oz)	30	8	tr	4
GROUPER					
cooked	3 oz	100	0	0	0
GUANABANA JUICE					
Libby					
Nectar	1 can (11.5 fl oz)	210	50	46	—
GUAVA JUICE					
Libby					
Nectar	1 can (11.5 fl oz)	220	54	47	—
GUINEA HEN					
w/ skin raw	½ hen (12.1 oz)	545	0	0	0
w/o skin raw	½ hen (9.3 oz)	292	0	0	0
HADDOCK					
FRESH					
cooked	3 oz	95	0	0	0

FOOD	PORTION	CALS.	CARB.	SUG.	FIB.
FROZEN					
Van De Kamp's					
Battered Fillets	2 (4 oz)	260	18	5	0
Breaded Fillets	2 (3.5 oz)	280	19	1	0
Lightly Breaded Fillets	1 (4 oz)	220	19	3	0
SMOKED					
smoked	1 oz	33	0	0	0
HAKE					
raw	3½ oz	84	0	0	0
HALIBUT					
FRESH					
atlantic & pacific cooked	3 oz	119	0	0	0
greenland baked	3 oz	203	0	0	0
FROZEN					
Van De Kamp's					
Battered Fillets	3 (4 oz)	300	16	4	0
HALVA					
(*see* SESAME)					
HAM					
(*see also* HAM DISHES, PORK, TURKEY)					
boneless 11% fat roasted	3 oz	151	0	0	0
canned extra lean roasted	3 oz	116	tr	—	0
canned extra lean roasted	1 cup	190	1	—	0
center slice country style lean roasted	4 oz	220	tr	—	0
chopped	1 oz	65	0	0	0
patty cooked	1 patty (2 oz)	203	1	—	0
steak boneless extra lean	1 (2 oz)	69	0	0	0
Alpine Lace					
Boneless Cooked	2 oz	60	1	1	0
Carl Buddig					
Ham	1 oz	50	1	—	0
Healthy Choice					
Baked Cooked	3 slices (2.2 oz)	70	1	1	0
Cooked	3 slices (2.2 oz)	70	1	1	0
Deli-Thin Baked Cooked With Natural Juices	6 slices (2 oz)	60	2	2	0
Deli-Thin Cooked	6 slices (2 oz)	60	1	1	0
Deli-Thin Honey With Natural Juices	6 slices (2 oz)	60	2	1	0
Deli-Thin Smoked With Natural Juices	6 slices (2 oz)	60	1	1	0

FOOD	PORTION	CALS.	CARB.	SUG.	FIB.
Healthy Choice (CONT.)					
Fresh-Trak Cooked	1 slice (1 oz)	30	1	0	0
Fresh-Trak Honey	1 slice (1 oz)	30	1	1	0
Honey Boneless	3 oz	100	5	5	0
Smoked	3 slices (2.2 oz)	70	1	1	0
Variety Pack Regular	3 slice (2.2 oz)	70	1	1	0
Hormel					
Black Label Canned (refrigerated)	3 oz	100	1	1	0
Black Label Canned (shelf stable)	3 oz	110	0	0	0
Cure 81 Half Ham	3 oz	100	0	1	0
Curemaster	3 oz	80	0	0	0
Deviled Ham	4 tbsp (2 oz)	150	2	2	0
Ham & Cheese Patties	1 patty (2 oz)	190	0	0	0
Ham Patties	1 (2 oz)	180	1	1	0
Light & Lean 97 Sliced	1 slice (1 oz)	25	0	0	0
Primissimo Proscuitti	2 oz	120	0	0	0
Spiral Cure 81	3 oz	150	1	1	0
Jordan's					
Healthy Trim 97% Fat Free Cooked	1 slice (1 oz)	30	2	0	0
Healthy Trim 97% Fat Free EZ Serve	1 slice (1 oz)	30	2	1	0
Healthy Trim 97% Fat Free Virginia	1 slice (1 oz)	30	2	1	0
Louis Rich					
Carving Board Baked	2 slices (1.6 oz)	50	1	tr	0
Carving Board Honey Glazed Thin	6 slices (2.1 oz)	70	2	2	0
Carving Board Honey Glazed Traditional	2 slices (1.6 oz)	50	1	1	0
Carving Board Smoked	1 slice (1.6 oz)	45	0	0	0
Dinner Slices Baked	1 slice (3.3 oz)	80	1	1	0
Oscar Mayer					
Baked	3 slices (2.2 oz)	70	2	2	0
Boiled	3 slices (2.2 oz)	60	0	0	0
Chopped	1 slice (1 oz)	50	1	tr	0
Dinner Slice	3 oz	80	0	0	0
Dinner Steaks	1 (2 oz)	60	0	0	0
Free Baked	3 slices (1.6 oz)	35	1	1	0
Free Honey	3 slices (1.6 oz)	35	2	1	0
Free Smoked	3 slices (1.6 oz)	35	1	tr	0
Ham & Cheese Loaf	1 slice (1 oz)	70	1	1	0

FOOD	PORTION	CALS.	CARB.	SUG.	FIB.
Oscar Mayer (CONT.)					
Honey	3 slices (2.2 oz)	70	2	2	0
Lower Sodium	3 slices (2.2 oz)	70	2	1	0
Lunchables Cookies/Ham/ Swiss	1 pkg (4.2 oz)	360	29	5	tr
Lunchables Dessert Chocolate Pudding/Ham/ American	1 pkg (6.2 oz)	390	34	17	tr
Lunchables Ham/Cheddar	1 pkg (4.5 oz)	340	19	4	0
Smoked	3 slices (2.2 oz)	60	0	0	0
Russer					
Baked	2 oz	70	4	4	—
Canadian Brand Maple	2 oz	70	4	4	—
Chopped	2 oz	130	5	4	—
Cooked Ham	2 oz	60	2	2	—
Ham & Cheese Loaf	2 oz	120	5	3	—
Honey & Maple Cured	2 oz	70	3	2	—
Honey Cured	2 oz	60	2	2	—
Hot	2 oz	70	3	2	—
Light Cooked	2 oz	60	2	2	—
Light Smoked	2 oz	60	2	2	—
Smoked Virginia	2 oz	70	3	4	—
Spiced	2 oz	160	5	4	—
Sara Lee					
Bavarian Brand Baked	2 oz	80	1	1	—
Bavarian Brand Baked Honey	2 oz	80	2	2	—
Golden Cure Smoked	2 oz	80	1	1	—
Honey Ham	2 oz	60	2	2	—
Honey Roasted	2 oz	90	3	3	—
Spam					
Spread	4 tbsp (2 oz)	140	1	1	0

HAM DISHES
Croissant Pocket

FOOD	PORTION	CALS.	CARB.	SUG.	FIB.
Stuffed Sandwich Ham & Cheddar	1 piece (4.5 oz)	360	39	5	5
Hot Pocket					
Stuffed Sandwich Ham & Cheese	1 (4.5 ox)	340	37	6	4

HAMBURGER
(*see also* BEEF)
Jimmy Dean

FOOD	PORTION	CALS.	CARB.	SUG.	FIB.
Burger	1 (2 oz)	220	0	0	0

FOOD	PORTION	CALS.	CARB.	SUG.	FIB.
Jimmy Dean (CONT.)					
Flamed Broiled Cheeseburger	1 (6.3 oz)	540	34	3	1
Mini Cheeseburger	2 (3 oz)	270	23	3	1
Kid Cuisine					
Beef Patty Sandwich w/ Cheese	1 (8.5 oz)	410	58	27	4
Rudy's Farm					
Mild Burger	1 (3 oz)	360	0	0	0
White Castle					
Cheeseburger	2 (3.6 oz)	310	23	0	6
Hamburger	2 (3.2 oz)	270	23	0	5

HAZELNUTS

FOOD	PORTION	CALS.	CARB.	SUG.	FIB.
oil roasted unblanched	1 oz	187	5	—	2
Crumpy					
Chocolate Hazelnut Spread	1 tbsp (0.5 oz)	80	8	8	0

HEART

FOOD	PORTION	CALS.	CARB.	SUG.	FIB.
pork braised	1 cup	215	1	—	0
pork braised	1	191	1	—	0

HERBAL TEA
(*see* TEA/HERBAL TEA)

HERBS/SPICES
(*see also individual names*)

FOOD	PORTION	CALS.	CARB.	SUG.	FIB.
Ac'cent					
Flavor Enhancer	½ tsp	5	0	0	0
Herbal All Purpose Seasoning	½ tsp	0	0	0	0
Chi-Chi's					
Seasoning Mix	1 tsp (3 g)	10	1	0	0
Ka-Me					
Five Spice Powder	¼ tsp (1 g)	0	1	0	0
Lawry's					
Seasoning Blend Sloppy Joe	1 pkg	126	28	—	1
McIlhenny					
Crab Boil	3 oz	378	40	4	32
Watkins					
Apple Bake Seasoning	¼ tsp (0.5 g)	0	0	0	0
Barbecue Spice	¼ tsp (0.5 g)	0	0	0	0
Bean Soup Seasoning	¾ tsp (2 g)	5	1	0	0
Beef Jerky Seasoning	2 tsp (6 g)	15	3	1	0
Chicken Seasoning	½ tsp (1 g)	0	0	0	0

FOOD	PORTION	CALS.	CARB.	SUG.	FIB.
Watkins (CONT.)					
Cole Slaw Seasoning	½ tsp (1.5 g)	5	1	0	0
Egg Sensations	1 tsp (3 g)	10	1	0	0
Fajita Seasoning	½ tsp (3 g)	10	2	0	0
Grill Seasoning	¼ tsp (1 g)	0	0	0	0
Ground Beef Seasoning	⅛ tsp (0.5 g)	0	0	0	0
Italian Blend	1 tsp (3 g)	1	2	1	0
Meat Tenderizer	⅛ tsp (0.5 g)	0	0	0	0
Meatloaf Seasoning	½ tsp (5 g)	15	4	1	0
Mexican Blend	½ tbsp (4 g)	15	3	0	0
Omelet & Souffle Seasoning	¾ tsp (2 g)	5	1	0	0
Oriental Ginger Garlic Liquid Spice Blend	1 tbsp (0.5 oz)	120	0	0	0
Potato Salad Seasoning	¼ tsp (1 g)	0	0	0	0
Pumpkin Pie Spice	¼ tsp (0.5 g)	0	0	0	0
Smokehouse Liquid Blend	1 tbsp (0.5 oz)	120	0	0	0
Soup & Vegetable Seasoning	¼ tsp (0.5 g)	0	0	0	0
Spanish Seasoning Blend	¼ tsp (0.5 oz)	0	0	0	0
HERRING					
atlantic cooked	3 oz	172	0	0	0
pacific baked	3 oz	213	0	0	0
smoked	3.5 oz	210	0	0	0
HOMINY					
CANNED					
white	1 cup (5.6 oz)	482	23	—	4
Allen					
Golden	½ cup (4.5 oz)	120	27	tr	4
Mexican	½ cup (4.5 oz)	120	25	0	3
White	½ cup (4.5 oz)	100	22	1	4
Uncle William					
Golden	½ cup (4.5 oz)	120	27	tr	4
Mexican	½ cup (4.5 oz)	120	25	0	3
White	½ cup (4.5 oz)	100	22	1	4
Van Camp's					
Golden	½ cup (4.3 oz)	80	17	—	1
White	½ cup (4.3 oz)	80	15	—	1
HONEY					
honey	1 cup (11.9 oz)	1031	279	270	—
honey	1 tbsp (0.7 oz)	64	17	17	—
Burleson's					
Clover	1 tbsp	60	16	—	0

FOOD	PORTION	CALS.	CARB.	SUG.	FIB.
Burleson's (CONT.)					
Creamed	1 tbsp	60	16	—	0
Natural	1 tbsp	60	16	—	0
Pure	1 tbsp	60	16	—	0
Raw	1 tbsp	60	16	—	0
Rocky Mountain Clover	1 tbsp	60	16	—	0
Golden Blossom					
Honey	1 tsp	20	5	4	—
Tree Of Life					
Alfalfa	1 tbsp (0.7 oz)	60	17	16	—
Avocado	1 tbsp (0.7 oz)	60	17	16	—
Buckwheat	1 tbsp (0.7 oz)	60	17	16	—
Clover	1 tbsp (0.7 oz)	60	17	16	—
Honeybear Wildflower	1 tbsp (0.7 oz)	60	17	16	—
Orange	1 tbsp (0.7 oz)	60	17	16	—
Tupelo	1 tbsp (0.7 oz)	60	17	16	—
Wildflower	1 tbsp (0.7 oz)	60	17	16	—

HONEYDEW
FRESH
Dole

FOOD	PORTION	CALS.	CARB.	SUG.	FIB.
Honeydew	1/10	50	12	—	1

FROZEN
Big Valley

FOOD	PORTION	CALS.	CARB.	SUG.	FIB.
Balls	3/4 cup (4.9 oz)	45	11	7	1

HORSE

FOOD	PORTION	CALS.	CARB.	SUG.	FIB.
roasted	3 oz	149	0	0	0

HORSERADISH
Heluva Good Cheese

FOOD	PORTION	CALS.	CARB.	SUG.	FIB.
Horseradish	1 tsp (5 g)	0	0	0	0
Ka-Me					
Wasabi Powder	1/4 tsp (1 g)	0	1	0	0
Kraft					
Cream Style	1 tsp (5 g)	0	0	0	0
Horseradish Sauce	1 tsp (5 g)	20	tr	tr	0
Prepared	1 tsp (5 g)	0	0	0	0
Rosoff's					
Red	1 tbsp (0.5 oz)	8	2	—	—

HOT CAKES
(*see* PANCAKES)

HOT COCOA
(*see* COCOA)

HOT DOG
(*see also* MEAT SUBSTITUTES, SAUSAGE, SAUSAGE SUBSTITUTES)
Applegate Farms

FOOD	PORTION	CALS.	CARB.	SUG.	FIB.
Chicken Natural Uncured	1 (1.5 oz)	120	1	0	0

FOOD	PORTION	CALS.	CARB.	SUG.	FIB.
Applegate Farms (CONT.)					
Natural Turkey	1 (1.5 oz)	120	1	0	0
Empire					
Chicken	1 (2 oz)	100	1	0	0
Turkey	1 (2 oz)	90	1	0	0
Health Valley					
Weiners	1	96	1	—	0
Weiners Turkey	1	96	1	—	0
Healthy Choice					
Beef	1 (1.8 oz)	60	5	2	0
Bunsize	1 (2 oz)	70	5	2	0
Franks	1 (1.6 oz)	50	4	2	0
Jumbo	1 (2 oz)	70	5	2	0
Hormel					
Fat Free	1 (1.8 oz)	45	5	3	0
Fat Free Beef	1 (1.8 oz)	45	5	2	0
Jordan's					
Healthy Trim Low Fat	1 (1.8 oz)	70	3	3	0
Healthy Trim Low Fat Skinless	1 (1.8 oz)	70	3	3	0
Louis Rich					
Bun Length	1 (2 oz)	110	3	1	0
Cheese	1 (1.6 oz)	90	2	tr	0
Franks	1 (1.6 oz)	80	2	tr	0
Oscar Mayer					
Beef	1 (1.6 oz)	140	1	tr	0
Big & Juicy Franks Deli Style	1 (2.7 oz)	230	1	0	0
Big & Juicy Franks Original	1 (2.7 oz)	240	1	1	0
Big & Juicy Franks Quarter Pound	1 (4 oz)	350	2	2	0
Big & Juicy Weiners Hot 'N Spicy	1 (2.7 oz)	220	1	tr	0
Big & Juicy Weiners Smokie Links	1 (2.7 oz)	220	1	tr	0
Big & Juicy Wieners Original	1 (2.7 oz)	240	1	tr	0
Bun-Length Beef	1 (2 oz)	180	2	1	0
Cheese	1 (1.6 oz)	140	1	tr	0
Free Beef	1 (1.8 oz)	40	3	2	0
Free Turkey & Beef	1 (1.8 oz)	35	2	1	0
Jumbo Beef	1 (2 oz)	180	2	1	0
Light Beef	1 (2 oz)	110	2	1	0
Wieners	1 (1.6 oz)	150	1	tr	0

FOOD	PORTION	CALS.	CARB.	SUG.	FIB.
Oscar Mayer (CONT.)					
Wieners Bun-Length	1 (2 oz)	190	2	1	0
Wieners Light	1 (2 oz)	110	2	1	0
Wieners Little	6 (2 oz)	180	2	1	0
Russer					
Lil'Salt Deli Franks	1 (2.67 oz)	160	3	5	—
Shofar					
Kosher Beef	1 (1.8 oz)	150	0	0	0
Kosher Beef Reduced Fat Reduced Sodium	1 (1.8 oz)	120	0	0	0

HUMMUS
Athenos

Roasted Red Pepper	2 tbsp (1.1 oz)	60	6	0	1
Casbah					
Mix as prep	¼ cup	120	15	0	1
Cedar's					
No Salt Added Hommus Tahini	2 tbsp (1 oz)	50	5	0	3

ICE CREAM AND FROZEN DESSERTS
(*see also* ICES AND ICE POPS, PUDDING POPS, SHERBET, YOGURT FROZEN)

FOOD	PORTION	CALS.	CARB.	SUG.	FIB.
chocolate	½ cup (4 fl oz)	143	19	13	—
dixie cup chocolate	1 (3.5 fl oz)	125	16	11	—
dixie cup strawberry	1 (3.5 fl oz)	112	16	9	—
dixie cup vanilla	1 (3.5 fl oz)	116	14	9	—
freeze dried ice cream chocolate strawberry & vanilla	1 pkg (0.75 oz)	158	24	10	1
strawberry	½ cup (4 fl oz)	127	18	10	—
vanilla	½ cup (4 fl oz)	132	16	10	—
vanilla light	½ cup (2.3 oz)	92	15	12	—
3 Musketeers					
Single Chocolate	1 (2 fl oz)	160	16	—	0
Single Vanilla	1 (2 fl oz)	160	16	—	0
Snack Chocolate	1 (0.72 fl oz)	60	6	—	0
Snack Vanilla	1 (0.72 fl oz)	60	6	—	0
Ben & Jerry's					
Banana Walnut	½ cup (3.9 oz)	290	26	26	1
Butter Pecan	½ cup (3.9 oz)	310	20	19	1
Cherry Garcia	½ cup (3.7 oz)	240	25	25	0
Cherry Vanilla	½ cup (3.9 oz)	240	26	26	0
Chocolate Chip Cookie Dough	½ cup (3.7 oz)	270	30	25	0
Chocolate Fudge Brownie	½ cup (3.7 oz)	250	31	22	2

FOOD	PORTION	CALS.	CARB.	SUG.	FIB.
Ben & Jerry's (CONT.)					
Chunky Monkey	½ cup (3.7 oz)	280	29	28	1
Coconut Almond	½ cup (3.7 oz)	260	19	18	1
Coconut Almond Fudge Chip	½ cup (3.8 oz)	320	24	21	2
Coffee Almond Fudge	½ cup (3.7 oz)	290	24	23	2
Coffee Toffee Crunch	½ cup (3.7 oz)	280	28	28	0
English Toffee Crunch	½ cup (4 oz)	310	30	30	0
Mint Chocolate Cookie	½ cup (3.8 oz)	260	27	23	1
New York Super Fudge Chunk	½ cup (3.7 oz)	290	28	25	2
No Fat Strawberry	½ cup (3.3 oz)	140	31	25	0
No Fat Vanilla Fudge Swirl	½ cup (3.1 oz)	150	32	24	0
Peanut Butter Cup	½ cup (4.1 oz)	370	30	27	2
Pop Chocolate Chip Cookie Dough	1 (4.1 oz)	450	48	38	1
Pop English Toffee Crunch	1 (3.7 oz)	340	35	34	0
Pop Vanilla	1 (3.9 oz)	360	30	27	0
Rain Forest Crunch	½ cup (3.7 oz)	300	24	22	0
Smooth Aztec Harvest Coffee	½ cup (3.8 oz)	230	22	21	0
Smooth Deep Dark Chocolate	½ cup (3.9 oz)	260	32	29	2
Smooth Double Chocolate Fudge	½ cup (4.1 oz)	280	35	31	3
Smooth Mocho Fudge	½ cup (4 oz)	270	30	28	1
Smooth Vanilla	½ cup (3.8 oz)	230	21	21	0
Smooth Vanilla Bean	½ cup (3.8 oz)	230	21	21	0
Smooth Vanilla Caramel Fudge	½ cup (4.1 oz)	280	33	30	1
Smooth White Russian	½ cup (3.8 oz)	240	23	22	0
Vanilla	½ cup (3.7 oz)	230	21	21	0
Wavy Gravy	½ cup (4.1 oz)	330	29	26	2
Bon Bons					
Vanilla With Milk Chocolate Coating	8 pieces	330	27	21	0
Vanilla With Milk Chocolate Coating	5 pieces	200	17	13	0
Bounty					
Cherry/Dark	1 (0.84 fl oz)	70	8	—	0
Coconut/Dark	1 (0.84 fl oz)	70	7	—	0
Coconut/Milk	1 (0.84 fl oz)	70	7	—	0
Breyers					
Butter Pecan	½ cup (2.4 oz)	180	14	14	0

FOOD	PORTION	CALS.	CARB.	SUG.	FIB.
Breyers (CONT.)					
Caramel Praline Crunch	½ cup (2.6 oz)	180	22	20	0
Cherry Vanilla	½ cup (2.4 oz)	150	17	13	0
Chocolate	½ cup (2.4 oz)	160	18	17	tr
Chocolate Chip	½ cup (2.4 oz)	170	17	17	0
Chocolate Chip Cookie Dough	½ cup (2.5 oz)	180	20	17	0
Chocolate Rainbow	½ cup (2.4 oz)	120	16	14	0
Coffee	½ cup (2.4 oz)	150	15	14	0
Cookies N Cream	½ cup (2.4 oz)	170	19	17	0
Creamsicle	½ cup (2.8 oz)	130	22	17	0
Double Chocolate Fudge	½ cup (2.6 oz)	150	23	15	tr
Fat Free Caramel Praline	½ cup (2.5 oz)	120	25	20	0
Fat Free Chocolate	½ cup (2.4 oz)	90	19	15	tr
Fat Free Mint Cookies N Cream	½ cup (2.4 oz)	100	21	16	0
Fat Free Strawberry	½ cup (2.4 oz)	90	19	13	0
Fat Free Take Two Vanilla Strawberry	½ cup (2.4 oz)	80	19	15	0
Fat Free Vanilla	½ cup (2.4 oz)	90	19	16	tr
Fat Free Vanilla Chocolate Strawberry	½ cup (2.4 oz)	90	19	15	0
Fat Free Vanilla Fudge Twirl	½ cup (2.5 oz)	100	22	18	tr
French Vanilla	½ cup (2.4 oz)	160	15	14	0
Fruit Rainbow	½ cup (2.4 oz)	140	16	14	0
Hershey w/ Almonds	½ cup (2.7 oz)	190	23	18	tr
Light Butter Pecan	½ cup (2.3 oz)	120	19	14	0
Light Caramel Praline Pecan	½ cup (3 oz)	180	30	25	0
Light French Chocolate	½ cup (2.4 oz)	150	22	18	tr
Light Mint Chocolate Chip	½ cup (2.4 oz)	140	21	18	0
Light Vanilla	½ cup (2.4 oz)	130	18	16	0
Light Vanilla Chocolate Strawberry	½ cup (2.4 oz)	120	19	16	0
Light Low Fat Brown Marble Fudge	½ cup (2.6 oz)	130	26	18	tr
Light Low Fat French Vanilla	½ cup (2.3 oz)	110	20	16	0
Light Low Fat Swiss Almond Fudge	½ cup (2.5 oz)	130	24	15	tr
Low Fat Butter Pecan	½ cup (2.6 oz)	150	21	16	0
Low Fat Vanilla	½ cup (2.6 oz)	120	22	17	0
Low Fat Vanilla Chocolate Strawberry	½ cup (2.6 oz)	120	22	17	0

FOOD	PORTION	CALS.	CARB.	SUG.	FIB.
Breyers (CONT.)					
Mint Chocolate Chip	½ cup (2.4 oz)	170	17	14	0
No Sugar Added Fudge Twirl	½ cup (2.6 oz)	100	14	6	0
No Sugar Added Mint Chocolate Chip	½ cup (2.4 oz)	100	12	6	0
No Sugar Added Vanilla	½ cup (2.4 oz)	90	11	6	0
No Sugar Added Vanilla Chocolate Strawberry	½ cup (2.4 oz)	90	11	6	0
Peach	½ cup (2.4 oz)	130	17	17	0
Peanut Butter Cup	½ cup (2.7 oz)	210	24	20	tr
Rocky Road	½ cup (2.5 oz)	180	24	21	tr
Soft'N Creamy Vanilla	½ cup (2.3 oz)	150	19	15	0
Soft'N Creamy Vanilla Chocolate Strawberry	½ cup (2.3 oz)	150	19	15	0
Strawberry	½ cup (2.4 oz)	130	15	11	0
Take Two Vanilla Chocolate	½ cup (2.5 oz)	160	17	16	0
Take Two Vanilla Orange Sherbet	½ cup (2.7 oz)	130	21	17	0
Vanilla	½ cup (2.4 oz)	150	15	15	0
Vanilla Chocolate Strawberry	½ cup (2.4 oz)	150	16	14	0
Vanilla Fudge Twirl	½ cup (2.6 oz)	160	19	16	tr
Viennetta Cappuccino	½ cup (2.4 oz)	190	19	16	0
Viennetta Chocolate	½ cup (2.4 oz)	190	18	15	0
Viennetta Vanilla	½ cup (2.4 oz)	190	19	16	0
Butterfinger					
Bar	1 (2.5 oz)	170	14	12	0
Nuggets	8	340	29	27	0
California Joe					
Soft Serve Chocolate	½ cup (2.5 oz)	72	11	10	1
Soft Serve Vanilla	½ cup (2.5 oz)	70	11	10	1
Carnation					
Sundae Cup Strawberry	1 (3.3 oz)	200	29	23	0
Cool Creations					
Cookies & Cream Sandwich	1 (3.5 oz)	240	34	18	1
Mini Sandwich	1 (2.3 oz)	110	16	8	0
DoveBar					
Almond	1 (3.67 fl oz)	335	30	—	0
Bite Size Almond Praline	1 (0.75 fl oz)	80	8	—	0
Bite Size Cherry Royale	1 (0.75 fl oz)	70	8	—	0
Bite Size Classic Vanilla	1 (0.75 fl oz)	70	7	—	0
Bite Size French Vanilla	1 (0.75 fl oz)	70	7	—	0
Bite Size Mint Supreme	1 (0.75 fl oz)	80	8	—	0

FOOD	PORTION	CALS.	CARB.	SUG.	FIB.
DoveBar (CONT.)					
Caramel Pecan	1 (3.67 fl oz)	350	35	—	0
Chocolate Milk Chocolate	1 (3.8 fl oz)	340	35	—	0
Coffee Cashew	1 (3.67 fl oz)	335	31	—	0
Crunchy Cookie	1 (3.8 fl oz)	340	35	—	0
Peanut	1 (3.8 fl oz)	380	35	—	0
Single Vanilla/Dark	1 (2 fl oz)	200	24	—	0
Vanilla Dark Chocolate	1 (3.8 fl oz)	340	34	—	0
Vanilla Milk Chocolate	1 (3.8 fl oz)	340	34	—	0
Drumstick					
Cone Chocolate	1 (4.6 oz)	340	37	20	2
Cone Chocolate Dipped	1 (4.6 oz)	340	41	21	1
Cone Vanilla	1 (4.6 oz)	350	36	21	2
Cone Vanilla Caramel	1 (4.6 oz)	360	39	24	6
Cone Vanilla Fudge	1 (4.6 oz)	370	40	25	2
Flintstones					
Cool Cream	1 (2.75 oz)	90	18	14	0
Push-Up	1 (2.75 oz)	100	20	14	0
Friendly's					
Black Raspberry	½ cup	150	17	17	0
Chocolate Almond Chip	½ cup	170	18	17	0
Forbidden Chocolate	½ cup	150	14	13	0
Fudge Nut Brownie	½ cup	200	23	17	0
Heath English Toffee	½ cup (2.7 oz)	190	24	19	0
Purely Pistachio	½ cup	160	16	15	0
Vanilla	½ cup	150	16	11	0
Vanilla Chocolate Strawberry	½ cup	150	16	16	tr
Vienna Mocha Chunk	½ cup	180	19	18	0
Good Humor					
Banana Bob	1 (3 fl oz)	155	22	14	0
Bar Classic Toasted Almond	1 (3.1 fl oz)	170	22	25	1
Bar Classic Vanilla	1 (3.1 fl oz)	190	22	19	0
Bar Classic Almond	1 (3.1 fl oz)	210	21	20	1
Bar Sidewalk Sundae	1	280	21	20	2
Bubble O'Bill	1 (3.6 fl oz)	170	20	19	1
Bubble Play	1	110	25	18	—
Chip Burrrger	1 (4.7 oz)	320	44	34	1
Chip Sandwich	1 (4.7 fl oz)	320	44	34	1
Choco Taco	1 (4.4 fl oz)	320	38	27	1
Chocolate Eclair Classic	1 (3.1 fl oz)	170	21	17	1
Classic Candy Center Crunch Vanilla	1	280	21	20	0
Colonel Crunch Chocolate	1 (3.1 oz)	160	21	15	1

FOOD	PORTION	CALS.	CARB.	SUG.	FIB.
Good Humor (CONT.)					
Colonel Crunch Strawberry	1 (3.1 oz)	170	22	15	0
Combo Cup	1 (6.2 fl oz)	200	25	25	1
Cone Olde Nut Sundae	1 (3.9 oz)	230	32	22	2
Cone Sidewalk Sundae	1 (4.2 oz)	270	31	17	1
Creamee Burrrger	1 (4.7 oz)	310	40	17	1
Crunch Classic Candy Center	1 (3.1 fl oz)	260	21	21	1
Dinosaur Bar	1	110	25	17	—
Far Frog	1 (3.6 fl oz)	150	19	12	1
Fun Box Ice Cream Sandwich	1 (3.1 oz)	160	27	14	1
King Cone	1 (5.7 fl oz)	300	38	28	2
King Cone Classic Vanilla	1 (4.8 oz)	300	48	25	1
King Cone Strawberry	1 (5.7 oz)	250	38	32	1
Light Chocolate Chocolate Chip	½ cup (2.4 oz)	130	20	13	tr
Light Chocolate Chip	½ cup (2.4 oz)	130	20	14	0
Light Coffee	½ cup (2.4 oz)	110	18	13	0
Light Cookies N'Cream	½ cup (2.4 oz)	130	21	13	0
Light Heavenly Hash	½ cup (2.4 oz)	140	23	13	tr
Light Praline Almond Crunch	½ cup (2.4 oz)	130	20	14	0
Light Toffee Bar Crunch	½ cup (2.4 oz)	130	20	14	0
Light Vanilla	½ cup (2.4 oz)	110	19	13	0
Light Vanilla Chocolate Strawberry	½ cup (2.4 oz)	110	19	13	0
Light Vanilla Fudge	½ cup (2.6 oz)	120	21	14	0
Magmun Almond	1 (4.2 fl oz)	270	35	34	5
Magnum Chocolate	1 (4.2 fl oz)	260	38	36	2
Number One Bar	1 (4.1 fl oz)	190	22	17	1
Popsicle Ice Cream Bar	1 (3.1 oz)	160	15	15	1
Popsicle Ice Cream Sandwich	1 (3.6 fl oz)	190	28	22	1
Sandwich Classic Chip Cookie	1 (4.1 fl oz)	300	43	26	1
Sandwich Giant Neapolitan	1 (5.2 fl oz)	260	39	26	1
Sandwich Giant Vanilla	1 (5.2 oz)	240	35	22	1
Sandwich Ice Cream	1	190	28	22	1
Sandwich Sidewalk Sundae	1 (3.1 oz)	160	27	14	1
Sandwich Sprinkle	1 (3.1 fl oz)	180	28	16	1
Strawberry Shortcake Bar Classic	1 (3.1 fl oz)	160	20	17	1
Sundae Twist Cup	1	160	33	29	0

FOOD	PORTION	CALS.	CARB.	SUG.	FIB.
Good Humor (CONT.)					
Toffee Taco	1 (4.4 fl oz)	300	35	25	1
WWF Bar	1 (3.7 fl oz)	200	24	18	1
X-Men Bar	1 (3 fl oz)	150	23	9	0
Haagen-Dazs					
Baileys Original Irish Cream	½ cup (3.6 oz)	280	23	22	0
Brownies A La Mode	½ cup (3.7 oz)	280	25	23	0
Butter Pecan	½ cup (3.7 oz)	320	20	19	tr
Cappuccino Commotion	½ cup (3.6 oz)	310	25	23	1
Caramel Cone Explosion	½ cup (3.6 oz)	310	27	23	tr
Chocolate	½ cup (3.7 oz)	270	22	21	1
Chocolate Chocolate Chip	½ cup (3.7 oz)	300	26	24	2
Coffee	½ cup (3.7 oz)	270	21	21	0
Cookie Dough Dynamo	½ cup (3.6 oz)	300	29	24	0
Cookies & Cream	½ cup (3.6 oz)	270	23	20	0
DiSaronno Amaretto	½ cup (3.6 oz)	260	26	23	0
Macadamia Brittle	½ cup (3.7 oz)	300	25	23	0
Multi Pack Bars Caramel Cone Explosion	1 (3.1 oz)	330	30	25	tr
Multi Pack Bars Chocolate & Dark Chocolate	1 (3.2 oz)	320	27	24	3
Multi Pack Bars Coffee & Almond Crunch	1 (3 oz)	290	22	21	tr
Multi Pack Bars Iced Cappuccino Explosion	1 (2.9 oz)	290	21	20	tr
Multi Pack Bars Triple Brownie Overload	1 (3 oz)	320	23	21	1
Multi Pack Bars Vanilla & Almonds	1 (3 oz)	300	21	19	1
Multi Pack Bars Vanilla & Dark Chocolate	1 (3.2 oz)	320	27	24	4
Multi Pack Bars Vanilla & Milk Chocolate	1 (3 oz)	280	20	20	0
Peanut Butter Burst	½ cup (3.6 oz)	330	26	23	1
Rum Raisin	½ cup (3.7 oz)	270	22	21	0
Single Pack Bars Caramel Cone Explosion	1 (3.3 oz)	350	32	27	tr
Single Pack Bars Chocolate & Dark Chocolate	1 (3.9 oz)	400	33	29	4
Single Pack Bars Coffee & Almond Crunch	1 (3.7 oz)	360	27	25	1
Single Pack Bars Cookie Dough Dynamo	1 (3.5 oz)	380	34	27	1

FOOD	PORTION	CALS.	CARB.	SUG.	FIB.
Haagen-Dazs (CONT.)					
Single Pack Bars Iced Cappuccino	1 (3.4 oz)	330	24	23	tr
Single Pack Bars Triple Brownie Overload	1 (3.5 oz)	380	28	25	1
Single Pack Bars Vanilla & Almonds	1 (3.7 oz)	370	26	24	1
Single Pack Bars Vanilla & Dark Chocolate	1 (3.9 oz)	400	33	29	4
Single Pack Bars Vanilla & Milk Chocolate	1 (3.5 oz)	330	24	24	tr
Strawberry	½ cup (3.7 oz)	250	23	21	tr
Strawberry Cheesecake Craze	½ cup (3.7 oz)	290	28	25	tr
Triple Brownie Overload	½ cup (3.5 oz)	300	26	24	0
Vanilla	½ cup (3.7 oz)	270	21	21	0
Vanilla Fudge	½ cup (3.7 oz)	280	25	25	0
Vanilla Swiss Almond	½ cup (3.7 oz)	310	23	21	1
Healthy Choice					
Black Forest	½ cup (2.5 oz)	120	23	16	1
Bordeaux Cherry Chocolate Chip	½ cup (2.5 oz)	110	19	19	tr
Butter Pecan Crunch	½ cup (2.5 oz)	120	22	21	1
Cappuccino Chocolate Chunk	½ cup (2.5 oz)	120	32	14	1
Cookies 'N Cream	½ cup (2.5 oz)	120	21	19	tr
Double Fudge Swirl	½ cup (2.5 oz)	120	21	20	1
Fudge Brownie	½ cup (2.5 oz)	120	22	15	2
Malt Caramel Cone	½ cup (2.5 oz)	120	22	15	1
Mint Chocolate Chip	½ cup (2.5 oz)	120	21	20	tr
Peanut Butter Cookie Dough 'N Fudge	½ cup (2.5 oz)	120	22	21	tr
Praline & Caramel	½ cup (2.5 oz)	130	25	24	tr
Rocky Road	½ cup (2.5 oz)	140	28	19	2
Vanilla	½ cup	100	18	17	1
Heath					
Bar	1 (2.5 oz)	160	13	12	0
Nuggets	8	180	18	14	0
Hood					
Bar Orange Cream	1 bar (1.8 oz)	90	18	18	0
Bar Vanilla	1 bar (1.6 oz)	160	11	11	0
Caramel Butterscotch Blast	½ cup (2.3 oz)	160	20	20	0
Chocolate	½ cup (2.3 oz)	140	17	16	0
Chocolate Chip	½ cup (2.3 oz)	160	18	18	0

FOOD	PORTION	CALS.	CARB.	SUG.	FIB.
Hood (CONT.)					
Chocolate Eclair	1 bar (1.6 oz)	150	14	11	0
Christmas Tree	½ cup (2.3 oz)	140	18	18	0
Coffee	½ cup (2.3 oz)	140	16	16	0
Cookie Dough Delight	½ cup (2.3 oz)	160	21	21	0
Cookies N Cream	½ cup (2.3 oz)	160	19	16	0
Cooler Cups	1 (2.1 oz)	80	18	17	0
Crispy Bar	1 (1.9 oz)	180	15	13	0
Egg Nog	½ cup (2.3 oz)	130	17	17	0
Fabulous Fudge & Peanut Butter Swirled Fudge Bars	1 bar (2.1 oz)	110	17	17	0
Fabulous Fudgies Assorted Bars	1 bar (2.1 oz)	100	19	18	0
Fat Free Chocolate Passion	½ cup (2.5 oz)	100	23	22	0
Fat Free Classic Harlequin	½ cup (2.5 oz)	100	23	22	0
Fat Free Double Brownie Sundae	½ cup (2.5 oz)	120	27	25	0
Fat Free Heavenly Hash	½ cup (2.5 oz)	120	27	25	0
Fat Free Mississippi Mud Pie	½ cup (2.5 oz)	130	29	25	0
Fat Free Praline Pecan Delight	½ cup (2.5 oz)	120	27	26	0
Fat Free Raspberry Blush	½ cup (2.5 oz)	120	26	24	0
Fat Free Super Strawberry Swirl	½ cup (2.5 oz)	100	23	22	0
Fat Free Vanilla Fudge Twist	½ cup (2.5 oz)	120	26	25	0
Fat Free Very Vanilla	½ cup (2.5 oz)	100	23	23	0
Fudge Bars	1 bar (2.7 oz)	100	21	20	0
Grasshopper Pie	½ cup (2.3 oz)	160	22	19	0
Heavenly Hash	½ cup (2.3 oz)	140	21	20	0
Hendrie's Cherry Chocolate Dips	1 bar (1.3 oz)	120	11	11	0
Hoodsie Cup Vanilla & Chocolate	1 (1.7 oz)	100	12	12	0
Light Almond Praline Delight	½ cup (2.4 oz)	110	23	22	0
Light Brownie Nut Sundae	½ cup (2.4 oz)	140	22	20	0
Light Caribbean Coffee Royale	½ cup (2.4 oz)	110	18	17	0
Light Chocolate Almond Chip Sundae	½ cup (2.4 oz)	140	22	20	0
Light Chocolate Chocolate Chip Cookie Dough	½ cup (2.4 oz)	140	21	21	0

FOOD	PORTION	CALS.	CARB.	SUG.	FIB.
Hood (CONT.)					
Light Cookies N Cream	½ cup (2.4 oz)	130	21	18	0
Light Heath Toffee Chunk Swirl	½ cup (2.4 oz)	140	23	22	0
Light Heavenly Hash	½ cup (2.4 oz)	130	22	21	0
Light Maple Sugar Shack	⅓ cup (2.4 oz)	130	23	21	0
Light Massachusetts Mud Pie	½ cup (2.4 oz)	140	20	19	0
Light Raspberry Swirl	½ cup (2.4 oz)	120	22	20	0
Light Strawberry Supreme	½ cup (2.4 oz)	110	19	19	0
Light Triple Nut Cluster Sundae	½ cup (2.4 oz)	140	22	19	0
Light Vanilla	½ cup (2.4 oz)	110	18	18	0
Light Vanilla Chocolate Strawberry	½ cup (2.4 oz)	110	18	18	0
Low Fat No Sugar Added Caramel Swirl	½ cup (2.4 oz)	120	18	4	0
Low Fat No Sugar Added Chocolate Supreme	½ cup (2.4 oz)	120	19	4	0
Low Fat No Sugar Added Mocha Fudge	½ cup (2.4 oz)	110	18	4	0
Low Fat No Sugar Added Raspberry Swirl	½ cup (2.4 oz)	110	17	4	0
Low Fat No Sugar Added Vanilla	½ cup (2.4 oz)	100	14	5	0
Maple Walnut	½ cup (2.3 oz)	160	16	16	0
Rockets	1 (2 oz)	120	18	17	1
Sandwich Light	1 (2.2 oz)	160	29	16	1
Sandwich Vanilla	1 (2.2 oz)	180	27	16	1
Sports Bar	1 (2.9 oz)	250	23	22	0
Spumoni	½ cup (2.3 oz)	140	17	17	0
Strawberry	½ cup (2.3 oz)	130	16	16	0
Super Sortment Chocolate & Banana Fudge Bar	1 bar (2.1 oz)	100	18	17	0
Super Sortment Root Beer Float & Orange Cream Bar	1 bar (1.5 oz)	70	12	12	0
Vanilla	½ cup (2.3 oz)	140	16	16	0
Vanilla Chocolate Patchwork	½ cup (2.3 oz)	140	17	16	0
Vanilla Chocolate Strawberry	½ cup (2.3 oz)	140	16	16	0
Vanilla Fudge	½ cup (2.3 oz)	140	20	19	0

FOOD	PORTION	CALS.	CARB.	SUG.	FIB.
Klondike					
Almond Bar	1 (5.2 fl oz)	310	26	19	3
Caramel Crunch	1 (5.2 fl oz)	300	31	30	tr
Chocolate Chocolate Bar	1 (5.2 fl oz)	280	22	17	tr
Coffee Bar	1 (5.2 fl oz)	290	25	21	0
Dark Chocolate Bar	1 (5.2 fl oz)	290	24	23	tr
Gold Bar	1 (5.2 fl oz)	340	30	28	1
Krispy Bar	1 (5.2 fl oz)	300	28	22	0
Krunch	1 (3.1 fl oz)	200	17	14	1
Lite Bar	1 (2.3 fl oz)	110	14	5	1
Lite Bar Caramel	1 (2.4 fl oz)	120	18	4	1
Movie Bites Chocolate	8 pieces (4.6 fl oz)	340	22	22	1
Movie Bites Vanilla	8 pieces (4.6 fl oz)	320	27	27	1
Original Bar	1 (5.2 fl oz)	290	24	24	0
Sandwich Chocolate	1 (5.2 fl oz)	270	41	29	2
Sandwich Lite	1 (2.9 fl oz)	100	18	11	1
Sandwich Vanilla	1 (5.2 fl oz)	250	37	24	1
Mars					
Almond Bar	1 (1.85 fl oz)	210	20	—	0
Milky Way					
Single Chocolate/Milk	1 (2 fl oz)	210	24	—	0
Snack Chocolate/Milk	1 (0.72 fl oz)	70	9	—	0
Snack Vanilla/Dark	1 (0.72 oz)	70	9	—	0
Mocha Mix					
Berry Berry Berry	½ cup	140	20	16	0
Dutch Chocolate	½ cup (2.3 oz)	140	16	12	0
Mocha Almond Fudge	½ cup (2.3 oz)	150	19	12	0
Neapolitan	½ cup (2.3 oz)	140	18	12	0
Strawberry Swirl	½ cup (2.3 oz)	140	20	16	0
Vanilla	½ cup (2.3 oz)	140	18	12	0
Nestle Crunch					
Chocolate	1 bar (3 oz)	200	18	15	0
Cones	1 (4.6 oz)	300	36	23	2
Crunch King	1 (4 oz)	270	21	16	0
Nuggets	8 pieces	140	12	9	0
Reduced Fat	1 (2.5 oz)	130	14	6	0
Vanilla	1 bar (3 oz)	200	17	14	0
Perry's					
No Fat No Sugar Added Caramel	½ cup (2.8 oz)	90	25	5	1
No Fat No Sugar Added Chocolate	½ cup (2.6 oz)	80	21	5	2
No Fat No Sugar Added Peach	½ cup (2.9 oz)	90	24	6	tr

FOOD	PORTION	CALS.	CARB.	SUG.	FIB.
Perry's (CONT.)					
No Fat No Sugar Added Strawberry	½ cup (2.8 oz)	90	23	6	tr
No Fat No Sugar Added Vanilla	½ cup (2.6 oz)	80	21	5	tr
Sealtest					
American Glory	½ cup (2.4 oz)	130	17	13	0
Butter Pecan	½ cup (2.4 oz)	160	16	12	0
Candy Cane Crunch	½ cup (2.4 oz)	150	21	15	0
Chocolate	½ cup (2.4 oz)	140	19	15	tr
Chocolate Butter Pecan	½ cup (2.4 oz)	150	17	13	0
Chocolate Chip	½ cup (2.4 oz)	150	18	14	0
Coconut Chocolate	½ cup (2.4 oz)	160	18	14	tr
Coffee	½ cup (2.4 oz)	140	16	12	0
Cupid's Scoops	½ cup (2.5 oz)	140	20	15	0
French Vanilla	½ cup (2.4 oz)	140	16	13	0
Fudge Royale	½ cup (2.5 oz)	150	19	14	0
Heavenly Hash	½ cup (2.4 oz)	150	20	14	tr
Maple Walnut	½ cup (2.4 oz)	160	16	12	0
Strawberry	½ cup (2.4 oz)	130	19	15	0
Triple Chocolate Passion	½ cup (2.5 oz)	160	21	16	tr
Vanilla	½ cup (2.4 oz)	140	16	13	0
Vanilla Chocolate Strawberry	½ cup (2.4 oz)	140	18	14	0
Vanilla With Orange Sherbet	½ cup (2.7 oz)	130	22	16	0
Snickers					
Single	1 (2 fl oz)	220	22	—	0
Snack	1 (1 fl oz)	110	11	—	0
Starbucks					
Frappuccino	1 bar (2.8 oz)	110	20	17	0
Turkey Hill					
Black Cherry	½ cup (2.3 oz)	140	18	16	0
Butter Pecan	½ cup (2.3 oz)	170	16	15	0
Choco Mint Chip	½ cup (2.3 oz)	160	17	16	0
Cookies 'N Cream	½ cup (2.3 oz)	160	19	17	0
Lite Butter Pecan	½ cup (2.3 oz)	130	17	16	0
Lite Choco Mint Chip	½ cup (2.3 oz)	140	19	18	0
Lite Cookies 'N Cream	½ cup (2.3 oz)	130	21	18	0
Lite Vanilla & Chocolate	½ cup (2.3 oz)	110	18	18	0
Lite Vanilla Bean	½ cup (2.3 oz)	110	18	17	0
Neapolitan	½ cup (2.3 oz)	150	18	17	0
Rocky Road	½ cup (2.3 oz)	170	23	19	0
Tin Roof Sundae	½ cup (2.3 oz)	160	19	18	0

FOOD	PORTION	CALS.	CARB.	SUG.	FIB.
Turkey Hill (CONT.)					
Vanilla	½ cup (2.3 oz)	140	16	16	0
Vanilla & Chocolate	½ cup (2.3 oz)	150	17	16	0
Vanilla Bean	½ cup (2.3 oz)	140	16	16	0
Ultra Slim-Fast					
Bar Fudge	1	90	17	—	2
Bar Vanilla Cookie Crunch	1	90	14	—	1
Chocolate	4 oz	100	19	—	2
Chocolate Fudge	4 oz	120	24	—	2
Peach	4 oz	100	22	—	2
Pralines & Caramel	4 oz	120	25	—	2
Sandwich Vanilla	1	140	28	—	1
Sandwich Vanilla Chocolate	1	140	28	—	1
Sandwich Vanilla Oatmeal	1	150	26	—	3
Vanilla	4 oz	90	19	—	2
Vanilla Fudge Cookie	4 oz	110	24	—	2
Weight Watchers					
Chocolate Dip	1 bar	100	11	6	0
Chocolate Mousse	1 bar	40	9	3	1
Chocolate Treat	1 bar	100	20	17	1
English Toffee Crunch	1 bar	110	12	10	1
Orange Vanilla Treat	1 bar	40	10	3	0
Vanilla Sandwich	1 bar	150	28	14	1

ICE CREAM CONES AND CUPS

FOOD	PORTION	CALS.	CARB.	SUG.	FIB.
sugar cone	1	40	8	—	tr
wafer cone	1	17	3	—	tr
Comet					
Cups	1 (5 g)	20	1	0	tr
Sugar Cones	1 (12 g)	50	11	3	tr
Waffle Cone	1 (17 g)	70	14	3	1
Dutch Mill					
Chocolate Covered Wafer Cups	1 (0.5 oz)	80	8	6	0
Oreo					
Chocolate Cones	1 (13 g)	50	10	4	tr
Teddy Grahams					
Cinnamon Cones	1 (0.5 oz)	60	13	5	tr

ICE CREAM TOPPINGS
(see also SYRUP*)*

FOOD	PORTION	CALS.	CARB.	SUG.	FIB.
Ben & Jerry's					
Hot Fudge	(1.3 oz)	140	19	8	2
Crumpy					
Chocolate Hazelnut Spread	1 tbsp (0.5 oz)	80	8	8	0

FOOD	PORTION	CALS.	CARB.	SUG.	FIB.
Hershey					
Chocolate Shoppe Candy Bar Sprinkles York	2 tbsp (1.1 oz)	170	22	17	2
Kraft					
Butterscotch	2 tbsp (1.4 oz)	130	28	18	0
Caramel	2 tbsp (1.4 oz)	120	28	20	0
Chocolate	2 tbsp (1.4 oz)	110	26	20	1
Hot Fudge	2 tbsp (1.4 oz)	140	24	17	tr
Pineapple	2 tbsp (1.4 oz)	110	28	19	0
Strawberry	2 tbsp (1.4 oz)	110	29	22	0
Marzetti					
Caramel Apple	2 tbsp	60	23	20	0
Caramel Apple Reduced Fat	2 tbsp	30	26	21	0
Peanut Butter Caramel	2 tbsp	60	21	14	1
Planters					
Nut	2 tbsp (0.5 oz)	100	3	tr	1

ICED TEA
(*see also* TEA/HERBAL TEA)

MIX

FOOD	PORTION	CALS.	CARB.	SUG.	FIB.
Crystal Light					
Decaffeinated as prep	1 serv (8 oz)	5	tr	0	0
Iced Tea as prep	1 serv (8 oz)	5	0	0	0
Peach Tea as prep	1 serv (8 oz)	5	0	0	0
Raspberry Tea as prep	1 serv (8 oz)	5	0	0	0
Lipton					
100% Tea Decaffeinated as prep	1 serv	0	0	0	0
100% Tea Unsweetened as prep	1 serv	0	0	0	0
100% Tea as prep	1 serv	0	0	0	0
Calorie Free as prep	1 serv	0	0	0	0
Decaffeinated Ice Tea Brew as prep	1 serv (8 oz)	0	0	0	0
Decaffeinated Lemon as prep	1 serv	90	22	22	—
Diet Decaffeinated Lemon as prep	1 serv	5	1	0	—
Diet Lemon as prep	1 serv	5	1	0	—
Diet Peach as prep	1 serv	5	1	0	—
Diet Raspberry as prep	1 serv	5	1	0	—
Diet Tea & Lemondage as prep	1 serv	10	2	0	—
Herbal Iced Collection	1 tea bag	0	tr	0	—

FOOD	PORTION	CALS.	CARB.	SUG.	FIB.
Lipton (CONT.)					
Ice Tea Brew as prep	1 serv (8 oz)	0	0	0	0
Lemon as prep	1 serv	90	22	22	—
Lemon as prep	1 pkg (0.5 oz)	50	13	13	—
Natrual Brew Tropical as prep	1 serv	90	22	22	—
Natural Brew 100% Tea Decaffeinated as prep	1 serv	0	0	0	0
Natural Brew 100% Tea as prep	1 serv	0	0	0	0
Natural Brew Diet Lemon as prep	1 serv	5	1	0	—
Natural Brew Diet Peach as prep	1 serv	5	1	0	—
Natural Brew Diet Tropical as prep	1 serv	5	1	0	—
Natural Brew Unsweetened Lemon as prep	1 serv	0	tr	0	—
Peach as prep	1 serv	90	22	22	—
Rasberry as prep	1 serv	90	22	22	—
Tea & Lemonade as prep	1 serv	90	22	22	—
Nestea					
100% Instant Tea as prep	8 oz	2	0	0	0
READY-TO-DRINK					
Arizona					
Raspberry	8 fl oz	95	25	24	—
Crystal Light					
Lemon	1 serv (8 oz)	5	0	0	0
Peach Tea	1 serv (8 oz)	5	0	0	0
Raspberry Tea	1 serv (8 oz)	5	0	0	0
Lipton					
Carribean Cooler	1 can (12 oz)	130	34	34	—
Diet Lemon	8 oz	0	0	0	0
Diet Lemon	1 bottle (16 oz)	10	0	0	0
Green Tea & Passion Fruit	1 bottle (16 oz)	160	38	38	—
Lemon	8 oz	80	20	20	—
Lemon	1 can (12 oz)	120	33	33	—
Lemon	1 bottle (16 oz)	180	42	42	—
Natural Lemon	1 box (8 oz)	100	25	24	—
Peach	8 oz	80	20	20	—
Peach	1 bottle (16 oz)	220	52	52	—
Raspberry	8 oz	80	20	20	—
Raspberry	1 bottle (16 oz)	220	52	52	—
Raspberry Blast	1 can (12 oz)	130	35	35	—

FOOD	PORTION	CALS.	CARB.	SUG.	FIB.
Lipton (CONT.)					
Southern Style Extra Sweet No Lemon	1 bottle (16 oz)	240	58	58	—
Southern Style Lemon	1 bottle (16 oz)	200	50	50	—
Southern Style Sweetened No Lemon	1 bottle (16 oz)	200	48	48	—
Sweet	8 oz	80	20	20	—
Sweetened No Lemon	1 bottle (16 oz)	140	36	36	—
Sweetened Lemon	8 oz	80	20	20	—
Tangerine Twist	1 can (12 oz)	120	33	33	—
Tea & Lemonade	1 bottle (16 oz)	220	52	52	—
Unsweetened No Lemon	1 bottle (16 oz)	0	0	0	0
Nestea					
With Sugar & Lemon	1 bottle (16 fl oz)	176	44	40	—
With Sugar & Lemon	1 can (11.5 fl oz)	127	32	29	—
Schweppes					
Ice Tea	8 fl oz	90	22	22	0
Snapple					
Lemon	8 fl oz	110	27	27	—
Tropicana					
Diet Lemon Fruit	8 fl oz	15	4	3	—
Lemon Fruit	8 fl oz	100	25	23	—
Peach Fruit	1 can (11.5 fl oz)	160	41	40	—
Peach Fruit	1 bottle (10 fl oz)	140	35	33	—
Peach Fruit	8 fl oz	120	28	26	—
Raspberry Fruit	1 can (11.5 fl oz)	160	41	40	—
Raspberry Fruit	8 fl oz	120	28	26	—
Raspberry Fruit	1 bottle (10 fl oz)	140	34	33	—
Tangerine Fruit	8 fl oz	110	27	25	—
Tangerine Fruit	1 bottle (10 fl oz)	140	34	31	—
Tangerine Fruit	1 can (11.5 fl oz)	170	42	41	—
Twister Apple Berry	8 fl oz	100	28	23	—
Twister Lemon Citrus	8 fl oz	110	28	25	—
Turkey Hill					
Diet Decaffeinated	1 cup (8 oz)	0	0	0	0
Raspberry Cooler	1 cup (8 oz)	110	28	28	—
Regular	1 cup (8 oz)	90	22	22	—

ICES AND ICE POPS

(*see also* ICE CREAM AND FROZEN DESSERTS, PUDDING POPS, SHERBET, YOGURT FROZEN)

FOOD	PORTION	CALS.	CARB.	SUG.	FIB.
fruit & juice bar	1 (3 fl oz)	75	19	17	—
gelatin pop	1 (1.5 oz)	31	7	7	—
Cool Creations					
10 Pack	1 pop (2 oz)	60	14	13	0

FOOD	PORTION	CALS.	CARB.	SUG.	FIB.
Cool Creations (CONT.)					
Lion King Cone	1 (4 oz)	280	36	24	1
Mickey Mouse Bar	1 (2.5 oz)	110	12	10	0
Mickey Mouse Bar	1 (4 oz)	170	17	10	0
Surprise Pops	1 (2 oz)	60	14	13	0
Dole					
Fruit 'N Juice Coconut	1 bar (4 oz)	210	33	30	0
Fruit 'N Juice Lemonade	1 bar (4 oz)	120	28	26	0
Fruit 'N Juice Lime	1 bar (4 oz)	110	28	24	0
Fruit 'N Juice Peach Passion	1 bar (2.5 oz)	70	17	15	0
Fruit 'N Juice Pineapple Coconut	1 bar (4 oz)	140	27	24	0
Fruit 'N Juice Pineapple Orange Banana	1 bar (2.5 oz)	70	16	15	0
Fruit 'N Juice Pineapple Orange Banana	1 bar (4 oz)	110	26	24	0
Fruit 'N Juice Raspberry	1 bar (2.5 oz)	70	16	13	0
Fruit 'N Juice Strawberry	1 bar (2.5 oz)	70	17	15	0
Fruit 'N Juice Strawberry	1 bar (4 oz)	110	26	24	0
Fruit Juice Grape	1 bar (1.75 oz)	45	11	10	0
Fruit Juice No Sugar Added Grape	1 bar (1.75 oz)	25	6	3	0
Fruit Juice No Sugar Added Strawberry	1 bar (1.75 oz)	25	6	3	0
Fruit Juice Raspberry	1 bar (1.75 oz)	45	11	10	0
Fruit Juice Raspberry	1 bar (1.75 oz)	25	6	3	0
Fruit Juice Strawberry	1 bar (1.75 oz)	45	11	10	0
Flintstones					
Rock Pops	1 (3.5 oz)	80	20	0	0
Frozfruit					
Banana Cream	1 bar (4 oz)	150	20	18	1
Cantaloupe	1 bar (4 oz)	60	35	14	0
Cappuccino Cream	1 bar (3 oz)	140	18	13	0
Cherry	1 bar (4 oz)	70	18	17	1
Coconut Cream	1 bar (4 oz)	170	17	15	2
Kiwi Strawberry	1 bar (4 oz)	90	23	21	2
Lemon	1 bar (4 oz)	90	22	20	0
Lemon Iced Tea	1 bar (4 oz)	80	19	14	0
Lime	1 bar (4 oz)	90	21	19	0
Orange	1 bar (4 oz)	90	21	19	0
Pina Colada Cream	1 bar (4 oz)	170	23	21	1
Pineapple	1 bar (4 oz)	80	19	18	0
Raspberry	1 bar (4 oz)	80	20	18	1

FOOD	PORTION	CALS.	CARB.	SUG.	FIB.
Frozfruit (CONT.)					
Strawberry	1 (4 oz)	80	20	18	1
Strawberry Banana Cream	1 bar (4 oz)	140	22	19	1
Strawberry Cream	1 bar (4 oz)	130	21	20	1
Tropical	1 bar (4 oz)	90	23	22	1
Watermelon	1 bar (4 oz)	50	13	12	0
Good Humor					
Big Stick Cherry Pineapple	1 (3.6 fl oz)	50	12	10	0
Big Stick Popsicle	1 (3.6 fl oz)	50	12	10	—
Calippo Cherry	1 (3.8 fl oz)	100	23	21	—
Calippo Grape Lemon	1 (3.9 fl oz)	90	22	18	—
Calippo Orange	1 (3.9 fl oz)	90	23	19	—
Citrus Bites	1 (1.8 fl oz)	35	9	7	—
Creamsicle Orange	1 (2.8 fl oz)	110	20	15	0
Creamsicle Orange	1 (1.8 fl oz)	70	13	12	0
Creamsicle Orange Raspberry	1 (2.6 fl oz)	100	19	14	0
Creamsicle Sugar Free	1 (1.8 fl oz)	25	5	1	—
Flinstones Push-Up Yabba Dabba Doo Orange	1 (2.75 fl oz)	90	20	—	—
Fudgsicle Bar	1 (2.8 fl oz)	90	17	14	1
Fudgsicle Pop	1 (1.8 fl oz)	60	12	10	0
Fudgsicle Sugar Free	1 (1.8 fl oz)	40	8	3	1
Fun Box Fudge Bar	1 (2.3 fl oz)	80	16	15	0
Fun Box Pops	1 (2 fl oz)	35	10	8	—
Fun Box Twin Box Cherry	1 (2.6 fl oz)	50	14	12	—
Fun Box Twin Pop Banana	1 (2.6 fl oz)	50	14	12	—
Fun Box Twin Pop Blue Raspberry	1 (2.6 fl oz)	50	14	12	—
Fun Box Twin Pop Cherry Lemon	1 (2.6 fl oz)	50	14	12	—
Fun Box Twin Pop Orange Cherry Grape	1 (2.6 oz)	50	14	12	—
Fun Box Twin Pop Root Beer	1 (2.6 fl oz)	50	14	12	—
Garfield Bar	1 (3.9 fl oz)	90	22	17	—
Great White	1 (3.1 fl oz)	70	18	14	—
Hyperstripe	1 (2.8 fl oz)	80	21	16	—
Ice Stripe Cherry Orange	1 (1.5 fl oz)	35	9	7	0
Jumbo Jet Star	1 (4.7 fl oz)	80	20	14	—
Laser Blazer	1 (2.6 oz)	70	16	13	—
Popsicle All Natural	1 (1.8 fl oz)	45	10	8	—
Popsicle Orange Cherry Grape	1 (1.8 fl oz)	45	11	11	—

FOOD	PORTION	CALS.	CARB.	SUG.	FIB.
Good Humor (CONT.)					
Popsicle Rainbow Pops	1 (1.8 fl oz)	45	11	11	—
Popsicle Rootbeer Banana Lime	1 (1.8 fl oz)	45	11	11	—
Popsicle Strawberry Raspberry Wildberry	1 (1.8 fl oz)	45	11	11	—
Popsicle Supersicle Traffic Signal	1	80	20	14	—
Popsicle Twin Pop Cherry	1 (2.6 fl oz)	70	16	13	—
Popsicle Twin Pop Orange Cherry Grape Lime	1 (2.6 fl oz)	70	16	13	—
Snow Cone	1	60	14	13	—
Snowfruit Coconut Bar	1 (3.75 fl oz)	150	27	21	1
Snowfruit Orange Bar	1	140	34	25	tr
Snowfruit Strawberry Bar	1	120	31	23	tr
Snowfruit Tropical Fruit Bar	1	110	28	21	—
Sugar Free Pop Orange Cherry Grape	1 (1.8 fl oz)	15	3	0	—
Super Mario Bar	1	120	27	18	—
Supersicle Cherry Banana	1 (4.7 fl oz)	80	20	14	—
Supersicle Cherry Cola	1 (4.7 fl oz)	80	20	14	—
Supersicle Double Fudge	1 (4.7 fl oz)	150	29	28	1
Supersicle Firecracker	1 (4.7 fl oz)	90	20	14	—
Supersicle Firecracker Jr.	1	72	10	7	—
Supersicle Sour Tower	1	80	20	14	—
Swirl Bubble Gum	1 (2.7 fl oz)	55	13	10	—
Swirl Cherry Banana	1 (2.7 fl oz)	55	13	10	—
Torpedo Cherry	1 (1.8 fl oz)	35	10	8	0
Twister Blue Raspberry Cherry Cherry Cola Cherry	1 (1.8 fl oz)	45	10	8	—
Twister Cherry Lemon Orange Lemon	1 (1.8 fl oz)	45	10	8	—
Vampire's Deadly Secret	1 (2.8 fl oz)	100	24	17	—
Watermelon Bar	1 (3.6 fl oz)	80	20	16	—
Haagen-Dazs					
Sorbet Banana Strawberry	½ cup (4 oz)	140	34	28	tr
Sorbet Chocolate	½ cup (4 oz)	130	30	22	2
Sorbet Manago	½ cup (4 oz)	120	30	27	tr
Sorbet Orchard Peach	½ cup (4 oz)	140	35	31	tr
Sorbet Raspberry	½ cup (4 oz)	120	29	26	1
Sorbet Strawberry	½ cup (4 oz)	130	33	30	1
Sorbet Zesty Lemon	½ cup (4 oz)	130	32	28	tr
Sorbet & Cream Orange	½ cup (3.7 oz)	200	27	24	0

FOOD	PORTION	CALS.	CARB.	SUG.	FIB.
Haagen-Dazs (CONT.)					
Sorbet & Cream Raspberry	½ cup (3.7 oz)	190	23	22	tr
Sorbet Bar Chocolate	1 (2.7 oz)	80	20	15	1
Sorbet Bar Wild Berry	1 (2.7 oz)	90	22	17	tr
Hershey					
Orange Blossom	1 bar (1.6 oz)	90	10	10	0
Hood					
Hendrie's Sizzle'N Sour Stix	1 bar (2 oz)	80	15	15	0
Hoodsie Pop	1 (3.3 oz)	60	16	16	—
Natural Blenders Pineappple	1 bar (1 oz)	60	16	16	—
Natural Blenders Raspberry	1 bar (1 oz)	60	16	16	—
Natural Blenders Strawberry	1 bar (1 oz)	60	16	16	—
Pop Banana	1 (3.3 oz)	60	16	16	—
Pop Blue Raspberry	1 (3.3 oz)	60	16	16	—
Pop Cherry	1 (3.3 oz)	60	16	16	—
Pop Grape	1 (3.3 oz)	60	16	16	—
Pop Orange	1 (3.3 oz)	60	16	16	—
Pop Root Beer	1 (3.3 oz)	60	16	16	—
Super Sortment Juice Bars	1 bar (1.9 oz)	40	10	10	—
Lifesavers					
Ice Pops	1	35	9	—	0
Ice Pops	1 (1.75 oz)	35	9	8	0
Mr. Freeze					
Assorted	2 bars (3 oz)	45	11	11	0
Tropical	2 bars (3 oz)	45	11	11	0
Sunkist					
Orange Juice Bar	1 (3.4 fl oz)	80	19	19	—
Wildberry	1 (3.4 fl oz)	120	27	20	—

ICING
(*see* CAKE ICING)

INSTANT BREAKFAST
(*see* BREAKFAST DRINKS)

JALAPENO
(*see* PEPPERS)

JAM/JELLY/PRESERVES

FOOD	PORTION	CALS.	CARB.	SUG.	FIB.
all flavors jam	1 tbsp (0.7 oz)	48	13	10	tr
all flavors jam	1 pkg (0.5 oz)	34	9	7	tr
all flavors jelly	1 tbsp (0.7 oz)	52	14	12	tr
all flavors jelly	1 pkg (0.5 oz)	38	10	9	tr
all flavors preserve	1 pkg (0.5 oz)	34	9	7	tr

FOOD	PORTION	CALS.	CARB.	SUG.	FIB.
all flavors preserve	1 tbsp (0.7 oz)	48	13	10	tr
apple jelly	1 tbsp (0.7 oz)	52	14	12	tr
apple jelly	1 pkg (0.5 oz)	38	10	9	tr
linganberry jam	0.5 oz	23	6	4	tr
strawberry jam	1 pkg (0.5 oz)	34	9	7	tr
strawberry jam	1 tbsp (0.7 oz)	48	13	10	tr
strawberry preserve	1 pkg (0.5 oz)	34	9	7	tr
strawberry preserve	1 tbsp (0.7 oz)	48	13	10	tr
Estee					
Apple Reduced Calorie	1 pkg (0.5 oz)	10	2	2	—
Apple Slice	1 tbsp (0.5 oz)	10	2	2	—
Apricot	1 tbsp (0.5 oz)	5	1	1	—
Blackberry	1 tbsp (0.5 oz)	5	1	1	—
Cherry	1 tbsp (0.5 oz)	5	1	1	—
Grape	1 tbsp (0.5 oz)	10	2	2	—
Orange	1 tbsp (0.5 oz)	10	2	2	—
Peach	1 tbsp (0.5 oz)	5	1	1	—
Red Raspberry	1 tbsp (0.5 oz)	5	1	1	—
Strawberry	1 tbsp (0.5 oz)	10	2	2	—
Harvest Moon					
Apricot Fruit Spread	1 tbsp (0.6 oz)	35	9	9	—
Blueberry Fruit Spread	1 tbsp (0.6 oz)	35	9	9	—
Cherry Fruit Spread	1 tbsp (0.6 oz)	35	9	9	—
Grape Fruit Spread	1 tbsp (0.6 oz)	35	9	9	—
Peach Fruit Spread	1 tbsp (0.6 oz)	35	9	9	—
Raspberry Fruit Spread	1 tbsp (0.6 oz)	35	9	9	—
Strawberry Fruit Spread	1 tbsp (0.6 oz)	35	9	9	—
Red Wing					
Apple Jelly	1 tbsp (0.7 oz)	50	13	9	0
Apple Blackberry Jelly	1 tbsp (0.7 oz)	50	13	9	0
Apple Cherry Jelly	1 tbsp (0.7 oz)	50	13	9	0
Apple Currant Jelly	1 tbsp (0.7 oz)	50	13	9	0
Apple Grape Jelly	1 tbsp (0.7 oz)	50	13	9	0
Apple Raspberry Jelly	1 tbsp (0.7 oz)	50	13	9	0
Apple Strawberry Jelly	1 tbsp (0.7 oz)	50	13	9	0
Black Raspberry Jelly	1 tbsp (0.7 oz)	50	13	10	0
Blackberry Jelly	1 tbsp (0.7 oz)	50	13	10	0
Cherry Jelly	1 tbsp (0.7 oz)	50	13	10	0
Concord Grape Jelly	1 tbsp (0.7 oz)	50	13	10	0
Crabapple Jelly	1 tbsp (0.7 oz)	50	13	10	0
Cranberry Jelly	1 tbsp (0.7 oz)	50	13	10	0
Cranberry Grape Jelly	1 tbsp (0.7 oz)	50	13	9	0
Currant Jelly	1 tbsp (0.7 oz)	50	13	10	0
Damson Plum Jelly	1 tbsp (0.7 oz)	50	13	10	0

FOOD	PORTION	CALS.	CARB.	SUG.	FIB.
Red Wing (CONT.)					
Elderberry Jelly	1 tbsp (0.7 oz)	50	13	10	0
Grape Jelly	1 tbsp (0.7 oz)	50	13	10	0
Mint Jelly	1 tbsp (0.7 oz)	50	13	10	0
Mint Apple Jelly	1 tbsp (0.7 oz)	50	13	10	0
Mixed Fruit Jelly	1 tbsp (0.7 oz)	50	13	9	0
Red Plum Jelly	1 tbsp (0.7 oz)	50	13	10	0
Red Raspberry Jelly	1 tbsp (0.7 oz)	50	13	10	0
Strawberry Jelly	1 tbsp (0.7 oz)	50	13	10	0
Strawberry Apple Jelly	1 tbsp (0.7 oz)	50	13	9	0
Tabasco					
Spicy Pepper Jelly	1 tbsp (0.6 oz)	50	12	11	0
Tree Of Life					
Apricot Fruit Spread	1 tbsp (0.6 oz)	45	12	12	—
Blueberry Fruit Spread	1 tbsp (0.6 oz)	35	9	9	—
Cherry Fruit Spread	1 tbsp (0.6 oz)	40	10	10	—
Grape Fruit Spread	1 tbsp (0.6 oz)	35	8	8	—
Peach Fruit Spread	1 tbsp (0.6 oz)	45	12	12	—
Raspberry Fruit Spread	1 tbsp (0.6 oz)	30	7	7	—
Strawberry Fruit Spread	1 tbsp (0.6 oz)	35	9	9	—
Whistling Wings					
Blueberry Jam	1 oz	50	12	—	tr
Raspberry Jam	1 oz	60	14	—	1
White House					
Apple Butter	1 oz	50	12	—	1

JAPANESE FOOD
(*see* ASIAN FOOD, SUSHI)

JELLY
(*see* JAM/JELLY/PRESERVES)

JERUSALEM ARTICHOKE
(*see* ARTICHOKE)

KETCHUP

FOOD	PORTION	CALS.	CARB.	SUG.	FIB.
ketchup	1 tbsp	16	4	—	tr
ketchup	1 pkg (0.2 oz)	6	2	—	tr
low sodium	1 tbsp	16	4	—	tr
Del Monte					
Ketchup	1 tbsp (0.5 oz)	15	4	4	0
Estee					
Imitation Sodium Free	1 pkg (0.5 oz)	15	3	2	—
Healthy Choice					
Ketchup	1 tbsp (0.5 oz)	9	2	2	tr

FOOD	PORTION	CALS.	CARB.	SUG.	FIB.
Hunt's					
Ketchup	1 tbsp (0.6 oz)	16	3	4	0
No Salt Added	1 tbsp (0.6 oz)	16	3	4	0
McIlhenny					
Spicy	1 tbsp (0.6 oz)	20	5	2	0
Muir Glen					
Organic	1 tbsp (0.6 oz)	15	3	3	0
Red Wing					
Extra Fancy	1 tbsp (0.6 oz)	20	5	3	0
Tree Of Life					
Ketchup	1 tbsp (0.5 oz)	10	3	3	—
Salsa Ketchup	1 tbsp (0.5 oz)	10	3	1	—

KIDNEY

FOOD	PORTION	CALS.	CARB.	SUG.	FIB.
beef simmered	3 oz	122	0	0	0
pork cooked	1 cup	211	0	0	0
pork cooked	3 oz	128	0	0	0
veal braised	3 oz	139	0	0	0

KIDNEY BEANS
CANNED

FOOD	PORTION	CALS.	CARB.	SUG.	FIB.
B&M					
Red Baked Beans	½ cup (4.6 oz)	170	32	10	6
Eden					
Organic	½ cup (4.6 oz)	100	18	—	10
Friend's					
Red Baked Beans	½ cup (4.6 oz)	160	32	10	6
Goya					
Spanish Style	7.5 oz	140	29	—	10
Green Giant					
Dark Red	½ cup (4.5 oz)	110	18	tr	5
Light Red	½ cup (4.5 oz)	110	20	2	6
Hunt's					
Red	½ cup (4.5 oz)	94	20	6	5
Progresso					
Red	½ cup (4.6 oz)	110	20	0	8
Trappey					
Dark Red	½ cup (4.5 oz)	130	22	1	8
Light Red	½ cup (4.5 oz)	120	22	2	8
Light Red New Orleans Style With Bacon	½ cup (4.5 oz)	110	20	3	6
Light Red With Jalapeno	½ cup (4.5 oz)	110	19	2	6
With Chili Gravy	½ cup (4.5 oz)	110	20	3	7
Van Camp's					
Dark Red	½ cup (4.6 oz)	90	20	—	6

FOOD	PORTION	CALS.	CARB.	SUG.	FIB.
Van Camp's (CONT.)					
Light Red	½ cup (4.6 oz)	90	20	—	6
DRIED					
Arrowhead					
Red	¼ cup (1.6 oz)	160	29	0	10
KIWI JUICE					
After The Fall					
Kiwi Bear	1 cup (8 oz)	100	24	23	0
KIWIS					
fresh	1 med	46	11	—	3
Dole					
Fresh	2	90	18	—	4
Sonoma					
Dried	7-8 pieces (1 oz)	90	19	—	2
KNISH					
Joshua's					
Coney Island Potato	1 (4.6 oz)	280	52	12	1
LAMB					
(*see also* LAMB DISHES)					
FRESH					
cubed lean only braised	3 oz	190	0	0	0
cubed lean only broiled	3 oz	158	0	0	0
ground broiled	3 oz	240	0	0	0
loin chop w/ bone lean & fat Choice broiled	1 chop (2.3 oz)	201	0	0	0
loin chop w/ bone lean only Choice broiled	1 chop (1.6 oz)	100	0	0	0
rib chop lean & fat Choice broiled	3 oz	307	0	0	0
rib chop lean only Choice broiled	3 oz	200	0	0	0
shank lean & fat Choice braised	3 oz	206	0	0	0
shank lean & fat Choice roasted	3 oz	191	0	0	0
shoulder chop w/ bone lean & fat Choice braised	1 chop (2.5 oz)	244	0	0	0
shoulder chop w/ bone lean only Choice braised	1 chop (1.9 oz)	152	0	0	0
sirloin lean & fat Choice roasted	3 oz	248	0	0	0

FOOD	PORTION	CALS.	CARB.	SUG.	FIB.
FROZEN					
New Zealand lean & fat cooked	3 oz	259	0	0	0
New Zealand lean only cooked	3 oz	175	0	0	0

LECITHIN
(see SOY)

LEMON
Dole

Fresh	1	18	4	—	0

LEMON CURD

lemon curd made w/ egg	2 tsp	29	4	—	0
lemon curd made w/ starch	2 tsp	28	6	—	0

LEMON GRASS

fresh	1 cup (2.4 oz)	66	17	—	0
fresh	1 tbsp (5 g)	5	1	—	0

LEMON JUICE
After The Fall

Spicy Lemon	1 can (12 oz)	150	37	35	0

LEMONADE
FROZEN
Bright & Early

Lemonade	8 fl oz	120	30	29	—

Minute Maid

Country Style	8 fl oz	120	30	28	—
Cranberry Lemonade	8 fl oz	80	30	28	—
Lemonade	8 fl oz	110	29	28	—
Pink	8 fl oz	120	30	28	—
Raspberry	8 fl oz	120	30	28	—

Seneca

as prep	8 fl oz	110	27	—	1

MIX
Country Time

Lem'n Berry Sippers Cranberry Raspberry Lemonade as prep	1 serv (8 oz)	90	21	21	0
Lem'n Berry Sippers Raspberry Lemonade as prep	1 serv (8 oz)	90	21	21	0
Lem'n Berry Sippers Strawberry Lemonade as prep	1 serv (8 oz)	90	21	21	0

FOOD	PORTION	CALS.	CARB.	SUG.	FIB.
Country Time (CONT.)					
Lem'n Berry Sippers Wildberry Lemonade as prep	1 serv (8 oz)	90	21	21	0
Lem'n Berry Sippers Sugar Free Strawberry Lemonade as prep	1 serv (8 oz)	5	0	0	0
Lemonade as prep	1 serv (8 oz)	70	17	17	0
Pink as prep	1 serv (8 oz)	70	17	17	0
Sugar Free Pink as prep	1 serv (8 oz)	5	0	0	0
Sugar Free as prep	1 serv (8 oz)	5	0	0	0
Crystal Light					
Lemonade as prep	1 serv (8 oz)	5	0	0	0
Pink as prep	1 serv (8 oz)	5	0	0	0
Kool-Aid					
Lemonade as prep	1 serv (8 oz)	70	17	17	0
Mix as prep w/ sugar	1 serv (8 oz)	100	25	25	0
Pink as prep w/ sugar	1 serv (8 oz)	100	25	25	0
Soarin' Strawberry Lemonade as prep	1 serv (8 oz)	70	17	17	0
Soarin' Strawberry Lemonade as prep w/ sugar	1 serv (8 oz)	100	25	25	0
Sugar Free Soarin' Strawberry Lemonade as prep	1 serv (8 oz)	5	0	0	0
Sugar Free Mix as prep	1 serv (8 oz)	5	0	0	0
READY-TO-DRINK					
After The Fall					
Apple Raspberry	1 bottle (10 oz)	120	29	28	—
Crystal Geyser					
Juice Squeeze Pink	1 bottle (12 fl oz)	140	34	27	—
Crystal Light					
Lemonade	1 serv (8 oz)	5	0	0	0
Pink	1 serv (8 oz)	5	0	0	0
Diet Rite					
Salt/Sodium Free	8 fl oz	2	1	—	—
Everfresh					
Lemonade	1 can (8 oz)	120	29	29	0
Ruby Red	1 can (8 oz)	110	27	27	0
Fruitopia					
Lemonade	8 fl oz	120	29	29	—
Minute Maid					
Chilled	8 fl oz	110	28	26	—

FOOD	PORTION	CALS.	CARB.	SUG.	FIB.
Minute Maid (CONT.)					
Cranberry Chilled	8 fl oz	120	31	29	—
Juices To Go	1 bottle (16 fl oz)	110	28	27	—
Juices To Go	1 can (11.5 fl oz)	160	40	38	—
Juices To Go Canberry Lemonade	1 bottle (16 fl oz)	110	29	28	—
Juices To Go Raspberry Lemonade	1 bottle (16 fl oz)	120	29	29	—
Pink Chilled	8 fl oz	110	28	26	—
Raspberry Chilled	8 fl oz	120	30	28	—
Mott's					
Lemonade	10 fl oz	160	41	35	0
Newman's Own					
Lemonade	1 bottle (10 oz)	140	34	34	0
Roadside Virginia	8 fl oz	110	27	27	0
Odwalla					
Honey	8 fl oz	70	26	25	0
Strawberry	8 fl oz	150	40	38	2
Santa Cruz					
Organic	8 oz	100	24	21	—
Shasta Plus					
Lemonade	1 can (11.5 oz)	160	40	40	0
Snapple					
Lemonade	8 fl oz	110	29	27	—
Tropicana					
Lemonade	1 can (11.5 oz)	160	39	36	—
Lemonade	8 fl oz	110	28	26	—
Twister Wild Berry	8 fl oz	120	30	25	—
Turkey Hill					
Lemonade	8 fl oz	110	29	29	—
Veryfine					
Chillers	1 can (11.5 oz)	190	48	48	0
Chillers Cherry	8 fl oz	120	29	29	0
Chillers Peach	8 fl oz	120	31	31	0
Chillers Pink	1 can (11.5 oz)	180	45	45	0
Chillers Strawberry	1 can (11.5 oz)	170	43	42	0

LENTILS
CANNED

FOOD	PORTION	CALS.	CARB.	SUG.	FIB.
Eden					
Organic w/ Sweet Onion & Bay Leaf	½ cup (4.6 oz)	90	13	0	4
Health Valley					
Fast Menu Hearty Lentils Garden Vegetables	7½ oz	150	16	—	16

FOOD	PORTION	CALS.	CARB.	SUG.	FIB.
Health Valley (CONT.)					
Fast Menu Organic Lentils With Tofu Weiner	7½ oz	170	15	—	15
FROZEN					
Natural Touch					
Lentil Rice Loaf	1 in slice (3.2 oz)	170	14	tr	4
MIX					
Casbah					
Pilaf as prep	1 cup	200	38	0	2

LETTUCE
(*see also* SALAD)

FOOD	PORTION	CALS.	CARB.	SUG.	FIB.
bibb	1 head (6 oz)	21	4	—	2
boston	2 leaves	2	tr	—	tr
boston	1 head (6 oz)	21	4	—	2
iceberg	1 leaf	3	tr	—	tr
iceberg	1 head (19 oz)	70	11	—	5
romaine shredded	½ cup	4	1	—	tr
Dole					
Butter	1 head	21	4	—	2
Iceberg	⅙ med head	20	4	—	1
Leaf shredded	1½ cup	12	1	—	1
Romaine shredded	1½ cups	18	2	—	1
Western Express					
Heart's Of Romaine	6 leaves (3 oz)	20	3	2	1

LIMA BEANS
CANNED

FOOD	PORTION	CALS.	CARB.	SUG.	FIB.
Allen					
Green	½ cup (4.5 oz)	120	23	0	8
Green & White	½ cup (4.5 oz)	110	20	tr	9
Del Monte					
Green	½ cup (4.4 oz)	80	15	0	4
East Texas Fair					
Green	½ cup (4.5 oz)	120	23	0	8
Seneca					
Limas	½ cup	80	15	—	5
Trappey					
Baby Green With Bacon	½ cup (4.5 oz)	120	22	2	6
DRIED					
baby cooked	1 cup	229	42	—	17
large cooked	1 cup	217	39	—	14
Hurst					
HamBeens Baby Limas w/ Ham	1 serv	120	22	1	9

FOOD	PORTION	CALS.	CARB.	SUG.	FIB.
Hurst (CONT.)					
HamBeens Large Limas w/ Ham	1 serv	120	22	1	9
FROZEN					
Birds Eye					
Baby	½ cup (3.3 oz)	130	24	2	6
Fordhook	½ cup (3.3 oz)	100	19	3	5
Fresh Like					
Baby	3.5 oz	138	25	—	2
Green Giant					
Butter Sauce	⅔ cup (3.6 oz)	120	18	1	6
Harvest Fresh Baby	½ cup (2.7 oz)	80	15	tr	4

LIME JUICE
After The Fall					
Caribbean Lime	1 can (12 oz)	170	42	41	0
Key West	1 cup (8 oz)	100	25	24	0
Odwalla					
Summertime Lime	8 fl oz	90	23	21	0
Realime					
Juice	1 oz	6	2	—	—

LING
fresh baked	3 oz	95	0	0	0

LINGCOD
baked	3 oz	93	0	0	0

LIQUOR/LIQUEUR
(*see also* BEER AND ALE, CHAMPAGNE, DRINK MIXERS, MALT, WINE, WINE COOLERS)

anisette	⅔ oz	74	7	—	0
apricot brandy	⅔ oz	64	6	—	0
aquavit	3.5 oz	229	0	0	0
benedictine	⅔ oz	69	7	—	0
bourbon & soda	4 oz	105	0	0	0
cognac	3.5 oz	233	1	0	0
curacao liqueur	⅔ oz	54	6	—	0
gin	1½ oz	110	0	0	0
long island ice tea	1 serv (7.5 oz)	159	14	13	0
mint julep	10 oz	210	3	—	0
old-fashioned	2½ oz	127	3	—	0
rum	1½ oz	97	0	0	0
sloe gin fizz	2½ oz	132	4	—	0
vodka	1½ oz	97	0	0	0

FOOD	PORTION	CALS.	CARB.	SUG.	FIB.

LIVER
(see also PATE)

pork braised	3 oz	140	3	—	0

LOBSTER
(see also CRAYFISH)
CANNED
Progresso

Rock Lobster Sauce	½ cup (4.3 oz)	100	6	3	2

LOX
(see SALMON)

LYCHEES
Ka-Me

Whole Pitted In Syrup	15 pieces (5 oz)	130	32	0	0

MACADAMIA NUTS
MacFarms of Hawaii

Chocolate Covered	¼ cup (1.3 oz)	210	18	15	2
Dry Roasted Salted	¼ cup (1.3 oz)	220	4	1	3
Kona Coffee Dark Chocolate Covered	¼ cup (1.3 oz)	210	18	15	2

MACARONI
(see PASTA)

MACKEREL
CANNED

jack	1 can (12.7 oz)	563	0	0	0
jack	1 cup	296	0	0	0

Empress

Jack	4 oz	140	0	0	0

FRESH

atlantic cooked	3 oz	223	0	0	0
jack baked	3 oz	171	0	0	0
king baked	3 oz	114	0	0	0
pacific baked	3 oz	171	0	0	0
spanish cooked	3 oz	134	0	0	0

MALT
Bartles & Jaymes

Malt Cooler Berry	12 fl oz	210	32	29	—
Malt Cooler Black Cherry	12 fl oz	190	30	27	—
Malt Cooler Light Berry	12 fl oz	140	29	27	—
Malt Cooler Mandarin Lemon	12 fl oz	210	34	30	—

FOOD	PORTION	CALS.	CARB.	SUG.	FIB.
Bartles & Jaymes (CONT.)					
Malt Cooler Margarita	12 fl oz	250	44	39	—
Malt Cooler Original	12 fl oz	180	27	23	—
Malt Cooler Peach	12 fl oz	200	31	29	—
Malt Cooler Pina Colada	12 fl oz	270	48	45	—
Malt Cooler Planter's Punch	12 fl oz	220	35	32	—
Malt Cooler Red Sangria	12 fl oz	190	29	26	—
Malt Cooler Strawberry	12 fl oz	200	31	29	—
Malt Cooler Strawberry Daiquiri	12 fl oz	220	35	32	—
Malt Cooler Tropical	12 fl oz	220	36	33	—

MALTED MILK
POWDER
Carnation

Chocolate	3 tbsp (0.7 oz)	90	18	14	tr
Original	3 tbsp (0.7 oz)	90	15	10	tr

MANGO
CANNED
Ka-Me

Mango	4 pieces (5 oz)	102	25	0	0

DRIED
Rainforest Farms

Slices	6 slices (1.3 oz)	140	33	30	2
Sonoma					
Pieces	8 pieces (2 oz)	180	44	44	0

MANGO JUICE
After The Fall

Hawaiian Mango	1 can (12 oz)	180	45	36	0
Mango Ginger	1 can (12 oz)	150	35	30	0
Fresh Samantha					
Mango Mama	1 cup (8 oz)	125	33	—	2
Libby					
Nectar	1 can (11.5 fl oz)	210	52	46	—
Tang					
Drink Mix as prep	1 serv (8 oz)	100	25	25	0

MARGARINE
(*see also* BUTTER BLENDS, BUTTER SUBSTITUTES)

stick corn	1 tsp	34	0	0	0
stick salted	1 tsp	39	0	0	0
stick unsalted	1 tsp	34	0	0	0
tub corn	1 tsp	34	0	0	0

FOOD	PORTION	CALS.	CARB.	SUG.	FIB.
tub diet	1 tsp	17	0	0	0
tub safflower	1 tsp	34	0	0	0
tub salted	1 tsp	34	0	0	0
tub soybean salted	1 tsp	34	0	0	0
tub soybean unsalted	1 tsp	34	0	0	0
tub unsalted	1 tsp	34	0	0	0
tub unsalted	1 cup	1626	0	0	0
Blue Bonnet					
Stick	1 tbsp	100	0	0	0
Tub	1 tbsp	100	0	0	0
Whipped	1 tbsp	80	0	0	0
Fleischmann's					
Stick	1 tbsp	100	0	0	0
Stick Light Corn Oil	1 tbsp	80	0	0	0
Stick Sweet Unsalted	1 tbsp	100	0	0	0
Hain					
Stick Safflower	1 tbsp	100	0	0	0
Stick Safflower Unsalted	1 tbsp	100	0	0	0
Tub Safflower	1 tbsp	100	0	0	0
Hollywood					
Safflower	1 tbsp	100	0	0	0
Safflower Unsalted Sweet	1 tbsp	100	0	0	0
Soft Spread	1 tbsp	90	1	—	0
Land O'Lakes					
Stick	1 tbsp (0.5 oz)	90	0	0	0
Stick With Sweet Cream	1 tbsp (0.5 oz)	90	0	0	0
Stick With Sweet Cream Unsalted	1 tbsp (0.5 oz)	90	0	0	0
Tub	1 tbsp (0.5 oz)	80	0	0	0
Tub With Sweet Cream	1 tbsp (0.5 oz)	80	0	0	0
Mazola					
Stick	1 tbsp (14 g)	100	0	0	0
Stick Unsalted	1 cup (229 g)	1635	0	0	0
Stick Unsalted	1 tbsp (14 g)	100	0	0	0
Tub Diet	1 tbsp (14 g)	50	0	0	0
Tub Light Corn Oil Spread	1 tbsp (14 g)	50	0	0	0
Nucanola					
Stick	1 tbsp	90	0	0	0
Parkay					
Squeeze	1 tbsp (0.5 oz)	80	0	0	0
Stick	1 tbsp (0.5 oz)	90	0	0	0
Stick ⅓ Less Fat	1 tbsp (0.5 oz)	70	0	0	0
Tub	1 tbsp (0.5 oz)	60	0	0	0
Tub Light	1 tbsp (0.5 oz)	50	0	0	0

FOOD	PORTION	CALS.	CARB.	SUG.	FIB.
Parkay (CONT.)					
Tub Soft	1 tbsp (0.5 oz)	100	0	0	0
Tub Soft Diet	1 tbsp (0.5 oz)	50	0	0	0
Whipped	1 tbsp (0.3 oz)	70	0	0	0
Smart Balance					
No Trans Fat	1 tbsp (0.5 oz)	120	0	0	0
No Trans Fat Light	1 tbsp (0.5 oz)	45	0	0	0
No Trans Fat Spread	1 tbsp (0.5 oz)	80	0	0	0
Smart Beat					
Light Unsalted	1 tbsp (0.5 oz)	25	0	0	0
Super Light Trans Fat Free	1 tbsp (0.5 oz)	20	0	0	0
Tub	1 tbsp	25	0	0	0
Tub Unsalted	1 tbsp	25	0	0	0
Tree Of Life					
Canola Soft	1 tbsp (0.5 oz)	100	0	0	0
Stick 100% Soy	1 tbsp (0.5 oz)	100	0	0	0
Stick 100% Soy Salt Free	1 tbsp (0.5 oz)	100	0	0	0
Stick Canola Soy	1 tbsp (0.5 oz)	100	0	0	0
Stick Canola Soy Salt Free	1 tbsp (0.5 oz)	100	0	0	0
Weight Watchers					
Light	1 tbsp	45	2	0	0
Light Sodium Free	1 tbsp	45	2	0	0

MARINADE
(*see* SAUCE)

MARSHMALLOW
Joyva

Twists Chocolate Covered	2 (1.5 oz)	190	21	23	0
Just Born					
Peeps	5 (1.5 oz)	160	40	36	—

MATZO

egg	1 (1 oz)	111	22	—	1
egg & onion	1 (1 oz)	111	22	—	1
plain	1 (1 oz)	112	24	—	1
whole wheat	1 (1 oz)	99	22	—	3
Goodman's					
Matzo Ball Mix 50% Less Salt	2 tbsp (0.5 oz)	50	11	0	0
Matzo Ball Mix as prep	2 tbsp (0.5 oz)	60	12	0	1
Horowitz Margareten					
Egg Milk Chocolate Coated	1 oz	97	16	15	1
Manischewitz					
Daily Thin Tea	1	103	22	—	tr

FOOD	PORTION	CALS.	CARB.	SUG.	FIB.
Manischewitz (CONT.)					
Dietetic Thins	1	91	19	—	tr
Egg Dark Chocolate Coated	½ matzo (1 oz)	97	17	16	1
Matzo Meal	1 cup	514	109	—	tr
Passover Egg	1	132	27	—	—
Salted Thin	1	100	21	—	tr
Unsalted	1	110	24	—	tr
Whole Wheat w/ Bran	1	110	21	—	1
Streit's					
Dietetic	1 (1 oz)	100	23	0	1
Lightly Salted	1 (1 oz)	110	23	1	1
Matzoh Meal	¼ cup (1 oz)	110	24	0	1
Passover	1 (1 oz)	110	25	0	1
Unsalted	1 (0.9 oz)	100	22	0	1
Whole Wheat	1 (1 oz)	110	24	1	4

MAYONNAISE

(*see also* MAYONNAISE TYPE SALAD DRESSING, RELISH)

FOOD	PORTION	CALS.	CARB.	SUG.	FIB.
Kraft					
Fat Free	1 tbsp (0.6 oz)	10	2	1	0
Light	1 tbsp (0.5 oz)	50	2	tr	0
Real	1 tbsp (0.5 oz)	100	0	0	0
McIlhenny					
Spicy	1 tbsp (0.5 oz)	108	1	tr	tr
Red Wing					
"H" Style	1 tbsp (0.5 oz)	110	1	0	0
Weight Watchers					
Fat Free	1 tbsp	10	3	2	0
Light	1 tbsp	25	1	1	0
Light Low Sodium	1 tbsp	25	1	0	0

MAYONNAISE TYPE SALAD DRESSING

(*see also* MAYONNAISE, RELISH)

FOOD	PORTION	CALS.	CARB.	SUG.	FIB.
Miracle Whip					
Free	1 tbsp (0.5 oz)	15	2	2	0
Light	1 tbsp (0.5 oz)	35	2	2	0
Salad Dressing	1 tbsp (0.6 oz)	70	2	1	0
Nayonaise					
Cholesterol Free	1 tbsp (0.5 oz)	35	1	1	tr
Fat Free	1 tbsp (0.5 oz)	11	2		tr
Weight Watchers					
Fat Free Whipped Dressing	1 tbsp	15	3	2	0

MEAT STICKS

FOOD	PORTION	CALS.	CARB.	SUG.	FIB.
Pemmican					
Original Tender Kippered Beef Steak	1	110	3	0	0

FOOD	PORTION	CALS.	CARB.	SUG.	FIB.
Pemmican (CONT.)					
Peppered Tender Kippered Beef Steak	1	110	3	0	0
Slim Jim					
Spicy	1 (4½ in) (0.3 oz)	50	0	0	0
Spicy Big	1 (.44 oz)	70	1	0	0
Spicy Giant	1 (0.97 oz)	150	2	0	1
Spicy Super	1 (0.64 oz)	100	1	0	0

MEAT SUBSTITUTES

(see also BACON SUBSTITUTES, CHICKEN SUBSTITUTES, SAUSAGE SUBSTITUTES, TURKEY SUBSTITUTES)

FOOD	PORTION	CALS.	CARB.	SUG.	FIB.
simulated sausage	1 link (25 g)	64	2	—	—
Amy's Organic					
Veggie Burger California	1 (2.5 oz)	100	17	1	3
Veggie Burger Chicago	1 (2.5 oz)	100	9	1	2
Veggie Burger Texas	1 (2.5 oz)	130	15	3	3
Whole Meals Veggie Loaf	1 pkg (10 oz)	260	47	9	7
Boca Burgers					
Chef Max's Original	1 patty (2.5 oz)	110	9	0	4
Hint of Garlic	1 patty (2.5 oz)	110	9	0	4
Vegan Original	1 patty (2.5 oz)	84	9	0	5
Gardenburger					
Classic Greek	1 (2.5 oz)	120	17	2	2
Fire Roasted Vegetable	1 (2.5 oz)	120	17	2	2
Hamburger Style	1 (2.5 oz)	90	7	0	3
Hamburger Style w/ Cheese	1 (2.5 oz)	110	7	0	3
Savory Mushroom	1 (2.5 oz)	120	18	1	4
Green Giant					
Southwestern Style	1 patty (3.2 oz)	140	9	1	5
Harvest Burgers					
For Recipes	⅔ cup (2.1 oz)	90	8	tr	4
Italian Style	1 patty (3.2 oz)	140	8	tr	5
Original	1 (3 oz)	140	8	tr	5
Harvest Direct					
TVP Beef Chunks	3.5 oz	280	32	—	18
TVP Beef Chunks Flavored	3.5 oz	250	30	—	17
TVP Beef Strips	3.5 oz	280	32	—	18
TVP Ground Beef	3.5 oz	280	32	—	18
TVP Ground Beef Flavored	3.5 oz	250	30	—	17
Knox Mountain Farm					
Wheat Balls Mix	1 serv (¹/₁₀ pkg)	110	9	—	2
Loma Linda					
Big Franks	1 (1.8 oz)	110	2	0	2

FOOD	PORTION	CALS.	CARB.	SUG.	FIB.
Loma Linda (CONT.)					
Big Franks Low Fat	1 (1.8 oz)	80	3	0	2
Corn Dogs	1 (2.5 oz)	200	18	1	3
Dinner Cuts	2 pieces (3.2 oz)	90	3	0	2
Nuteena	⅜ in slice (1.9 oz)	160	6	tr	2
Patty Mix not prep	⅓ cup (0.9 oz)	90	7	0	5
Redi-Burger	⅝ in slice (3 oz)	120	7	1	4
Sandwich Spread	¼ cup (1.9 oz)	80	7	tr	3
Savory Dinner Loaf Mix not prep	⅓ cup (0.9 oz)	90	7	0	5
Swiss Stake	1 piece (3.2 oz)	120	8	tr	4
Tender Bits	6 pieces (3 oz)	110	7	0	3
Tender Rounds	6 pieces (2.8 oz)	120	5	tr	3
Vege-Burger	¼ cup (1.9 oz)	70	2	0	2
Vita Burger Chunks not prep	¼ cup (0.7 oz)	70	6	1	3
Vita Burger Granules	3 tbsp (0.7 oz)	70	6	1	3
Midland Harvest					
Burger n' Loaf Chili w/o Beans	0.8 oz	90	7	—	2
Burger n' Loaf Herbs & Spice	3.2 oz	140	7	—	4
Burger n' Loaf Italian	3.2 oz	140	7	—	4
Burger n' Loaf Original	3.2 oz	140	7	—	4
Burger n' Loaf Sloppy Joe w/o Sauce	0.8 oz	80	9	—	1
Burger n' Loaf Taco	2.7 oz	90	7	—	1
Morningstar Farms					
Better'n Burger	1 (2.7 oz)	70	6	0	3
Burger Style Recipe Crumbles	⅔ cup (1.9 oz)	90	4	0	2
Deli Franks	1 (1.6 oz)	110	3	1	2
Garden Grille	1 patty (2.5 oz)	120	18	1	4
Garden Veggie Patties	1 patty (2.4 oz)	100	9	1	4
Ground Meatless	½ cup (1.9 oz)	60	4	0	2
Prime Patties	1 (2.7 oz)	110	5	tr	3
Quarter Prime	1 patty (3.4 oz)	140	6	1	3
Southwestern Veggie Burger Kit	¼ pkg (0.9 oz)	90	9	tr	4
Spicy Black Bean Burger	1 (2.7 oz)	110	16	2	5
Natural Touch					
Dinner Entree	1 patty (3 oz)	220	2	0	2
Garden Veggie Pattie	1 (2.4 oz)	110	8	0	3
Loaf Mix not prep	4 tbsp (1 oz)	100	10	tr	7

FOOD	PORTION	CALS.	CARB.	SUG.	FIB.
Natural Touch (CONT.)					
Okara Pattie	1 (2.2 oz)	110	4	0	3
Original Veggie Burger Kit not prep	¼ pkg (0.8 oz)	80	6	0	4
Southwestern Veggie Burger Kit not prep	¼ pkg (0.9 oz)	90	9	tr	4
Spicy Black Bean Burger	1 (2.7 oz)	100	15	2	5
Stroganoff Mix not prep	4 tbsp (0.8 oz)	90	10	1	3
Taco Mix not prep	3 tbsp (0.6 oz)	90	5	tr	3
Vegan Burger	1 (2.7 oz)	70	6	0	3
Vegan Burger Crumbles	½ cup (1.9 oz)	60	4	0	2
Vege Frank	1 (1.6 oz)	100	2	0	2
NewMenu					
VegiBurger	1 patty (3 oz)	110	12	2	1
VegiDogs	1 (1.5 oz)	45	1	0	0
Quorn					
Burger	1 patty (3 oz)	100	9	—	4
Sovex					
Better Than Burger?	½ cup (1.9 oz)	165	25	2	9
Soy Is Us					
Beef Not!	½ cup (1.75 oz)	140	15	4	9
Trader Joe's					
French Village Burger Champignon No Soy No Preservatives	1 patty (3.4 oz)	190	29	0	6
Veggie Patch					
Burgeriffics	1 (2.5 oz)	110	8	—	4
Perfectly Franks	1 (1.7 oz)	70	2	—	1
Veggie Rounds	1 (2.5 oz)	120	15	—	4
Veggitinos Meatballs	5 (2.8 oz)	120	10	—	3
White Wave					
Meatless Healthy Franks	1 (1.5 oz)	90	6	0	0
Meatless Jumbo Franks	1 (3 oz)	170	11	2	0
Meatless Sandwich Slices Beef	2 slices (1.6 oz)	90	8	2	1
Meatless Sandwich Slices Bologna	2 slices (1.6 oz)	120	5	0	1
Meatless Sandwich Slices Pastrami	2 slices (1.6 oz)	90	8	2	1
Veggie Burger	1 patty (2.5 oz)	110	16	1	2
Worthington					
Beef Style Meatless	⅜ in slice (1.9 oz)	110	4	tr	3
Bolono	3 slices (2 oz)	80	2	0	2
Choplets	2 slices (3.2 oz)	90	3	0	2

FOOD	PORTION	CALS.	CARB.	SUG.	FIB.
Worthington (CONT.)					
Corn Beef Meatless	4 slices (2 oz)	140	5	tr	2
Country Stew	1 cup (8.4 oz)	210	20	2	5
Dinner Roast	¾ in slice (3 oz)	180	5	1	3
FriPats	1 patty (2.2 oz)	60	4	0	3
Granburger not prep	3 tbsp (0.6 oz)	60	3	0	2
Multigrain Cutlet	2 slices (3.2 oz)	100	5	0	4
Numete	⅜ in slice (1.9 oz)	130	5	tr	3
Prime Stakes	1 piece (3.2 oz)	140	4	0	4
Prosage Patties	1 (1.3 oz)	100	3	0	2
Prosage Roll	⅝ in slice (1.9 oz)	140	2	0	2
Protose	⅜ in slice (1.9 oz)	130	5	tr	3
Salami Meatless	3 slices (2 oz)	130	2	0	2
Savory Slices	3 slices (2.9 oz)	150	6	0	3
Smoked Beef Meatless	6 slices (2 oz)	120	6	1	3
Stakelets	1 piece (2.5 oz)	140	6	0	2
Veelets	1 patty (2.5 oz)	180	10	tr	5
Vegetable Skallops	½ cup (3 oz)	90	3	0	2
Vegetable Steaks	2 pieces (2.5 oz)	80	3	0	3
Vegetarian Burger	¼ cup (1.9 oz)	60	2	0	1
Veja Links Low Fat	1 (1.1 oz)	40	1	0	0
Wham	2 slices (1.6 oz)	80	1	1	0
Zoglo's					
Crispy Vegetarian Cutlets	1 (3.5 oz)	200	10	1	2
Savory Vegetarian Kebabs	1 serv (2.8 oz)	135	5	1	2
Tender Vegetarian Burgers	1 (2.6 oz)	150	5	1	2
Vegetable Patties	1 (2.6 oz)	130	10	1	2
Vegetarian Franks	1 (2.6 oz)	125	5	1	2

MELON
(*see also individual names*)

FROZEN
Big Valley

Mixed	¾ cup (4.9 oz)	40	10	7	1

MEXICAN FOOD
(*see* SALSA, SAUCE, SPANISH FOODS, TORTILLA)

MILK
(*see also* CHOCOLATE, COCOA, MILK DRINKS, MILKSHAKE)

CANNED
Carnation

Evaporated	2 tbsp	40	3	3	—
Evaporated Lowfat	2 tbsp	25	3	3	—

FOOD	PORTION	CALS.	CARB.	SUG.	FIB.
Carnation (CONT.)					
Sweetened Condensed	2 tbsp	130	22	22	—
DRIED					
Carnation					
Nonfat	⅓ cup dry	80	12	12	—
Saco					
Cultured Buttermilk	4 tbsp (0.8 oz)	80	13	12	0
Sanalac					
As Prep	8 oz	80	12	—	0
REFRIGERATED					
BodyWise					
Nonfat	8 fl oz	100	14	14	0
CaliMilk					
CalciMilk	8 fl oz	102	12	—	0
Cool Cow					
Low Fat	1 cup (8 oz)	110	12	12	0
Farmland					
1%	8 fl oz	100	12	12	0
2%	8 fl oz	130	12	12	0
Skim	8 fl oz	80	12	12	0
Skim Plus	8 fl oz	110	17	16	0
Friendship					
Buttermilk	8 fl oz	120	12	12	0
Hood					
1%	1 cup (8 oz)	110	13	12	0
Better Taste 2%	1 cup (8 oz)	130	13	12	0
Buttermilk	1 cup (8 oz)	90	13	12	0
Whole	1 cup (8 oz)	150	12	12	0
Lactaid					
1%	8 fl oz	102	12	—	0
Nonfat	8 fl oz	86	12	—	0
Nuform					
1%	1 cup (8 oz)	120	15	14	0
Skim	1 cup (8 oz)	100	15	14	0
Silovet					
Skim	1 cup (8 oz)	90	13	12	0
Weight Watchers					
Skim	1 cup	90	13	13	0
SHELF-STABLE					
Parmalat					
1%	1 cup (8 oz)	110	13	13	0
2%	1 cup (8 oz)	130	13	12	0
Skim	1 cup (8 oz)	90	13	12	0

FOOD	PORTION	CALS.	CARB.	SUG.	FIB.
Parmalat (CONT.)					
Whole	1 cup (8 oz)	160	13	12	0

MILK DRINKS

(*see also* BREAKFAST DRINKS, CHOCOLATE, COCOA, MILKSHAKES)

FOOD	PORTION	CALS.	CARB.	SUG.	FIB.
Body Wise					
Chocolate Nonfat Milk	1 cup (8 fl oz)	180	35	32	1
Hood					
Chocolate Lowfat	1 cup (8 oz)	150	27	25	0
Lactaid					
Chocolate Milk 1%	8 fl oz	158	26	—	tr
Parmalat					
Chocolate 2%	1 box (8 oz)	180	28	27	1
Quik					
Banana Powder	2 tbsp (0.8 oz)	90	27	20	0
Cookies n Cream Powder	2 tbsp (0.8 oz)	100	21	14	1
Strawberry Powder	2 tbsp (0.8 oz)	90	22	21	0

MILK SUBSTITUTES

(*see also* COFFEE WHITENERS)

FOOD	PORTION	CALS.	CARB.	SUG.	FIB.
EdenBlend					
Original	8 fl oz	120	16	12	0
Edensoy					
Carob	8 fl oz	150	23	14	0
Extra Original	8 oz	130	13	7	0
Extra Original	8 fl oz	130	12	7	0
Extra Vanilla	8 fl oz	150	23	15	0
Original	8 oz	130	13	7	0
Vanilla	8 oz	150	32	15	0
Health Valley					
Soo Moo	1 cup	120	12	—	0
Vitamite					
Non-Dairy 2% Fat	1 cup (8 oz)	110	14	3	0
Non-Diary Nonfat	1 cup (8 oz)	90	21	6	0
Vitasoy					
Carob Supreme	8 fl oz	210	32	21	1
Cocoa Light	8 fl oz	130	25	17	1
Original Creamy	8 fl oz	160	14	9	1
Original Light	8 fl oz	90	15	9	1
Rich Cocoa	8 fl oz	210	32	19	1
Vanilla Light	8 fl oz	110	20	15	1
Vanilla Delite	8 fl oz	190	27	21	1

MILKSHAKE

FOOD	PORTION	CALS.	CARB.	SUG.	FIB.
D'Frosta Shake					
Vanilla	1 serv (13.5 oz)	340	57	48	1

FOOD	PORTION	CALS.	CARB.	SUG.	FIB.
Freeze Flip					
Fruit Shake No Fat Lactose Free Black Raspberry	1 serv (6 oz)	150	37	29	1
Hood					
Shake Up Chocolate	1 cup (8 oz)	240	38	35	0
Shake Up Strawberry	1 cup (8 oz)	220	36	34	0
Shake Up Vanilla	1 cup (8 oz)	220	36	33	0
Milky Way					
Shake	1 (10 fl oz)	390	54	—	0
Parmalat					
Shake A Shake Chocolate	1 box (6 oz)	180	29	27	1
Shake A Shake Orange Vanilla	1 box (6 oz)	110	14	14	0
Shake A Shake Vanilla	1 box (6 oz)	170	28	27	0
Weight Watchers					
Chocolate Fudge Shake Mix as prep	1 pkg	80	12	6	2

MILLET
cooked	1 cup (6.1 oz)	207	41	—	2

MINERAL WATER
(*see* WATER)

MISO
miso	½ cup	284	39	—	7
Eden					
Genmai Miso Organic	1 tbsp (0.5 oz)	25	3	1	tr
Hacho Miso Organic	1 tbsp (0.5 oz)	35	2	0	1
Kome Miso Organic	1 tbsp (0.6 oz)	25	3	1	tr
Mugi Miso Organic	1 tbsp (0.6 oz)	25	3	tr	1
Shiro Miso Organic	1 tbsp (0.6 oz)	35	5	3	1

MOLASSES
molasses	1 tbsp (0.7 oz)	53	14	12	—
molasses	1 cup (11.5 oz)	873	226	195	—
McIlhenny					
Molasses	1 tbsp (0.7 oz)	66	16	12	tr
Tree Of Life					
Blackstrap	1 tbsp (0.5 oz)	45	11	8	—

MONKFISH
baked	3 oz	82	0	0	0

MOOSE
roasted	3 oz	114	0	0	0

FOOD	PORTION	CALS.	CARB.	SUG.	FIB.
MOUSSE					
FROZEN					
Sara Lee					
Chocolate Mint Mousse	⅕ pkg (4.3 oz)	440	40	29	2
Weight Watchers					
Chocolate Mousse	1 (2.75 oz)	190	31	6	3
MUFFIN					
FROZEN					
Health Valley					
Almond & Date Oat Bran Fancy Fruit	1	180	31	—	8
Fat Free Apple Spice	1	140	30	—	5
Fat Free Banana	1	130	29	—	5
Fat Free Raisin Spice	1	140	32	—	5
Oat Bran Fancy Fruit Blueberry	1	140	32	—	8
Oat Bran Fancy Fruit Raisin	1	180	5	—	8
Rice Bran Fancy Fruit Raisin	1	210	7	—	6
Pepperidge Farm					
Blueberry	1	170	27	—	1
Cinnamon Swirl	1	190	30	—	1
Sara Lee					
Blueberry	1 (2.2 oz)	220	27	12	tr
Corn	1 (2.2 oz)	260	30	14	1
Weight Watchers					
Chocolate Chocolate Chip	1 (2.5 oz)	190	39	14	4
Fat Free Banana	1 (2.5 oz)	170	41	17	3
Fat Free Blueberry	1 (2.5 oz)	160	38	15	2
MIX					
Arrowhead					
Bran	⅓ cup (1.4 oz)	150	26	tr	7
Oat Bran Wheat Free	⅓ cup (1.5 oz)	160	23	0	7
Flako					
Corn	⅓ cup (1.4 oz)	160	29	8	1
Hain					
Oat Bran Apple Cinnamon	1	140	28	—	5
Oat Bran Banana Nut	1	140	26	—	4
Oat Bran Raspberry Spice	1	140	27	—	4
Jiffy					
Apple Cinnamon as prep	1	190	28	13	1
Banana Nut as prep	1	180	25	11	1
Blueberry as prep	1	190	28	13	1

FOOD	PORTION	CALS.	CARB.	SUG.	FIB.
Jiffy (CONT.)					
Bran With Dates as prep	1	170	26	12	3
Corn as prep	1	180	28	8	1
Honey Date as prep	1	170	27	11	1
Oatmeal as prep	1	180	26	10	2
Wanda's					
Blue Corn	¼ cup mix per serv (1.2 oz)	130	25	8	1
READY-TO-EAT					
blueberry	1 (2 oz)	158	27	—	2
oat bran wheat free	1 (2 oz)	154	28	—	4
Arnold					
Bran'nola	1 (2.3 oz)	160	30	—	2
Raisin	1 (2.3 oz)	160	33	—	2
Dutch Mill					
Apple Oat Bran	1 (2 oz)	180	31	5	1
Banana Walnut	1 (2 oz)	220	33	15	1
Carrot	1 (2 oz)	190	31	19	1
Corn	1 (2 oz)	190	31	14	1
Cranberry Orange	1 (2 oz)	170	26	14	1
Raisin Bran	1 (2 oz)	230	37	12	3
Freihofer's					
Corn Toasters	1 (1.3 oz)	130	18	7	0
Hostess					
Mini Apple Cinnamon	5 (2 oz)	260	28	14	3
Mini Banana Nut	5 (2 oz)	260	28	14	tr
Mini Blueberry	5 (2 oz)	240	30	14	tr
Mini Chocolate Chip	5 (2 oz)	260	29	15	1
Muffin Loaf Blueberry	1 (3.8 oz)	440	62	34	2
Oat Bran	1 (1.5 oz)	160	22	10	tr
Oat Bran Banana Nut	1 (1.5 oz)	150	22	9	1
Otis Spunkmeyer					
Chocolate Chocolate Chip Low Fat	1 (2.25 oz)	210	41	26	1
Weight Watchers					
Fat Free Apple Crisp	1 (2.5 oz)	160	37	16	1
Fat Free Cranberry Orange	1 (2.5 oz)	160	38	14	1
Fat Free Double Chocolate	1 (2.5 oz)	180	40	26	2
Fat Free Wild Blueberry	1 (2.5 oz)	160	36	15	1
Low Fat Apple Cinnamon	1 (2.5 oz)	170	35	20	2
Low Fat Blueberry	1 (2.5 oz)	180	37	20	2
Low Fat Carrot	1 (2.5 oz)	160	34	16	2
Low Fat Chocolate Chip	1 (2.5 oz)	180	38	21	2
Low Fat Cranberry Orange	1 (2.5 oz)	180	38	20	2

FOOD	PORTION	CALS.	CARB.	SUG.	FIB.
Weight Watchers (CONT.)					
Low Fat Lemon Poppy	1 (2.5 oz)	190	38	20	2
MULLET					
striped cooked	3 oz	127	0	0	0
MUSHROOMS					
CANNED					
chanterelle	3½ oz	12	tr	—	6
straw	1 cup (6.4 oz)	58	8	—	5
BinB					
Pieces & Stems	1 can (4.2 oz)	30	4	1	2
Sliced	1 can (4.2 oz)	30	4	1	2
Sliced With Garlic	1 can (4.2 oz)	35	4	1	1
Whole	1 can (4.2 oz)	30	4	1	2
Green Giant					
Pieces & Stems	½ cup (4.2 oz)	30	4	1	2
Sliced	½ cup (4.2 oz)	30	3	1	2
Whole	½ cup (4.2 oz)	30	4	1	2
Ka-Me					
Stir Fry	½ cup (4.5 oz)	20	3	0	2
Straw Whole Peeled	½ cup (4.5 oz)	20	3	0	2
Seneca					
Mushrooms	½ cup	25	3	—	2
DRIED					
chanterelle	3½ oz	89	2	—	60
cloud ear	1 (5 g)	13	3	—	3
cloud ears	1 cup (1 oz)	80	20	—	20
straw	1 piece (6 g)	2	tr	—	tr
FRESH					
chanterelle	3½ oz	11	tr	—	6
morel	3½ oz	9	0	—	7
oyster raw	1 sm (0.5 oz)	6	1	—	tr
oyster raw	1 lg (5.2 oz)	55	9	—	4
raw	1 (½ oz)	5	1	—	tr
raw sliced	½ cup	9	2	—	tr
sliced cooked	½ cup	21	4	—	1
Mother Earth					
Organic	4 oz	35	5	—	tr
FROZEN					
Empire					
Breaded	7 (2.8 oz)	90	16	4	1
Fresh Like					
Mushrooms	3.5 oz	28	4	—	1

FOOD	PORTION	CALS.	CARB.	SUG.	FIB.
MUSKRAT					
roasted	3 oz	199	0	0	0
MUSTARD					
Blanchard & Blanchard					
Mustard	1 tsp (5 g)	0	0	0	0
Estee					
Sodium Free	1 pkg (0.5 oz)	5	tr	0	—
Grey Poupon					
Country Dijon	1 tsp	6	0	0	0
Dijon	1 tsp	6	0	0	0
Parisian	1 tsp	6	0	0	0
Ka-Me					
Hot Mustard Powder Chinese Style	¼ tsp (1 g)	5	1	0	1
Kraft					
Horseradish Mustard	1 tsp (5 g)	0	0	0	0
Mustard	1 tsp (5 g)	0	0	0	0
McIlhenny					
Coarse Ground	1 tsp (0.2 oz)	4	tr	tr	tr
Spicy	1 tsp (0.2 oz)	6	tr	tr	1
Russer					
Deli	1 tsp (5 g)	4	0	0	0
Watkins					
Country Mill	1 tsp (7 g)	15	2	2	0
Dusseldorf	1 tsp (7 g)	10	1	0	0
Horseradish	1 tsp (7 g)	10	1	0	0
Jalapeno	1 tsp (7 g)	10	1	0	0
Onion	1 tsp (7 g)	10	1	0	0
Parisienne	1 tsp (7 g)	10	1	0	0
MUSTARD GREENS					
Allen					
Mustard Greens	½ cup (4.1 oz)	30	5	tr	3
Birds Eye					
Chopped	1 cup (3 oz)	30	2	1	2
Sunshine					
Mustard Greens	½ cup (4.1 oz)	30	5	tr	3
NAVY BEANS					
CANNED					
Allen					
Navy Beans	½ cup (4.5 oz)	110	19	tr	6
Eden					
Organic	½ cup (4.3 oz)	100	18	0	7

FOOD	PORTION	CALS.	CARB.	SUG.	FIB.
Eden (CONT.)					
Organic	½ cup (4.6 oz)	110	20	—	7
Trappey					
With Bacon	½ cup (4.5 oz)	110	17	3	7
With Bacon & Jalapeno	½ cup (4.5 oz)	110	17	3	7
DRIED					
Hurst					
HamBeens w/ Ham	3 tbsp (1.2 oz)	120	20	1	11

NECTARINE

FOOD	PORTION	CALS.	CARB.	SUG.	FIB.
fresh	1	67	16	—	2
Dole					
Nectarine	1	70	16	—	3

NEUFCHATEL

FOOD	PORTION	CALS.	CARB.	SUG.	FIB.
Philadelphia					
Neufchatel	1 oz	70	tr	tr	0
WisPride					
Garden Vegetable Cup	2 tbsp (1.1 oz)	60	2	0	0
Garlic & Herb Cup	2 tbsp (1.1 oz)	60	2	0	0

NON-DAIRY CREAMERS
(*see* COFFEE WHITENERS)

NON-DAIRY WHIPPED TOPPINGS
(*see* WHIPPED TOPPINGS)

NOODLE DISHES
(*see also* NOODLES AND PASTA DINNERS)

CANNED

FOOD	PORTION	CALS.	CARB.	SUG.	FIB.
Van Camp's					
Noodlee Weenee	1 can (8 oz)	230	34	—	1
FROZEN					
Luigino's					
Stroganoff	1 pkg (8 oz)	310	25	1	2
MIX					
Kraft					
Noodle Classics Cheddar Cheese as prep	1 cup (7.4 oz)	400	47	8	1
Noodle Classics Savory Chicken as prep	1 cup (8.5 oz)	340	46	5	2
La Choy					
Ramen Noodles Beef as prep	1 cup	200	33	—	4
Ramen Noodles Chicken as prep	1 cup	200	29	—	4

FOOD	PORTION	CALS.	CARB.	SUG.	FIB.
Lipton					
Noodles & Sauce Alfredo Broccoli as prep	1 cup (2.2 oz)	340	43	5	2
Noodles & Sauce Alfredo as prep	1 cup (2.2 oz)	330	42	5	2
Noodles & Sauce Beef as prep	1 cup (2.1 oz)	280	43	2	2
Noodles & Sauce Butter as prep	1 cup (2.2 oz)	310	41	4	2
Noodles & Sauce Butter & Herb as prep	1 cup (2.2 oz)	300	42	4	2
Noodles & Sauce Chicken Broccoli as prep	1 cup (2.1 oz)	310	44	4	2
Noodles & Sauce Chicken Tetrazzini as prep	1 cup (2 oz)	300	41	4	2
Noodles & Sauce Chicken as prep	1 cup (2.1 oz)	290	42	2	2
Noodles & Sauce Creamy Chicken as prep	1 cup (2.1 oz)	320	42	5	2
Noodles & Sauce Parmesan as prep	1 cup (2.1 oz)	330	40	5	2
Noodles & Sauce Sour Cream & Chives as prep	1 cup (2.2 oz)	310	41	4	2
Noodles & Sauce Stroganoff as prep	1 cup (2 oz)	300	40	5	2
Noodles By Leonardo					
Macaroni & Cheese as prep	1 cup (2.5 oz)	250	49	6	2
Ultra Slim-Fast					
Noodles & Alfredo Sauce	2.3 oz	240	47	—	4
Noodles & Beef	2.3 oz	230	45	—	4
Noodles & Cheese	2.3 oz	230	44	—	4
Noodles & Chicken Sauce	2.3 oz	220	45	—	4
Noodles & Tomato Herb Sauce	2.3 oz	220	46	—	5
SHELF-STABLE					
Hormel					
Microcup Meals Noodles & Chicken	1 cup (7.5 oz)	200	20	2	1

NOODLES

FOOD	PORTION	CALS.	CARB.	SUG.	FIB.
chow mein	1 cup (1.6 oz)	237	25	—	2
egg cooked	1 cup (5.6 oz)	213	40	—	2
rice cooked	1 cup (6.2 oz)	192	44	—	2
spinach/egg cooked	1 cup (5.6 oz)	211	39	—	4

FOOD	PORTION	CALS.	CARB.	SUG.	FIB.
Golden Grain					
Egg	2 oz	210	39	—	2
Herb's					
Egg Fine	2 oz	220	42	1	2
Egg Medium	2 oz	220	42	1	2
Kluski Medium	2 oz	220	42	1	2
Kluski Wide	2 oz	220	42	1	2
Hodgson Mill					
Veggie Egg	2 oz	200	37	0	2
Whole Wheat Egg	2 oz	190	34	0	4
Whole Wheat Spinach Egg	2 oz	190	32	0	5
Ka-Me					
Chinese Egg	½ cup (2 oz)	210	40	0	2
Chinese Plain	½ cup (2 oz)	200	45	0	1
Chuka Soba Curly Noodles	2 oz	200	42	0	1
Lo Mein Wide Chinese	½ cup (2 oz)	200	45	0	1
Py Mai Fun Rice Sticks	2 oz	193	48	0	0
Sai Fun Bean Thread	1 cup (2 oz)	190	50	0	1
Soba Shin Shu Japanese Buckwheat	2 oz	200	40	6	2
Tomoshiraga Somen Noodles	2 oz	190	41	0	1
Udon Japanese Thick	2 oz	190	41	0	1
La Choy					
Chow Mein Narrow	½ cup	150	16	—	tr
Chow Mein Wide	½ cup	150	16	—	tr
Rice	½ cup	130	21	—	tr
Noodles By Leonardo					
Egg Fine	2 oz	210	39	1	2
Egg Medium	2 oz	210	39	1	2
Egg Wide	2 oz	210	39	1	2
Shofar					
No Yolks	2 oz	210	41	3	3

NUTMEG

FOOD	PORTION	CALS.	CARB.	SUG.	FIB.
Watkins					
Ground	¼ tsp (0.5 g)	0	0	0	0

NUTRITIONAL SUPPLEMENTS

(*see also* BREAKFAST BAR, BREAKFAST DRINKS, SPORTS DRINKS)

FOOD	PORTION	CALS.	CARB.	SUG.	FIB.
BeneFit					
Chocolate	1 serv	120	15	—	1
Nutrition Bar	1 (2 oz)	240	33	—	tr
Vanilla	1 serv	120	15	—	tr

FOOD	PORTION	CALS.	CARB.	SUG.	FIB.
Boost					
Chocolate	1 can (8 oz)	240	40	27	0
Vanilla	8 oz	240	40	23	0
California Joe					
All Natural Protein Drink Mix as prep	1 serv (8 oz)	165	21	18	0
Calorie Shed					
Shake Fat Free No Sugar Caramel Ripple	½ cup (4 fl oz)	70	21	3	2
Shake Fat Free No Sugar Chocolate	½ cup (4 fl oz)	70	21	3	2
Shake Fat Free No Sugar Marshmellow Nougat	½ cup (4 fl oz)	70	21	3	2
Dynatrim					
Dutch Chocolate as prep w/ 1% milk	8 oz	220	33	—	6
Strawberry Royale as prep w/ 1% milk	8 oz	220	33	—	6
Vanilla as prep w/ 1% milk	8 oz	220	33	—	6
Ensure					
Honey Graham Crunch	1 bar (2.23 oz)	130	21	11	2
Essential					
Protein Powder	1 serv (0.6 oz)	70	6	5	tr
Fat Burner					
Diet Fruit Punch	8 fl oz	0	0	0	0
Fi-Bar					
Apple	1 (1 oz)	90	15	—	5
Cocoa Almond	1	130	21	—	4
Cocoa Peanut	1	130	20	—	4
Cranberry & Wild Berries	1 (1 oz)	100	13	—	4
Lemon	1 (1 oz)	90	15	—	5
Mandarin Orange	1 (1 oz)	99	15	—	5
Raspberry	1 (1 oz)	100	13	—	4
Strawberry	1 (1 oz)	100	13	—	4
Treat Yourself Right Almond	1	152	22	—	5
Treat Yourself Right Peanutty Butter	1	152	18	—	5
Vanilla Almond	1	130	21	—	4
Vanilla Peanut	1	130	20	—	4
Gatorade					
GatorBar	1 (1.17 oz)	110	13	11	1
GatorLode	1 can (11.6 fl oz)	280	71	24	—
GatorPro	1 can (11 fl oz)	360	59	24	0

FOOD	PORTION	CALS.	CARB.	SUG.	FIB.
Gatorade (CONT.)					
ReLode	1 pkt (0.75 oz)	80	17	3	—
GeniSoy					
Soy Protein Shake Chocolate	1 scoop (1.2 oz)	120	17	15	2
Soy Protein Shake Vanilla	1 scoop (1.2 oz)	130	18	13	—
Soy Protein Bar Chocolate	1 bar (2.2 oz)	210	36	18	1
Soy Protein Bar Chocolate Coated	1 bar (2.2 oz)	220	33	19	1
Meal On The Go					
Apple	1 bar (3 oz)	294	50	—	5
Banana w/ Pecans	1 bar (3 oz)	289	50	—	8
Original	1 bar (3 oz)	286	52	—	7
Nancy Grey's					
Shake Hi-Protein Black Raspberry	1 cup (8 fl oz)	340	40	35	0
Shake Hi-Protein Chocolate	1 cup (8 fl oz)	340	42	37	—
Shake Hi-Protein Vanilla	1 cup (8 fl oz)	340	40	35	0
NiteBite					
Chocolate Fudge	1 bar (0.9 oz)	100	15	10	0
Peanut Butter	1 bar (0.9 oz)	100	15	10	0
Power Bar					
Malt-Nut	1 bar (2.3 oz)	230	45	18	3
Resource					
Fructose Sweetened	1 pkg (8 oz)	250	23	—	3
Slim-Fast					
Powder Chocolate as prep w/ skim milk	8 oz	190	32	—	2
Powder Chocolate Malt as prep w/ skim milk	8 oz	190	32	—	2
Powder Strawberry as prep w/ skim milk	8 oz	190	32	—	2
Powder Vanilla as prep w/ skim milk	8 oz	190	32	—	2
Sustacal					
Vanilla	8 oz	240	33	26	tr
Sweet Success					
Chewy Bar Chocolate Brownie	1 (1.6 oz)	120	28	10	3
Chewy Bar Chocolate Peanut Butter	1 (1.6 oz)	120	23	10	3
Chewy Bar Chocolate Raspberry	1 (1.6 oz)	120	23	10	3
Chewy Bar Chocolate Chip	1 (1.6 oz)	120	23	10	3

FOOD	PORTION	CALS.	CARB.	SUG.	FIB.
Sweet Success (CONT.)					
Chewy Bar Oatmeal Raisin	1 (1.6 oz)	120	23	10	3
Chocolate Raspberry Truffle	1 can (10 fl oz)	200	38	30	6
Chocolate Raspberry as prep w/ skim milk	9 fl oz	180	30	—	6
Chocolate Mocha Supreme	1 can (10 fl oz)	200	38	30	6
Chocolate Mocha Supreme as prep w/ skim milk	9 fl oz	180	30	—	6
Classic Chocolate Chip as prep w/ skim milk	9 fl oz	180	30	—	6
Creamy Milk Chocolate	1 carton (12 fl oz)	220	45	37	6
Creamy Milk Chocolate	1 can (10 fl oz)	200	38	30	6
Creamy Milk Chocolate as prep w/ skim milk	9 fl oz	180	30	—	6
Creamy Vanilla Delight as prep w/ skim milk	9 fl oz	180	33	—	6
Dark Chocolate Fudge	1 can (10 fl oz)	200	38	30	6
Dark Chocolate Fudge	1 carton (12 fl oz)	220	45	37	6
Dark Chocolate Fudge as prep w/ skim milk	9 fl oz	180	30	—	6
Rich Chocolate Almond	1 carton (12 fl oz)	220	45	37	6
Rich Chocolate Almond	1 can (10 fl oz)	200	38	30	6
Rich Chocolate Almond as prep w/ skim milk	9 fl oz	180	30	—	6
Smooth Vanilla Creme	1 can (10 fl oz)	200	38	30	6
The Pumper					
Body Building Milkshake Banana	1 serv (13.5 oz)	390	82	64	3
Body Building MilkShake Chocolate	1 serv (13.5 oz)	390	80	66	5
Think!					
Apple Spice Chocolate Coated	1 bar (2 oz)	205	40	15	7
Ultra Slim-Fast					
Cafe Mocha as prep w/ skim milk	8 oz	200	38	—	6
Chocolate Royale as prep w/ skim milk	8 oz	200	36	—	5
Crunch Bar Cocoa Almond	1	110	19	—	3
Crunch Bar Cocoa Raspberry	1	100	21	—	3
Crunch Bar Vanilla Almond	1	110	18	—	3
Dutch Chocolate as prep w/ water	8 oz	220	40	—	5

FOOD	PORTION	CALS.	CARB.	SUG.	FIB.
Ultra Slim-Fast (CONT.)					
French Vanilla as prep w/ skim milk	8 oz	190	36	—	4
French Vanilla as prep w/ water	8 oz	220	40	—	4
Fruit Juice Mix as prep w/ fruit juice	8 oz	200	43	—	6
Nutrition Bar Dutch Chocolate	1	130	17	—	6
Nutrition Bar Peanut Butter	1	140	15	—	7
Pina Colada as prep w/ skim milk	8 oz	180	36	—	6
Ready-To-Drink Chocolate Royale	12 oz	250	45	—	5
Ready-To-Drink Chocolate Royale	11 oz	230	42	—	5
Ready-To-Drink French Vanilla	12 oz	220	38	—	5
Ready-To-Drink French Vanilla	11 oz	230	38	—	5
Ready-To-Drink Strawberry Supreme	12 oz	220	38	—	5
Strawberry Supreme as prep w/ water	8 oz	220	40	—	4
Strawberry as prep w/ skim milk	8 oz	190	36	—	4
NUTS MIXED					
(see also individual names)					
Planters					
Cashews & Peanuts Honey Roasted	1 oz	150	10	5	2
Deluxe Oil Roasted	1 oz	170	6	tr	2
Dry Roasted	1 oz	170	7	1	2
Honey Roasted	1 oz	140	9	5	2
Lightly Salted Oil Roasted	1 oz	170	6	0	2
No Brazils Lightly Salted Oil Roasted	1 oz	170	6	0	2
No Brazils Oil Roasted	1 oz	170	6	0	2
Oil Roasted	1 oz	170	5	1	2
Select Mix Cashews Almonds & Macadamias Oil Roasted	1 oz	170	6	tr	2
Select Mix Cashews Almonds & Pecans Oil Roasted	1 oz	170	7	tr	2

FOOD	PORTION	CALS.	CARB.	SUG.	FIB.
Planters (CONT.)					
Unsalted Oil Roasted	1 oz	170	6	tr	3
OIL					
(*see also* FAT)					
almond	1 cup	1927	0	0	0
almond	1 tbsp	120	0	0	0
apricot kernel	1 cup	1927	0	0	0
apricot kernel	1 tbsp	120	0	0	0
avocado	1 cup	1927	0	0	0
avocado	1 tbsp	124	0	0	0
babassu palm	1 tbsp	120	0	0	0
butter oil	1 tbsp	112	0	0	0
butter oil	1 cup	1795	0	0	0
canola	1 tbsp	124	0	0	0
canola	1 cup	1927	0	0	0
coconut	1 tbsp	117	0	0	0
corn	1 tbsp	120	0	0	0
corn	1 cup	1927	0	0	0
cottonseed	1 cup	1927	0	0	0
cottonseed	1 tbsp	120	0	0	0
cupu assu	1 tbsp	120	0	0	0
grapeseed	1 tbsp	120	0	0	0
hazelnut	1 cup	1927	0	0	0
hazelnut	1 tbsp	120	0	0	0
mustard	1 cup	1927	0	0	0
mustard	1 tbsp	124	0	0	0
oat	1 tbsp	120	0	0	0
olive	1 tbsp	119	0	0	0
olive	1 cup	1909	0	0	0
palm	1 tbsp	120	0	0	0
palm	1 cup	1927	0	0	0
palm kernel	1 cup	1879	0	0	0
palm kernel	1 tbsp	117	0	0	0
peanut	1 tbsp	119	0	0	0
peanut	1 cup	1909	0	0	0
poppyseed	1 tbsp	120	0	0	0
poppyseed	3.5 fl oz	900	0	0	0
pumpkin seed	3.5 oz	925	0	0	0
rice bran	1 tbsp	120	0	0	0
safflower	1 tbsp	120	0	0	0
safflower	1 cup	1927	0	0	0
sesame	1 tbsp	120	0	0	0
sheanut	1 tbsp	120	0	0	0

FOOD	PORTION	CALS.	CARB.	SUG.	FIB.
soybean	1 tbsp	120	0	0	0
soybean	1 cup	1927	0	0	0
sunflower	1 cup	1927	0	0	0
sunflower	1 tbsp	120	0	0	0
teaseed	1 tbsp	120	0	0	0
tomatoseed	1 tbsp	120	0	0	0
vegetable soybean & cottonseed	1 cup	1927	0	0	0
vegetable soybean & cottonseed	1 tbsp	120	0	0	0
walnut	1 cup	1927	0	—	1
walnut	1 tbsp	120	0	0	0
wheat germ	1 tbsp	120	0	0	0
Arrowhead					
Flax Seed	1 tbsp (0.5 fl oz)	120	0	0	0
Hazelnut	1 tbsp (0.5 fl oz)	120	0	0	0
Crisco					
Corn Canola	1 tbsp (0.5 fl oz)	120	0	0	0
Oil	1 tbsp (0.5 fl oz)	120	0	0	0
Puritan Canola	1 tbsp (0.5 fl oz)	120	0	0	0
Eden					
Hot Pepper Sesame	1 tbsp (0.5 oz)	130	0	0	0
Safflower	1 tbsp (0.5 oz)	120	0	0	0
Sesame	1 tbsp (0.5 oz)	140	0	0	0
Toasted Sesame	1 tbsp (0.5 oz)	130	0	0	0
Hain					
All Blend	1 tbsp	120	0	0	0
Almond	1 tbsp	120	0	0	0
Apricot Kernel	1 tbsp	120	0	0	0
Avocado	1 tbsp	120	0	0	0
Canola	1 tbsp	120	0	0	0
Canola Organic	1 tbsp	120	0	0	0
Coconut	1 tbsp	120	0	0	0
Corn	1 tbsp	120	0	0	0
Garlic & Oil	1 tbsp	120	0	0	0
Olive	1 tbsp	120	0	0	0
Peanut	1 tbsp	120	0	0	0
Rice Bran	1 tbsp	120	0	0	0
Safflower	1 tbsp	120	0	0	0
Safflower Hi-Oleic	1 tbsp	120	0	0	0
Safflower Organic	1 tbsp	120	0	0	0
Sesame	1 tbsp	120	0	0	0
Soy	1 tbsp	120	0	0	0
Sunflower	1 tbsp	120	0	0	0

FOOD	PORTION	CALS.	CARB.	SUG.	FIB.
Hain (CONT.)					
Sunflower Organic	1 tbsp	120	0	0	0
Walnut	1 tbsp	120	0	0	0
Hollywood					
Canola	1 tbsp	120	0	0	0
Peanut	1 tbsp	120	0	0	0
Safflower	1 tbsp	120	0	0	0
Soy	1 tbsp	120	0	0	0
Sunflower	1 tbsp	120	0	0	0
House Of Tsang					
Hot Chili Sesame	1 tsp (5 g)	45	0	0	0
Mongolian Fire	1 tsp (5 g)	45	0	0	0
Pure Sesame	1 tsp (5 g)	45	0	0	0
Singapore Curry	1 tsp (5 g)	45	0	0	0
Wok Oil	1 tbsp (0.5 oz)	130	0	0	0
Italica					
Olive Oil	1 tbsp	120	0	0	0
Ka-Me					
Chili Hot	1 tbsp (0.5 fl oz)	130	0	0	0
Sesame	1 tbsp (0.5 fl oz)	130	0	0	0
Sesame Tempura	1 tbsp (0.5 fl oz)	130	0	0	0
Mazola					
No Stick	2.5 sec spray (0.2 g)	2	0	0	0
Oil	1 cup (221 g)	1955	0	0	0
Oil	1 tbsp (14 g)	120	0	0	0
Orville Redenbacher's					
Oil	1 tbsp	120	0	0	0
Pam					
Butter	⅓ sec spray (0.3 g)	0	0	0	0
Cooking Spray	⅓ sec spray (0.3 g)	0	0	0	0
Olive Oil	⅓ sec spray (0.3 g)	0	0	0	0
Planters					
Peanut	1 tbsp (0.5 oz)	120	0	0	0
Popcorn	1 tbsp (0.5 oz)	120	0	0	0
Progresso					
Olive Extra Light	1 tbsp	119	0	0	0
Olive Extra Mild	1 tbsp (0.5 oz)	120	0	0	0
Olive Extra Virgin	1 tbsp (0.5 oz)	120	0	0	0
Olive Riviera Blend	1 tbsp (0.5 oz)	120	0	0	0
Smart Beat					
Canola	1 tbsp	120	0	0	0
Oil	1 tbsp	120	0	0	0

FOOD	PORTION	CALS.	CARB.	SUG.	FIB.
Tree Of Life					
Almond	1 tbsp (0.5 g)	130	0	0	0
Apricot Kernel	1 tbsp (0.5 g)	130	0	0	0
Avocado	1 tbsp (0.5 g)	130	0	0	0
Macademia Nut	1 tbsp (0.5 g)	130	0	0	0
Olive Extra Virgin Organic	1 tbsp (0.5 g)	130	0	0	0
Sesame	1 tbsp (0.5 g)	130	0	0	0
Toasted Sesame	1 tbsp (0.5 oz)	130	0	0	0
Weight Watchers					
Butter Spray	⅓ sec spray	0	0	0	0
Cooking Spray	⅓ sec spray	0	0	0	0
Wesson					
Canola	1 tbsp	120	0	0	0
Cooking Spray Lite	0.5 sec spray	0	0	0	0
Corn	1 tbsp	120	0	0	0
Olive	1 tbsp	120	0	0	0
Sunflower	1 tbsp	120	0	0	0
Vegetable	1 tbsp	120	0	0	0
FISH OIL					
cod liver	1 tbsp	123	0	0	0
herring	1 tbsp	123	0	0	0
menhaden	1 tbsp	123	0	0	0
salmon	1 tbsp	123	0	0	0
sardine	1 tbsp	123	0	0	0
shark	3.5 oz	945	0	0	0
whale	3.5 oz	945	0	0	0
Hain					
Cod Liver	1 tbsp	120	0	0	0
Cod Liver Cherry	1 tbsp	120	0	0	0
Cod Liver Mint	1 tbsp	120	0	0	0
OKRA					
CANNED					
Allen					
Cut	½ cup (4.4 oz)	25	6	1	3
McIlhenny					
Pickled	2 pieces (1 oz)	7	1	tr	1
Trappey					
Cocktail Hot	2 pieces (1 oz)	8	2	tr	1
Cocktail Mild	1 piece (1 oz)	9	1	tr	1
Creole Gumbo	½ cup (4.2 oz)	35	6	1	3
Cut	½ cup (4.4 oz)	25	6	1	3
FROZEN					
Birds Eye					
Cut	¾ cup (2.9 oz)	25	5	1	3

FOOD	PORTION	CALS.	CARB.	SUG.	FIB.
Birds Eye (CONT.)					
Whole	9 pods (3 oz)	25	5	1	3
Fresh Like					
Cut	3.5 oz	26	6	—	1
Whole	3.5 oz	32	7	—	1
OLIVES					
green	3 extra lg	15	tr	—	tr
green	4 med	15	tr	—	tr
ripe	1 sm	4	tr	—	tr
ripe	1 lg	5	tr	—	tr
spanish stuffed	5 (0.5 oz)	15	1	0	0
Progresso					
Oil Cured	6 (0.5 oz)	80	3	0	1
Olive Salad (drained)	2 tbsp (0.8 oz)	25	1	1	1
ONION					
CANNED					
Watkins					
Liquid Spice	1 tbsp (0.5 oz)	120	0	0	0
DRIED					
Watkins					
Flakes	¼ tsp (1 g)	0	0	0	0
FRESH					
raw chopped	1 tbsp	4	1	—	tr
scallions raw chopped	1 tbsp	2	tr	—	tr
scallions raw sliced	½ cup	16	4	—	1
Antioch Farms					
Vidalia	1 med	60	14	—	3
Dole					
Green Chopped	1 tbsp	2	tr	—	tr
Medium	1	60	14	—	3
FROZEN					
Birds Eye					
Diced	⅔ cup (3 oz)	30	6	5	1
Pearl Onions In Cream Sauce	½ cup (4.4 oz)	60	8	6	1
Fresh Like					
Diced	3.5 oz	29	7	—	0
Whole	3.5 oz	37	8	—	1
Kineret					
Rings	6 (3 oz)	200	25	3	0
Ore Ida					
Chopped	¾ cup (3 oz)	25	6	5	1
Onion Ringers	6 pieces (3 oz)	240	26	5	2

FOOD	PORTION	CALS.	CARB.	SUG.	FIB.
OPOSSUM					
roasted	3 oz	188	0	0	0
ORANGE					
CANNED					
Del Monte					
Mandarin In Heavy Syrup	½ cup (4.4 oz)	80	19	19	tr
Dole					
Mandarin Segments	½ cup	70	19	—	—
Pineapple Mandarin Segments	½ cup	80	19	—	—
Empress					
Mandarin	5.5 oz	100	25	—	—
Mandarin From Japan	5.5 oz	35	8	—	—
S&W					
Mandarin Natural Style	½ cup	60	15	—	—
Mandarin Selected Sections in Heavy Syrup	½ cup	76	20	—	—
Mandarin Unsweetened	½ cup	28	7	—	—
FRESH					
california navel	1	65	16	—	3
california valencia	1	59	14	—	3
florida	1	69	17	—	4
peel	1 tbsp	6	2	—	—
sections	1 cup	85	21	—	4
Dole					
Orange	1	50	13	—	6
ORANGE JUICE					
canned	1 cup	104	25	—	—
chilled	1 cup	110	25	—	—
fresh	1 cup	111	26	—	—
frzn as prep	1 cup	112	27	—	1
frzn not prep	6 oz	339	81	—	2
mandarin orange	3.5 oz	47	10	—	—
orange drink	6 oz	94	24	—	—
After The Fall					
Juice	1 bottle (10 oz)	110	26	26	—
Bright & Early					
Chilled	8 fl oz	120	30	27	—
Frozen	8 fl oz	120	30	28	—
Capri Sun					
Drink	1 pkg (7 oz)	100	25	25	0
Del Monte					
Juice	8 fl oz	110	27	22	tr

FOOD	PORTION	CALS.	CARB.	SUG.	FIB.
Everfresh					
Juice	1 can (8 oz)	100	24	24	0
Ruby Red Orange Drink	1 can (8 oz)	130	33	33	0
Fresh Samantha					
Juice	1 cup (8 oz)	109	24	—	1
Hi-C					
Box	8.45 fl oz	130	33	32	—
Drink	8 fl oz	130	32	31	—
Drink	1 can (11.5 fl oz)	180	45	44	—
Hood					
From Concentrate	1 cup (8 oz)	120	30	30	—
Select	1 cup (8 oz)	120	30	30	—
With Calcium	1 cup (8 oz)	120	30	30	—
Kool-Aid					
Drink Mix Orange as prep	1 serv (8 oz)	60	16	16	0
Orange Drink as prep w/ sugar	1 serv (8 oz)	100	25	25	0
Libby					
Juice	6 fl oz	80	20	—	—
Minute Maid					
Box	8.45 fl oz	120	28	24	—
Calcium Rich Chilled	8 fl oz	120	27	24	—
Calcium Rich frzn	8 fl oz	120	27	24	—
Chilled	8 fl oz	110	27	24	—
Country Style Chilled	8 fl oz	110	27	24	—
Country Style frzn	8 fl oz	110	27	24	—
Juices To Go	1 can (11.5 fl oz)	160	39	35	—
Juices To Go	1 bottle (16 fl oz)	110	27	24	—
Juices To Go	1 bottle (10 fl oz)	140	34	30	—
Orange Punch Box	8.45 fl oz	130	33	32	—
Premium Choice Chilled	8 fl oz	110	27	24	—
Pulp Free Chilled	8 fl oz	110	27	24	—
Pulp Free frzn	8 fl oz	110	27	24	—
Reduced Acid frzn	8 fl oz	110	27	24	—
Mott's					
From Concentrate	10 fl oz	130	29	22	0
Ocean Spray					
100% Juice	8 fl oz	120	31	31	0
Odwalla					
Juice	8 fl oz	110	25	24	1
S&W					
100% Unsweetened	6 oz	83	18	—	—
Shasta Plus					
Orange Drink	1 can (11.5 oz)	160	40	40	0

FOOD	PORTION	CALS.	CARB.	SUG.	FIB.
Sippin' Pak					
100% Pure	8.45 fl oz	110	26	—	—
Snapple					
Juice	10 fl oz	130	29	—	—
Orangeade	8 fl oz	120	31	—	—
Tang					
Orange Drink as prep	1 serv (8 oz)	90	23	23	0
Sugar Free Orange as prep	1 serv (8 oz)	5	0	0	0
Tree Of Life					
Juice	8 fl oz	110	27	23	0
Tree Top					
Juice	6 oz	90	22	—	—
Tropicana					
Double Vitamin C with Vitamin E	8 fl oz	110	26	—	—
Frozen as prep	6 fl oz	110	27	23	—
Juice	1 container (6 fl oz)	80	20	17	—
Juice	1 container (8 fl oz)	110	27	23	—
Juice	8 fl oz	110	27	23	—
Juice	1 container (10 fl oz)	130	33	28	—
Prue Premium Calcium & Extra Vitamin C	8 fl oz	110	26	—	—
Prue Premium Vitamins C& E	8 fl oz	110	26	—	—
Season's Best	1 bottle (7 fl oz)	90	23	20	—
Season's Best	1 bottle (10 fl oz)	130	33	28	—
Season's Best	1 can (11.5 fl oz)	140	36	31	—
Season's Best Homestyle	8 fl oz	110	27	23	—
Veryfine					
100% Juice	1 bottle (10 oz)	150	37	35	2
Chillers Arctic Orange	8 fl oz	130	33	32	0
Juice Blend	1 can (11.5 oz)	160	39	34	0
Orange Drink	1 bottle (10 oz)	160	41	36	0

OREGANO

FOOD	PORTION	CALS.	CARB.	SUG.	FIB.
ground	1 tsp	5	1	—	—
Watkins					
Liquid Spice	1 tbsp (0.5 oz)	120	0	0	0

ORGAN MEATS

(*see* BRAINS, GIBLETS, GIZZARD, HEART, KIDNEY, LIVER, SWEETBREADS)

FOOD	PORTION	CALS.	CARB.	SUG.	FIB.

ORIENTAL FOOD
(*see* ASIAN FOOD, EGG ROLLS, DINNER, NOODLES, RICE, SUSHI)

OYSTERS
CANNED
eastern	1 cup	170	10	—	—
eastern	3 oz	58	3	—	—
Bumble Bee					
Whole	½ cup (3.5 oz)	100	6	—	0
Empress					
Whole	4 oz	100	8	—	—
S&W					
Fancy Whole	2 oz	95	4	—	—
FRESH					
eastern cooked	3 oz	117	7	—	—
eastern cooked	6 med	58	3	—	—
eastern raw	6 med	58	3	—	—
eastern raw	1 cup	170	10	—	—
pacific raw	3 oz	69	4	—	—
pacific raw	1 med	41	2	—	—
steamed	3 oz	138	8	—	—
steamed	1 med	41	2	—	—

PANCAKE/WAFFLE SYRUP
(*see also* SYRUP)

low calorie	1 tbsp	12	3	—	0
maple	1 cup (11.1 oz)	824	212	191	—
maple	1 tbsp (0.8 oz)	52	13	12	—
pancake syrup	1 tbsp (0.7 oz)	57	15	—	—
pancake syrup	1 cup (11 oz)	903	238	—	—
pancake syrup light	1 oz	46	13	—	—
pancake syrup w/ butter	1 tbsp (0.7 oz)	59	15	—	—
pancake syrup w/ butter	1 cup (11 oz)	933	234	—	—
Aunt Jemima					
Butter Rich	¼ cup (2.8 oz)	210	52	29	—
Butterlite	¼ cup (2.5 oz)	100	26	26	—
Lite	¼ cup (2.5 oz)	100	27	—	—
Syrup	¼ cup (2.8 oz)	210	53	38	—
Brer Rabbit					
Dark	2 tbsp	120	31	—	—
Light	2 tbsp	120	31	—	—
Estee					
Lite Maple	¼ cup (2.4 oz)	80	20	20	—
Golden Griddle					
Syrup	1 cup (321 g)	885	229	—	—

FOOD	PORTION	CALS.	CARB.	SUG.	FIB.
Golden Griddle (CONT.)					
Syrup	1 tbsp (20 g)	50	14	—	—
Karo					
Syrup	1 tbsp (21 g)	60	15	—	—
Log Cabin					
Country Kitchen	1 oz	103	27	21	—
Lite	1 oz	49	13	13	—
Mrs. Butter-worth's					
Original	¼ cup (2 oz)	230	56	35	—
Mrs.Richardson's					
Lite	¼ cup (2.5 oz)	100	26	25	—
Original Recipe	¼ cup (2.8 oz)	210	52	23	—
Red Wing					
Lite	¼ cup (2 oz)	100	26	25	0
Syrup	¼ cup (2 oz)	210	53	27	0
Tree Of Life					
Maple	¼ cup (2.1 oz)	200	53	53	—

PANCAKES

FROZEN

FOOD	PORTION	CALS.	CARB.	SUG.	FIB.
buttermilk	1 4 in diam (1.3 ox)	83	16	—	—
plain	1 4 in diam (1.3 oz)	83	16	—	—
Aunt Jemima					
Blueberry	3 (3.4 oz)	210	40	—	2
Buttermilk	3 (3 oz)	180	34	—	2
Lowfat	3 (3.4 oz)	130	33	—	8
Original	3 (3.4 oz)	200	40	—	2
Downyflake					
Blueberry	3	290	48	—	—
Buttermilk	3	280	45	—	—
Pancakes And Sausages	1 pkg (5.5 oz)	430	47	—	—
Regular	3	280	45	—	—
Eggo					
Buttermilk	3 (4.1 oz)	270	44	10	1
Great Starts					
Pancakes And Sausages	6 oz	460	52	—	—
Pancakes With Bacon	4½ oz	400	43	—	—
Silver Dollar Pancakes And Sausage	3¾ oz	310	37	—	—
Whole Wheat Pancakes With Lite Links	5½ oz	350	39	—	—
Healthy Starts					
Pancakes w/ LeanLinks	6 oz	360	48	—	—
Jimmy Dean					
Flapstick	1 (2.5 oz)	240	22	9	1

FOOD	PORTION	CALS.	CARB.	SUG.	FIB.
Jimmy Dean (CONT.)					
Flapstick Blueberry	1 (2.5 oz)	260	23	8	1
Pillsbury					
Buttermilk Microwave	3	260	51	—	—
Harvest Wheat Microwave	3	240	48	—	—
Microwave	3	250	49	—	—
Original Microwave	3	240	47	—	—
Quaker					
Lite Pancakes & Lite Links	1 pkg (6 oz)	310	43	—	—
Lite Pancakes & Lite Syrup	1 pkg (6 oz)	260	53	—	—
Pancakes & Sausages	1 pkg (6 oz)	420	57	—	—
HOME RECIPE					
plain	1 (4 in diam)	86	11	—	—
MIX					
buckwheat	1 (4 in diam)	62	9	—	—
buttermilk	1 4 in diam (1.3 oz)	74	14	—	tr
plain	1-4 in diam (1.3 oz)	74	14	—	tr
sugar free low sodium	1 (3 in diam)	44	9	—	—
whole wheat	1 (4 in diam)	92	13	—	—
Arrowhead					
Multigrain Pancake & Waffle Mix	¼ cup (1.2 oz)	120	24	2	3
Aunt Jemima					
Buckwheat Pancake & Waffle Mix	¼ cup (1.4 oz)	120	28	2	4
Buttermilk Pancake & Waffle Mix	⅓ cup (1.9 oz)	190	38	6	2
Original Pancake & Waffle Mix	⅓ cup (1.6 oz)	150	34	5	1
Pancake & Waffle Mix Regular	⅓ cup (1.9 oz)	190	39	8	1
Pancake & Waffle Mix Whole Wheat	¼ cup (1.4 oz)	130	28	4	3
Betty Crocker					
Buttermilk	3 (4 in diam)	280	39	—	—
Bisquick					
Apple Cinnamon Shake 'N Pour	3 (4 in diam)	240	47	—	—
Blueberry Shake 'N Pour	3 (4 in diam)	270	54	—	—
Buttermilk Shake 'N Pour	3 (4 in diam)	250	49	—	—
Original Shake 'N Pour	3 (4 in diam)	250	49	—	—
Estee					
Pancake Mix Fat Free as prep	4 (4 in diam)	180	40	tr	1

FOOD	PORTION	CALS.	CARB.	SUG.	FIB.
Fast Shake					
Blueberry	1 serv (2.5 oz)	251	50	—	—
Buttermilk	1 serv (2.5 oz)	258	50	—	—
Original	1 serv (2.5 oz)	266	50	—	—
Health Valley					
Pancake Mix not prep	1 oz	100	20	—	3
Hodgson Mill					
Buckwheat	⅓ cup (1.8 oz)	160	35	2	1
Hungry Jack					
Potato as prep	3 (3 in diam)	90	16	tr	1
Stone-Buhr					
Buckwheat	¼ cup (1.4 oz)	130	29	0	3
Oat Bran	¼ cup (1.4 oz)	130	30	0	2
Whole Wheat	¼ cup (1.4 oz)	120	25	0	3
Wanda's					
Blue Corn	⅓ cup mix per serv (1.7 oz)	170	32	9	2

PANCREAS
(*see* SWEETBREADS)

PAPAYA

fresh	1	117	30	—	—
fresh cubed	1 cup	54	14	—	—
Ka-Me					
Papaya	¾ cup	120	29	29	1
Sonoma					
Dried Pieces	2 pieces (2 oz)	200	41	35	6

PAPAYA JUICE

nectar	1 cup	142	36	—	—
Everfresh					
Premium Drink	1 can (8 oz)	140	35	35	0
Goya					
Nectar	6 oz	110	27	—	—
Kern's					
Nectar	6 fl oz	110	27	—	—
Libby					
Nectar	1 can (11.5 fl oz)	210	51	47	—

PAPRIKA

paprika	1 tsp	6	1	—	—
Watkins					
Ground	¼ tsp (0.5 oz)	0	0	0	0

PARSLEY

dry	1 tsp	1	tr	—	—

FOOD	PORTION	CALS.	CARB.	SUG.	FIB.
dry	1 tbsp	1	tr	—	—
fresh chopped	½ cup	11	2	—	—
Dole					
Chopped	1 tbsp	10	1	—	tr

PARSNIPS
fresh cooked	1 (5.6 oz)	130	31	—	—
fresh sliced cooked	½ cup	63	15	—	—
raw sliced	½ cup	50	12	—	—

PASSION FRUIT
purple fresh	1	18	4	—	—

PASSION FRUIT JUICE
purple	1 cup	126	34	—	—
yellow	1 cup	149	36	—	—
Snapple					
Passion Supreme	10 fl oz	160	39	—	—

PASTA
(*see also* NOODLES, PASTA DINNERS, PASTA SALAD)
DRY
corn cooked	1 cup (4.9 oz)	176	39	—	7
elbows cooked	1 cup (4.9 oz)	197	40	—	2
shells small cooked	1 cup (4 oz)	162	33	—	2
shells small protein fortified cooked	1 cup (4 oz)	189	36	—	—
spaghetti cooked	1 cup (4.9 oz)	197	40	—	2
spaghetti protein fortified cooked	1 cup (4.9 oz)	230	44	—	2
spinach spaghetti cooked	1 cup (4.9 oz)	182	37	—	—
spirals cooked	1 cup (4.7 oz)	189	38	—	2
vegetable cooked	1 cup (4.7 oz)	172	36	—	6
whole wheat cooked	1 cup (4.9 oz)	174	37	—	4
whole wheat spaghetti cooked	1 cup (4.9 oz)	174	37	—	6
Anthony					
Pasta	2 oz	210	42	0	tr
Barilla					
Conchiglie Rigate	1 cup (2 oz)	200	40	1	2
Gemelli as prep	1 cup (2 oz)	200	42	1	2
Pennette Rigate	1⅓ cups (2 oz)	200	42	1	2
Bella Via					
Angel Hair	2 oz	200	40	—	—
Artichoke Angel Hair as prep	⅝ cup	200	40	—	—
Artichoke Spaghetti as prep	⅝ cup	200	40	—	—

FOOD	PORTION	CALS.	CARB.	SUG.	FIB.
Bella Via (CONT.)					
Elbows	2 oz	200	40	—	—
Fettucini as prep	⅝ cup	200	40	—	—
Linguini	2 oz	200	40	—	—
Penne as prep	⅝ cup	200	40	—	—
Rotelli	2 oz	200	40	—	—
Shells	2 oz	200	40	—	—
Spaghetti	2 oz	200	40	—	—
Ziti	2 oz	200	40	—	—
Classico					
Gnocchi Di Toscana	1 cup (2 oz)	210	42	3	2
Creamette					
Elbow Macaroni not prep	2 oz	210	42	—	—
Spaghetti not prep	2 oz	210	42	—	—
Spinach Ribbons not prep	2 oz	210	42	—	—
Cuore					
Capellini cooked	1⅓ cup (2 oz)	190	39	1	3
Fusilli cooked	1⅓ cup (2 oz)	190	39	1	3
Tortiglioni cooked	1⅓ cup (2 oz)	190	39	1	3
De Bole's					
Whole Wheat Organic Elbows	2 oz	210	40	2	5
DeCecco					
Whole Wheat Linguine cooked	2 oz	180	33	1	7
DeFino					
Lasagna No Boil	1 oz	102	20	—	—
Ribbons No Boil	2 oz	204	40	—	—
Delverde					
Spaghetti Whole Wheat	2 oz	206	42	—	5
Eden					
Elbows Whole Wheat Organic	2 oz	210	39	2	6
Elbows Whole Wheat Vegetable Organic	2 oz	210	39	2	6
Kudzu And Sweet Potato Pasta	2 oz	190	47	0	0
Kudzu Kiri Pasta	2 oz	190	47	0	0
Mung Bean Pasta Harusame	2 oz	190	47	0	0
Organic Endless Tubes	½ cup (1.9 oz)	210	41	2	4
Ribbons Durum Wheat Curry Organic	2 oz	220	44	tr	3
Ribbons Durum Wheat Organic	2 oz	220	44	tr	3

FOOD	PORTION	CALS.	CARB.	SUG.	FIB.
Eden (cont.)					
Ribbons Durum Wheat Paella Organic	2 oz	220	44	tr	3
Ribbons Durum Wheat Parsley Garlic Organic	2 oz	220	44	tr	3
Ribbons Durum Wheat Pesto Organic	2 oz	220	44	tr	3
Ribbons Whole Wheat Spinach Organic	2 oz	200	40	tr	7
Rice Pasta Bifun	2 oz	200	44	0	0
Shells Durum Wheat Vegetable Organic	2 oz	210	42	1	2
Soba	2 oz	200	38	3	2
Soba 100% Buckwheat	2 oz	200	41	5	3
Soba Lotus Root	2 oz	190	37	2	4
Soba Mugwort	2 oz	190	37	2	2
Soba Wild Yam Jinenjo	2 oz	190	37	2	2
Somen	2 oz	200	38	1	3
Spaghetti Durum Wheat Organic	2 oz	210	42	1	2
Spaghetti Kamut Organic	2 oz	210	38	2	6
Spaghetti Parsley Garlic Organic	2 oz	210	42	1	2
Spaghetti Whole Wheat Organic	2 oz	210	39	2	6
Spirals Durum Wheat Vegetable Organic	2 oz	210	42	1	2
Spirals Kamut Organic	2 oz	210	38	2	6
Spirals Sesame Rice Organic	2 oz	200	37	1	6
Spirals Whole Wheat Vegetable Organic	2 oz	210	39	2	6
Udon	2 oz	200	38	1	3
Udon Brown Rice	2 oz	200	38	1	3
Gioia					
Pasta	2 oz	210	42	0	tr
Golden Grain					
Pasta	2 oz	203	41	—	0
Health Valley					
Lasagna Whole Wheat	2 oz	170	40	—	7
Lasagna Spinach Whole Wheat	2 oz	170	40	—	7
Spaghetti Amaranth	2 oz	170	40	—	9
Spaghetti Oat Bran	2 oz	120	23	—	4

FOOD	PORTION	CALS.	CARB.	SUG.	FIB.
Health Valley (CONT.)					
Spaghetti Spinach Whole Wheat	2 oz	170	40	—	7
Spaghetti Whole Wheat	2 oz	170	40	—	7
Hodgson Mill					
Spaghetti Whole Wheat Spinach not prep	2 oz	190	35	0	5
Veggie Bows not prep	2 oz	200	41	0	1
Veggie Rotini not prep	2 oz	200	41	0	1
Veggie Wagon Wheels not prep	2 oz	200	41	0	1
Whole Wheat Spirals not prep	2 oz	190	34	0	6
La Molisana					
Radiatori	2 oz	230	48	—	—
Lupini					
Elbow uncooked	½ cup (2 oz)	190	37	tr	5
Spaghetti Light uncooked	½ cup (2 oz)	190	37	tr	5
Spaghetti With Triticale	⅟₇ pkg (2 oz)	190	38	<2	6
Luxury					
Pasta	2 oz	210	42	0	tr
Merlino's					
Pasta	2 oz	210	42	0	tr
Mueller's					
Dinosaurs	2 oz (57 g)	210	42	—	—
Jungle Animals	2 oz (57 g)	210	42	—	—
Lasagne	2 oz (57 g)	210	42	—	—
Monsters	2 oz (57 g)	210	42	—	—
Outer Space	2 oz	210	42	—	—
Spaghetti	2 oz (57 g)	210	42	—	—
Teddy Bears	2 oz (57 g)	210	42	—	—
Twists Tri Color	2 oz (57 g)	210	41	—	—
Noodles By Leonardo					
Capellini	2 oz	200	40	2	2
Elbows not prep	½ cup (2 oz)	200	40	2	2
Fettucini	2 oz	200	40	2	2
Linguine not prep	½ cup (2 oz)	200	40	2	2
Rigatoni	2 oz	200	40	2	2
Rotini	2 oz	200	40	2	2
Shells not prep	½ cup (2 oz)	200	40	2	2
Spaghetti not prep	½ cup (2 oz)	200	40	2	2
Spaghettini	2 oz	200	40	2	2
Vermicelli not prep	½ cup (2 oz)	200	40	2	2

FOOD	PORTION	CALS.	CARB.	SUG.	FIB.
Penn Dutch					
Pasta	2 oz	210	42	0	tr
Pomi					
Capellini	2 oz	210	41	—	—
Prince					
Egg	2 oz	221	40	0	1
Pasta	2 oz	210	42	0	tr
Rainbow	2 oz	210	42	0	1
Spinach Egg	2 oz	220	40	0	1
Pritikin					
Spaghetti Whole Wheat	⅛ box (2 oz)	190	40	—	—
Spiral	⅔ cup (2 oz)	190	40	—	—
Red Cross					
Pasta	2 oz	210	42	0	tr
Ronco					
Pasta	2 oz	210	42	0	tr
Ronzoni					
Elbows	¾ cup (2 oz)	210	40	—	—
Fettucini	¾ cup (2 oz)	210	40	—	—
Fusilli	¾ cup (2 oz)	210	40	—	—
Lasagne	¾ cup (2 oz)	210	40	—	—
Manicotti	¾ cup (2 oz)	210	40	—	—
Mostaccioli	¾ cup (2 oz)	210	40	—	—
Rigatoni	¾ cup (2 oz)	210	40	—	—
Rotelle uncooked	¾ cup (2 oz)	210	40	—	—
Rotini uncooked	¾ cup (2 oz)	210	40	—	—
Shells uncooked	¾ cup (2 oz)	210	40	—	—
Shells Jumbo	¾ cup (2 oz)	210	40	—	—
Spaghetti not prep	¾ cup (2 oz)	210	40	—	—
Tubettini	¾ cup (2 oz)	210	40	—	—
San Giorgio					
Bowties Egg	2 oz	210	38	—	—
Capellini	2 oz	210	40	2	2
Elbow Macaroni	2 oz	210	40	2	2
Fettuccine Egg	2 oz	210	38	—	—
Fettuccini Florentine	2 oz	210	38	—	—
Lasagne	2 oz	210	40	2	2
Linguini	2 oz	210	40	2	2
Manicotti	2 oz	210	40	2	2
Rigatoni	2 oz	210	40	2	2
Rotini	2 oz	210	40	2	2
Shells	2 oz	210	40	2	2
Spaghetti	2 oz	210	40	2	2
Spaghetti Thin	2 oz	210	40	2	2

FOOD	PORTION	CALS.	CARB.	SUG.	FIB.
San Giorgio (CONT.)					
Vermicelli	2 oz	210	40	2	2
Ziti Cut	2 oz	210	40	2	2
Tree Of Life					
Cajun as prep	⅝ cup (4.9 oz)	200	40	0	1
Confetti as prep	⅝ cup (4.9 oz)	200	40	0	1
Garlic & Parsley as prep	⅝ cup (4.9 oz)	200	40	0	1
Jamaican Spice as prep	⅝ cup (4.9 oz)	200	40	0	1
Lemon Pepper as prep	⅝ cup (4.9 oz)	200	40	0	1
Spinach as prep	⅝ cup (4.9 oz)	200	40	0	1
Tex Mex as prep	⅝ cup (4.9 oz)	200	40	0	1
Thai as prep	⅝ cup (4.9 oz)	200	40	0	1
Tomato Basil as prep	⅝ cup (4.9 oz)	200	40	0	1
Vimco					
Pasta	2 oz	210	42	0	tr
FRESH					
cooked	2 oz	75	14	—	—
spinach cooked	2 oz	74	14	—	—
Contadina					
Angel's Hair	1¼ cup (2.8 oz)	240	43	1	2
Fettuccine	1¼ cup (2.9 oz)	250	45	1	2
Fettuccine Cholesterol Free	1 cup (2.9 oz)	240	46	2	2
Light Ravioli Cheese	1 cup (3.1 oz)	240	35	4	2
Light Ravioli Garden Vegetable	1¼ cup (3.8 oz)	290	43	5	3
Light Tortellini Garlic & Cheese	1 cup (3.6 oz)	280	50	3	3
Linguine	1¼ cup (3 oz)	260	47	1	2
Linguine Cholesterol Free	1¼ cup (3.1 oz)	250	49	2	2
Ravioli Beef And Garlic	1¼ cup (4 oz)	350	39	3	3
Ravioli Cheese	1 cup (3.1 oz)	280	31	3	2
Ravioli Chicken And Rosemary	1¼ cup (4 oz)	330	43	5	3
Tagliatelli Spinach	1¼ cup (3.1 oz)	270	46	1	4
Tortellini Spinach Three Cheese	¾ cup (3.1 oz)	280	38	2	3
Tortelloni Cheese	¾ cup (3 oz)	260	39	2	3
Tortelloni Cheese And Basil	1 cup (4 oz)	360	49	5	3
Tortelloni Chicken And Prosciutto	1 cup (3.8 oz)	360	46	3	3
Tortelloni Chicken And Vegetable	¾ cup (2.9 oz)	260	39	2	2
Tortelloni Spicy Italian Sausage And Bell Pepper	1 cup (3.6 oz)	330	47	4	3

FOOD	PORTION	CALS.	CARB.	SUG.	FIB.
Di Giorno					
Angel's Hair	1 cup	160	31	1	2
Beef & Roasted Garlic Tortellini	1 cup	340	46	2	1
Fettuccine	1 cup	200	38	1	2
Four Cheese Ravioli	1 cup	350	40	1	2
Herb Linguine	1 cup	200	38	1	2
Italian Sausage Ravioli In Green Bell Pepper Pasta	1¼ cup	350	45	3	3
Lemon Chicken Tortellini In Cracked Black Pepper Pasta	1 cup	270	42	2	1
Light Cheese Ravioli	1 cup	280	40	1	2
Linguine	1 cup	200	38	1	2
Mozzarella Garlic Tortelloni	1 cup	300	42	1	1
Pesto Tortelloni	1 cup	320	46	1	3
Portabello Mushroom Tortelloni	1 cup	310	48	1	3
Red Bell Pepper Fettuccine	1 cup	200	38	1	2
Spinach Fettuccine	1 cup	190	38	tr	2
Sun-Dried Tomato Ravioli	1⅛ cup	380	48	5	3
Three Cheese Tortellini	¾ cup	250	37	2	2
Herb's					
Fettucine Bell Pepper Basil	2 oz	220	42	1	2
Fettucine Parsley Garlic	2 oz	220	42	1	2
Fettucine Spinach	2 oz	220	42	1	2
Ribbons Vegetable	2 oz	220	42	1	2
Ribbons Whole Wheat	2 oz	200	40	1	7
Rotini Mixed Vegetable	2 oz	210	42	1	2
Shells Mixed Vegetable	2 oz	210	42	1	2
Trios					
Ravioli Cracked Pepper Garlic Cheese	1 cup (4.3 oz)	340	48	4	0
HOME RECIPE					
made w/o egg cooked	2 oz	71	14	—	—
plain made w/ egg cooked	2 oz	74	13	—	—

PASTA DINNERS

(*see also* DINNER, PASTA SALAD)

CANNED

Chef Boyardee					
ABC's & 1,2,3's In Cheese Flavor Sauce	7.5 oz	180	37	—	—
ABC's & 1,2,3's w/ Mini Meatballs	7.5 oz	?60	32	—	2

FOOD	PORTION	CALS.	CARB.	SUG.	FIB.
Chef Boyardee (CONT.)					
Beef Ravioli	7.5 oz	190	31	—	2
Beef Ravioli 99% Fat Free	1 cup (8.6 oz)	210	41	6	3
Beefaroni	7.5 oz	220	31	—	2
Cheese Ravioli In Meat Sauce	7.5 oz	200	37	—	—
Dinosaurs In Cheese Flavor Sauce	7.5 oz	180	36	—	—
Dinosaurs w/ Meatballs	7.5 oz	240	32	—	4
Elbows In Beef Sauce	7.5 oz	210	29	—	—
Lasagna	7.5 oz	230	31	—	—
Lasagna In Garden Vegetable Sauce	7.5 oz	170	34	—	—
Macaroni & Cheese	7.5 oz	180	27	—	1
Pasta Rings & Meatballs	7.5 oz	220	33	—	4
Rigatoni	7.5 oz	210	31	—	—
Rings & Franks	7.5 oz	190	31	—	3
Shells In Meat Sauce	7.5 oz	210	32	—	—
Shells In Mushroom Sauce	7.5 oz	170	35	—	—
Spaghetti & Meat Balls	7.5 oz	230	29	—	—
Tic Tac Toes In Cheese Flavor Sauce	7.5 oz	170	36	—	3
Tic Tac Toes w/ Mini Meatballs	7.5 oz	250	32	—	3
Turtles In Sauce	7.5 oz	160	33	—	2
Turtles w/ Meatballs	7.5 oz	210	30	—	2
Franco-American					
Beef RavioliO's In Meat Sauce	½ can (7½ oz)	250	35	—	—
CircusO's Pasta In Tomato & Cheese Sauce	½ can (7⅜ oz)	170	33	—	—
CircusO's Pasta With Meatballs In Tomato Sauce	½ can (7⅜ oz)	210	25	—	—
Macaroni & Cheese	½ can (7⅜ oz)	170	24	—	—
Spaghetti In Tomato Sauce w/ Cheese	½ can (7⅜ oz)	180	36	—	—
Spaghetti w/ Meatballs In Tomato Sauce	½ can (7⅜ oz)	220	28	—	—
SpaghettiO's With Meatballs	½ can (7⅜ oz)	220	25	—	—
SpaghettiO's With Sliced Franks	½ can (7⅜ oz)	220	26	—	—
SpaghettiO's In Tomato & Cheese Sauce	½ can (7⅜ oz)	170	33	—	—

FOOD	PORTION	CALS.	CARB.	SUG.	FIB.
Franco-American (CONT.)					
SportyO's In Tomato & Cheese Sauce	½ can (7½ oz)	170	33	—	—
SportyO's Pasta With Meatballs In Tomato Sauce	½ can (7⅜ oz)	210	25	—	—
TeddyO's In Tomato & Cheese Sauce	½ can (7½ oz)	170	33	—	—
TeddyO's Pasta With Meatballs	½ can (7⅜ oz)	210	25	—	—
Hormel					
Spaghetti & Meatballs	1 can (7.5 oz)	210	28	8	2
Kid's Kitchen					
Microwave Meals Cheezy Mac & Beef	1 cup (7.5 oz)	260	33	7	1
Microwave Meals Noodle Rings & Chicken	1 cup (7.5 oz)	150	17	2	1
Microwave Meals Spaghetti Rings & Franks	1 cup (7.5 oz)	240	32	11	1
Progresso					
Beef Ravioli	1 cup (9.1 oz)	260	45	9	4
Cheese Ravioli	1 cup (9.1 oz)	220	43	9	4
Van Camp's					
Spaghetti Weenee	1 can (8 oz)	230	34	—	1
FROZEN					
Amy's Organic					
Macaroni & Cheese	1 pkg (9 oz)	390	50	6	4
Macaroni & Soy Cheese	1 pkg (9 oz)	360	42	2	4
Pasta Primavera	1 pkg (9.5 oz)	320	39	7	3
Ravioli w/ Sauce	1 pkg (9.5 oz)	340	44	7	6
Tofu Vegetable Lasagna	1 pkg (9.5 oz)	300	41	6	4
Vegetable Lasagna	1 pkg (9.5 oz)	300	39	7	5
Whole Meals Cannelloni	1 pkg (9 oz)	260	32	9	5
Armour					
Classics Chicken Fettucini	1 meal (10 oz)	230	25	7	6
Banquet					
Family Entree Lasagna w/ Meat Sauce	1 serv (8 oz)	240	32	4	5
Family Entree Macaroni & Beef	1 serv (8 oz)	230	31	3	3
Family Entree Macaroni & Cheese	1 serv (8 oz)	300	39	2	2
Family Entree Noodles & Chicken	1 serv (8 oz)	210	24	2	2

FOOD	PORTION	CALS.	CARB.	SUG.	FIB.
Banquet (CONT.)					
Family Entree Noodles & Beef	1 serv (7.47 oz)	140	16	1	2
Birds Eye					
Easy Recipe Meal Starter Cheesy Cheese	1 serv	280	30	5	2
Easy Recipe Meal Starter Chicken Primavera as prep	1 serv	280	30	4	2
Easy Recipe Meal Starter Chicken Alfredo as prep	1 serv	280	30	4	2
Pasta Secrets Creamy Peppercorn	2⅓ cups (6.6 oz)	300	29	8	2
Pasta Secrets Italian Pesto	2⅓ cups (6.4 oz)	240	32	6	2
Pasta Secrets Primavera	2⅓ cups (6.6 oz)	230	26	4	3
Pasta Secrets Three Cheese	2 cups (6.1 oz)	230	31	8	2
Pasta Secrets White Cheddar	2 cups (6.3 oz)	240	30	7	2
Pasta Secrets Zesty Garlic	2 cups (5.9 oz)	240	31	6	2
Budget Gourmet					
Cheese Ravioli	1 meal (9.5 oz)	290	34	—	—
Lasagna Italian Sausage	1 meal (10 oz)	430	34	—	—
Lasagna Vegetable	1 meal (10.5 oz)	390	36	—	—
Lasagne Three Cheese	1 meal (10 oz)	390	26	—	—
Lasagne With Meat Sauce	1 meal (9.4 oz)	290	30	—	—
Linguini With Shrimp & Clams	1 meal (9.5 oz)	280	34	—	—
Linguini With Shrimp And Clams	1 meal (10 oz)	270	35	—	—
Macaroni & Cheese	1 meal (5.75 oz)	230	22	—	—
Macaroni & Cheese With Cheddar & Parmesan	1 meal (10.5 oz)	330	49	—	—
Manicotti Cheese	1 meal (10 oz)	440	36	—	—
Pasta Alfredo With Broccoli	1 meal (5.5 oz)	210	22	—	—
Penne Pasta With Chunky Tomato Sauce & Italian Sausage	1 meal (10 oz)	320	34	—	—
Rigatoni In Cream Sauce With Broccoli & Chicken	1 meal (10.8 oz)	290	44	—	—
Spaghetti With Chunky Tomato & Meat Sauce	1 meal (10 oz)	300	44	—	—
Tortellini Cheese	1 meal (5.5 oz)	200	25	—	—
Ziti In Marinara Sauce	1 meal (6.25 oz)	200	23	—	—
Dining Light					
Cheese Cannelloni	9 oz	310	38	—	—

FOOD	PORTION	CALS.	CARB.	SUG.	FIB.
Formagg					
Penne Pasta Alfredo	⅔ cup (5 oz)	190	35	2	0
Penne Pasta Primavera	⅔ cup (5 oz)	190	35	2	0
Vegetable Pasta & Caesar Italian Garden	⅔ cup (5 oz)	190	35	2	0
Green Giant					
Create A Meal Creamy Alfredo as prep	1¼ cups (10 oz)	380	33	9	4
Create A Meal Creamy Cheddar as prep	1½ cups (10 oz)	290	29	8	4
Create A Meal Creamy Chicken Noodle as prep	1¼ cups (10 oz)	350	34	8	3
Pasta Accents Alfredo	2 cups (5.6 oz)	210	25	5	4
Pasta Accents Creamy Cheddar	2⅓ cups (6.7 oz)	250	36	6	5
Pasta Accents Florentine	2 cups (7.3 oz)	310	44	5	5
Pasta Accents Garden Herb Seasoning	2 cups (6.8 oz)	230	32	4	7
Pasta Accents Garlic Seasoning	2 cups (6.6 oz)	260	36	5	5
Pasta Accents Primavera	2¼ cups (7 oz)	320	40	5	7
Pasta Accents White Cheddar Sauce	1¾ cups (5.6 oz)	300	38	7	4
Healthy Choice					
Beef Macaroni Casserole	1 meal (8.5 oz)	200	34	4	5
Cheese Ravioli Parmigiana	1 meal (9 oz)	250	44	14	6
Chicken Broccoli Alfredo	1 meal (12.1 oz)	370	53	35	6
Chicken Fettucini Alfredo	1 meal (8.5 oz)	250	34	0	3
Classics Pasta Shells Marinara	1 meal (12 oz)	360	59	5	5
Classics Turkey Fettuccine Alla Crema	1 meal (12.5 oz)	350	50	3	5
Fettucini Alfredo	1 meal (8 oz)	240	39	1	3
Lasagna Roma	1 meal (13.5 oz)	390	60	11	9
Macaroni & Cheese	1 meal (9 oz)	290	45	3	4
Spaghetti Bolognese	1 meal (10 oz)	260	43	7	5
Three Cheese Manicotti	1 meal (11 oz)	310	41	11	7
Vegetable Pasta Italiano	1 meal (10 oz)	220	44	3	6
Zucchini Lasagna	1 meal (14 oz)	330	58	11	11
Kid Cuisine					
Macaroni & Cheese	1 pkg (10.6 oz)	420	68	34	3
Mini Cheese Ravioli	1 pkg (9.82 oz)	320	63	35	6
Le Menu					
Entree LightStyle Garden Vegetables Lasagna	10½ oz	260	35	—	—

FOOD	PORTION	CALS.	CARB.	SUG.	FIB.
Le Menu (CONT.)					
Entree LightStyle Lasagna With Meat Sauce	10 oz	290	36	—	—
Entree LightStyle Meat Sauce & Cheese Tortellini	8 oz	250	34	—	—
Entree LightStyle Spaghetti With Beef Sauce And Mushrooms	9 oz	280	45	—	—
LightStyle 3-Cheese Stuffed Shells	10 oz	280	34	—	—
LightStyle Cheese Tortellini	10 oz	230	35	—	—
Manicotto With Three Cheeses	11¾ oz	390	44	—	—
Lean Cuisine					
Alfredo Pasta Primavera	1 pkg (10 oz)	290	46	6	3
Angel Hair Pasta	1 pkg (10 oz)	220	41	11	6
Bow Tie Pasta & Creamy Tomato Sauce	1 pkg (9.5 oz)	260	43	9	6
Cafe Classics Bow Tie Pasta & Chicken	1 pkg (9.5 oz)	250	34	7	3
Cafe Classics Cheese Lasagna w/ Chicken Scaloppini	1 pkg (10 oz)	290	33	8	3
Cheddar Bake With Pasta	1 pkg (9 oz)	220	30	8	3
Cheese Cannelloni	1 pkg (9.1 oz)	230	28	9	3
Cheese Lasagna Casserole	1 pkg (10 oz)	270	40	6	5
Cheese Ravioli	1 pkg (8.5 oz)	270	40	10	5
Cheese Stuffed Shells	1 serv (8.9 oz)	230	34	10	3
Chicken Fettucini	1 pkg (9.25 oz)	280	36	6	4
Chicken Lasagna	1 pkg (10 oz)	270	30	7	5
Classic Cheese Lasagna	1 pkg (11.5 oz)	270	41	10	6
Fettucini Alfredo	1 pkg (9 oz)	300	47	7	2
Fettucini Primavera	1 pkg (10 oz)	270	38	8	4
Five Cheese Lasagna	1 serv (8 oz)	210	31	8	4
Lasagne With Meat Sauce	1 pkg (10.5 oz)	290	37	9	4
Macaroni & Beef	1 pkg (10 oz)	270	43	9	4
Macaroni & Cheese	1 pkg (10 oz)	290	43	6	4
Penne Pasta Bolognese	1 pkg (9.5 oz)	270	39	9	4
Penne Pasta w/ Tomato Basil Sauce	1 pkg (10 oz)	270	52	10	5
Spaghetti w/ Meat Sauce	1 pkg (11.5 oz)	290	50	10	7
Spaghetti w/ Meatballs	1 pkg (9.5 oz)	280	40	6	4
Vegetable Lasagna	1 pkg (10.5 oz)	260	35	9	5

FOOD	PORTION	CALS.	CARB.	SUG.	FIB.
Life Choice					
Linguini Roma	1 meal (13.2 oz)	230	48	8	6
Sun Dried Tomato Manicotti	1 meal (11.65 oz)	220	39	9	7
Vegetable Lasagna Primavera	1 meal (11.2 oz)	170	30	7	8
Luigino's					
& Pomodoro Sauce With Meatballs	1 pkg (9 oz)	320	43	3	2
& Pomodoro Sauce With Meatballs	1 cup (6.3 oz)	270	36	2	2
Cheese Ravioli & Alfredo With Broccoli Sauce	1 pkg (8.5 oz)	420	30	2	2
Cheese Tortellini & Alfredo Sauce With Broccoli	1 pkg (8 oz)	390	28	2	2
Fettuccine Alfredo	1 cup (7.5 oz)	330	36	1	3
Fettuccine Alfredo	1 pkg (9.4 oz)	390	45	1	4
Fettuccine Alfredo With Broccoli	1 pkg (9.2 oz)	360	39	1	4
Fettuccine Carbonara	1 pkg (9 oz)	360	47	1	3
Lasagna Alfredo	1 pkg (9 oz)	360	30	1	2
Lasagna Alfredo	1 cup (6.3 oz)	300	25	1	2
Lasagna Pollo	1 pkg (9 oz)	320	33	1	3
Lasagna With Meat Sauce	1 pkg (9 oz)	290	36	2	2
Lasagna With Meat Sauce	1 cup (7.2 oz)	240	30	2	2
Lasagna With Vegetables	1 pkg (9 oz)	290	35	2	2
Linguini With Clams & Sauce	1 pkg (9 oz)	270	42	1	2
Linguini With Red Sauce &	1 pkg (9 oz)	260	41	3	3
Linguini With Seafood	1 pkg (9 oz)	290	45	3	4
Macaroni & Cheese	1 pkg (9 oz)	370	45	0	3
Macaroni & Cheese	1 cup (7.2 oz)	310	37	0	2
Marinara Sauce Penne Pasta Italian Sausage & Peppers	1 pkg (9 oz)	350	32	1	2
Marinara Sauce Penne Pasta Italian Sausage & Peppers	1 cup (7.4 oz)	290	27	1	2
Meat Ravioli & Pomodoro Sauce	1 pkg (8.5 oz)	320	37	4	3
Minestrone With Penne Pasta	1 cup (6.3 oz)	180	21	1	1
Penne Pollo	1 pkg (9 oz)	330	36	1	3
Penne Primavera	1 pkg (9 oz)	350	50	1	3

FOOD	PORTION	CALS.	CARB.	SUG.	FIB.
Luigino's (CONT.)					
Rigatoni Pomodoro Italiano	1 pkg (9 oz)	290	40	3	4
Shells & Cheese With Jalapenos	1 pkg (8.5 oz)	360	41	1	2
Spaghetti Bolognese	1 pkg (9 oz)	270	38	2	4
Spaghetti Marinara	1 pkg (10 oz)	250	49	3	3
Spinach Ravioli & Primavera Sauce	1 pkg (8.5 oz)	360	36	2	2
Morton					
Macaroni & Cheese	1 serv (8 oz)	220	34	2	2
Mrs. Paul's					
Entrees Light Seafood Lasagne	9½ oz	290	39	—	—
Entrees Light Seafood Rotini	9 oz	240	34	—	—
Seafood Rotini	9 oz	240	34	—	—
Palmazone					
Macaroni 'n Cheese	½ pkg (6 oz)	260	36	—	—
Pasta Favorites					
Chicken Pasta Primavera	1 pkg (10.5 oz)	330	40	10	6
Fettuccini Alfredo	1 pkg (10.5 oz)	370	39	5	4
Italian Sausage & Peppers	1 pkg (10.5 oz)	340	43	10	7
Lasagna	1 pkg (10.5 oz)	290	39	11	6
Macaroni & Cheese	1 pkg (10.5 oz)	350	47	6	5
Pasta Primavera	1 pkg (10.5 oz)	320	40	13	7
Spaghetti w/ Meatballs	1 pkg (10.5 oz)	370	40	10	6
Vegetable Lasagna	1 pkg (10.5 oz)	260	41	10	7
White Cheddar & Rotini	1 pkg (10.5 oz)	350	48	5	6
Senor Felix's					
Lasagna Southwestern	1 serv (6 oz)	160	15	4	2
Stouffer's					
Cheddar Pasta w/ Beef & Tomatoes	1 pkg (11 oz)	450	45	7	3
Cheese Manicotti	1 pkg (9 oz)	380	38	10	4
Cheese Ravioli	1 pkg (10.6 oz)	380	51	11	6
Chicken Lasagna	1 serv (7.8 oz)	320	29	5	4
Fettucini Alfredo	1 pkg (10 oz)	520	17	5	4
Fettucini Primavera	1 pkg (10 oz)	430	49	6	5
Five Cheese Lasagna	1 pkg (10.75 oz)	360	40	10	6
Grilled Chicken & Angel Hair Pasta	1 pkg (10.9 oz)	380	40	6	5
Homestyle Chicken Fettucini	1 pkg (10.5 oz)	390	32	8	3
Homestyle Chicken Parmigiana w/ Spaghetti	1 pkg (12 oz)	460	54	9	5

FOOD	PORTION	CALS.	CARB.	SUG.	FIB.
Stouffer's (CONT.)					
Homestyle Veal Parmigiana w/ Spaghetti	1 pkg (11.9 oz)	430	49	10	6
Lasagna Bake	1 pkg (10.25 oz)	370	47	9	6
Lasagna w/ Meat Sauce	1 pkg (10.5 oz)	370	39	6	4
Macaroni & Cheese	1 cup (6 oz)	320	31	5	3
Macaroni & Cheese w/ Broccoli	1 pkg (10.5 oz)	360	37	7	5
Macaroni & Beef	1 pkg (11.5 oz)	420	40	12	5
Noodles Romanoff	1 pkg (12 oz)	490	48	7	4
Pasta Shells w/ American Cheese	1 cup (6 oz)	260	31	8	2
Salisbury Steak w/ Macaroni & Cheese	1 serv (11.3 oz)	410	34	4	2
Spaghetti w/ Meat Sauce	1 pkg (10 oz)	350	46	7	5
Spaghetti w/ Meatballs	1 pkg (12.6 oz)	440	56	8	5
Tuna Noodle Casserole	1 pkg (10 oz)	320	37	7	0
Turkey Tettrazini	1 pkg (10 oz)	360	33	5	1
Vegetable Lasagna	1 pkg (10.5 oz)	440	43	9	5
Swanson					
Homestyle Lasagne With Meat Sauce	10½ oz	400	39	—	—
Homestyle Macaroni & Cheese	10 oz	390	37	—	—
Homestyle Spaghetti With Italian Style Meatballs	13 oz	490	60	—	—
Macaroni & Cheese	12¼ oz	370	48	—	—
Macaroni & Cheese	7 oz	200	24	—	—
Spaghetti & Meatballs	12½ oz	390	46	—	—
Tabatchnick					
Macaroni & Cheese	7.5 oz	280	30	1	2
Tyson					
Parmigiana	1 pkg (11.25 oz)	380	37	—	—
Ultra Slim-Fast					
Pasta Primavera	12 oz	340	52	—	5
Spaghetti With Beef & Mushroom Sauce	12 oz	370	49	—	0
Weight Watchers					
Smart Ones Angel Hair Pasta	1 pkg (9 oz)	170	29	5	4
Smart Ones Bowtie Pasta & Mushrooms Marsala	1 pkg (9.65 oz)	280	36	3	5
Smart Ones Chicken Fettucini	1 pkg (10 oz)	290	39	3	4

FOOD	PORTION	CALS.	CARB.	SUG.	FIB.
Weight Watchers (CONT.)					
Smart Ones Creamy Rigatoni w/ Broccoli & Chicken	1 pkg (9 oz)	230	40	5	4
Smart Ones Fettucini Alfredo w/ Broccoli	1 pkg (8.5 oz)	230	34	8	3
Smart Ones Lasagna Florentine	1 pkg (10 oz)	200	34	5	5
Smart Ones Lasagna Alfredo	1 pkg (9 oz)	300	45	3	2
Smart Ones Lasagna w/ Meat Sauce	1 pkg (9 oz)	240	43	5	4
Smart Ones Lasagna w/ Meat Sauce	1 pkg (10.25 oz)	270	38	6	6
Smart Ones Macaroni & Cheese	1 pkg (9 oz)	220	42	5	4
Smart Ones Pasta & Spinach Romano	1 pkg (10.4 oz)	240	32	10	4
Smart Ones Pasta w/ Tomato Basil Sauce	1 pkg (9.6 oz)	260	33	3	5
Smart Ones Penne Pasta w/ Sun-Dried Tomatoes	1 pkg (10 oz)	290	41	2	4
Smart Ones Penne Pollo	1 pkg (10 oz)	290	40	8	3
Smart Ones Ravioli Florentine	1 pkg (8.5 oz)	220	43	5	4
Smart Ones Spaghetti Marinara	1 pkg (9 oz)	280	46	3	5
Smart Ones Spaghetti w/ Meat Sauce	1 pkg (10 oz)	290	41	8	4
Smart Ones Spicy Penne & Ricotta	1 pkg (10.2 oz)	280	45	5	5
Smart Ones Tuna Noodle Casserole	1 pkg (9.5 oz)	270	39	7	4
Smart Ones Zita Mozzarella	1 pkg (9 oz)	280	45	2	4
HOME RECIPE					
macaroni & cheese	1 cup	430	40	—	—
spaghetti w/ meatballs & tomato sauce	1 cup	330	39	—	—
MIX					
Casbah					
Pasta Fasul	1 pkg (1.6 oz)	150	10	0	2
Golden Grain					
Macaroni & Cheese	½ cup	310	36	—	—

FOOD	PORTION	CALS.	CARB.	SUG.	FIB.
Hain					
Pasta & Sauce Creamy Parmesan	¼ pkg	150	22	—	—
Pasta & Sauce Creamy Swiss	¼ pkg	170	26	—	—
Pasta & Sauce Fettuccine Alfredo	¼ pkg	180	27	—	—
Pasta & Sauce Italian Herb	¼ pkg	110	17	—	—
Pasta & Sauce Primavera	¼ pkg	140	20	—	—
Pasta & Sauce Tangy Cheddar	¼ pkg	180	24	—	—
Kraft					
Deluxe Macaroni & Cheese Four Cheese Blend as prep	1 cup (6.2 oz)	320	44	4	1
Deluxe Macaroni & Cheese Original as prep	1 cup (6.1 oz)	320	44	4	1
Light Deluxe Macaroni & Cheese as prep	1 cup (6.5 oz)	290	48	7	1
Macaroni & Cheese All Shapes as prep	1 cup (6.9 oz)	410	49	8	1
Macaroni & Cheese Original as prep	1 cup (6.9 oz)	410	49	8	1
Macaroni & Cheese Original as prep light recipe	1 cup (6.4 oz)	290	48	8	2
Premium Macaroni & Cheese Cheesy Alfredo as prep	1 cup (6.9 oz)	410	49	8	2
Premium Macaroni & Cheese Mild White Cheddar as prep	1 cup (6.8 oz)	410	49	8	1
Premium Macaroni & Cheese Thick 'N Creamy as prep	1 cup (7.6 oz)	420	50	9	2
Premium Macaroni & Cheese Three Cheese as prep	1 cup (6.9 oz)	410	49	8	2
Spaghetti Classics Mild Italian as prep	1 cup (9.1 oz)	240	46	9	3
Spaghetti Classics Tangy Italian as prep	1 cup (8.9 oz)	240	46	7	3
Spaghetti Classics Zesty Cheese as prep	1 cup (8.6 oz)	240	46	9	3

FOOD	PORTION	CALS.	CARB.	SUG.	FIB.
Kraft (CONT.)					
Spaghetti Classics w/ Meat Sauce as prep	1 cup (8.2 oz)	330	47	7	3
Lipton					
Pasta & Sauce Angel Hair Chicken Broccoli as prep	1 cup	260	43	2	2
Pasta & Sauce Angel Hair Parmesan as prep	1 cup	280	41	3	2
Pasta & Sauce Bow Tie Chicken Primavera as prep	1 cup	290	43	6	2
Pasta & Sauce Bow Tie Italian Cheese as prep	1 cup	300	41	4	tr
Pasta & Sauce Butter & Herbs as prep	1 cup	270	40	3	2
Pasta & Sauce Cheddar Broccoli as prep	1 cup	340	49	7	1
Pasta & Sauce Chicken Herb Parmesan as prep	1 cup	80	43	3	2
Pasta & Sauce Chicken Stir-Fry as prep	1 cup	270	43	3	2
Pasta & Sauce Creamy Garlic as prep	1 cup	350	50	6	1
Pasta & Sauce Creamy Mushroom as prep	1 cup	320	46	4	0
Pasta & Sauce Garlic & Butter Linguine as prep	1 cup	260	40	3	2
Pasta & Sauce Mild Cheddar Cheese as prep	1 cup	290	41	4	tr
Pasta & Sauce Roasted Garlic Chicken as prep	1 cup	290	43	3	tr
Pasta & Sauce Roasted Garlic & Olive Oil w/ Tomato as prep	1 cup	270	42	3	2
Pasta & Sauce Rotini Primavera as prep	1 cup	320	45	4	2
Pasta & Sauce Savory Herb w/ Garlic as prep	1 cup	280	52	3	2
Pasta & Sauce Three Cheese Rotini as prep	1 cup	320	44	5	tr
Melting Pot					
Terrazza Black Beans & Penne	1 cup	180	36	5	2
Terrazza Florentine Red Beans & Fusilli	1 cup	220	43	6	2

FOOD	PORTION	CALS.	CARB.	SUG.	FIB.
Melting Pot (CONT.)					
Terrazza Red Lentils & Bow Ties	1 cup	240	42	7	5
Terrazza Tuscan White Beans & Gemell	1 cup	220	44	6	3
Nile Spice					
Pasta'n Sauce Mediterranean	1 pkg	210	33	tr	2
Pasta'n Sauce Parmesan	1 pkg	200	36	3	1
Pasta'n Sauce Primavera	1 pkg	200	34	1	2
Ultra Slim-Fast					
Macaroni & Cheese	2.3 oz	230	46	—	4
Uncle Ben					
Country Inn Pasta & Sauce Angel Hair Parmesan	1 serv (2.2 oz)	245	39	—	3
Country Inn Pasta & Sauce Broccoli & White Cheddar	1 serv (2.2 oz)	240	40	—	2
Country Inn Pasta & Sauce Butter & Herb	1 serv (2 oz)	230	36	—	1
Country Inn Pasta & Sauce Creamy Garlic	1 serv (2.4 oz)	261	45	—	2
Country Inn Pasta & Sauce Fettuccine Alfredo	1 serv (2.2 oz)	310	41	—	2
Country Inn Pasta & Sauce Herb Linguine	1 serv (2.2 oz)	240	43	—	2
Country Inn Pasta & Sauce Mushroom Fettuccine	1 serv (2.2 oz)	250	41	—	2
Country Inn Pasta & Sauce Vegetable Alfredo	1 serv (2.2 oz)	240	42	—	2
Velveeta					
Rotini & Cheese w/ Broccoli as prep	1 cup (7.2 oz)	400	47	5	2
Shells & Cheese Bacon as prep	1 cup (6.8 oz)	360	43	4	1
Shells & Cheese Original as prep	1 cup (6.6 oz)	360	44	4	1
Shells & Cheese Salsa as prep	1 cup (7.5 oz)	380	47	5	2
SHELF-STABLE					
Chef Boyardee					
Microwave Main Meal Beans & Pasta	10.5 oz	200	44	—	10
Microwave Main Meal Beef Ravioli Suprema	10.5 oz	290	52	—	5

FOOD	PORTION	CALS.	CARB.	SUG.	FIB.
Chef Boyardee (CONT.)					
Microwave Main Meal Cheese Ravioli Suprema	10.5 oz	290	52	—	5
Microwave Main Meal Fettuccine	10.5 oz	290	46	—	6
Microwave Main Meal Lasagna	10.5 oz	290	41	—	5
Microwave Main Meal Meat Tortellini	10.5 oz	220	53	—	6
Microwave Main Meal Noodles w/ Chicken	10.5 oz	170	27	—	3
Microwave Main Meal Peas & Pasta	10.5 oz	190	39	—	6
Microwave Main Meal Spaghetti Suprema	10.5 oz	200	37	—	7
Microwave Main Meal Zesty Macaroni	10.5 oz	290	40	—	5
Microwave Main Meal Ziti In Sauce	10.5 oz	210	52	—	7
Hormel					
Microcup Meals Lasagna	1 cup (7.5 oz)	250	24	6	1
Microcup Meals Macaroni & Cheese	1 cup (7.5 oz)	260	30	3	1
Microcup Meals Ravioli w/ Tomato Sauce	1 cup (7.5 oz)	220	34	12	2
Microcup Meals Spaghetti & Meatballs	1 cup (7.5 oz)	220	28	10	1
Kid's Kitchen					
Microwave Meals Beefy Macaroni	1 cup (7.5 oz)	190	23	4	2
Microwave Meals Macaroni & Cheese	1 cup (7.5 oz)	260	30	3	1
Microwave Meals Mini Ravioli	1 cup (7.5 oz)	240	34	6	1
Microwave Meals Spaghetti & Meatballs	1 cup (7.5 oz)	220	28	10	1
Microwave Meals Spaghetti Ring & Meatballs	1 cup (7.5 oz)	250	35	12	3
Lunch Bucket					
Elbows In Tomato Sauce	1 pkg (7.5 oz)	190	38	—	—
Lasagna With Meatsauce	1 pkg (7.5 oz)	220	38	—	—
Light'n Healthy Italian Style Pasta	1 pkg (7.5 oz)	130	23	—	—
Light'n Healthy Pasta In Wine Sauce	1 pkg (7.5 oz)	130	21	—	—

FOOD	PORTION	CALS.	CARB.	SUG.	FIB.
Lunch Bucket (CONT.)					
Light'n Healthy Pasta'n Garden Vegetables	1 pkg (7.5 oz)	150	30	—	—
Macaroni'n Cheese	1 pkg (7.5 oz)	210	24	—	—
Pasta'n Chicken	1 pkg (7.5 oz)	180	22	—	—
Spaghetti'n Meatsauce	1 pkg (7.5 oz)	240	39	—	—
My Own Meal					
Cheese Tortellini	1 pkg (10 oz)	340	49	6	6

PASTA MACHINE MIX
Wanda's

FOOD	PORTION	CALS.	CARB.	SUG.	FIB.
Dried Tomato	⅓ cup mix per serv (1.9 oz)	202	42	0	1
Durum & Semolina	⅓ cup mix per serv (1.9 oz)	199	42	0	1
Semolina Blend	⅓ cup mix per serv (1.9 oz)	202	42	0	1
Spinach	⅓ cup mix per serv (1.9 oz)	202	42	0	1
Whole Wheat & Semolina	⅓ cup mix per serv (1.9 oz)	198	41	0	4

PASTA SALAD
MIX
Kraft

FOOD	PORTION	CALS.	CARB.	SUG.	FIB.
Herb & Garlic as prep	¾ cup (4.9 oz)	280	34	5	2
Pasta Salad Classic Ranch w/ Bacon as prep	¾ cup (4.7 oz)	350	32	3	2
Pasta Salad Creamy Ceasar as prep	¾ cup (4.8 oz)	340	31	5	2
Pasta Salad Garden Primavera as prep	¾ cup (5 oz)	240	35	3	2
Pasta Salad Italian 97% Fat Free as prep	¾ cup (4.9 oz)	190	3534	5	2
Pasta Salad Parmesan Peppercorn as prep	¾ cup (4.9 oz)	360	29	3	2
Suddenly Salad					
Classic Pasta Low Fat Recipe as prep	¾ cup	180	34	3	1
Classic Pasta as prep	¾ cup	220	34	3	1
Garden Italian 98% Fat Free as prep	¾ cup	140	29	4	2

PASTRY
(*see* BROWNIE, CAKE, DANISH PASTRY)

PATE

FOOD	PORTION	CALS.	CARB.	SUG.	FIB.
antipasto pate	1 can (2.25 oz)	110	3	1	1

FOOD	PORTION	CALS.	CARB.	SUG.	FIB.
chicken liver canned	1 tbsp (13 g)	109	1	—	—
chicken liver canned	1 oz	238	2	—	—
duck pate	1 oz	96	1	tr	—
fish pate	1 oz	76	1	—	—
goose liver smoked canned	1 oz	131	1	—	—
goose liver smoked canned	1 tbsp (13 g)	60	1	—	—
liver canned	1 oz	90	tr	—	—
liver canned	1 tbsp (13 g)	41	tr	—	—
mushroom anchovy pate	1 can (2.25 oz)	130	7	1	1
pate foie gras	1 oz	127	1	—	—
pork pate	1 oz	107	1	1	0
pork pate en croute	1 oz	91	3	tr	tr
rabbit pate	1 oz	66	1	—	—
salmon pate	1 can (2.25 oz)	140	6	1	0
shrimp	1 can (2.25 oz)	140	7	1	0
smoked turkey	1 can (2.25 oz)	170	7	1	0
Sells					
Liver	2.08 oz	190	4	—	—

PEACH
CANNED

FOOD	PORTION	CALS.	CARB.	SUG.	FIB.
halves in heavy syrup	1 half	60	16	—	—
halves in light syrup	1 half	44	12	—	—
halves juice pack	1 half	34	9	—	—
halves water pack	1 half	18	5	—	—
spiced in heavy syrup	1 fruit	66	18	—	—
spiced in heavy syrup	1 cup	180	49	—	—
Del Monte					
Halves Cling In Heavy Syrup	½ cup (4.5 oz)	100	24	23	1
Halves Cling Lite	½ cup (4.4 oz)	60	15	14	1
Halves Cling Melba In Heavy Syrup	½ cup (4.5 oz)	100	24	23	1
Halves Freestone In Heavy Syrup	½ cup (4.5 oz)	100	24	23	1
Sliced Cling Fruit Naturals	½ cup (4.4 oz)	60	15	14	1
Sliced Cling In Heavy Syrup	½ cup (4.5 oz)	100	24	23	1
Sliced Cling Lite	½ cup (4.4 oz)	60	15	14	1
Sliced Freestone In Heavy Syrup	½ cup (4.5 oz)	100	24	23	1
Sliced Freestone Lite	½ cup (4.4 oz)	60	14	13	1
Snack Cups Diced Fruit Naturals	1 serv (4.5 oz)	60	16	15	1
Snack Cups Diced Fruit Naturals EZ-Open Lid	1 serv (4.2 oz)	60	15	14	1

FOOD	PORTION	CALS.	CARB.	SUG.	FIB.
Del Monte (CONT.)					
Snack Cups Diced In Heavy Syrup	1 serv (4.5 oz)	100	24	23	1
Snack Cups Diced In Heavy Syrup EZ-Open Lid	1 serv (4.2 oz)	90	23	22	1
Snack Cups Diced Lite	1 serv (4.5 oz)	60	16	15	1
Snack Cups Diced Lite EZ-Open Lid	1 serv (4.2 oz)	60	15	14	1
Whole Cling In Heavy Syrup	½ cup (4.2 oz)	100	24	23	tr
Hunt's					
Halves	½ cup (4.5 oz)	100	24	23	1
Slices	½ cup (4.5 oz)	100	24	23	1
Libby					
Halves Yellow Cling Lite	½ cup (4.4 oz)	60	13	12	1
Sliced Yellow Cling Lite	½ cup (4.4 oz)	60	13	12	1
S&W					
Halves Clingstone	½ cup	100	25	—	—
Halves Clingstone Diet	½ cup	30	8	—	—
Halves Clingstone Unsweetened	½ cup	30	8	—	—
Halves Freesstone Diet	½ cup	30	7	—	—
Halves Freestone In Heavy Syrup	½ cup	100	26	—	—
Sliced Clingstone Diet	½ cup	30	8	—	—
Sliced Clingstone Unsweetened	½ cup	30	8	—	—
Sliced Freestone Diet	½ cup	30	7	—	—
Sliced Freestone In Heavy Syrup	½ cup	100	26	—	—
Sliced Yellow Cling Natural Style	½ cup	90	20	—	—
Sliced Yellow Cling Premium In Heavy Syrup	½ cup	100	25	—	—
Whole Yellow Cling Spiced In Heavy Syrup	½ cup	90	23	—	—
Yellow Cling Natural Lite	½ cup	50	13	—	—
DRIED					
halves	1 cup	383	98	—	13
halves	10	311	80	—	11
halves cooked w/ sugar	½ cup	139	36	—	—
halves cooked w/o sugar	½ cup	99	25	—	—
Del Monte					
Sun Dried	⅓ cup (1.4 oz)	90	28	21	5

FOOD	PORTION	CALS.	CARB.	SUG.	FIB.
Sonoma					
Pieces	3-5 pieces (1.4 oz)	120	31	—	1
FRESH					
peach	1	37	10	—	1
sliced	1 cup	73	19	—	—
Dole					
Peach	2	70	19	—	1
FROZEN					
slices sweetened	1 cup	235	60	—	—
Big Valley					
Freestone	⅔ cup (4.9 oz)	50	13	9	1
PEACH JUICE					
nectar	1 cup	134	35	—	—
Goya					
Nectar	6 oz	110	27	—	—
Kern's					
Nectar	6 fl oz	110	26	—	—
Libby					
Nectar	1 can (11.5 fl oz)	210	52	46	—
Mott's					
Fruit Basket Orchard Peach Juice Cocktail as prep	8 fl oz	130	32	29	0
Smucker's					
Juice	8 oz	120	30	—	—
Snapple					
Dixie Peach	10 fl oz	140	39	—	—
PEANUT BUTTER					
chunky	2 tbsp	188	7	—	2
chunky	1 cup	1520	56	—	17
chunky w/o salt	2 tbsp	188	7	—	2
chunky w/o salt	1 cup	1520	56	—	17
smooth	2 tbsp	188	7	—	2
smooth	1 cup	1517	53	—	15
smooth w/o salt	2 tbsp	188	7	—	2
smooth w/o salt	1 cup	1517	53	—	15
Arrowhead					
Creamy	2 tbsp (1.1 oz)	200	6	1	1
Crunchy	2 tbsp (1.1 oz)	200	6	1	1
BAMA					
Creamy	2 tbsp	200	6	—	—
Crunchy	2 tbsp	200	6	—	—
Jelly & Peanut Butter	2 tbsp	150	20	—	—

FOOD	PORTION	CALS.	CARB.	SUG.	FIB.
Crazy Richard's					
Natural Creamy	2 tbsp (1.1 oz)	190	6	2	2
Erewhon					
Chunky	2 tbsp (32 g)	190	7	—	—
Chunky Unsalted	2 tbsp (32 g)	190	7	—	—
Creamy	2 tbsp (32 g)	190	7	—	—
Creamy Unsalted	2 tbsp (32 g)	190	7	—	—
Estee					
Chunky Sodium Free	2 tbsp (1 oz)	190	7	2	2
Chunky Sodium Free Sorbitol Sweetened	2 tbsp (1 oz)	190	7	2	2
Creamy Sodium Free	2 tbsp (1 oz)	190	7	2	2
Creamy Sodium Free Sorbitol Sweetened	2 tbsp (1 oz)	190	7	2	2
Health Valley					
Chunky No Salt	2 tbsp	170	6	—	2
Creamy No Salt	2 tbsp	170	6	—	3
Hollywood					
Creamy	1 tbsp	35	1	—	1
Crunchy	1 tbsp	35	1	—	1
Unsalted	1 tbsp	35	1	—	1
Jif					
Creamy	2 tbsp (1.1 oz)	190	7	3	2
Extra Crunchy	2 tbsp (1.1 oz)	190	7	3	2
Reduced Fat	2 tbsp (1.3 oz)	190	15	4	2
Simply Creamy	2 tbsp (1.1 oz)	190	6	2	2
Simply Extra Crunchy	2 tbsp (1.1 oz)	190	6	2	2
Peter Pan					
Creamy	2 tbsp	190	6	—	2
Creamy Salt Free	2 tbsp	190	5	—	2
Crunchy	2 tbsp	190	6	—	2
Crunchy Salt Free	2 tbsp	190	5	—	2
Red Wing					
Creamy	2 tbsp (1.1 oz)	200	6	3	2
Crunchy	2 tbsp (1.1 oz)	200	6	3	2
Reese's					
Peanut Butter Chips	¼ cup (1.5 oz)	230	19	—	—
Skippy					
Creamy	1 cup (263 g)	1540	38	—	—
Creamy w/ 2 slices white bread	1 sandwich	340	33	—	—
Reduced Fat Creamy	2 tbsp	190	13	3	1
Super Chunk	1 cup (260 g)	1540	36	—	—
Super Chunk	2 tbsp (32 g)	190	4	—	—

FOOD	PORTION	CALS.	CARB.	SUG.	FIB.
Skippy (CONT.)					
Super Chunk w/ slices white bread	1 sandwich	340	32	—	—
Smucker's					
Goober Grape	2 tbsp	180	18	—	—
Honey Sweetened	2 tbsp	200	7	—	—
Natural	2 tbsp	200	6	—	—
Natural No-Salt Added	2 tbsp	200	6	—	—
Tree Of Life					
Creamy	2 tbsp (1 oz)	190	7	—	1
Creamy No Salt	2 tbsp (1 oz)	190	7	—	1
Creamy Organic	2 tbsp (1 oz)	190	7	—	1
Creamy Organic No Salt	2 tbsp (1 oz)	190	7	—	1
Crunchy	2 tbsp (1 oz)	190	7	—	1
Crunchy No Salt	2 tbsp (1 oz)	190	7	—	1
Crunchy Organic	2 tbsp (1 oz)	190	7	—	1
Crunchy Organic No Salt	2 tbsp (1 oz)	190	7	—	1
Peanut Wonder 78% Less Fat	2 tbsp (1 oz)	100	11	7	1

PEANUTS

FOOD	PORTION	CALS.	CARB.	SUG.	FIB.
chocolate coated	10 (1.4 oz)	208	20	—	—
chocolate coated	1 cup (5.2 oz)	773	74	—	—
cooked	½ cup	102	7	—	—
dry roasted	1 cup	855	31	—	12
dry roasted	1 oz	164	6	—	2
oil roasted	1 oz	163	5	—	2
oil roasted	1 cup	837	27	—	13
oil roasted w/o salt	1 cup	837	27	—	13
oil roasted w/o salt	1 oz	163	5	—	2
spanish oil roasted	1 oz	162	5	—	2
spanish oil roasted w/o salt	1 oz	162	5	—	2
unroasted	1 oz	159	5	—	—
valencia oil roasted	1 cup	848	23	—	9
valencia oil roasted	1 oz	165	5	—	2
valencia oil roasted w/o salt	1 oz	165	5	—	2
valencia oil roasted w/o salt	1 cup	848	23	—	9
virginia oil roasted	1 cup	826	28	—	—
virginia oil roasted	1 oz	161	5	—	—
Beer Nuts					
Peanuts	1 pkg (1 oz)	180	7	—	—
Fisher					
Salted-In-Shell shelled	1 oz	170	6	—	—

FOOD	PORTION	CALS.	CARB.	SUG.	FIB.
Fisher (CONT.)					
Spanish Roasted	1 oz	180	6	—	—
Frito Lay					
Dry Roasted	1.2 oz	190	7	—	—
Salted	1 oz	170	6	—	—
Guy's					
Dry Roasted	1 oz	170	3	—	—
Spanish Salted	1 oz	170	3	—	—
Lance					
Honey Toasted	1 pkg (39 g)	230	11	—	—
Roasted w/ Shell	1 pkg (50 g)	190	8	—	—
Salted	1 pkg (32 g)	190	7	—	—
Salted Tube	1 pkg (42 g)	240	9	—	—
Little Debbie					
Salted	1 pkg (1.2 oz)	230	3	1	2
Pennant					
Oil Roasted	1 oz	170	6	1	3
Planters					
Cocktail Lightly Salted Oil Roasted	1 oz	170	5	0	2
Cocktail Oil Roasted	1 oz	170	6	1	3
Cocktail Unsalted Oil Roasted	1 oz	170	6	1	2
Dry Roasted	1 oz	160	6	1	3
Fun Size! Oil Roasted	2 pkg (1 oz)	170	6	1	2
Heat Hot Spicy Oil Roasted	1 pkg (1.7 oz)	290	9	2	4
Heat Hot Spicy Oil Roasted	1 oz	160	5	1	2
Heat Hot Spicy Oil Roasted	1 pkg (2 oz)	330	10	2	5
Heat Mild Spicy Oil Roasted	1 oz	160	5	1	2
Honey Roasted	1 oz	160	8	5	2
Honey Roasted Dry Roasted	1 pkg (1.7 oz)	260	17	11	3
Lightly Salted Dry Roasted	1 oz	160	5	1	3
Lightly Salted Dry Roasted	1 pkg (1.75 oz)	290	9	2	4
Lightly Salted Oil Roasted	1 pkg (1.8 oz)	300	8	2	4
Munch'N Go Singles Heat Hot Spicy Oil Roasted	1 pkg (2.5 oz)	410	13	3	6
Reduced Fat Honey Roasted	⅓ cup (1 oz)	130	12	9	2
Salted Oil Roasted	1 pkg (1 oz)	170	5	1	2
Spanish Oil Roasted	1 oz	170	5	1	2
Spanish Raw	1 oz	150	6	1	3
Sweet N Crunchy	1 oz	140	16	14	2

FOOD	PORTION	CALS.	CARB.	SUG.	FIB.
Planters (CONT.)					
Unsalted Dry Roasted	1 oz	160	6	1	3
Weight Watchers					
Honey Roasted	1 pkg (0.7 oz)	100	7	3	2

PEAR
CANNED

FOOD	PORTION	CALS.	CARB.	SUG.	FIB.
halves in heavy syrup	1 cup	188	49	—	—
halves in heavy syrup	1 half	68	15	—	—
halves in light syrup	1 half	45	12	—	—
halves juice pack	1 cup	123	32	—	—
halves water pack	1 half	22	6	—	—
Del Monte					
Halves Fruit Naturals	½ cup (4.4 oz)	60	15	14	1
Halves In Heavy Syrup	½ cup (4.5 oz)	100	24	33	1
Halves Lite	½ cup (4.4 oz)	60	15	14	1
Sliced In Heavy Syrup	½ cup (4.5 oz)	100	24	23	1
Sliced Lite	½ cup (4.4 oz)	60	15	14	1
Snack Cups Diced In Heavy Syrup	1 serv (4.5 oz)	100	24	23	1
Snack Cups Diced In Heavy Syrup EZ-Open Lid	1 serv (4.2 oz)	90	23	22	1
Snack Cups Diced Lite	1 serv (4.5 oz)	60	15	14	1
Snack Cups Diced Lite EZ-Open Lid	1 serv (4.2 oz)	60	15	14	1
Libby					
Halves Lite	½ cup (4.3 oz)	60	13	12	1
Sliced Lite	½ cup (4.3 oz)	60	13	12	1
S&W					
Halves Bartlett In Heavy Syrup	½ cup	100	25	—	—
Halves Bartlett Peeled Unsweetened	½ cup	35	10	—	—
Halves Peeled Diet	½ cup	35	10	—	—
Quartered Peeled Diet	½ cup	35	10	—	—
Sliced Natural Light Bartlett	½ cup	60	15	—	—
Sliced Natural Style	½ cup	80	20	—	—

DRIED

FOOD	PORTION	CALS.	CARB.	SUG.	FIB.
halves	10	459	122	—	—
halves	1 cup	472	125	—	—
halves cooked w/ sugar	½ cup	196	52	—	—
halves cooked w/o sugar	½ cup	163	43	—	—
Sonoma					
Pieces	3-4 pieces (1.4 oz)	120	33	—	3

FOOD	PORTION	CALS.	CARB.	SUG.	FIB.
FRESH					
asian	1 (4.3 oz)	51	13	—	—
pear	1	98	25	—	4
sliced w/ skin	1 cup	97	25	—	4
Dole					
Pear	1	100	25	—	4
PEAR JUICE					
nectar	1 cup	149	39	—	—
Goya					
Nectar	6 oz	120	29	—	—
Kern's					
Nectar	6 fl oz	120	28	—	—
Libby					
Nectar	1 can (11.5 fl oz)	220	54	45	3
PEAS					
CANNED					
green	½ cup	59	11	—	—
green low sodium	½ cup	59	11	—	—
Allen					
Crowder	½ cup (4.5 oz)	110	19	0	8
Purple Hull	½ cup (4.4 oz)	120	21	tr	6
Crest Top					
Early June	½ cup (4.5 oz)	100	20	1	6
Del Monte					
Sweet	½ cup (4.4 oz)	60	11	6	4
Sweet 50% Less Salt	½ cup (4.4 oz)	60	11	6	4
Sweet No Salt Added	½ cup (4.4 oz)	60	11	6	4
Sweet Very Young	½ cup (4.4 oz)	60	10	5	4
East Texas Fair					
Cream Peas	½ cup (4.4 oz)	120	20	0	5
Crowder	½ cup (4.5 oz)	110	19	0	8
Lady Peas With Snaps	½ cup (4.3 oz)	100	17	tr	4
Peas 'n Pork	½ cup (4.5 oz)	110	19	tr	5
Pepper Peas	½ cup (4.5 oz)	120	22	0	6
Purple Hull	½ cup (4.4 oz)	120	21	tr	6
White Acre	½ cup (4.3 oz)	100	17	tr	5
Green Giant					
Sweet	½ cup (4.3 oz)	60	11	3	4
Sweet 50% Less Sodium	½ cup (4.3 oz)	60	11	2	3
Homefolks					
Crowder	½ cup (4.5 oz)	110	19	0	8
Purple Hull	½ cup (4.4 oz)	120	21	tr	6

FOOD	PORTION	CALS.	CARB.	SUG.	FIB.
LeSueur					
Early Peas	½ cup (4.2 oz)	60	12	4	3
Early Peas 50% Less Sodium	½ cup (4.2 oz)	60	11	3	4
Sweet	½ cup (4.2 oz)	60	12	4	3
Sweet 50% Less Sodium	½ cup (4.2 oz)	60	11	3	4
S&W					
Petit Pois	½ cup	70	12	—	—
Sweet	½ cup	70	12	—	—
Sweet Water Pack	½ cup	40	8	—	—
Veri-Green Sweet	½ cup	70	14	—	—
Seneca					
Natural Pack	½ cup	60	9	—	4
Peas	½ cup	50	9	—	5
Sunshine					
Field Peas	½ cup (4.4 oz)	120	21	tr	6
Lady Peas	½ cup (4.3 oz)	100	17	tr	5
Trappey					
Field Peas With Bacon	½ cup (4.5 oz)	90	15	0	5
Field Peas With Snaps And Bacon	½ cup (4.5 oz)	110	19	0	4
DRIED					
split cooked	1 cup	231	41	—	—
Bascom's					
Yellow Split as prep	½ cup	110	20	1	—
Hurst					
HamBeens Green Split Peas w/ Ham	1 serv	120	21	1	4
FRESH					
green cooked	½ cup	67	13	—	—
green raw	½ cup	58	11	—	—
snap peas cooked	½ cup	34	6	—	2
snap peas raw	½ cup	30	5	—	2
Dole					
Sugar Peas	½ cup	30	5	—	2
FROZEN					
green cooked	½ cup	63	11	—	—
snap peas cooked	½ cup	42	7	—	—
snap peas cooked	1 pkg (10 oz)	132	23	—	—
Birds Eye					
Baby Pea Blend	¾ cup (2.6 oz)	40	7	3	2
Baby Sweet	⅔ cup (3.1 oz)	70	12	6	4
Field Peas w/ Snaps	⅔ cup (3.4 oz)	130	24	1	4
Purple Hull Peas	½ cup (2.8 oz)	110	21	1	4

FOOD	PORTION	CALS.	CARB.	SUG.	FIB.
Chun King					
Snow Pea Pods	½ pkg (3 oz)	35	4	2	2
Fresh Like					
Green	3.5 oz	85	14	—	2
Tiny Green	3.5 oz	63	12	—	1
Green Giant					
Butter Sauce	¾ cup (4 oz)	100	16	4	5
Butter Sauce LeSueur Baby Peas	¾ cup (4 oz)	100	16	4	4
Harvest Fresh LeSueur Baby	⅔ cup (3.2 oz)	70	13	4	4
Harvest Fresh Sugar Snap	⅔ cup (3.2 oz)	50	10	5	3
Harvest Fresh Sweet	⅔ cup (3.3 oz)	60	12	6	4
LaSueur Baby Sweet	⅔ cup (2.8 oz)	60	11	3	5
LaSueur Early June	⅔ cup (2.8 oz)	80	11	3	5
LaSueur Early June w/ Mushrooms	¾ cup (3 oz)	60	10	2	4
Select Sugar Snap	¾ cup (2.8 oz)	35	7	3	3
Sweet	⅔ cup (3.1 oz)	70	13	2	4
Le Seur					
Early In Butter Sauce	½ cup	80	14	—	3
Early Select	½ cup	60	13	—	4
Tree Of Life					
Peas	⅔ cup (3.1 oz)	70	12	6	4
SPROUTS					
raw	½ cup	77	17	—	—
PECANS					
dried	1 oz	190	5	—	2
dry roasted	1 oz	187	6	—	—
dry roasted salted	1 oz	187	6	—	—
halves dried	1 cup	721	20	—	7
oil roasted	1 oz	195	5	—	—
oil roasted salted	1 oz	195	5	—	—
Planters					
Chips	1 pkg (2 oz)	390	9	1	7
Gold Measure Halves	1 pkg (2 oz)	390	9	1	3
Halves	1 oz	190	4	tr	2
Honey Roasted	1 oz	180	9	5	2
Pieces	1 oz	190	4	tr	2
Pieces	1 pkg (2 oz)	390	9	1	3
PECTIN					
powder	1 pkg (1.75 oz)	163	45	—	—
powder	¼ pkg (0.4 oz)	39	11	—	—

FOOD	PORTION	CALS.	CARB.	SUG.	FIB.
Slim Set					
Packet	1 pkg	208	44	—	14
Powder	1 tbsp	3	1	—	tr
Sure Jell					
For Lower Sugar Recipes	¼ tsp (0.7 g)	5	1	1	0
Pectin	¼ tsp (0.9 g)	5	1	1	0
PEPEAO					
pepeao dried	½ cup	36	10	—	—
pepeao raw sliced	1 cup	25	7	—	—
PEPPER					
black	1 tsp	5	1	—	—
cayenne	1 tsp	6	1	—	—
red	1 tsp	6	1	—	—
white	1 tsp	7	2	—	—
Ac'cent					
Lemon	½ tsp	0	0	0	0
Seasoned	½ tsp	0	0	0	0
Lawry's					
Lemon	1 tsp	6	1	—	tr
Watkins					
Black	¼ tbsp (0.5 g)	0	0	0	0
Cajun	¼ tbsp (0.5 g)	0	0	0	0
Cracked Black	¼ tbsp (0.5 g)	0	0	0	0
Dijon	¼ tbsp (0.5 g)	0	0	0	0
Garlic Peppercorn Blend	¼ tbsp (1 g)	0	0	0	0
Herb	¼ tbsp (0.5 g)	0	0	0	0
Italian	¼ tbsp (0.5 g)	0	0	0	0
Lemon	¼ tbsp (1 g)	0	0	0	0
Mexican	¼ tbsp (0.5 g)	0	0	0	0
Red Pepper Flakes	¼ tsp (0.5 oz)	0	0	0	0
Royal Pepper Blend	¼ tbsp (0.5 g)	0	0	0	0
PEPPERS					
CANNED					
chili green	1 cup (5.5 oz)	29	6	—	2
chili green hot chopped	½ cup	17	4	—	—
chili red hot	1 (2.6 oz)	18	4	—	—
chili red hot chopped	½ cup	17	4	—	—
green halves	½ cup	13	3	—	—
jalapeno chopped	½ cup	17	3	—	—
red halves	½ cup	13	3	—	—
Chi-Chi's					
Chilies Diced Green	2 tbsp (1.2 oz)	10	1	0	0

FOOD	PORTION	CALS.	CARB.	SUG.	FIB.
Chi-Chi's (CONT.)					
Chilies Green Whole	¾ pepper (1 oz)	10	1	0	0
Del Monte					
Chilpotle In Spice Sauce	2 tbsp (1.1 oz)	20	4	3	1
Hot Chili	4 (1 oz)	10	3	2	tr
Jalapeno Nacho Pickled Sliced	2 tbsp (1 oz)	5	1	tr	tr
Jalapeno Pickled Sliced	2 tbsp (1.1 oz)	5	1	0	tr
Jalapeno Pickled Whole	2 tbsp (1.1 oz)	5	1	0	tr
Jalapeno Whole	1 (0.7 oz)	3	tr	tr	tr
Hebrew National					
Filet	¼ pepper (1 oz)	9	2	—	—
Hot Cherry	⅓ pepper (1 oz)	11	2	—	—
Red Filet	¼ pepper (1 oz)	9	2	—	—
McIlhenny					
Jalapeno Nacho Slices	12 slices (1.1 oz)	7	1	tr	1
Old El Paso					
Green Chilies Chopped	2 tbsp (1 oz)	5	1	0	1
Green Chilies Whole	1 (1.2 oz)	10	2	0	1
Jalapenos Peeled	3 (1 oz)	10	1	0	1
Jalapenos Pickled	2 (0.9 oz)	5	1	0	0
Jalapenos Slices	2 tbsp (1.1 oz)	15	3	0	1
Progresso					
Cherry (drained)	2 tbsp (0.9 oz)	30	2	1	1
Fried (drained)	2 tbsp (0.9 oz)	60	3	2	1
Hot Cherry	1 (1 oz)	15	0	0	0
Pepper Salad (drained)	2 tbsp (0.9 oz)	25	1	0	1
Roasted	½ piece (1 oz)	10	1	1	0
Tuscan (drained)	3 (1 oz)	10	1	0	1
Rosoff's					
Sweet	¼ pepper (1 oz)	9	2	—	—
Schorr's					
Filet Peppers	1 oz	9	2	—	—
Trappey					
Banana Mild	3 peppers (1 oz)	6	1	tr	1
Banana Sliced Rings	21 slices (1 oz)	6	1	tr	1
Cherry Hot	2 peppers (1 oz)	7	1	tr	1
Cherry Mild	2 peppers (1 oz)	10	2	tr	1
Dulcito Italian Pepperoncini	4 peppers (1 oz)	8	2	tr	1
In Vinegar Hot	15 peppers (1 oz)	9	2	tr	tr
Jalapeno Hot Sliced	21 slices (1 oz)	4	1	tr	1
Jalapeno Whole	2 peppers (1 oz)	11	2	tr	1
Serano	7 peppers (1 oz)	7	1	tr	tr
Tempero Golden Greek Pepperoncini	4 peppers (1 oz)	7	1	tr	1

FOOD	PORTION	CALS.	CARB.	SUG.	FIB.
Trappey (CONT.)					
Torrido Santa Fe Grande	3 peppers (1 oz)	10	2	tr	tr
Vlasic					
Hot Banana Pepper Rings	1 oz	4	1	—	—
Hot Cherry	1 oz	10	2	—	—
Jalapeno Mexican Hot	1 oz	8	2	—	—
Mexican Tiny Hot	1 oz	6	2	—	—
Mild Cherry	1 oz	8	2	—	—
Mild Greek Pepperoncini Salad Peppers	1 oz	4	1	—	—
DRIED					
ancho	1 (0.6 oz)	48	9	—	4
green	1 tbsp	1	tr	—	—
pasilla	1 (7 g)	24	4	—	2
red	1 tbsp	1	tr	—	—
FRESH					
banana raw	1 cup (4.4 oz)	33	7	—	4
banana raw	1 (4 in) (1.2 oz)	9	2	—	1
chili green hot raw	1	18	4	—	—
chili green hot raw chopped	½ cup	30	7	—	—
chili red hot raw	1 (1.6 oz)	18	4	—	—
chili red raw chopped	½ cup	30	7	—	—
green chopped cooked	½ cup	19	5	—	—
green cooked	1 (2.6 oz)	20	5	—	—
green raw	1 (2.6 oz)	20	5	—	1
green raw chopped	½ cup	13	3	—	1
hungarian raw	1 (0.9 oz)	8	2	—	0
jalapeno raw	1 (0.5 oz)	4	1	—	tr
jalapeno raw sliced	1 cup (3.2 oz)	27	5	—	3
red chopped cooked	½ cup	19	5	—	—
red cooked	1 (2.6 oz)	20	5	—	—
red raw	1 (2.6 oz)	20	5	—	1
red raw chopped	½ cup	13	3	—	1
serrano raw	1 (6 g)	2	tr	—	tr
serrano raw chopped	1 cup (3.7 oz)	34	7	4	4
yellow raw	1 (6.5 oz)	50	12	—	—
yellow raw	10 strips	14	3	—	—
Dole					
Medium	1	25	5	—	2
FROZEN					
green chopped not prep	1 oz	6	1	—	—
red chopped	1 oz	6	1	—	—

FOOD	PORTION	CALS.	CARB.	SUG.	FIB.
Birds Eye					
Diced Green	¾ cup (2.9 oz)	20	4	3	2
PERCH					
FRESH					
cooked	3 oz	99	0	0	0
cooked	1 fillet (1.6 oz)	54	0	0	0
ocean perch atlantic cooked	3 oz	103	0	0	0
ocean perch atlantic cooked	1 fillet (1.8 oz)	60	0	0	0
ocean perch atlantic raw	3 oz	80	0	0	0
raw	3 oz	77	0	0	0
red raw	3½ oz	114	0	0	0
FROZEN					
Gorton's					
Fishmarket Fresh Ocean Perch	5 oz	140	2	—	—
Van De Kamp's					
Battered Fillets	2 (4 oz)	300	19	2	0
PERSIMMONS					
dried japanese	1	93	25	—	—
fresh	1	32	8	—	—
fresh japanese	1	118	31	—	—
Sonoma					
Dried	6-8 pieces (1.4 oz)	140	35	26	3
PHEASANT					
breast w/o skin raw	½ breast (6.4 oz)	243	0	0	0
leg w/o skin raw	1 (3.6 oz)	143	0	0	0
roasted	3.5 oz	215	0	0	0
w/ skin raw	½ pheasant (14 oz)	723	0	0	0
w/o skin raw	½ pheasant (12.4 oz)	470	0	0	0
PHYLLO DOUGH					
phyllo dough	1 oz	85	15	—	—
sheet	1	57	10	—	—
Ekizian					
Sheets	½ lb	865	151	3	—
PICANTE					
(*see* SALSA)					
PICKLES					
dill	1 (2.3 oz)	12	3	—	—
dill low sodium	1 (2.3 oz)	12	3	—	1
dill low sodium sliced	1 slice	1	tr	—	tr

FOOD	PORTION	CALS.	CARB.	SUG.	FIB.
dill sliced	1 slice	1	tr	—	tr
gerkins	3½ oz	21	4	—	—
kosher dill	1 (2.3 oz)	12	3	—	1
polish dill	1 (2.3 oz)	12	3	—	1
quick sour	1 (1.2 oz)	4	1	—	—
quick sour low sodium	1 (1.2 oz)	4	1	—	—
quick sour sliced	1 slice	1	tr	—	—
sweet	1 (1.2 oz)	41	11	—	tr
sweet gherkin	1 sm (½ oz)	20	5	—	—
sweet low sodium	1 (1.2 oz)	41	11	—	tr
sweet sliced	1 slice	7	2	—	tr
Del Monte					
Dill Halves	¼ pickle (1 oz)	5	tr	0	tr
Dill Hamburger Chips	5 pieces (1 oz)	5	1	0	0
Dill Sweet Chips	5 pieces (1 oz)	40	10	10	tr
Dill Sweet Gherkin	2 pickles (1 oz)	40	10	10	tr
Dill Sweet Midgets	3 pickles (1 oz)	40	10	10	tr
Dill Sweet Whole	2 pickles (1 oz)	40	10	10	tr
Dill Tiny Kosher	1½ pickle (1 oz)	5	1	0	tr
Dill Whole Pickles	1½ pickle (1 oz)	5	tr	0	tr
Hebrew National					
Half Sour	½ pickle (1 oz)	4	1	—	—
Kosher	⅓ pickle (1 oz)	4	1	—	—
Kosher Barrel Cured Dill	1 pkg	23	4	—	—
Kosher Barrel Cured Hot Dill	1 pkg	23	4	—	—
Kosher Chips	3 slices (1 oz)	4	1	—	—
Kosher Halves	⅓ pickle (1 oz)	4	1	—	—
Kosher Large	⅕ pickle (1 oz)	4	1	—	—
Kosher Spears	½ spear (1 oz)	4	1	—	—
Sour Garlic	⅓ pickle (1 oz)	3	1	—	—
McIlhenny					
Hot N' Sweet	4 (1 oz)	42	10	10	tr
Rosoff's					
Half Sour	⅓ pickle (1 oz)	4	1	—	—
Half Sour Spears	½ spear (1 oz)	4	1	—	—
Kosher	⅓ pickle (1 oz)	4	1	—	—
Kosher Halves	⅓ pickle (1 oz)	4	1	—	—
Schorr's					
Garlic	⅓ pickle (1 oz)	3	1	—	—
Half Sour	½ spear (1 oz)	4	1	—	—
Half Sour	⅓ pickle (1 oz)	4	1	—	—
Kosher Deli	½ pickle (1 oz)	4	1	—	—
Kosher Halves	⅓ pickle (1 oz)	4	1	—	—

FOOD	PORTION	CALS.	CARB.	SUG.	FIB.
Schorr's (CONT.)					
Kosher Spears	½ spear (1 oz)	4	1	—	—
Kosher Whole	⅓ pickle (1 oz)	4	1	—	—
Vlasic					
Bread & Butter Chips	1 oz	30	7	—	—
Bread & Butter Chunks	1 oz	25	6	—	—
Bread & Butter Stixs	1 oz	18	5	—	—
Deli Bread & Butter	1 oz	25	6	—	—
Deli Dill Halves	1 oz	4	1	—	—
Half-The-Salt Hamburger Dill Chips	1 oz	2	1	—	—
Half-The-Salt Kosher Crunchy Dills	1 oz	4	1	—	—
Half-The-Salt Kosher Dill Spears	1 oz	4	1	—	—
Half-The-Salt Sweet Butter Chips	1 oz	30	7	—	—
Hot & Spicy Garden Mix	1 oz	4	1	—	—
Kosher Baby Dills	1 oz	4	1	—	—
Kosher Crunchy Dills	1 oz	4	1	—	—
Kosher Dill Gherkins	1 oz	4	1	—	—
Kosher Dill Spears	1 oz	4	1	—	—
Kosher Snack Chunks	1 oz	4	1	—	—
No Garlic Dill Spears	1 oz	4	1	—	—
Original Dills	1 oz	2	1	—	—
Polish Snack Chunk Dills	1 oz	4	1	—	—
Zesty Crunchy Dills	1 oz	4	1	—	—
Zesty Dill Snack Chunks	1 oz	4	1	—	—
Zesty Dill Spears	1 oz	4	1	—	—

PIE
(*see also* PIE CRUST)
CANNED FILLING

FOOD	PORTION	CALS.	CARB.	SUG.	FIB.
apple	⅛ can (2.6 oz)	74	19	18	1
apple	1 can (21 oz)	599	156	143	6
cherry	⅛ can (2.6 oz)	85	22	—	—
cherry	1 can (21 oz)	683	175	—	—
pumpkin pie mix	1 cup	282	71	—	—
Libby					
Pumpkin Pie Mix	½ cup	100	25	22	2
None Such					
Mincemeat Condensed	¼ pkg	220	50	—	—
Mincemeat Ready-to-Use	⅓ cup	200	48	—	—
Mincemeat Ready-to-Use With Brandy & Rum	⅓ cup	220	48	—	—

FOOD	PORTION	CALS.	CARB.	SUG.	FIB.
S&W					
Mincemeat Old Fashioned	½ cup	206	49	—	—
FROZEN					
apple	⅛ of 9 in pie (4.4 oz)	297	43	—	2
blueberry	⅛ of 9 in pie (4.4 oz)	289	44	—	—
cherry	⅛ of 9 in pie (4.4 oz)	325	50	—	1
chocolate creme	⅙ of 8 in pie (4 oz)	344	38	—	—
coconut creme	⅙ of 7 in pie (2.2 oz)	191	24	—	1
lemon meringue	⅙ of 8 in pie (4.5 oz)	303	53	—	1
peach	⅙ of 8 in pie (4.1 oz)	261	39	—	—
Amy's Organic					
Apple	1 serv (8 oz)	280	42	—	—
Banquet					
Apple	⅕ pie (4 oz)	300	41	22	2
Banana Cream	⅓ pie (4.7 oz)	350	39	28	1
Cherry	⅕ pie (4 oz)	290	39	14	2
Chocolate Cream	⅓ pie (4.7 oz)	360	43	33	3
Coconut Cream	⅓ pie (4.7 oz)	350	39	30	2
Lemon Cream	⅓ pie (4.7 oz)	360	43	31	2
Mincemeat	⅕ pie (4 oz)	310	46	26	2
Peach	⅕ pie (4 oz)	260	36	17	2
Pumpkin	⅙ pie (4 oz)	250	40	21	3
Kineret					
Apple Homestyle	⅙ pie (4 oz)	313	41	20	1
McMillin's					
Apple	4 oz	430	51	—	—
Berry	4 oz	430	52	—	—
Cherry	4 oz	430	51	—	—
Chocolate Pudding	4 oz	420	54	—	—
Coconut Pudding	4 oz	450	50	—	—
Lemon	4 oz	450	52	—	—
Peach	4 oz	430	52	—	—
Strawberry	4 oz	400	50	—	—
Mrs. Smith's					
Apple	⅛ of 9 in pie (4.6 oz)	370	50	27	2
Apple	⅒ of 10 in pie (4.6 oz)	280	43	22	1

FOOD	PORTION	CALS.	CARB.	SUG.	FIB.
Mrs. Smith's (CONT.)					
Apple	1/6 of 8 in pie (4.3 oz)	270	41	20	1
Apple Cranberry	1/6 of 8 in pie (4.3 oz)	280	43	22	1
Apple Lattice Ready To Serve	1/5 of 8 in pie (4.6 oz)	310	45	23	2
Banana Cream	1/4 of 8 in pie (3.4 oz)	250	40	28	1
Berry	1/6 of 8 in pie (4.3 oz)	280	44	22	0
Blackberry	1/6 of 8 in pie (4.3 oz)	280	43	21	1
Blueberry	1/6 of 8 in pie	260	39	17	1
Boston Cream	1/8 of 8 in pie (2.4 oz)	170	29	19	0
Cherry	1/6 of 8 in pie	270	41	19	1
Cherry	1/8 of 9 in pie (4.6 oz)	320	48	24	1
Cherry Lattice Ready To Serve	1/5 of 8 in pie (4.6 oz)	320	47	22	1
Chocolate Cream	1/4 of 8 in pie (3.4 oz)	290	37	25	1
Coconut Cream	1/4 of 8 in pie (3.4 oz)	280	36	25	0
Coconut Custard	1/5 of 8 in pie (5 oz)	280	35	18	0
Dutch Apple	1/10 of 10 in pie (4.6 oz)	320	50	23	1
Dutch Apple	1/6 of 8 in pie	310	48	21	1
Dutch Apple	1/9 of 9 in pie (4.5 oz)	300	48	27	2
French Silk Cream	1/5 of 8 in pie (4.8 oz)	410	55	42	1
Hearty Pumpkin	1/5 of 8 in pie (5.2 oz)	280	46	26	2
Lemon Cream	1/4 of 8 in pie (3.4 oz)	270	36	25	0
Lemon Meringue	1/5 of 8 in pie (4.8 oz)	300	54	37	0
Mince	1/6 of 8 in pie (4.3 oz)	300	48	23	2
Peach	1/6 of 8 in pie	260	38	17	1
Peach	1/8 of 9 in pie (4.6 oz)	310	46	25	1

FOOD	PORTION	CALS.	CARB.	SUG.	FIB.
Mrs. Smith's (CONT.)					
Pecan	⅛ of 10 in pie (4.5 oz)	500	68	40	1
Pumpkin	⅑ of 10 in pie (5.1 oz)	250	42	24	1
Pumpkin	⅕ of 8 in pie (5.2 oz)	270	44	24	1
Red Raspberry	⅙ of 8 in pie (4.3 oz)	280	43	21	0
Strawberry Rhubarb	⅕ of 8 in pie (4.8 oz)	520	73	45	1
Strawberry Rhubarb	⅙ of 8 in pie (4.3 oz)	280	44	22	0
Pepperidge Farm					
Hyannis Boston Cream Pie	1	230	34	—	2
Mississippi Mud	1	310	23	—	—
Pet-Ritz					
Apple	⅙ pie (4.33 oz)	330	53	—	—
Banana Cream	⅙ pie (2.33 oz)	170	22	—	—
Blueberry	⅙ pie (4.33 oz)	370	50	—	—
Cherry	⅙ pie (4.33 oz)	300	48	—	—
Chocolate Cream	⅙ pie (2.33 oz)	190	27	—	—
Coconut Cream	⅙ pie (2.33 oz)	190	27	—	—
Egg Custard	⅙ pie (4.0 oz)	200	28	—	—
Lemon Cream	⅙ pie (2.33 oz)	190	26	—	—
Mince	⅙ pie (4.33 oz)	280	48	—	—
Neapolitan Cream	⅙ pie (2.33 oz)	180	17	—	—
Peach	⅙ pie (4.33 oz)	320	51	—	—
Pumpkin Custard	⅙ pie (4.33 oz)	250	39	—	—
Strawberry Cream	⅙ pie (2.33 oz)	170	20	—	—
Sweet Potato	⅙ pie (3.33 oz)	150	21	—	—
Sara Lee					
Chocolate Silk	⅕ pie (4.8 oz)	500	49	35	2
Coconut Cream	⅕ pie (4.8 oz)	480	47	35	2
Fruit's Of The Forest	⅛ pie (4.6 oz)	340	40	15	3
Homestyle Apple	⅛ pie (4.6 oz)	340	46	26	1
Homestyle Blueberry	⅛ pie (4.6 oz)	360	54	26	2
Homestyle Cherry	⅛ pie (4.6 oz)	330	46	27	2
Homestyle Dutch Apple	⅛ pie (4.6 oz)	350	53	30	2
Homestyle Mince	⅛ pie (4.6 oz)	390	56	30	3
Homestyle Peach	⅛ pie (4.6 oz)	330	50	30	2
Homestyle Pecan	⅛ pie (4.2 oz)	520	70	28	3
Homestyle Pumpkin	⅛ pie (4.6 oz)	260	37	18	2
Homestyle Raspberry	⅛ pie (4.6 oz)	380	48	20	2

FOOD	PORTION	CALS.	CARB.	SUG.	FIB.
Sara Lee (CONT.)					
Lemon Meringue	⅙ pie (5 oz)	350	59	42	5
Slice Lemon Icebox	1 (3.5 oz)	260	41	37	2
Slice Southern Pecan	1 (4 oz)	470	62	31	2
Weight Watchers					
Mississippi Mud	1 piece (2.45 oz)	160	24	13	5
HOME RECIPE					
pecan	⅛ of 9 in pie (4.3 oz)	502	64	—	4
pumpkin	⅛ of 9 in pie (5.4 oz)	316	41	—	4
MIX					
banana cream no-bake	⅛ of 9 in pie (3.2 oz)	231	29	—	—
chocolate mousse no-bake	⅛ of 9 in pie (3.3 oz)	247	28	—	—
coconut creme no-bake	⅛ of 9 in pie (3.3 oz)	259	27	—	—
Betty Crocker					
Boston Cream Classic Dessert	⅛ pie	270	50	—	—
Jell-O					
No Bake Chocolate Silk as prep	⅙ pie (4.4 oz)	320	37	20	tr
Royal					
Key Lime Pie Filling	mix for 1 serv	50	13	—	—
Lemon Pie Filling	mix for 1 serv	50	13	—	0
Lemon Meringue No-Bake	⅛ pie	210	38	—	—
READY-TO-EAT					
Entenmann's					
Apple Homestyle	1 serv (2.1 oz)	140	21	—	—
Coconut Custard	1 serv (1.8 oz)	140	16	—	—
SNACK					
apple	1 (3 oz)	266	33	—	—
apple fried	1 (6.4 oz)	404	55	—	3
blueberry fried	1 (6.4 oz)	404	55	—	3
cherry	1 (3 oz)	266	33	—	—
cherry fried	1 (6.4 oz)	404	55	—	3
lemon	1 (3 oz)	266	33	—	—
lemon fried	1 (6.4 oz)	404	55	—	3
peach fried	1 (6.4 oz)	404	55	—	3
strawberry fried	1 (6.4 oz)	404	55	—	3
Drake's					
Apple	1 (2 oz)	210	29	—	—

FOOD	PORTION	CALS.	CARB.	SUG.	FIB.
Drake's (CONT.)					
Blueberry	1 (2 oz)	210	30	—	—
Cherry	1 (2 oz)	220	30	—	—
Lemon	1 (2 oz)	210	27	—	—
Lance					
Pecan	1 (38 g)	350	51	—	—
Little Debbie					
Marshmallow Banana	1 pkg (1.4 oz)	160	27	17	0
Marshmallow Banana	1 pkg (2.7 oz)	320	54	33	0
Marshmallow Banana	1 pkg (2 oz)	240	40	25	0
Marshmallow Chocolate	1 pkg (1.4 oz)	160	27	16	1
Marshmallow Chocolate	1 pkg (2 oz)	240	40	24	1
Marshmallow Chocolate	1 pkg (2.7 oz)	320	53	32	1
Oatmeal Creme	1 pkg (1.3 oz)	170	25	16	1
Oatmeal Creme	1 pkg (3 oz)	360	58	36	2
Oatmeal Creme	1 pkg (2.5 oz)	300	48	30	1
Raisin Creme	1 pkg (1.2 oz)	140	23	16	1
Raisin Creme	1 pkg (2.5 oz)	290	47	32	0
Tastykake					
Apple	1 pkg (113 g)	300	46	—	2
Banana Creme	1 pkg (120 g)	380	54	—	2
Blueberry	1 pkg (113 g)	310	55	—	2
Cherry	1 pkg (113 g)	300	49	—	2
Coconut Creme	1 pkg (113 g)	380	46	—	2
French Apple	1 pkg (120 g)	350	63	—	2
Lemon	1 pkg (113 g)	320	48	—	2
Lemon Lime	1 pkg (113 g)	320	49	—	1
Peach	1 pkg (113 g)	300	47	—	—
Pineapple Cheese	1 pkg (120 g)	340	54	—	2
Pumpkin	1 pkg (4 oz)	320	46	—	2
Strawberry	1 pkg (113 g)	340	57	—	1
Tasty Klair	1 pkg (113 g)	400	51	—	2
PIE CRUST					
(*see also* PIE)					
FROZEN					
baked	⅛ of 9 in pie (0.6 oz)	82	8	—	—
baked	9 in shell (4.4 oz)	647	63	—	—
puff pastry baked	1 shell (1.4 oz)	223	18	—	—
Oronoque					
Deep Dish	⅙ pie (1.41 oz)	200	16	—	—
Pie Crust	⅙ pie (1.23 oz)	170	14	—	—
Pepperidge Farm					
Patty Shells	1	210	16	—	—

FOOD	PORTION	CALS.	CARB.	SUG.	FIB.
Pepperidge Farm (CONT.)					
Puff Pastry Sheets	¼ sheet	260	22	—	—
Pet-Ritz					
Deep Dish	⅙ pie (1 oz)	130	12	—	—
Graham Cracker	⅙ pie (0.83 oz)	110	8	—	—
Regular	⅙ pie (0.83 oz)	110	11	—	—
Tart Shells	1	150	12	—	—
HOME RECIPE					
9-inch crust	1	900	79	—	—
baked	9 in shell (6.3 oz)	949	86	—	—
baked	⅛ of 9 in crust (0.8 oz)	119	11	—	—
MIX					
as prep	9 in crust (5.6 oz)	801	81	—	—
as prep	⅛ of 9 in pie (0.7 oz)	100	10	—	—
Betty Crocker					
Pie Crust	1/16 pkg	120	10	—	—
Sticks	1/16 pkg	120	10	—	—
Flako					
Mix	¼ cup (0.9 oz)	130	13	0	1
Jiffy					
As prep	1/7 crust	180	19	0	tr
Pillsbury					
Mix	⅙ of 2 crust pie	270	25	—	—
Stick	⅙ of a 2 crust pie	270	25	—	—
READY-TO-EAT					
chocolate cookie crumb baked	⅛ of 9 in pie (1 oz)	139	15	—	—
chocolate cookie crumb baked	9 in crust (7.7 oz)	1130	122	—	—
chocolate cookie crumb chilled	9 in crust (7.8 oz)	1127	121	—	—
chocolate cookie crumb chilled	⅛ of 9 in pie (1 oz)	142	15	—	—
graham cracker baked	⅛ of 9 in pie (1 oz)	148	20	—	—
graham cracker baked	9 in crust (8.4 oz)	1181	156	—	—
graham cracker chilled	⅛ of 9 in pie (1 oz)	150	20	—	—
graham cracker chilled	9 in crust (8.6 oz)	1182	155	—	—
vanilla wafer cracker crumbs baked	9 in crust (6.1 oz)	937	89	—	—
vanilla wafer cracker crumbs baked	⅛ of 9 in pie (0.8 oz)	119	11	—	—
vanilla wafer cracker crumbs chilled	⅛ of 9 in pie (0.8 oz)	117	11	—	—

FOOD	PORTION	CALS.	CARB.	SUG.	FIB.
vanilla wafer cracker crumbs chilled	9 in crust (6.2 oz)	934	88	—	—
Generic Label					
Graham	⅛ pie (0.7 oz)	110	14	6	1
Honey Maid					
Graham	⅙ crust (1 oz)	140	18	8	tr
Nabisco					
Nilla	⅙ crust (1 oz)	140	18	11	0
Oreo					
Crumb Crust	⅙ crust (1 oz)	140	18	9	tr
Ready Crust					
Chocolate	1 (3 in diam)	110	15	—	—
Chocolate	⅛ pie 9 in	100	14	—	—
Graham	⅛ pie 9 in	100	13	—	—
Graham	1 (3 in diam)	110	15	—	—
REFRIGERATED					
Pillsbury					
All Ready	⅛ of 2 crust pie	240	24	—	—

PIEROGI

FOOD	PORTION	CALS.	CARB.	SUG.	FIB.
pierogi	¾ cup (4.4 oz)	307	24	—	—
Empire					
Potato Cheese	3 (4.6 oz)	260	40	6	5
Potato Onion	3 (4.6 oz)	250	43	9	4
Golden					
Potato Cheese	3 (4 oz)	250	38	—	—
Potato Onion	3 (4 oz)	210	36	—	—
Mrs. T's					
Potato And Cheddar Cheese	1 (1.3 oz)	60	11	—	—
Potato And Onion	1 (1.3 oz)	50	10	—	—

PIG'S EARS AND FEET

FOOD	PORTION	CALS.	CARB.	SUG.	FIB.
ear simmered	1	184	tr	—	0
feet pickled	1 oz	58	tr	—	0
feet pickled	1 lb	921	tr	—	0
feet simmered	3 oz	165	0	0	0
Hormel					
Pickled Feet	2 oz	80	0	0	0
Pickled Hocks	2 oz	110	0	0	0

PIGEON

FOOD	PORTION	CALS.	CARB.	SUG.	FIB.
w/ skin & bone	3.5 oz	169	0	0	0

PIGEON PEAS

FOOD	PORTION	CALS.	CARB.	SUG.	FIB.
dried cooked	½ cup	102	20	—	—
dried cooked	1 cup	204	39	—	—

FOOD	PORTION	CALS.	CARB.	SUG.	FIB.
PIGNOLIA					
(*see* PINE NUTS)					
PIKE					
northern cooked	3 oz	96	0	0	0
northern cooked	½ fillet (5.4 oz)	176	0	0	0
northern raw	3 oz	75	0	0	0
roe raw	3½ oz	130	2	—	—
walleye baked	3 oz	101	0	0	0
walleye fillet baked	4.4 oz	147	0	0	0
PILLNUTS					
pillnuts- canarytree dried	1 oz	204	1	—	—
PIMIENTOS					
canned	1 tbsp	3	1	—	—
canned	1 slice	0	tr	—	—
Dromedary					
Pimientos	1 oz	10	2	—	—
PINE NUTS					
pignolia dried	1 tbsp	51	1	—	—
pignolia dried	1 oz	146	4	—	—
pinyon dried	1 oz	161	5	—	—
Progresso					
Pignoli	1 jar (1 oz)	170	2	0	0
PINEAPPLE					
CANNED					
chunks in heavy syrup	1 cup	199	52	—	—
chunks juice pack	1 cup	150	39	—	—
crushed in heavy syrup	1 cup	199	52	—	—
slices in heavy syrup	1 slice	45	12	—	—
slices in light syrup	1 slice	30	8	—	—
slices juice pack	1 slice	35	9	—	—
slices water pack	1 slice	19	5	—	—
tidbits in heavy syrup	1 cup	199	52	—	—
tidbits in juice	1 cup	150	19	—	—
tidbits in water	1 cup	79	20	—	—
Del Monte					
Chunks In Heavy Syrup	½ cup (4.3 oz)	90	24	22	1
Chunks In Its Own Juice	½ cup (4.4 oz)	70	17	15	1
Crushed In Heavy Syrup	½ cup (4.4 oz)	90	24	22	1
Crushed In Its Own Juice	½ cup (4.3 oz)	70	17	15	1
Sliced In Heavy Syrup	½ cup (4.1 oz)	90	23	21	1
Sliced In Its Own Juice	½ cup (4 oz)	60	16	14	1

FOOD	PORTION	CALS.	CARB.	SUG.	FIB.
Del Monte (CONT.)					
Snack Cups Tidbits In Juice	1 serv (4.5 oz)	70	18	16	1
Snack Cups Tidbits In Juice EZ-Open Lid	1 serv (4.2 oz)	60	17	15	1
Spears In Its Own Juice	½ cup (4.3 oz)	70	17	15	1
Tidbits In Its Own Juice	½ cup (4.3 oz)	70	17	15	1
Wedges In Its Own Juice	½ cup (4.3 oz)	70	17	15	1
Dole					
All Cuts Juice Pack	½ cup	70	18	—	—
All Cuts Syrup Pack	½ cup	90	23	—	—
Empress					
Chunk	4 oz	70	18	—	—
Crushed	4 oz	70	18	—	—
Sliced	4 oz	70	18	—	—
Libby					
Crushed	1 cup with juice	140	35	—	—
Sliced In Unsweetened Juice	1 cup with juice	140	35	—	—
S&W					
Hawaiian Slice In Heavy Syrup	½ cup	90	23	—	—
Hawaiian Slice Juice Pack	½ cup	70	17	—	—
Sliced Unsweetened	½ cup	60	15	—	—
DRIED					
Sonoma					
Pieces	2 pieces (1.4 oz)	140	30	26	2
FRESH					
diced	1 cup	77	19	—	2
slice	1 slice	42	10	—	1
Dole					
Pineapple	2 slices	90	21	—	2
FROZEN					
chunks sweetened	½ cup	104	27	—	—
PINEAPPLE JUICE					
canned	1 cup	39	34	—	—
frzn as prep	1 cup	129	32	—	—
frzn not prep	6 oz	387	96	—	—
After The Fall					
Mandarin Pineapple	1 can (12 oz)	150	37	35	0
Bright & Early					
Frozen	8 fl oz	120	30	29	—
Del Monte					
Juice	1 serv (11.5 oz)	190	45	39	1

FOOD	PORTION	CALS.	CARB.	SUG.	FIB.
Del Monte (CONT.)					
Juice	6 fl oz	80	20	17	0
Juice	8 fl oz	110	26	23	0
Dole					
100% frzn as prep	8 fl oz	130	30	25	0
Chilled	6 fl oz	90	22	—	—
Minute Maid					
Box	8.45 fl oz	130	33	31	—
Frozen	8 fl oz	110	28	28	—
S&W					
Unsweetened	6 oz	100	25	—	—
Tree Top					
Juice	6 oz	100	24	—	—

PINK BEANS
CANNED

Goya					
Spanish Style	7.5 oz	140	32	—	10
DRIED					
cooked	1 cup	252	47	—	—

PINTO BEANS
CANNED

pinto	1 cup	186	35	—	—
Allen					
Pinto Beans	½ cup (4.5 oz)	110	20	1	7
Brown Beauty					
Pinto Beans	½ cup (4.5 oz)	110	20	1	7
Chi-Chi's					
Pinto Beans	½ cup (4.3 oz)	100	18	1	3
East Texas Fair					
Pinto Beans	½ cup (4.5 oz)	110	20	1	7
Eden					
Organic	½ cup (4.6 oz)	100	18	—	6
Organic Spicy w/ Jalapeno & Red Peppers	½ cup (4.6 oz)	125	24	2	7
Gebhardt					
Pinto Beans	4 oz	100	19	—	5
Goya					
Spanish Style	7.5 oz	140	31	—	10
Green Giant					
Pinto Beans	½ cup (4.4 oz)	110	20	2	5
Old El Paso					
Pinto Beans	½ cup (4.6 oz)	110	19	0	7

FOOD	PORTION	CALS.	CARB.	SUG.	FIB.
Progresso					
Pinto Beans	½ cup (4.6 oz)	110	18	0	7
Trappey					
Jalapinto With Bacon	½ cup (4.5 oz)	120	22	3	8
With Bacon	½ cup (4.5 oz)	120	20	tr	7
DRIED					
cooked	1 cup	235	44	—	—
Arrowhead					
Dried	¼ cup (1.5 oz)	150	27	0	8
Hurst					
HamBeens w/ Ham	3 tbsp (1.2 oz)	120	20	1	6
FROZEN					
cooked	3 oz	152	29	—	—
SPROUTS					
cooked	3½ oz	22	4	—	—
raw	3½ oz	62	12	—	—

PINYON
(*see* PINE NUTS)

PISTACHIOS

FOOD	PORTION	CALS.	CARB.	SUG.	FIB.
dried	1 oz	164	7	—	3
dried	1 cup	739	32	—	14
dry roasted	1 oz	172	8	—	—
dry roasted salted	1 oz	172	8	—	—
dry roasted salted	1 cup	776	35	—	—
Dole					
Shelled	1 oz	163	7	—	—
Shells On	1 oz	90	3	—	—
Fisher					
Red Tint	1 oz	170	6	—	—
Lance					
Pistachios	1 pkg (32 g)	100	4	—	—
Planters					
Munch'N Go Singles Shelled Dry Roasted	1 pkg (2 oz)	330	14	4	6
Red Salted Dry Roasted	1 pkg	160	7	2	3
Uncolored Dry Roasted	½ cup	160	7	2	3
Sonoma					
Salted Shelled	¼ cup (1 oz)	190	9	3	3

PITANGA

FOOD	PORTION	CALS.	CARB.	SUG.	FIB.
fresh	1 cup	57	13	—	—
fresh	1	2	1	—	—

FOOD	PORTION	CALS.	CARB.	SUG.	FIB.
PIZZA					
DOUGH					
Boboli					
Shell + Sauce	⅛ lg shell (2.6 oz)	170	28	2	1
Shell + Sauce	⅙ sm shell (2.6 oz)	170	29	2	1
House of Pasta					
Frozen	⅛ of 14 in pie (1.9 oz)	140	27	1	1
Jiffy					
As prep	¼ crust	180	33	2	2
Sassafras					
Cornmeal Pizza Crust	1 slice (1.4 oz)	140	30	1	1
Italian Pizza Crust Mix	1 slice (1.4 oz)	140	30	1	1
Wanda's					
Crust Mix Oregano & Basil	⅒ pie (1.4 oz)	149	32	4	1
Crust Mix Oregano & Basil Whole Wheat	⅒ pie (1.4 oz)	141	30	4	5
Watkins					
Crust Mix	⅛ pkg (1.8 oz)	180	36	5	2
FROZEN					
Amy's Organic					
Cheese	1 (13 oz)	310	39	5	2
Pocket Sandwich Cheese Pizza	1 (4.5 oz)	290	38	4	3
Pocket Sandwich Veggie Pepperoni Pizza	1 (4.5 oz)	220	28	5	3
Roasted Vegetable	1 (12 oz)	270	43	5	3
Spinach	1 (14 oz)	320	40	5	2
Celeste					
Italian Bread Deluxe	1 (5.1 oz)	290	36	—	3
Italian Bread Garlic & Herb Zesty Chicken	1 (5 oz)	260	34	—	3
Italian Bread Pepperoni	1 (5 oz)	320	37	—	3
Italian Bread Zesty Four Cheese	1 (4.6 oz)	300	32	—	3
Large Cheese	¼ pie (4.4 oz)	320	32	—	3
Large Deluxe	¼ pie (5.5 oz)	350	35	—	4
Large Pepperoni	¼ pie (4.7 oz)	350	33	—	3
Large Suprema With Meat	⅕ pie (4.6 oz)	290	27	—	3
Large Zesty Four Cheese	¼ pie (4.4 oz)	330	34	—	3
Small Cheese	1 (7.5 oz)	540	60	—	4
Small Deluxe	1 (8.2 oz)	540	53	—	6
Small Hot & Zesty Four Cheese	1 (7 oz)	530	50	—	4

FOOD	PORTION	CALS.	CARB.	SUG.	FIB.
Celeste (CONT.)					
Small Original Four Cheese	1 (7 oz)	540	47	—	4
Small Pepperoni	1 (6.7 oz)	520	53	—	4
Small Sausage	1 (7.5 oz)	530	52	—	5
Small Suprema Vegetable	1 (7.5 oz)	480	52	—	5
Small Suprema With Meat	1 (9 oz)	580	56	—	7
Small Zesty Four Cheese	1 (7 oz)	530	50	—	4
Croissant Pocket					
Stuffed Sandwich Pepperoni Pizza	1 piece (4.5 oz)	350	39	7	3
Di Giorno					
Rising Crust 12 inch Four Cheese	⅙ pie (4.9 oz)	320	39	6	3
Rising Crust 12 inch Italian Sausage	⅙ pie (5.3 oz)	360	40	6	3
Rising Crust 12 inch Pepperoni	⅙ pie (5.2 oz)	370	40	6	3
Rising Crust 12 inch Supreme	⅙ pie (5.8 oz)	380	40	7	3
Rising Crust 12 inch Three Meat	⅙ pie (5.4 oz)	380	40	6	3
Rising Crust 12 inch Vegetable	⅙ pie (5.6 oz)	310	41	7	3
Rising Crust 8 inch Chicken Supreme	⅓ pie (4.8 oz)	270	33	5	2
Rising Crust 8 inch Four Cheese	⅓ pie (4 oz)	260	33	5	2
Rising Crust 8 inch Italian Sausage	⅓ pie (4.4 oz)	300	33	5	2
Rising Crust 8 inch Pepperoni	⅓ pie (4.2 oz)	300	33	5	2
Rising Crust 8 inch Spinach	⅓ pie (4.3 oz)	250	33	5	3
Rising Crust 8 inch Supreme	⅓ pie (4.7 oz)	310	34	5	2
Rising Crust 8 inch Three Meat	⅓ pie (4.4 oz)	310	34	5	2
Rising Crust 8 inch Vegetable	⅓ pie (4.6 oz)	250	33	6	2
Empire					
3 Pack	1 (3 oz)	210	23	1	7
Bagel	1 (2 oz)	150	15	1	0
English Muffin	1 (2 oz)	130	15	2	1
Pizza	½ pie (5 oz)	340	38	3	2
Fox					
Deluxe Golden Topping	½ pizza	240	25	—	—

FOOD	PORTION	CALS.	CARB.	SUG.	FIB.
Fox (CONT.)					
Deluxe Hamburger	½ pizza	260	26	—	—
Deluxe Pepperoni	½ pizza	250	26	—	—
Deluxe Sausage	½ pizza	260	26	—	—
Deluxe Sausage & Pepperoni	½ pizza	260	26	—	—
Healthy Choice					
French Bread Cheese	1 (5.6 oz)	310	49	3	6
French Bread Pepperoni	1 (6 oz)	360	48	1	5
French Bread Sausage	1 (6 oz)	330	52	5	6
French Bread Supreme	1 (6.35 oz)	340	49	4	5
Hot Pocket					
Stuffed Sandwich Pepperoni & Sausage Pizza	1 (4.5 oz)	340	38	7	3
Stuffed Sandwich Pepperoni Pizza	1 (4.5 oz)	350	38	5	2
Jack's					
Great Combinations 12 inch Bacon Cheeseburger	¼ pie (4.7 oz)	360	31	4	2
Great Combinations 12 inch Double Cheese	¼ pie (4.9 oz)	380	32	5	2
Great Combinations 12 inch Pepperoni	¼ pie (5.2 oz)	410	42	5	3
Great Combinations 12 inch Pepperoni & Mushrooms	¼ pie (4.8 oz)	340	32	5	2
Great Combinations 12 inch Sausage	¼ pie (5.4 oz)	390	40	5	3
Great Combinations 12 inch Sausage & Mushroom	¼ pie (4.9 oz)	310	29	5	3
Great Combinations 12 inch Sausage & Pepperoni	¼ pie (4.8 oz)	350	29	4	2
Great Combinations 12 inch Supreme	¼ pie (5.2 oz)	350	30	3	5
Great Combinations 9 inch Double Cheese	½ pie (5.5 oz)	430	38	5	3
Great Combinations 9 inch Pepperoni & Sausage	½ pie (5.1 oz)	380	36	5	3
Naturally Rising 12 inch Bacon Cheeseburger	⅙ pie (5 oz)	350	35	7	2

FOOD	PORTION	CALS.	CARB.	SUG.	FIB.
Jack's (CONT.)					
Naturally Rising 12 inch Canadian Bacon	⅙ pie (4.9 oz)	280	34	7	2
Naturally Rising 12 inch Cheese	⅙ pie (4.5 oz)	290	35	7	2
Naturally Rising 12 inch Combination w/ Sausage & Pepperoni	⅙ pie (5.2 oz)	360	34	7	2
Naturally Rising 12 inch Pepperoni	⅙ pie (4.9 oz)	350	35	7	2
Naturally Rising 12 inch Pepperoni Supreme	⅙ pie (5.1 oz)	340	34	11	2
Naturally Rising 12 inch Sausage	⅙ pie (5.1 oz)	340	34	7	2
Naturally Rising 12 inch Spicy Italian Sausage	⅙ pie (5.1 oz)	330	34	11	2
Naturally Rising 12 inch The Works	⅙ pie (5.3 oz)	330	34	7	2
Naturally Rising 9 inch Cheese	⅓ pie (4.7 oz)	300	38	7	2
Naturally Rising 9 inch Combination w/ Sausage & Pepperoni	¼ pie (4.2 oz)	300	29	5	2
Naturally Rising 9 inch Pepperoni	⅓ pie (5.2 oz)	360	38	7	2
Naturally Rising 9 inch Sausage	⅓ pie (5.4 oz)	360	38	7	2
Naturally Rising 9 inch The Works	¼ pie (4.5 oz)	280	29	6	2
Original 12 inch Canadian Bacon	¼ pie (4.4 oz)	280	31	5	2
Original 12 inch Cheese	⅓ pie (5 oz)	360	41	6	3
Original 12 inch Hamburger	¼ pie (4.4 oz)	300	28	4	2
Original 12 inch Pepperoni	¼ pie (4.3 oz)	330	31	4	2
Original 12 inch Sausage	¼ pie (4.3 oz)	300	28	4	2
Original 12 inch Spicy Italian Sausage	¼ pie (4.3 oz)	290	29	5	2
Original 9 inch Pepperoni	½ pie (5 oz)	380	37	5	3
Original 9 inch Sausage	½ pie (5.1 oz)	360	36	5	3
Pizza Bursts Combination Sausage & Pepperoni	6 pieces (3 oz)	250	26	3	2
Pizza Bursts Pepperoni	6 pieces (3 oz)	260	25	3	2
Pizza Bursts Sausage	6 pieces (3 oz)	250	25	3	2
Pizza Bursts Supercheese	6 pieces (3 oz)	250	25	3	2

FOOD	PORTION	CALS.	CARB.	SUG.	FIB.
Jack's (CONT.)					
Pizza Bursts Supreme	6 pieces (3 oz)	250	26	3	2
Jeno's					
4-Pack Cheese	1 pizza	160	17	—	—
4-Pack Combination	1 pizza	180	17	—	—
4-Pack Hamburger	1 pizza	180	17	—	—
4-Pack Pepperoni	1 pizza	170	17	—	—
4-Pack Sausage	1 pizza	180	17	—	—
Crisp 'n Tasty Canandian Bacon	½ pizza	250	27	—	—
Crisp 'n Tasty Cheese	½ pizza	270	28	—	—
Crisp 'n Tasty Hamburger	½ pizza	290	28	—	—
Crisp 'n Tasty Pepperoni	½ pizza	280	27	—	—
Crisp 'n Tasty Sausage	½ pizza	300	28	—	—
Crisp 'n Tasty Sausage & Pepperoni	½ pizza	300	27	—	—
Microwave Pizza Rolls Pepperoni & Cheese	6	240	23	—	—
Microwave Pizza Rolls Sausage & Cheese	6	250	24	—	—
Pizza Rolls Cheese	6	240	23	—	—
Pizza Rolls Hamburger	6	240	21	—	—
Pizza Rolls Pepperoni & Cheese	6	230	22	—	—
Pizza Rolls Sausage & Pepperoni	6	230	22	—	—
Kid Cuisine					
Cheese	1 (8 oz)	430	71	34	5
Hamburger	1 (8.30 oz)	400	61	28	6
Kineret					
Bagel Pizza	2 (4 oz)	300	39	2	1
Slice	1 (4.9 oz)	490	93	2	2
Lean Cuisine					
French Bread Cheese	1 pkg (6 oz)	300	49	6	4
French Bread Deluxe	1 pkg (6.1 oz)	300	46	5	4
French Bread Pepperoni	1 pkg (5.25 oz)	310	46	5	3
Lean Pockets					
Stuffed Sandwich Pizza Deluxe	1 (4.5 oz)	270	37	7	2
MicroMagic					
Deep Dish Combination	1 (6.5 oz)	605	60	—	—
Deep Dish Pepperoni	1 (6.5 oz)	615	65	—	—
Deep Dish Sausage	1 (6.5 oz)	590	62	—	—

FOOD	PORTION	CALS.	CARB.	SUG.	FIB.
Mrs. P's					
Combination	½ pizza	260	26	—	—
Golden Topping	½ pizza	240	25	—	—
Hamburger	½ pizza	260	26	—	—
Pepperoni	½ pizza	250	26	—	—
Sausage	½ pizza	260	26	—	—
Old El Paso					
Pizza Burrito Cheese	1 (3.5 oz)	320	27	3	0
Pizza Burrito Pepperoni	1 (3.5 oz)	260	31	3	0
Pizza Burrito Sausage	1 (3.5 oz)	260	32	2	0
Pappalo's					
French Bread Cheese	1 pizza	360	40	—	—
French Bread Combination	1 pizza	430	41	—	—
French Bread Pepperoni	1 pizza	410	41	—	—
French Bread Sausage	1 pizza	410	41	—	—
Pan Combination	⅙ pizza	340	34	—	—
Pan Hamburger	⅙ pizza	310	34	—	—
Pan Pepperoni	⅙ pizza	330	34	—	—
Pan Sausage	⅙ pizza	360	34	—	—
Thin Crust Combination	⅙ pizza	260	29	—	—
Thin Crust Hamburger	⅙ pizza	240	28	—	—
Thin Crust Pepperoni	⅙ pizza	270	28	—	—
Thin Crust Sausage	⅙ pizza	250	28	—	—
Pepperidge Farm					
Croissant Pastry Cheese	1	430	41	—	—
Croissant Pastry Deluxe	1	440	43	—	—
Croissant Pastry Pepperoni	1	420	43	—	—
Pillsbury					
Microwave Cheese	½ pizza	240	28	—	—
Microwave Combination	½ pizza	310	29	—	—
Microwave French Bread	1 pizza	370	41	—	—
Microwave French Bread Pepperoni	1 pizza	430	46	—	—
Microwave French Bread Sausage	1 pizza	410	48	—	—
Microwave French Bread Sausage & Pepperoni	1 pizza	450	47	—	—
Microwave Pepperoni	½ pizza	300	29	—	—
Microwave Sausage	½ pizza	280	29	—	—
Small World					
Four Cheese	1 (4 oz)	240	38	3	1
Special Delivery					
Organic	⅓ pizza (5.3 oz)	320	46	2	1
Organic Soy Kaas	⅓ pizza (5.3 oz)	320	47	2	1

FOOD	PORTION	CALS.	CARB.	SUG.	FIB.
Stouffer's					
French Bread Bacon Cheddar	1 piece (5.7 oz)	430	46	4	4
French Bread Cheese	1 piece (5.2 oz)	370	43	4	3
French Bread Cheeseburger	1 piece (6 oz)	420	44	3	3
French Bread Deluxe	1 piece (6.2 oz)	430	49	5	3
French Bread Double Cheese	1 piece (5.9 oz)	400	49	4	4
French Bread Pepperoni	1 piece (5.6 oz)	430	46	5	3
French Bread Pepperoni & Mushroom	1 piece (6.1 oz)	440	49	4	5
French Bread Sausage	1 piece (6 oz)	420	48	5	3
French Bread Sausage & Pepperoni	1 piece (6.25 oz)	470	47	4	3
French Bread Three Meat	1 piece (6.25 oz)	460	48	4	5
French Bread Vegetable Deluxe	1 piece (6.4 oz)	380	46	4	4
French Bread White Pizza	1 piece (5.1 oz)	460	45	1	5
Tombstone					
Double Top Pepperoni	1/6 pie (4.5 oz)	340	24	5	2
Double Top Sausage	1/6 pie (4.6 oz)	320	25	6	2
Double Top Sausage & Pepperoni	1/6 pie (4.6 oz)	340	25	5	2
Double Top Supreme	1/6 pie (4.7 oz)	330	25	5	2
Double Top Two Cheese	1/6 pie (5.2 oz)	380	29	6	2
For One 1/2 Less Fat Cheese	1 pie (6.5 oz)	460	43	8	3
For One 1/2 Less Fat Vegetable	1 pie (7.2 oz)	360	48	11	5
For One Extra Cheese	1 pie (6.9 oz)	520	47	8	3
For One Pepperoni	1 pie (6.9 oz)	550	41	8	3
For One Supreme	1 pie (7.5 oz)	550	42	8	3
Light Supreme	1/5 pie (4.8 oz)	270	30	6	3
Light Vegetable	1/5 pie (4.6 oz)	240	31	5	3
Original 12 inch Canadian Bacon	1/4 pie (5.5 oz)	350	36	7	3
Original 12 inch Deluxe	1/5 pie (4.8 oz)	310	29	6	3
Original 12 inch Extra Cheese	1/4 pie (5.1 oz)	350	35	7	3
Original 12 inch Hamburger	1/5 pie (4.4 oz)	310	29	5	2
Original 12 inch Pepperoni	1/4 pie (5.3 oz)	400	35	7	3
Original 12 inch Sausage	1/5 pie (4.4 oz)	300	29	6	2
Original 12 inch Sausage & Mushroom	1/5 pie (4.6 oz)	300	29	6	3
Original 12 inch Sausage & Pepperoni	1/5 pie (4.4 oz)	320	29	6	2

FOOD	PORTION	CALS.	CARB.	SUG.	FIB.
Tombstone (CONT.)					
Original 12 inch Supreme	⅕ pie (5.1 oz)	320	29	6	2
Original 9 inch Deluxe	⅓ pie (4.4 oz)	280	27	5	2
Original 9 inch Extra Cheese	½ pie (5.6 oz)	380	40	8	3
Original 9 inch Hamburger	⅓ pie (4 oz)	280	27	5	2
Original 9 inch Pepperoni	⅓ pie (4 oz)	300	27	5	2
Original 9 inch Pepperoni & Sausage	⅓ pie (4.1 oz)	300	27	5	2
Original 9 inch Sausage	⅓ pie (4 oz)	280	27	5	2
Original 9 inch Supreme	⅓ pie (4.4 oz)	310	27	5	2
Oven Rising Italian Sausage	⅙ pie (5.1 oz)	320	35	12	2
Oven Rising Pepperoni	⅙ pie (4.9 oz)	340	34	7	2
Oven Rising Supreme	⅙ pie (5.1 oz)	320	34	8	2
Oven Rising Three Cheese	⅙ pie (4.8 oz)	320	34	7	2
Oven Rising Three Meat	⅙ pie (5.1 oz)	340	34	7	2
Thin Crust Four Meat Combo	¼ pie (5 oz)	380	26	5	2
Thin Crust Italian Sausage	¼ pie (5 oz)	370	26	5	2
Thin Crust Pepperoni	¼ pie (4.8 oz)	400	25	5	2
Thin Crust Supreme	¼ pie (5 oz)	380	26	5	2
Thin Crust Supreme Taco	¼ pie (5.1 oz)	370	27	5	2
Thin Crust Three Cheese	¼ pie (4.7 oz)	360	25	5	2
Totino's					
Microwave Cheese	1 pizza	250	34	—	—
Microwave Pepperoni	1 pizza	280	34	—	—
Microwave Sausage	1 pizza	320	33	—	—
Microwave Sausage Pepperoni Combination	1 pizza	310	31	—	—
My Classic Deluxe Cheese	⅙ pizza	210	23	—	—
My Classic Deluxe Combination	⅙ pizza	270	23	—	—
My Classic Deluxe Pepperoni	⅙ pizza	260	23	—	—
Pan Pepperoni	⅙ pizza	330	34	—	—
Pan Sausage	⅙ pizza	320	34	—	—
Pan Sausage & Pepperoni Combination	⅙ pizza	340	34	—	—
Pan Three Cheese	⅙ pizza	290	33	—	—
Party Bacon	½ pizza	370	35	—	—
Party Canadian Bacon	½ pizza	310	35	—	—
Party Cheese	½ pizza	340	34	—	—
Party Combination	½ pizza	380	35	—	—

FOOD	PORTION	CALS.	CARB.	SUG.	FIB.
Totino's (CONT.)					
Party Hamburger	½ pizza	370	35	—	—
Party Mexican Style	½ pizza	380	35	—	—
Party Pepperoni	½ pizza	370	35	—	—
Party Sausage	½ pizza	390	35	—	—
Party Vegetable	½ pizza	300	36	—	—
Slices Cheese	1	170	20	—	—
Slices Combination	1	200	20	—	—
Slices Pepperoni	1	190	20	—	—
Slices Sausage	1	200	20	—	—
Weight Watchers					
Smart Ones Deluxe Combo	1 (6.57 oz)	380	47	4	6
Smart Ones Pepperoni	1 (5.56 oz)	390	46	3	4
SAUCE					
Boboli					
Sauce	¼ cup (2.5 oz)	40	9	2	1
Sauce	1 pkg (1.2 oz)	20	4	1	1
Contadina					
Flavored With Pepperoni	¼ cup	40	6	1	1
Pizza Sauce	¼ cup	35	6	1	1
Squeeze	¼ cup	35	6	1	1
With Italian Cheeses	¼ cup	40	6	1	1
Eden					
Pizza Pasta Sauce	½ cup (4.4 oz)	80	12	6	3
Muir Glen					
Organic	¼ cup (2.2 oz)	40	6	3	2
Progresso					
Pizza Sauce	¼ cup (2.2 oz)	35	5	2	1
Ragu					
Quick Traditional	3 tbsp (1.7 oz)	35	3	—	—
Tree Of Life					
Sauce	¼ cup (1.9 oz)	30	5	4	—
PLANTAINS					
fresh uncooked	1 (6.3 oz)	218	57	—	—
sliced cooked	½ cup	89	24	—	—
Chifles					
Plantain Chips	1 pkg (2 oz)	170	17	tr	2
PLUMS					
CANNED					
purple in heavy syrup	3	119	31	—	—
purple in heavy syrup	1 cup	320	60	—	—
purple in light syrup	1 cup	158	41	—	—
purple in light syrup	3	83	22	—	—

FOOD	PORTION	CALS.	CARB.	SUG.	FIB.
purple juice pack	3	55	14	—	—
purple juice pack	1 cup	146	38	—	—
purple water pack	1 cup	102	27	—	—
purple water pack	3	39	10	—	—
S&W					
Halves Purple Fancy Unpeeled In Extra Heavy Syrup	½ cup	135	35	—	—
Whole Purple Fancy Unpeeled In Extra Heavy Syrup	½ cup	135	35	—	—
Whole Unpeeled Diet	½ cup	52	13	—	—
FRESH					
plum	1	36	9	—	—
sliced	1 cup	91	21	—	—
Dole					
Plums	2	70	17	—	1
POI					
poi	½ cup	134	33	—	—
POKEBERRY SHOOTS					
cooked	½ cup	16	3	—	—
raw	½ cup	18	3	—	—
Allen					
Pokeberry Shoots	½ cup (4.1 oz)	35	5	0	3
POLENTA					
(*see* CORNMEAL)					
POLLACK					
altantic fillet baked	5.3 oz	178	0	0	0
atlantic baked	3 oz	100	0	0	0
Mrs. Paul's					
Fillets Light frzn	1 fillet (4.5 oz)	240	18	—	—
POMEGRANATES					
pomegranate	1	104	26	—	—
POMPANO					
florida cooked	3 oz	179	0	0	0
florida raw	3 oz	140	0	0	0
POPCORN					
(*see also* CHIPS, POPCORN CAKES, PRETZELS, SNACKS)					
air-popped	1 cup (0.3 oz)	31	6	—	2
air-popped	1 oz	108	22	—	4
caramel coated	1 oz	122	22	11	1

FOOD	PORTION	CALS.	CARB.	SUG.	FIB.
caramel coated	1 cup (1.2 oz)	152	28	14	2
carmel coated w/ peanuts	⅔ cup (1 oz)	114	23	11	1
cheese	1 cup (0.4 oz)	58	6	—	1
cheese	1 oz	149	15	—	3
oil popped	1 oz	142	16	tr	3
oil popped	1 cup (0.4 oz)	55	6	tr	1
Barrel O' Fun					
Baked Curl	1 oz	150	17	0	0
Caramel Corn	1 oz	115	25	5	1
Corn Pop	1 oz	190	10	0	0
Popcorn	1 oz	160	13	0	1
White Cheddar Pops	1 oz	170	11	0	0
Cheetos					
Cheddar Cheese	0.5 oz	80	6	—	—
Chesters					
Microwave	3 cups	110	13	—	—
Microwave Butter	3 cups	120	13	—	—
Microwave Cheese	3 cups	110	11	—	—
Popcorn	0.5 oz	70	9	—	—
Cracker Jack					
Original	1 oz	120	22	—	—
Estee					
No Sugar Added Caramel	1 cup (1 oz)	120	26	1	1
Greenfield					
Caramel	1 cup (1 oz)	120	22	—	—
Herr's					
Regular	3 cups (1 oz)	140	11	1	3
Jiffy Pop					
Bag Butter	3 cups	90	11	—	2
Bag Lite	3 cups	70	11	—	2
Bag Regular	3 cups	100	11	—	2
Glazed Popcorn Clusters	1 oz	120	25	—	1
Microwave Butter	4 cup	140	17	—	3
Microwave Regular	4 cup	140	17	—	3
Pan Butter	4 cup	130	16	—	2
Pan Regular	4 cup	130	16	—	2
Lance					
Cheese	1 pkg (25 g)	130	13	—	—
Plain	1 pkg (25 g)	140	13	—	—
White Cheddar Cheese	1 pkg (25 g)	140	12	—	—
Louise's					
Fat-Free Apple Cinnamon	1 oz	100	24	17	1
Fat-Free Buttery Toffee	1 oz	100	24	17	1
Fat-Free Caramel	1 oz	100	24	17	1

FOOD	PORTION	CALS.	CARB.	SUG.	FIB.
Newman's Own					
Microwave Butter Flavor	3½ cups	170	16	0	3
Microwave Light Butter	3½ cups	110	20	0	3
Microwave Light Natural	3½ cups	110	20	0	3
Microwave Natural	3½ cups	170	16	0	3
Popcorn unpopped	3 tbsp	110	27	0	7
Orville Redenbacher's					
Gourmet Hot Air	3 cups	40	10	—	3
Gourmet Original	3 cups	80	10	—	3
Gourmet White	3 cups	80	10	—	3
Microwave Gourmet	3 cups	100	11	—	3
Microwave Gourmet Butter	3 cups	100	11	—	3
Microwave Gourmet Butter Toffee	2½ cups	210	26	—	2
Microwave Gourmet Caramel	2½ cups	240	29	—	2
Microwave Gourmet Cheddar Cheese	3 cups	130	14	—	3
Microwave Gourmet Frozen	3 cups	100	11	—	3
Microwave Gourmet Frozen Butter	3 cups	100	11	—	3
Microwave Gourmet Light	3 cups	70	8	—	3
Microwave Gourmet Light Butter	3 cups	70	8	—	3
Microwave Gourmet Salt Free	3 cups	100	11	—	3
Microwave Gourmet Salt Free Butter	3 cups	100	11	—	3
Microwave Gourmet Sour Cream 'n Onion	3 cups	160	12	—	3
Pillsbury					
Microwave Butter	3 cups	210	20	—	—
Microwave Original	3 cups	210	20	—	—
Microwave Salt Free	3 cups	170	23	—	—
Planters					
Fiddle Faddle Caramel Fat Free	1 cup (1 oz)	110	28	16	1
Pop Secret					
Microwave 94% Fat Free Butter	6 cups	110	23	—	4
Microwave Light Butter	6 cups	120	20	—	4
Pop Chips	1½ cups (1 oz)	130	23	3	1
Smartfood					
Cheddar Cheese	0.5 oz	80	7	—	—

FOOD	PORTION	CALS.	CARB.	SUG.	FIB.
Smartfood (CONT.)					
Lowfat Toffee Crunch	¾ cup	110	24	16	1
Reduced Fat White Cheddar	¾ cup	130	17	1	3
Snyder's					
Butter	1 oz	140	13	—	3
Ultra Slim-Fast					
Lite N' Tasty	½ oz	60	10	—	2
Weight Watchers					
Butter	1 pkg (0.66 oz)	90	14	0	3
Butter Toffee	1 pkg (0.9 oz)	110	21	11	1
Caramel	1 pkg (0.9 oz)	100	22	11	1
Microwave	1 pkg (1 oz)	100	22	0	7
White Cheddar Cheese	1 pkg (0.66 oz)	90	12	0	2
Wise					
Tender Eating	0.5 oz	70	4	—	—
With Real Premium White Cheddar Cheese	0.5 oz	70	4	—	—

POPCORN CAKES

FOOD	PORTION	CALS.	CARB.	SUG.	FIB.
popcorn cake	1 (0.3 oz)	38	8	—	—
General Mills					
Popcorn Bars Caramel	1 (0.6 oz)	70	16	11	0
Lundberg					
Organic Lightly Salted	1	60	12	—	—
Organic Unsalted	1	60	12	—	—
Rye With Caraway Lightly Salted	1	59	14	—	—
Mother's					
Butter Flavor	1 (0.3 oz)	35	7	0	0
Unsalted	1 (0.3 oz)	35	7	0	0
Orville Redenbacher's					
Chocolate Peanut Crunch Mini	6 pieces (0.5 oz)	60	12	4	1
Peanut Caramel Crunch	6 (0.5 oz)	60	13	4	1
Quaker					
Blueberry Crunch	1 (0.5 oz)	50	11	—	—
Butter Mini	6 (0.5 oz)	50	11	—	2
Butter Popped	1 (0.3 oz)	35	7	—	—
Caramel	1 (0.5 oz)	50	12	—	—
Caramel Mini	5 (0.5 oz)	50	12	4	1
Cheddar Cheese Mini	6 (0.5 oz)	50	11	1	1
Lightly Salted Mini	7 (0.5 oz)	50	12	—	2
Monterey Jack	1 (0.4 oz)	40	8	—	—
Strawberry Crunch	1 (0.5 oz)	50	11	—	—

FOOD	PORTION	CALS.	CARB.	SUG.	FIB.
Quaker (CONT.)					
White Cheddar	1 (0.4 oz)	40	8	—	—

POPOVER

FOOD	PORTION	CALS.	CARB.	SUG.	FIB.
home recipe as prep w/ 2% milk	1 (1.4 oz)	87	11	—	—
home recipe as prep w/ whole milk	1 (1.4 oz)	90	11	—	—
mix as prep	1 (1.2 oz)	67	10	—	—

POPPY SEEDS

FOOD	PORTION	CALS.	CARB.	SUG.	FIB.
poppy seeds	1 tsp	15	1	—	—

PORK

(*see also* BACON, BACON SUBSTITUTES, CANADIAN BACON, DELI MEATS/COLD CUTS, HAM, PORK DISHES, SAUSAGE)

CANNED

FOOD	PORTION	CALS.	CARB.	SUG.	FIB.
Hormel					
Pickled Tidbits	2 oz	100	0	0	0
FRESH					
boston blade roast lean & fat cooked	3 oz	229	0	0	0
boston blade steak lean & fat cooked	3 oz	220	0	0	0
center loin roast lean bone in cooked	3 oz	169	0	0	0
center loin chop lean bone in cooked	3 oz	172	0	0	0
center rib chop lean & fat bone in cooked	3 oz	213	0	0	0
center rib roast lean & fat bone in cooked	3 oz	217	0	0	0
fresh ham rump lean roasted	3 oz	175	0	0	0
fresh ham rump lean & fat roasted	3 oz	214	0	0	0
fresh ham shank lean roasted	3 oz	183	0	0	0
fresh ham shank lean & fat roasted	3 oz	246	0	0	0
fresh ham whole lean roasted	3 oz	179	0	0	0
fresh ham whole lean roasted diced	1 cup	285	0	0	0
fresh ham whole lean & fat roasted	3 oz	232	0	0	0
fresh ham whole lean & fat roasted diced	1 cup	369	0	0	0

FOOD	PORTION	CALS.	CARB.	SUG.	FIB.
ground cooked	3 oz	252	0	0	0
loin chop lean bone in braised	3 oz	191	0	0	0
loin chop lean bone in broiled	3 oz	199	0	0	0
loin roast lean bone in roasted	3 oz	210	0	0	0
loin whole lean & fat braised	3 oz	203	0	0	0
loin whole lean & fat broiled	3 oz	206	0	0	0
loin whole lean & fat roasted	3 oz	211	0	0	0
lungs braised	3 oz	84	0	0	0
pancreas cooked	3 oz	186	0	0	0
ribs country style lean & fat braised	3 oz	252	0	0	0
shoulder arm picnic lean & fat roasted	3 oz	269	0	0	0
shoulder whole lean & fat roasted	3 oz	248	0	0	0
shoulder whole lean & fat roasted diced	1 cup	394	0	0	0
shoulder whole lean roasted	3 oz	196	0	0	0
shoulder whole lean roasted diced	1 cup	311	0	0	0
sirloin chop lean & fat bone in braised	3 oz	208	0	0	0
sirloin roast lean & fat bone in cooked	3 oz	222	0	0	0
spareribs braised	3 oz	338	0	0	0
spleen braised	3 oz	127	0	0	0
tail simmered	3 oz	336	0	0	0
tenderloin lean roasted	3 oz	139	0	0	0
top loin chop boneless lean & fat cooked	3 oz	198	0	0	0
top loin roast boness lean & fat cooked	3 oz	192	0	0	0
Oscar Mayer					
Sweet Morsel Smoked Boneless Pork Shoulder Butt	3 oz	180	0	0	0

PORK DISHES
Jimmy Dean

| BBQ Pork Rib Sandwich | 1 (5.4 oz) | 440 | 36 | 7 | 1 |

POSOLE
(*see* HOMINY)

POT PIE
Amy's Organic

| Broccoli | 1 (7.5 oz) | 430 | 46 | 3 | 4 |

FOOD	PORTION	CALS.	CARB.	SUG.	FIB.
Amy's Organic (CONT.)					
Country Vegetable	1 (7.5 oz)	370	47	5	4
Shepard's	1 (8 oz)	160	27	5	5
Vegetable	1 (7.5 oz)	360	44	3	4
Vegetable Non-Dairy	1 (7.5 oz)	320	50	3	4
Award Brand					
Beef	1 (7 oz)	350	37	2	3
Chicken	1 (7 oz)	350	39	2	3
Banquet					
Family Entree Chicken Pie	1 serv (8 oz)	450	39	—	6
Macaroni & Cheese	1 pkg (6.5 oz)	200	35	2	2
Vegetable & Cheese	1 (7 oz)	390	49	2	3
Vegetable Pie w/ Beef	1 (7 oz)	330	38	2	3
Vegetable Pie w/ Chicken	1 (7 oz)	350	36	2	3
Vegetable Pie w/ Turkey	1 (7 oz)	370	38	3	3
Empire					
Chicken	1 (8.1 oz)	440	41	1	11
Turkey	1 (8.1 oz)	470	46	2	11
Great Value					
Beef	1 (7 oz)	390	38	6	3
Chicken	1 (7 oz)	380	39	6	2
Turkey	1 (7 oz)	400	42	6	3
Lean Cuisine					
Chicken Pie	1 pkg (9.5 oz)	290	35	15	5
Turkey & Country Vegetable	1 pkg (9.5 oz)	320	40	13	4
Morton					
Beef	1 (7 oz)	310	34	—	2
Chicken	1 (7 oz)	320	32	—	3
Macaroni & Cheese	1 (6 oz)	160	30	2	3
Turkey	1 (7 oz)	300	29	2	2
Ozark Valley					
Chicken	1 (7 oz)	330	32	2	2
Macaroni & Cheese	1 (6.5 oz)	160	29	0	0
Turkey	1 (7 oz)	280	29	2	2
Stouffer's					
Beef Pie	1 pkg (10 oz)	450	36	10	3
Chicken Pie	1 pkg (10 oz)	540	38	11	4
Turkey	1 pkg (10 oz)	530	36	11	3
Swanson					
Beef	7 oz	370	36	—	—
Beef Hungry Man	16 oz	610	58	—	—
Chicken	7 oz	380	35	—	—
Chicken Homestyle	8 oz	410	41	—	—
Hungry Man Chicken	16 oz	630	57	—	—

FOOD	PORTION	CALS.	CARB.	SUG.	FIB.
Swanson (CONT.)					
Hungry Man Turkey	16 oz	650	57	—	—
Turkey	7 oz	380	36	—	—
POTATO					
(*see also* CHIPS, KNISH, PANCAKES)					
CANNED					
potatoes	½ cup	54	12	—	—
Allen					
Refried Potatoes	½ cup (4.5 oz)	150	24	1	11
Butterfield					
Diced	⅔ cup (5.7 oz)	100	22	0	3
Sliced	½ cup (5.7 oz)	100	22	0	4
Whole	2½ pieces (5.6 oz)	90	20	0	2
Del Monte					
New Sliced	⅔ cup (5.4 oz)	60	13	0	2
New Whole	⅔ cup (5.5 oz)	60	13	0	2
Hormel					
Au Gratin & Bacon	1 can (7.5 oz)	250	23	1	2
S&W					
New Potatoes Extra Small	½ cup	45	9	—	—
Seneca					
Potatoes	½ cup	80	15	—	2
Sunshine					
Whole	2½ pieces (5.6 oz)	90	20	0	2
FRESH					
baked skin only	1 skin (2 oz)	115	27	—	2
baked w/ skin	1 (6.5 oz)	220	51	—	—
baked w/o skin	1 (5 oz)	145	34	—	2
baked w/o skin	½ cup	57	13	—	1
boiled	½ cup	68	16	—	1
microwaved	1 (7 oz)	212	49	—	—
microwaved w/o skin	½ cup	78	18	—	—
raw w/o skin	1 (3.9 oz)	88	20	—	—
FROZEN					
french fries	10 strips	111	17	—	2
french fries thick cut	10 strips	109	17	—	—
hashed brown	½ cup	170	22	—	—
potato puffs	½ cup	138	19	—	—
potato puffs as prep	1	16	2	—	—
Birds Eye					
Whole	3 (2.6 oz)	50	13	0	1
Budget Gourmet					
Baked With Broccoli And Cheese	1 pkg (10.5 oz)	300	40	—	—

FOOD	PORTION	CALS.	CARB.	SUG.	FIB.
Budget Gourmet (CONT.)					
Cheddared Potatoes	1 pkg (5.5 oz)	260	22	—	—
Cheddared Potatoes With Broccoli	1 pkg (5 oz)	150	14	—	—
Three Cheese Potatoes	1 pkg (5.75 oz)	220	23	—	—
Empire					
Crinkle Cut French Fries	½ cup (3 oz)	90	18	0	7
Latkes Potato Pancakes	1 (2 oz)	80	15	0	8
Latkes Mini Potato Pancakes	2 (2 oz)	90	16	0	6
Golden					
Potato Pancakes	1 (1.33 oz)	71	10	—	—
Healthy Choice					
Cheddar Broccoli Potatoes	1 meal (10.5 oz)	310	53	8	8
Garden Potato Casserole	1 meal (9.25 oz)	200	30	5	6
Kineret					
Crinkle Cut	18 pieces (3 oz)	120	20	1	2
Kugel	1 piece (2.5 oz)	150	13	1	1
Latkes	1 (1.5 oz)	90	9	1	2
Latkes Mini	10 (3 oz)	160	18	tr	2
Lean Cuisine					
Deluxe Cheddar	1 pkg (10.4 oz)	270	40	7	6
Roasted Potatoes w/ Broccoli & Cheddar Cheese Sauce	1 pkg (10.25 oz)	260	39	7	7
MicroMagic					
French Fries Low Fat	1 pkg (3 oz)	130	23	0	3
Skinny Fries	1 pkg (3 oz)	350	49	—	—
Oh Boy!					
Stuffed With Cheddar Cheese	1 (6 oz)	130	20	—	4
Stuffed With Real Bacon	1 (6 oz)	120	20	—	4
Ore Ida					
Cheddar Browns	1 patty (3 oz)	90	14	1	1
Cottage Fries	14 pieces (3 oz)	130	21	tr	1
Crispers!	17 pieces (3 oz)	220	24	2	2
Crispers! Nacho	10 pieces (3 oz)	170	21	tr	2
Crispers! Texas	3 oz	170	19	3	2
Crispy Crowns!	12 pieces (3 oz)	100	21	tr	2
Crispy Crunchies	12 pieces (3 oz)	160	18	tr	2
Deep Fries Crinkle Cuts	18 pieces (3 oz)	160	23	tr	2
Deep Fries French Fries	22 pieces (3 oz)	160	22	tr	2
Dinner Fries Country Style	8 pieces (3 oz)	110	19	tr	1
Fast Fries	23 pieces (3 oz)	140	20	tr	2

FOOD	PORTION	CALS.	CARB.	SUG.	FIB.
Ore Ida (CONT.)					
Fast Fries Ranch	22 pieces (3 oz)	150	21	tr	1
Golden Crinkles	16 pieces (3 oz)	120	20	tr	2
Golden Fries	16 pieces (3 oz)	120	20	tr	1
Golden Patties	1 (2.5 oz)	140	16	tr	1
Golden Twirls	28 pieces (3 oz)	160	22	tr	2
Hash Browns Country Style	1 cup (2.6 oz)	60	13	tr	1
Hash Browns Shredded	1 patty (3 oz)	70	15	tr	1
Hash Browns Southern Style	¾ cup (3 oz)	70	17	tr	2
Hot Tots	9 pieces (3 oz)	150	21	tr	2
Mashed Natural Butter	½ cup (2.1 oz)	80	14	tr	tr
Microwave Crinkle Cuts	1 pkg (3.5 oz)	180	26	1	2
Microwave Hash Browns	1 patty (2 oz)	110	13	tr	tr
Microwave Tater Tots	1 pkg (3.75 oz)	190	26	tr	2
O'Brien Potatoes	¾ cup (3 oz)	60	13	1	2
Pixie Crinkles	33 pieces (3 oz)	140	21	tr	3
Shoestrings	38 pieces (3 oz)	150	22	tr	2
Snackin' Fries	1 pkg (5 oz)	180	36	3	3
Snackin' Fries Extra Zesty	1 pkg (5 oz)	180	35	tr	4
Tater ABC's	10 pieces (3 oz)	190	20	2	2
Tater Tots	9 pieces (3 oz)	160	21	tr	2
Tater Tots Bacon	9 pieces (3 oz)	150	20	tr	1
Tater Tots Onion	9 pieces (3 oz)	150	20	tr	2
Toaster Hash Browns	2 patties (3.5 oz)	190	21	tr	1
Topped Broccoli & Cheese	½ (6 oz)	150	24	6	4
Topped Salsa & Cheese	½ (5.5 oz)	160	25	6	3
Topped Vegetable Primavera	1 (6.13 oz)	160	23	—	—
Twice Baked Butter	1 (5 oz)	200	27	tr	4
Twice Baked Cheddar Cheese	1 (5 oz)	190	27	tr	3
Twice Baked Ranch	1 (5 oz)	180	27	3	3
Twice Bakes Sour Cream & Chives	1 (5 oz)	180	28	tr	3
Waffle Fries	15 pieces (3 oz)	140	22	tr	2
Wedges With Skin	9 pieces (3 oz)	110	19	tr	2
Zesties!	12 pieces (3 oz)	160	21	3	1
Stouffer's					
Au Gratin	½ cup (5.75 oz)	130	15	3	1
Scalloped	1 serv (5 oz)	140	19	4	2
Scalloped	½ cup (5.75 oz)	140	17	3	2
Weight Watchers					
Smart Ones Baked Broccoli & Cheese	1 pkg (10 oz)	250	35	3	6

FOOD	PORTION	CALS.	CARB.	SUG.	FIB.
HOME RECIPE					
au gratin	½ cup	160	14	—	—
mashed w/ whole milk & margarine	⅓ cup	66	13	—	—
scalloped	½ cup	105	13	—	—
MIX					
au gratin as prep	4½ oz	127	18	—	—
instant mashed flakes as prep w/ whole milk & butter	½ cup	118	16	—	—
instant mashed flakes not prep	½ cup	78	18	—	—
instant mashed granules as prep w/ whole milk & butter	½ cup	114	15	—	—
instant mashed granules not prep	½ cup	372	86	—	—
scalloped as prep	4½ oz	127	18	—	—
Barbara's					
Mashed not prep	⅓ cup (0.8 oz)	70	17	0	1
Betty Crocker					
Au Gratin as prep	½ cup	110	22	1	1
Cheddar & Bacon as prep	½ cup	120	21	2	1
Cheddar & Sour Cream as prep	½ cup	130	25	3	1
Chicken & Vegetable as prep	⅔ cup	140	24	3	1
Chicken & Vegetable as prep	⅔ cup	130	24	3	1
Creamy Garlic as prep	⅔ cup	150	24	3	1
Hash Browns as prep	½ cup	200	31	0	2
Homestyle Broccoli Au Gratin as prep	½ cup	110	21	2	2
Homestyle Broccoli Au Gratin Stove Top Recipe as prep	½ cup	130	21	2	2
Homestyle Cheddar Cheese Stove Top Recipe as prep	½ cup	140	21	2	1
Homestyle Cheddar Cheese as prep	½ cup	120	21	2	1
Homestyle Cheesy Scalloped Stove Top Recipe as prep	½ cup	130	20	3	1
Homestyle Cheesy Scalloped as prep	½ cup	120	20	3	1
Julienne as prep	½ cup	110	20	4	1

FOOD	PORTION	CALS.	CARB.	SUG.	FIB.
Betty Crocker (CONT.)					
Mashed Butter & Herb Reduced Fat Recipe as prep	½ cup	130	20	2	1
Mashed Butter & Herb as prep	½ cup	160	20	2	1
Mashed Potato Buds Reduced Fat Recipe as prep	⅔ cup	120	19	2	1
Mashed Potato Buds Sour Cream 'N Chive as prep	⅔ cup	190	23	2	1
Mashed Potato Buds Sour Cream 'N Chive Reduced Fat as prep	⅔ cup	160	23	2	1
Mashed Potato Buds as prep	⅔ cup	160	19	2	1
Mashed Roasted Garlic Reduced Fat Recipe as prep	½ cup	130	19	2	1
Mashed Roasted Garlic as prep	½ cup	160	19	2	◄
Mashed Sour Cream & Chives Reduced Fat Recipe as prep	½ cup	130	21	2	1
Mashed Sour Cream & Chives as prep	½ cup	160	21	2	1
Potato Shakers Original Low Fat Recipe as prep	⅔ cup	120	23	2	2
Potato Shakers Original as prep	⅔ cup	140	23	2	2
Potato Shakers Parmesan & Herb Low Fat Recipe as prep	⅔ cup	120	23	2	2
Potato Shakers Parmesan & Herb as prep	⅔ cup	140	23	2	2
Potato Shakers Zesty Cheddar Low Fat Recipe as prep	⅔ cup	120	22	2	2
Potato Shakers Zesty Cheddar as prep	⅔ cup	140	22	2	2
Ranch as prep	½ cup	130	25	3	1
Scalloped Potatoes & Ham as prep	½ cup	120	21	2	1

FOOD	PORTION	CALS.	CARB.	SUG.	FIB.
Betty Crocker (CONT.)					
Scalloped as prep	½ cup	130	23	3	1
Smokey Cheddar as prep	½ cup	120	22	2	1
Sour Cream 'n Chive as prep	½ cup	120	22	3	1
Three Cheese as prep	½ cup	120	23	2	1
Twice Baked Cheddar & Bacon Low Fat Recipe as prep	⅔ cup	130	22	6	1
Twice Baked Cheddar & Bacon as prep	⅔ cup	210	22	6	1
White Cheddar as prep	½ cup	120	22	3	1
Country Store					
Mashed not prep	⅓ cup	70	15	—	—
French's					
Cheddar & Bacon Casserole	½ cup	130	18	—	—
Creamy Italian Scalloped	½ cup	120	19	—	—
Creamy Stroganoff	½ cup	130	20	—	—
Crispy Top Scalloped With Savory Onion	½ cup	140	20	—	—
Real Cheese Scalloped	½ cup	140	19	—	—
Real Sour Cream & Chives	½ cup	150	19	—	—
Spuds Mashed	½ cup	140	17	—	—
Tangy Au Gratin	½ cup	130	20	—	—
Hungry Jack					
Au Gratin as prep	½ cup	150	24	3	1
Cheddar & Bacon as prep	½ cup	150	24	3	2
Chessy Scalloped as prep	½ cup	150	24	3	1
Creamy Scalloped as prep	½ cup	150	24	3	2
Mashed Butter Flavored as prep	½ cup	150	19	2	1
Mashed Flakes as prep	½ cup	160	20	2	1
Mashed Garlic Flavored as prep	½ cup	150	19	2	1
Mashed Parsley Butter as prep	½ cup	150	19	2	1
Mashed Sour Cream 'n Chives as prep	½ cup	150	19	2	1
Sour Cream & Chives as prep	½ cup	160	23	3	1
Idaho					
Mashed Potato Flakes as prep	½ cup	150	20	2	1

FOOD	PORTION	CALS.	CARB.	SUG.	FIB.
Idaho (CONT.)					
Mashed Potato Granules as prep	½ cup	160	22	2	2
Shake 'N Bake					
Perfect Potatoes Crispy Cheddar	⅙ pkg (7 g)	30	2	tr	0
Perfect Potatoes Herb & Garlic	⅙ pkg (7 g)	20	5	1	0
Perfect Potatoes Home Fries	⅙ pkg (7 g)	20	5	1	0
Perfect Potatoes Parmesan Peppercorn	⅙ pkg (7 g)	25	3	1	0
Perfect Potatoes Savory Onion	⅙ pkg (7 g)	20	5	1	0
REFRIGERATED					
Simply Potatoes					
Au Gratin	¼ pkg (3 oz)	130	13	—	—
Hash Browns	⅕ pkg (4 oz)	100	23	—	—
Hash Browns Onion	⅕ pkg (4 oz)	120	26	—	—
Hash Browns Southwest Style	⅕ pkg (4 oz)	100	23	—	—
Mashed	⅕ pkg (4 oz)	90	15	—	—
Scalloped	¼ pkg (3 oz)	100	11	—	—
SHELF-STABLE					
Lunch Bucket					
Scalloped	1 pkg (7.5 oz)	160	20	—	—
Micro Cup Meals					
Microcup Meals Scalloped Potatoes w/ Ham	1 cup (7.5 oz)	240	20	1	2
Pantry Express					
Augratin	½ cup	120	17	—	2

POTATO STARCH

FOOD	PORTION	CALS.	CARB.	SUG.	FIB.
potato starch	3½ oz	335	83	—	—
Manischewitz					
Potato Starch	1 cup	570	137	—	—

POUT

FOOD	PORTION	CALS.	CARB.	SUG.	FIB.
ocean baked	3 oz	86	0	0	0
ocean fillet baked	4.8 oz	139	0	0	0

PRESERVE

(*see* JAM/JELLY/PRESERVES)

PRETZELS

(*see also* CHIPS, POPCORN, SNACKS)

FOOD	PORTION	CALS.	CARB.	SUG.	FIB.
chocolate covered	1 (0.4 oz)	50	8	—	—

FOOD	PORTION	CALS.	CARB.	SUG.	FIB.
chocolate covered	1 oz	130	20	—	—
dutch twist	4 (2.1 oz)	229	48	—	2
pretzels	1 oz	108	23	—	1
rods	4 (2 oz)	229	48	—	2
sticks	10	10	2	—	—
sticks	120 (2 oz)	229	48	—	2
twist	1 (½ oz)	65	13	—	—
twists	10 (2.1 oz)	229	48	—	2
whole wheat	2 sm (1 oz)	103	23	—	—
whole wheat	2 med (2 oz)	205	46	—	—
Barrel O' Fun					
Mini	1 oz	110	23	0	1
Sticks	1 oz	110	23	0	1
Twists	1 oz	110	23	0	1
Estee					
Dutch Unsalted	2 (1.1 oz)	130	26	1	1
Nuggets Ranch Reduced Sodium	23 (1 oz)	130	24	1	tr
Nuggets Reduced Sodium	30 (1 oz)	120	24	3	1
Unsalted	23 (1 oz)	120	25	tr	1
Formagg					
Pretzel Nuts	1 oz	120	21	tr	tr
Herr's					
Hard Sourdough	1 (1 oz)	100	23	0	2
J&J					
Soft	1 (2.25 oz)	170	37	—	—
Soft Bites	5 bites	110	23	—	—
Lance					
Twist	1 pkg (42 g)	150	30	—	—
Manischewitz					
Bagel Pretzels Original	4 (1 oz)	110	22	tr	1
Mister Salty					
Chips	16 (1 oz)	110	21	2	tr
Dutch	2 (1.1 oz)	120	25	tr	1
Fat Free Chips	16 (1 oz)	100	22	2	1
Mini	22 (1 oz)	110	22	tr	1
Sticks Fat Free	47 (1 oz)	110	23	tr	1
Twist Fat Free	9 (1 oz)	110	23	1	1
Mr. Phipps					
Chips Lower Sodium	16 (1 oz)	120	21	2	tr
Chips Original	16 (1 oz)	120	21	2	tr
Chips Original Fat Free	16 (1 oz)	100	22	2	tr
Nabisco					
Air Crisps Fat Free	23 pieces (1 oz)	110	23	2	tr

FOOD	PORTION	CALS.	CARB.	SUG.	FIB.
Nestle					
Flipz Milk Chocolate Covered	9 pieces (1 oz)	130	19	10	tr
Flipz White Fudge Covered	9 pieces (1 oz)	130	19	11	0
Newman's Own					
Salted Rounds Organic	1 pkg (1.4 oz)	150	31	2	1
Planters					
Twists	1 oz	100	23	1	1
Twists	1 pkg (1.5 oz)	160	35	2	1
Quinlan					
Beers	1 oz	110	22	1	1
Hard Sourdough	1 oz	110	22	1	1
Logs	1 oz	110	22	1	1
Nuggets	1 oz	110	22	1	1
Rods	1 oz	110	22	1	1
Sticks	1 oz	110	22	1	1
Thins	1 oz	110	22	1	1
Rold Gold					
Bavarian	3 pieces (1 oz)	120	22	—	—
Fat Free Hard Sour Dough	1	80	19	1	1
Fat Free Thins	12 pieces (1 oz)	110	23	1	1
Fat Free Tiny Twists	18 pieces (1 oz)	110	23	1	1
Pretzel Chips	1 oz	110	22	—	—
Pretzel Chips Cheese	1 oz	120	22	—	—
Rods	3 pieces (1 oz)	110	23	—	—
Snack Mix	½ cup (1 oz)	140	18	—	—
Sticks	50 pieces (1 oz)	110	23	—	—
Seyfart's					
Butter Rods	1 oz	110	21	—	—
Snyder's					
Logs	1 oz	310	22	—	—
Minis	1 oz	310	22	—	—
Minis Unsalted	1 oz	310	22	—	—
Nibblers	1 oz	310	22	—	—
Oat Bran	1 oz	120	14	—	—
Old Fashioned Hard	1 oz	111	23	—	—
Old Fashioned Hard Unsalted	1 oz	100	23	—	—
Old Tyme	1 oz	310	22	—	—
Old Tyme Unsalted	1 oz	110	22	—	—
Rods	1 oz	310	22	—	—
Sourdough Hard Buttermilk Ranch	1 oz	130	19	tr	0
Sourdough Hard Cheddar Cheese	1 oz	160	13	tr	0

FOOD	PORTION	CALS.	CARB.	SUG.	FIB.
Snyder's (CONT.)					
Sourdough Hard Honey Mustard & Onion	1 oz	130	19	3	0
Stix	1 oz	310	22	—	—
Very Thins	1 oz	310	22	—	—
Sunshine					
California Pretzels	1 oz	110	22	1	1
Ultra Slim-Fast					
Lite N' Tasty	1 oz	100	21	—	4
Wege					
Sourdough	1 oz	102	23	—	—
Unsalted	1 oz	102	23	—	—
Whole Wheat	1 oz	109	21	—	—
Weight Watchers					
Oat Bran Nuggets	1 pkg (1.5 oz)	170	33	0	3

PRICKLYPEAR

FOOD	PORTION	CALS.	CARB.	SUG.	FIB.
fresh	1	42	10	—	—

PRUNE JUICE

FOOD	PORTION	CALS.	CARB.	SUG.	FIB.
canned	1 cup	181	45	—	3
Del Monte					
Juice	8 fl oz	170	43	27	1
Ocean Spray					
100% Juice	8 fl oz	180	44	42	0
S&W					
Unsweetened	6 oz	120	31	—	—

PRUNES
CANNED

FOOD	PORTION	CALS.	CARB.	SUG.	FIB.
in heavy syrup	5	90	24	—	—
in heavy syrup	1 cup	245	65	—	—
DRIED					
cooked w/ sugar	½ cup	147	39	—	7
cooked w/o sugar	½ cup	113	30	—	6
dried	10	201	53	—	6
dried	1 cup	385	101	—	12
Del Monte					
Pitted	¼ cup (1.4 oz)	120	29	14	3
Unpitted	⅓ cup (1.4 oz)	110	12	13	1
Sonoma					
Pitted	¼ cup (1.4 oz)	120	29	15	3
Sunsweet					
Orange Essence Pitted Prunes	6 (1.4 oz)	100	26	11	3

FOOD	PORTION	CALS.	CARB.	SUG.	FIB.

PUDDING
(*see also* CUSTARD, PUDDING POPS)
HOME RECIPE

FOOD	PORTION	CALS.	CARB.	SUG.	FIB.
bread pudding	1 recipe 6 serv (26.4 oz)	1266	185	—	—
chocolate as prep w/ whole milk	½ cup (5.5 oz)	221	40	—	—
corn	⅔ cup	181	21	—	—
cornstarch	½ cup (4.4 oz)	137	20	—	—
rice	½ cup (5.3 oz)	217	40	—	—
yorkshire as prep w/ skim milk	3.5 oz	93	12	—	1
yorkshire as prep w/ whole milk	3.5 oz	104	12	—	1

MIX

FOOD	PORTION	CALS.	CARB.	SUG.	FIB.
banana as prep w/ 2% milk	½ cup (4.9 oz)	142	26	—	—
banana as prep w/ whole milk	½ cup (4.9 oz)	157	25	—	—
chocolate as prep w/ 2% milk	½ cup (5 oz)	150	28	—	—
chocolate as prep w/ whole milk	½ cup (5 oz)	158	26	—	—
coconut cream as prep w/ 2% milk	½ cup (4.9 oz)	148	25	—	—
coconut cream as prep w/ whole milk	½ cup (4.9 oz)	160	25	—	—
instant banana as prep w/ 2% milk	½ cup (5.2 oz)	152	29	—	—
instant banana as prep w/ whole milk	½ cup (5.2 oz)	167	27	—	—
instant chocolate as prep w/ 2% milk	½ cup (5.2 oz)	149	28	—	—
instant chocolate as prep w/ whole milk	½ cup (5.2 oz)	164	28	—	—
instant coconut cream as prep w/ 2% milk	½ cup (5.2 oz)	157	28	—	—
instant coconut cream as prep w/ whole milk	½ cup (5.2 oz)	172	28	—	—
instant lemon as prep w/ 2% milk	½ cup (5.2 oz)	155	30	—	—
instant lemon as prep w/ whole milk	½ cup (5.2 oz)	169	30	—	—
instant vanilla as prep w/ 2% milk	½ cup (5 oz)	147	28	—	—
instant vanilla as prep w/ whole milk	½ cup (5 oz)	181	28	—	—

FOOD	PORTION	CALS.	CARB.	SUG.	FIB.
lemon	½ cup (5.1 oz)	163	36	—	—
rice as prep w/ 2% milk	½ cup (5.1 oz)	161	30	—	—
rice as prep w/ whole milk	½ cup (5.1 oz)	175	30	—	—
tapioca as prep w/ 2% milk	½ cup (5 oz)	147	28	—	—
tapioca as prep w/ whole milk	½ cup (5 oz)	161	28	—	—
vanilla as prep w/ 2% milk	½ cup (4.9 oz)	141	26	—	—
vanilla as prep w/ whole milk	½ cup (4.9 oz)	155	26	—	—
Emes					
Dietetic as prep w/ skim milk	½ cup (4 fl oz)	71	13	—	—
Jell-O					
Americana Rice as prep w/ skim milk	½ cup (5.2 oz)	140	29	19	0
Americana Tapioca as prep w/ skim milk	½ cup (5.1 oz)	130	28	21	0
Banana Cream as prep w/ 2% milk	½ cup (5.1 oz)	140	26	21	0
Butterscotch as prep w/ 2% milk	½ cup (5.2 oz)	160	30	25	0
Chocolate as prep w/ 2% milk	½ cup (5.2 oz)	150	28	21	tr
Chocolate Fudge as prep w/ 2% milk	½ cup (5.2 oz)	150	28	21	1
Coconut Cream as prep w/ 2% milk	½ cup (5.1 oz)	150	24	19	tr
Fat Free Chocolate as prep w/ skim milk	½ cup (5.2 oz)	130	29	21	0
Fat Free Vanilla as prep w/ skim milk	½ cup (5.1 oz)	130	28	22	0
Instant Banana Cream as prep w/ 2% milk	½ cup (5.2 oz)	150	29	24	0
Instant Butterscotch as prep w/ 2% milk	½ cup (5.2 oz)	150	29	24	0
Instant Chocolate as prep w/ 2% milk	½ cup (5.2 oz)	160	31	25	tr
Instant Chocolate Fudge as prep w/ 2% milk	½ cup (4.2 oz)	160	31	23	tr
Instant Coconut Cream as prep w/ 2% milk	½ cup (4.2 oz)	160	27	22	tr
Instant French Vanilla as prep w/ 2% milk	½ cup (4.2 oz)	150	29	24	0
Instant Lemon as prep w/ 2% milk	½ cup (4.2 oz)	150	29	25	0
Instant Pistachio as prep w/ 2% milk	½ cup (4.2 oz)	160	29	24	0

FOOD	PORTION	CALS.	CARB.	SUG.	FIB.
Jell-O (CONT.)					
Instant Vanilla as prep w/ 2% milk	½ cup (4.2 oz)	150	29	25	0
Instant Fat Free Chocolate as prep w/ skim milk	½ cup (5.3 oz)	140	31	25	tr
Instant Fat Free Devil's Food as prep w/ skim milk	½ cup (5.3 oz)	140	31	25	tr
Instant Fat Free Sugar Free Banana as prep w/ skim milk	½ cup (4.6 oz)	70	12	6	0
Instant Fat Free Sugar Free Butterscotch as prep w/ skim milk	½ cup (4.6 oz)	70	12	6	0
Instant Fat Free Sugar Free Chocolate Fudge as prep w/ skim milk	½ cup (4.7 oz)	80	14	6	tr
Instant Fat Free Sugar Free Chocolate as prep w/ skim milk	½ cup (4.6 oz)	80	14	6	tr
Instant Fat Free Sugar Free Vanilla as prep w/ skim milk	½ cup (4.6 oz)	70	12	6	0
Instant Fat Free Sugar Free White Chocolate as prep w/ skim milk	½ cup (4.6 oz)	70	12	6	0
Instant Fat Free Vanilla as prep w/ skim milk	½ cup (5.2 oz)	140	29	25	0
Instant Fat Free White Chocolate as prep w/ skim milk	½ cup (5.2 oz)	140	29	25	0
Lemon as prep	½ cup (4.4 oz)	140	29	23	0
Milk Chocolate as prep w/ 2% milk	½ cup (5.2 oz)	150	28	22	tr
Sugar Free Chocolate as prep w/ 2% milk	½ cup (4.6 oz)	90	13	6	tr
Sugar Free Vanilla as prep w/ 2% milk	½ cup (4.5 oz)	80	11	6	0
Vanilla as prep w/ 2% milk	½ cup (5.1 oz)	140	26	21	0
Knorr					
Creme Caramel Flan & Sauce as prep	½ cup + 1 tbsp sauce	190	34	—	—
My*T*Fine					
Butterscotch	mix for 1 serv	90	22	—	—

FOOD	PORTION	CALS.	CARB.	SUG.	FIB.
My*T*Fine (CONT.)					
Chocolate	mix for 1 serv	100	23	—	0
Chocolate Almond	mix for 1 serv	100	23	—	—
Chocolate Fudge	mix for 1 serv	100	24	—	1
Lemon	mix for 1 serv	90	22	—	—
Vanilla	mix for 1 serv	90	22	—	0
Vanilla Tapioca	mix for 1 serv	80	19	—	—
Royal					
Banana Cream	mix for 1 serv	80	20	—	0
Banana Cream Instant	mix for 1 serv	90	22	—	—
Butterscotch	mix for 1 serv	90	25	—	0
Butterscotch Instant	mix for 1 serv	90	22	—	—
Cherry Vanilla Instant	mix for 1 serv	90	23	—	0
Chocolate	mix for 1 serv	90	22	—	0
Chocolate Almond Instant	mix for 1 serv	120	26	—	—
Chocolate Chocolate Chip Instant	mix for 1 serv	110	26	—	0
Chocolate Instant	mix for 1 serv	110	23	—	0
Chocolate Peanut Butter Instant	mix for 1 serv	110	26	—	0
Chocolate Sugar Free Instant	mix for 1 serv	50	11	—	—
Dark 'n Sweet Chocolate	mix for 1 serv	90	22	—	1
Dark 'N Sweet Instant	mix for 1 serv	110	25	—	0
Lemon Instant	mix for 1 serv	90	23	—	—
Pistachio Instant	mix for 1 serv	90	22	—	0
Strawberry Instant	mix for 1 serv	100	24	—	—
Toasted Coconut Instant	mix for 1 serv	100	22	—	—
Vanilla	mix for 1 serv	80	20	—	0
Vanilla Chocolate Chip Instant	mix for 1 serv	90	22	—	0
Vanilla Instant	mix for 1 serv	90	23	—	—
READY-TO-EAT					
banana	1 pkg (5 oz)	180	30	23	—
chocolate	1 pkg (5 oz)	189	32	23	—
lemon	1 pkg (5 oz)	177	36	—	—
rice	1 pkg (5 oz)	231	31	—	—
tapioca	1 pkg (5 oz)	169	28	—	—
vanilla	1 pkg (4 oz)	146	25	—	—
Del Monte					
Snack Cups Banana	1 serv (4 oz)	140	25	19	0
Snack Cups Butterscotch	1 serv (4 oz)	140	25	19	0
Snack Cups Chocolate	1 serv (4 oz)	160	27	20	0
Snack Cups Chocolate Fudge	1 serv (4 oz)	150	25	19	0

FOOD	PORTION	CALS.	CARB.	SUG.	FIB.
Del Monte (CONT.)					
Snack Cups Chocolate Peanut Butter	1 serv (4 oz)	160	28	21	0
Snack Cups Lite Chocolate	1 serv (4 oz)	100	19	13	0
Snack Cups Lite Vanilla	1 serv (4 oz)	90	18	14	0
Snack Cups Tapioca	1 serv (4 oz)	140	23	15	0
Snack Cups Vanilla	1 serv (4 oz)	150	26	19	0
Handi-Snacks					
Banana	1 serv (3.5 oz)	120	22	16	0
Butterscotch	1 serv (3.5 oz)	120	22	17	0
Chocolate	1 serv (3.5 oz)	130	23	18	tr
Chocolate Fudge	1 serv (3.5 oz)	130	23	18	tr
Fat Free Chocolate	1 serv (3.5 oz)	90	21	16	0
Fat Free Vanilla	1 serv (3.5 oz)	90	21	16	0
Tapioca	1 serv (3.5 oz)	120	21	14	0
Vanilla	1 serv (3.5 oz)	120	21	17	0
Hunt's					
Snack Pack Banana	1 (4 oz)	158	25	15	0
Snack Pack Butterscotch	1 (4 oz)	153	24	17	0
Snack Pack Chocolate	1 (4 oz)	167	25	20	0
Snack Pack Chocolate Fudge	1 (4 oz)	167	26	18	0
Snack Pack Chocolate Marshmallow	1 (4 oz)	155	23	18	0
Snack Pack Fat Free Chocolate	1 (4 oz)	96	21	16	0
Snack Pack Fat Free Tapioca	1 (4 oz)	95	21	16	0
Snack Pack Fat Free Vanilla	1 (4 oz)	93	21	17	0
Snack Pack Lemon	1 (4 oz)	162	33	27	0
Snack Pack Swirl Chocolate Caramel	1 (4 oz)	168	26	19	0
Snack Pack Swirl Chocolate Peanut Butter	1 (4 oz)	166	25	20	0
Snack Pack Swirl Milk Chocolate	1 (4 oz)	164	26	19	0
Snack Pack Swirl Smores	1 (4 oz)	154	25	19	0
Snack Pack Tapioca	1 (4 oz)	151	23	16	0
Snack Pack Vanilla	1 (4 oz)	163	25	19	0
Imagine Foods					
Lemon Dream	1 (4 oz)	120	30	—	—
Jell-O					
Chocolate	1 serv (4 oz)	160	28	23	0
Chocolate Marshmallow	1 serv (4 oz)	160	27	22	0

FOOD	PORTION	CALS.	CARB.	SUG.	FIB.
Jell-O (CONT.)					
Chocolate Vanilla Swirls	1 serv (4 oz)	160	27	22	0
Free Chocolate	1 serv (4 oz)	100	23	17	tr
Free Chocolate Vanilla Swirl	1 serv (4 oz)	100	23	17	tr
Free Devil's Food	1 serv (4 oz)	100	23	18	tr
Free Rocky Road	1 serv (4 oz)	100	23	17	tr
Free Vanilla	1 serv (4 oz)	100	23	18	0
Tapioca	1 serv (4 oz)	140	26	21	0
Tapioca	1 serv (4 oz)	100	23	17	0
Vanilla	1 serv (4 oz)	160	25	21	0
Kozy Shack					
Banana	1 pkg (4 oz)	130	22	17	1
Chocolate	1 pkg (4 oz)	140	24	19	1
Light Chocolate	1 pkg (4 oz)	110	22	21	1
Light Vanilla	1 pkg (4 oz)	110	22	22	0
Rice	1 pkg (4 oz)	130	23	16	1
Tapioca	1 pkg (4 oz)	140	25	20	0
Vanilla	1 pkg (4 oz)	130	22	17	1
Matthew Walker					
Plum	3.5 oz	290	60	—	1
Snack Pack					
Banana	4.25 oz	145	22	—	0
Butterscotch	4.25 oz	170	27	—	0
Chocolate	4.25 oz	170	26	—	0
Chocolate Marshmallow	4.25 oz	165	26	—	0
Chocolate Fudge	4.25 oz	165	27	—	0
Lemon	4.25 oz	150	30	—	tr
Light Chocolate	4.25 oz	100	20	—	0
Light Tapioca	4.25 oz	100	18	—	0
Tapioca	4.25 oz	150	23	—	0
Vanilla	4.25 oz	170	27	—	0
Swiss Miss					
Butterscotch	4 oz	180	29	—	0
Chocolate	4 oz	180	29	—	0
Chocolate Fudge	4 oz	220	38	—	0
Chocolate Sundae	4 oz	220	36	—	0
Light Chocolate	4 oz	100	20	—	0
Light Chocolate Fudge	4 oz	100	20	—	0
Light Vanilla	4 oz	100	20	—	0
Light Vanilla Chocolate Parfait	4 oz	100	20	—	0
Tapioca	4 oz	160	27	—	0
Vanilla	4 oz	190	30	—	0
Vanilla Parfait	4 oz	180	29	—	0

FOOD	PORTION	CALS.	CARB.	SUG.	FIB.
Swiss Miss (CONT.)					
Vanilla Sundae	4 oz	200	36	—	0
Ultra Slim-Fast					
Butterscotch	4 oz	100	21	—	2
Chocolate	4 oz	100	21	—	2
Vanilla	4 oz	100	21	—	2

PUDDING POPS
(see also ICE CREAM AND FROZEN DESSERTS, PUDDING)

chocolate	1 (1.6 oz)	72	12	10	—
vanilla	1 (1.6 oz)	75	13	11	—

PUMMELO

fresh	1	228	59	—	—
sections	1 cup	71	18	—	—

PUMPKIN
CANNED

pumpkin	½ cup	41	10	—	—
Libby					
Solid Pack	½ cup	60	15	4	4

FRESH

cooked mashed	½ cup	24	6	—	—
flowers cooked	½ cup	10	2	—	—
flowers raw	1	0	tr	—	—
leaves cooked	½ cup	7	1	—	—
leaves raw	½ cup	4	tr	—	—
raw cubed	½ cup	15	4	—	—

SEEDS

dried	1 oz	154	5	—	—
roasted	1 cup	1184	31	—	—
roasted	1 oz	148	4	—	—
salted & roasted	1 cup	1184	31	—	—
salted & roasted	1 oz	148	4	—	—
whole roasted	1 oz	127	15	—	—
whole roasted	1 cup	285	34	—	—
whole salted roasted	1 cup	285	34	—	—
whole salted roasted	1 oz	127	15	—	—

PURSLANE

cooked	1 cup	21	4	—	—
raw	1 cup	7	1	—	—

QUAHOGS
(see CLAM)

QUAIL

breast w/o skin raw	1 (2 oz)	69	0	0	0

FOOD	PORTION	CALS.	CARB.	SUG.	FIB.
w/ skin raw	1 quail (3.8 oz)	210	0	0	0
w/o skin raw	1 quail (3.2 oz)	123	0	0	0
QUINCE					
fresh	1	53	14	—	—
QUINOA					
quinoa not prep	1 cup (6 oz)	636	117	—	10
Arrowhead					
Quinoa	¼ cup (1.4 oz)	140	25	0	4
Eden					
Not Prep	¼ cup (1.6 oz)	170	31	1	3
RABBIT					
domestic w/o bone roasted	3 oz	167	0	0	0
wild w/o bone stewed	3 oz	147	0	0	0
RACCOON					
roasted	3 oz	217	0	0	0
RADICCHIO					
leaf	3.5 oz	18	3	0	1
raw shredded	½ cup	5	1	—	—
RADISHES					
DRIED					
chinese	½ cup	157	37	—	—
daikon	½ cup	157	37	—	—
FRESH					
chinese raw	1 (12 oz)	62	14	—	—
chinese raw sliced	½ cup	8	2	—	—
chinese sliced cooked	½ cup	13	3	—	—
daikon raw	1 (12 oz)	62	14	—	—
daikon raw sliced	½ cup	8	2	—	—
daikon sliced cooked	½ cup	13	3	—	—
red raw	10	7	2	—	—
red sliced	½ cup	10	2	—	—
white icicle raw	1 (½ oz)	2	tr	—	—
white icicle raw sliced	½ cup	7	1	—	—
Dole					
Radishes	7	20	3	—	0
SPROUTS					
raw	½ cup	8	1	—	—
RAISINS					
chocolate coated	10 (0.4 oz)	39	7	—	—
chocolate coated	1 cup (6.7 oz)	741	130	—	—
golden seedless	1 cup	437	115	—	8

FOOD	PORTION	CALS.	CARB.	SUG.	FIB.
seedless	1 cup	434	115	—	8
seedless	1 tbsp	27	7	—	—
sultanas	1 oz	88	23	—	2
Del Monte					
Golden	¼ cup (1.4 oz)	130	31	29	2
Raisins	1 box (1.5 oz)	140	33	31	3
Raisins	1 box (1 oz)	90	22	20	2
Raisins	1 box (0.5 oz)	45	11	10	tr
Raisins	¼ cup (1.4 oz)	130	31	29	2
Yogurt Raisins Strawberry	1 pkg (0.9 oz)	110	20	17	tr
Yogurt Raisins Vanilla	1 pkg (0.9 oz)	110	20	17	tr
Yogurt Raisins Vanilla	1 pkg (1 oz)	120	22	17	tr
Yogurt Raisins Vanilla	3 tbsp (1 oz)	130	23	19	1
Dole					
Golden	½ cup	250	66	—	—
Seedless	½ cup	250	66	—	—
Sonoma					
Monukka Thompson	¼ cup (1.4 oz)	130	31	29	2
Tree Of Life					
Organic	¼ cup (1.4 oz)	130	31	29	2

RASPBERRIES
CANNED
in heavy syrup	½ cup	117	30	—	—

FRESH
raspberries	1 cup	61	14	—	—
raspberries	1 pint	154	36	—	—
Dole					
Raspberries	1 cup	45	10	—	9

FROZEN
sweetened	1 cup	256	65	—	—
sweetened	1 pkg (10 oz)	291	74	—	—
Big Valley					
Raspberries	⅔ cup (4.9 oz)	80	18	7	3
Birds Eye					
Red	½ cup (4.4 oz)	90	22	22	5

RASPBERRY JUICE
Crystal Geyser					
Juice Squeeze Mountain Raspberry	1 bottle (12 fl oz)	135	32	29	—
Crystal Light					
Raspberry Ice Drink	1 serv (8 oz)	5	0	0	0
Raspberry Ice Drink Mix as prep	1 serv (8 oz)	5	0	0	0

FOOD	PORTION	CALS.	CARB.	SUG.	FIB.
Fresh Samantha					
Raspberry Dream	1 cup (8 oz)	120	30	—	2
Kool-Aid					
Drink Mix as prep	1 serv (8 oz)	60	17	17	0
Raspberry Drink as prep w/ sugar	1 serv (8 oz)	100	25	25	0
Splash Blue Raspberry Drink	1 serv (8 oz)	120	30	30	0
Smucker's					
Juice	8 oz	120	30	—	—
Juice Sparkler	10 oz	130	32	—	—

RED BEANS
CANNED
Allen

Red Beans	½ cup (4.5 oz)	160	19	1	9
Green Giant					
Red Beans	½ cup (4.5 oz)	100	19	2	6
Hunt's					
Small	½ cup (4.5 oz)	89	19	4	6
Van Camp's					
Red Beans	½ cup (4.6 oz)	90	20	—	5

MIX
Bean Cuisine

Pasta & Beans Barcelona Red With Radiatore	½ cup	170	170	—	—
Mahatma					
Red Beans & Rice	1 cup	190	40	2	7

RED KIDNEY BEANS
DRIED
Hurst

HamBeens w/ Ham	1 serv	120	20	1	10

RELISH

cranberry orange	½ cup	246	64	—	—
hamburger	1 tbsp	19	5	—	—
hamburger	½ cup	158	42	—	—
hot dog	½ cup	111	28	—	—
hot dog	1 tbsp	14	4	—	—
piccalilli	1.4 oz	13	2	—	1
sweet	½ cup	159	43	—	—
sweet	1 tbsp	19	5	—	—
Del Monte					
Hamburger	1 tbsp (0.5 oz)	20	6	5	tr

FOOD	PORTION	CALS.	CARB.	SUG.	FIB.
Del Monte (CONT.)					
Hot Dog	1 tbsp (0.5 oz)	15	4	3	tr
Sweet Pickle	1 tbsp (0.5 oz)	20	5	5	0
Green Giant					
Corn	1 tbsp (0.6 oz)	20	5	2	0
Hellman's					
Sandwich Spread	1 tbsp (15 g)	55	2	—	—
Old El Paso					
Jalapeno	1 tbsp (0.5 oz)	5	1	0	0
Vlasic					
Dill	1 oz	2	1	—	—
Hamburger	1 oz	40	9	—	—
Hot Dog	1 oz	40	8	—	—
Hot Piccalilli	1 oz	35	8	—	—
India	1 oz	30	8	—	—
Sweet	1 oz	30	8	—	—

RENNIN

FOOD	PORTION	CALS.	CARB.	SUG.	FIB.
tablet	1 (0.9 g)	1	tr	—	—

RHUBARB

FOOD	PORTION	CALS.	CARB.	SUG.	FIB.
fresh	½ cup	13	3	—	—
frzn	½ cup	60	3	—	—
frzn as prep w/ sugar	½ cup	139	37	—	—

RICE

(*see also* BRAN, CEREAL, FLOUR, RICE CAKES, WILD RICE)

FOOD	PORTION	CALS.	CARB.	SUG.	FIB.
brown long grain cooked	1 cup (6.8 oz)	216	45	—	4
brown medium grain cooked	1 cup (6.8 oz)	218	46	—	4
glutinous cooked	1 cup (6.1 oz)	169	37	—	2
starch	3½ oz	343	85	—	—
white long grain cooked	1 cup (5.5 oz)	205	45	—	1
white long grain instant cooked	1 cup (5.8 oz)	162	35	—	1
white medium grain cooked	1 cup (6.5 oz)	242	53	—	1
white short grain cooked	1 cup (6.5 oz)	242	53	—	—
Arrowhead					
Basmati Brown	¼ cup (1.5 oz)	150	33	0	2
Basmati White	¼ cup (1.5 oz)	150	34	0	tr
Brown Quick Regular	⅓ cup (1.5 oz)	150	32	0	2
Brown Quick Spanish Style	¼ pkg (1.4 oz)	150	30	0	2
Brown Quick Vegetable Herb	¼ pkg (1.4 oz)	150	30	0	3
Brown Quick Wild Rice & Herb	¼ pkg (1.3 oz)	140	28	0	3

FOOD	PORTION	CALS.	CARB.	SUG.	FIB.
Birds Eye					
Rice & Broccoli In Cheese Sauce	1 pkg (10 oz)	290	44	4	2
White & Wild	1 cup (6.6 oz)	180	31	2	2
Budget Gourmet					
Oriental Rice With Vegetables	1 pkg (5.75 oz)	230	28	—	—
Rice Pilaf With Green Beans	1 pkg (5.5 oz)	230	30	—	—
Carolina					
Red Beans & Rice as prep	¼ pkg	190	40	1	6
Casbah					
Basmati as prep	1 cup	158	36	—	—
Jambalaya	1 pkg (1.4 oz)	130	27	0	1
La Fiesta	1 pkg (1.59 oz)	170	34	4	0
Nutted Pilaf as prep	1 cup	220	40	0	1
Pilaf as prep	1 cup	200	44	0	tr
Spanish Pilaf as prep	1 cup	200	44	0	1
Thai Yum	1 pkg (1.7 oz)	180	33	7	1
Chun King					
Fried Rice	1 pkg (8 oz)	290	48	11	5
Fried Rice With Chicken	1 pkg (8 oz)	270	44	9	4
Goodman's					
Rice & Vermicelli For Beef	¾ cup	160	33	4	0
Rice & Vermicelli For Chicken	¾ cup	160	33	3	1
Goya					
Arroz Amarillo	¼ cup (1.6 oz)	170	37	0	1
Green Giant					
Rice & Broccoli	1 pkg (10 oz)	320	44	1	2
Rice Medley	1 pkg (10 oz)	240	46	3	2
Rice Pilaf	1 pkg (10 oz)	230	44	3	3
White & Wild	1 pkg (10 oz)	250	45	3	3
Hain					
Almondine	½ cup	130	17	—	—
Oriental 3-Grain Goodness	½ cup	120	15	—	—
Kitchen Del Sol					
Mediterranean Paella Costa Brave as prep	½ cup (1.2 oz)	130	23	1	1
Mediterranean Sunny Lemon Pilaf as prep	½ cup (1.2 oz)	110	22	1	1
Mediterranean Tomato & Basil With Pine Nuts	½ cup (1 oz)	110	18	0	1

FOOD	PORTION	CALS.	CARB.	SUG.	FIB.
Knorr					
Risotto Milanese With Saffron	½ cup	130	24	—	—
Risotto Tomato	½ cup	110	23	—	—
Risotto With Mushrooms	½ cup	110	24	—	—
Risotto With Onion	½ cup	110	24	—	—
Risotto With Peas And Corn	½ cup	110	23	—	—
La Choy					
Chinese Fried Rice	¾ cup	190	41	—	tr
Lipton					
Golden Saute Onion Mushroom	½ cup (2.1 oz)	240	45	2	2
Oriental Stir Fry as prep	1 cup	270	47	2	1
Rice & Sauce Alfredo Broccoli as prep	1 cup	320	46	4	1
Rice & Sauce Beef as prep	1 cup	270	47	1	1
Rice & Sauce Cajun Style as prep	1 cup	270	46	1	1
Rice & Sauce Cajun Style w/ Beans as prep	1 cup	310	52	1	7
Rice & Sauce Cheddar Broccoli as prep	1 cup	280	46	1	1
Rice & Sauce Chicken & Parmesan Risotto as prep	1 cup	270	43	0	tr
Rice & Sauce Chicken Broccoli as prep	1 cup	280	46	1	2
Rice & Sauce Chicken Flavor as prep	1 cup	280	45	1	1
Rice & Sauce Creamy Chicken as prep	1 cup	290	45	2	1
Rice & Sauce Herb & Butter as prep	1 cup	280	43	0	tr
Rice & Sauce Medley as prep	1 cup	270	44	1	2
Rice & Sauce Mushroom as prep	1 cup	270	45	1	1
Rice & Sauce Mushroom & Herb as prep	1 cup	290	49	0	1
Rice & Sauce Oriental as prep	1 cup	280	48	2	2
Rice & Sauce Pilaf as prep	1 cup	260	44	1	1
Rice & Sauce Scampi Style as prep	1 cup	270	44	1	1

FOOD	PORTION	CALS.	CARB.	SUG.	FIB.
Lipton (CONT.)					
Rice & Sauce Spanish as prep	1 cup	270	47	2	2
Rice & Sauce Teriyaki as prep	1 cup	270	45	2	1
Roasted Chicken as prep	1 cup	260	46	1	1
Salsa Style as prep	1 cup	220	37	1	2
Southwestern Chicken Flavor as prep	1 cup	260	47	1	1
Luigino's					
Fried Rice Chicken	1 pkg (8 oz)	250	38	2	2
Fried Rice Pork	1 pkg (8 oz)	250	37	2	2
Fried Rice Pork & Shrimp	1 pkg (8 oz)	250	39	2	2
Fried Rice Shrimp	1 pkg (8 oz)	220	38	2	2
Luigino's					
Fried Rice Shrimp	1 pkg (8 oz)	220	38	2	2
Risotto Parmesano	1 pkg (8 oz)	360	30	1	2
Mahatma					
Broccoli & Cheese	1 cup	200	41	1	2
Jambalaya	1 cup (2 oz)	190	43	1	tr
Long Grain & Wild	1 cup (2 oz)	190	41	0	2
Pilaf	1 cup (2 oz)	190	43	0	tr
Spanish	1 cup (2 oz)	180	42	1	2
Yellow Rice Mix	1 cup	190	43	1	tr
Melting Pot					
Risotto Melanese w/ Saffron	1 cup	210	48	1	0
Risotto Primavera	1 cup	200	44	3	1
Risotto Sun-Dried Tomatoes & Peas	1 cup	200	45	2	1
Risotto Three Cheese	1 cup	200	44	1	0
Risotto Wild Mushroom	1 cup	200	44	3	2
Minute					
Boil-In-Bag White as prep	1 cup (5.7 oz)	190	42	0	tr
Instant Brown as prep	1 cup (5.2 oz)	170	34	0	2
Instant White as prep	1 cup (5.7 oz)	160	36	0	tr
Long Grain & Wild Seasoned w/ Herbs as prep	1 cup (7.8 oz)	230	50	2	1
Near East					
Barley Pilaf as prep	1 cup	220	41	1	5
Beef Pilaf as prep	1 cup	220	42	1	1
Curry Rice as prep	1 cup	220	42	1	1

FOOD	PORTION	CALS.	CARB.	SUG.	FIB.
Near East (CONT.)					
Lentil Pilaf as prep	1 cup	210	37	5	0
Long Grain & Wild as prep	1 cup	220	42	0	2
Pilaf Brown Rice as prep	1 cup	220	41	1	2
Pilaf Chicken as prep	1 cup	220	42	2	1
Pilaf Kosher as prep	1 cup	220	42	0	1
Spanish Pilaf as prep	1 cup	230	42	1	1
Old El Paso					
Mexican	½ cup (4 oz)	410	90	3	3
Spanish	1 cup (8.6 oz)	130	28	2	2
Pritikin					
Mexican	⅓ cup (2 oz)	200	43	—	—
Oriental	⅓ cup (2 oz)	190	43	—	—
Rice-A-Roni					
Beef	½ cup	140	24	—	—
Beef & Mushroom	½ cup	150	26	—	—
Chicken	½ cup	150	26	—	—
Chicken & Broccoli	½ cup	150	25	—	—
Chicken & Mushroom	½ cup	180	26	—	—
Chicken & Vegetables	½ cup	140	25	—	—
Fried Rice	½ cup	110	21	—	—
Herb & Butter	½ cup	130	22	—	—
Long Grain & Wild Chicken w/ Almonds	½ cup	140	24	—	—
Long Grain & Wild Original	½ cup	130	23	—	—
Long Grain & Wild Pilaf	½ cup	130	23	—	—
Pilaf	½ cup	150	25	—	—
Risotto	½ cup	200	32	—	—
Spanish	½ cup	150	25	—	—
Stroganoff	½ cup	200	27	—	—
Yellow Rice	½ cup	140	25	—	—
S&W					
Brown Quick Natural Long Grain	3.5 oz	110	25	—	—
Brown Quick Natural Long Grain cooked	3.5 oz	119	26	—	—
Long Grain cooked	3.5 oz	106	23	—	—
Success					
Beef Oriental	½ cup	190	43	2	2
Broccoli & Cheese	½ cup	200	41	4	2
Brown & Wild	½ cup	190	40	1	3
Classic Chicken	½ cup	150	32	0	1

FOOD	PORTION	CALS.	CARB.	SUG.	FIB.
Success (CONT.)					
Long Grain & Wild	½ cup	190	42	2	1
Pilaf	½ cup	200	44	3	2
Spanish	½ cup	190	43	2	1
Superfino					
Arborio	½ cup	100	22	—	—
Ultra Slim-Fast					
Oriental Style	2.3 oz	240	58	—	4
Rice & Chicken Sauce	2.3 oz	240	56	—	4
Uncle Ben					
Boil-In-Bag	1 serv (0.9 oz)	94	22	—	tr
Brown	1 serv (1.6 oz)	158	34	—	1
Brown & Wild Fast Cooking	1 serv (1.3 oz)	120	26	—	1
Country Inn Broccoli Almondine	1 serv (1.2 oz)	124	25	—	1
Country Inn Broccoli & White Cheddar	1 serv (1.2 oz)	131	24	—	1
Country Inn Broccoli Au Gratin	1 serv (1.1 oz)	116	22	—	1
Country Inn Chicken Stock	1 serv (1.2 oz)	123	24	—	1
Country Inn Chicken With Wild Rice	1 serv (1.1 oz)	108	23	—	1
Country Inn Creamy Chicken & Mushroom	1 serv (1.3 oz)	138	24	—	1
Country Inn Creamy Chicken & Wild Rice	1 serv (1.3 oz)	135	27	—	1
Country Inn Green Bean Almondine	1 serv (1.2 oz)	128	25	—	1
Country Inn Herbed Au Gratin	1 serv (1.2 oz)	119	24	—	1
Country Inn Homestyle Chicken & Vegetables	1 serv (1.3 oz)	139	24	—	1
Country Inn Rice Florentine	1 serv (1.2 oz)	212	24	—	1
Country Inn Vegetable Pilaf	1 serv (1.2 oz)	115	25	—	1
In An Instant	1 serv (1.1 oz)	111	25	—	tr
Long Grain & Wild Chicken Stock Sauce	1 serv (1.3 oz)	133	25	—	1
Long Grain & Wild Fast Cooking	1 serv (1 oz)	101	22	—	1
Long Grain & Wild Garden Vegetable Blend	1 serv (1.3 oz)	128	26	—	1
Long Grain & Wild Original	1 serv (1 oz)	96	21	—	1
White Converted	1 serv (1.2 oz)	123	27	—	tr
Van Camp's					
Spanish	1 cup (9 oz)	180	37	—	3

FOOD	PORTION	CALS.	CARB.	SUG.	FIB.
Watkins					
Brown & Wild	¼ cup (1.6 oz)	160	34	0	3
Calico Medley	¼ cup (1.6 oz)	160	37	0	4
East/West Medley	¼ cup (1.6 oz)	160	33	0	5
Heartland Medley	¼ cup (1.6 oz)	160	35	0	4
Minnesota Medley	¼ cup (1.6 oz)	160	34	0	2
White & Wild	¼ cup (1.6 oz)	160	34	0	1

RICE CAKES
 (*see also* POPCORN CAKES)

FOOD	PORTION	CALS.	CARB.	SUG.	FIB.
brown rice	1 (0.3 oz)	35	7	—	tr
brown rice & buckwheat	1 (0.3 oz)	34	7	—	tr
brown rice & buckwheat unsalted	1 (0.3 oz)	34	7	—	tr
brown rice & corn	1 (0.3 oz)	35	7	—	—
brown rice & rye	1 (0.3 oz)	35	7	—	tr
brown rice & sesame seed	1 (0.3 oz)	35	7	—	—
brown rice multigrain	1 (0.3 oz)	35	7	—	—
brown rice multigrain unsalted	1 (0.3 oz)	35	7	—	—
brown rice unsalted	1 (0.3 oz)	35	7	—	tr
Hain					
5-Grain	1	40	8	—	—
Mini Apple Cinnamon	½ oz	60	12	—	0
Mini Barbeque	½ oz	70	10	—	0
Mini Cheese	½ oz	60	10	—	0
Mini Honey Nut	½ oz	60	11	—	0
Mini Nacho Cheese	½ oz	70	10	—	—
Mini Plain	½ oz	60	12	—	0
Mini Plain No Salt Added	½ oz	60	12	—	0
Mini Ranch	½ oz	70	9	—	—
Mini Teriyaki	½ oz	50	12	—	0
Plain	1	40	8	—	—
Plain No Salt Added	1	40	8	—	—
Sesame	1	40	8	—	—
Sesame No Salt	1	40	8	—	—
Ka-Me					
Cheese	16 pieces (1 oz)	120	24	0	0
Onion	16 pieces (1 oz)	120	25	0	0
Plain	16 pieces (1 oz)	120	25	0	0
Seaweed	16 pieces (1 oz)	120	25	0	0
Sesame	16 pieces (1 oz)	120	24	0	0
Unsalted	16 pieces (1 oz)	120	26	0	0
Lundberg					
Organic Lightly Salted	1	60	14	—	—

FOOD	PORTION	CALS.	CARB.	SUG.	FIB.
Lundberg (CONT.)					
Organic Unsalted	1	60	14	—	—
Premium Lightly Salted	1	60	14	—	—
Premium Unsalted	1	60	14	—	—
Sesame Lightly Salted	1	59	16	—	—
Mother's					
Mini Apple	5 (0.5 oz)	50	12	3	0
Mini Caramel	5 (0.5 oz)	50	12	3	0
Mini Cinnamon	5 (0.5 oz)	50	12	3	0
Mini Plain Unsalted	7 (0.5 oz)	60	12	0	0
Multigrain Lightly Salted	1 (0.3 oz)	35	7	0	0
Rye Unsalted	1 (0.3 oz)	35	7	0	1
Wheat Unsalted	1 (0.3 oz)	35	7	0	1
Pritikin					
Mini Apple Crisp	5 (0.5 oz)	50	12	—	—
Multigrain	1 (0.3 oz)	35	7	—	—
Multigrain Unsalted	1 (0.3 oz)	35	7	—	—
Plain	1 (0.3 oz)	35	7	—	—
Plain Unsalted	1 (0.3 oz)	35	7	—	—
Sesame Low Sodium	1 (0.3 oz)	35	7	—	—
Sesame Unsalted	1 (0.3 oz)	35	7	—	—
Quaker					
Apple Cinnamon	1 (0.5 oz)	50	11	—	—
Banana Crunch	1 (0.5 oz)	50	11	—	—
Cinnamon Crunch	1 (0.5 oz)	50	11	—	—
Mini Apple Cinnamon	5 (0.5 oz)	50	12	—	—
Mini Banana Nut	5 (0.5 oz)	50	12	—	—
Mini Butter Popped Corn	6 (0.5 oz)	50	12	—	—
Mini Caramel Corn	5 (0.5 oz)	50	12	—	—
Mini Chocolate Crunch	5 (0.5 oz)	50	12	—	—
Mini Cinnamon Crunch	5 (0.5 oz)	50	12	—	—
Mini Honey Nut	5 (0.5 oz)	50	12	—	—
Mini Monterey Jack	6 (0.5 oz)	50	11	—	—
Mini White Cheddar	6 (0.5 oz)	50	11	—	—
Salt-Free	1 (0.3 oz)	35	7	—	—
Salted	1 (0.3 oz)	35	7	—	—
Tree Of Life					
Fat Free Mini Apple Cinnamon	15	60	13	12	0
Fat Free Mini Caramel	15	60	13	12	0
Fat Free Mini Honey Nut	15	60	13	12	0
Fat Free Mini Jalapeno	15	60	13	12	0
Fat Free Mini Plain	15	50	12	12	0

FOOD	PORTION	CALS.	CARB.	SUG.	FIB.
ROCKFISH					
pacific cooked	1 fillet (5.2 oz)	180	0	0	0
pacific cooked	3 oz	103	0	0	0
pacific raw	3 oz	80	0	0	0
ROE					
(see also individual fish names)					
fish	3.5 oz	39	tr	—	—
fresh baked	1 oz	58	1	—	—
fresh baked	3 oz	173	2	—	—
ROLL					
(see also BISCUIT, CROISSANT, ENGLISH MUFFIN, MUFFIN, POPOVER, SCONE)					
FROZEN					
New York					
Garlic	1 (2 oz)	210	26	1	1
Pepperidge Farm					
Cinnamon Roll	1 (2¼ oz)	220	34	—	—
Sara Lee					
Deluxe Cinnamon Rolls w/ Icing	1 (2.7 oz)	370	53	30	1
Deluxe Cinnamon Rolls w/o Icing	1 (2.7 oz)	320	41	21	1
HOME RECIPE					
dinner as prep w/ 2% milk	1 (2½ in)	111	19	—	—
dinner as prep w/ whole milk	1 (2½ in)	112	19	—	—
raisin & nut	1 (2 oz)	196	30	—	—
MIX					
Dromedary					
Hot Roll Mix	2	239	41	—	—
Natural Ovens					
German Hard	1 (2.1 oz)	138	36	0	1
Gourmet Dinner	1 (1 oz)	50	15	0	2
Hearty Sandwich	1 (1.8 oz)	110	30	0	2
Pillsbury					
Hot Roll Mix	2	240	42	—	—
READY-TO-EAT					
brioche sweet roll	1 (3.5 oz)	410	41	5	3
brown & serve	1 (1 oz)	85	14	—	—
cheese	1 (2.3 oz)	238	29	—	—
cinnamon raisin	1 (2¾ in)	223	31	—	1
dinner	1 (1 oz)	85	14	—	—
egg	1 (2½ in)	107	18	—	1
french	1 (1.3 oz)	105	19	—	—

FOOD	PORTION	CALS.	CARB.	SUG.	FIB.
hamburger	1 (1½ oz)	123	22	—	—
hamburger multi-grain	1 (1½ oz)	113	19	—	2
hamburger reduced calorie	1 (1½ oz)	84	18	—	3
hard	1 (3½ in)	167	30	—	—
hot cross bun	1	202	38	—	1
hotdog	1 (1½ oz)	123	22	—	—
hotdog multi-grain	1 (1½ oz)	113	19	—	2
hotdog reduced calorie	1 (1½ oz)	84	18	—	3
kaiser	1 (3½ in)	167	30	—	—
oat bran	1 (1.2 oz)	78	13	—	1
rye	1 (1 oz)	81	15	—	—
submarine	1 (4.7 oz)	155	30	—	—
wheat	1 (1 oz)	77	13	—	—
whole wheat	1 (1 oz)	75	15	—	—
Alvarado St. Bakery					
Burger Buns	1 (2.2 oz)	140	27	4	3
Hot Dog Buns	1 (2.2 oz)	140	28	4	3
Arnold					
8-inch Francisco	1 (2.5 oz)	210	39	—	—
Augusto Pan Cubano	1	230	43	—	2
Bakery Light	1 (1.5 oz)	80	21	—	4
Bran'nola Buns	1 (1.5 oz)	100	20	—	3
Deli Kaiser	1	170	34	—	—
Deli Onion	1	170	34	—	—
Dinner Plain	1 (0.7 oz)	50	9	—	1
Dinner Sesame	1 (0.7 oz)	50	9	—	1
Dutch Egg	1	130	21	—	2
French Francisco	1 (2.5 oz)	210	39	—	—
French Mini Francisco	1	130	24	—	—
Hamburger	1	120	20	—	2
Hot Dog	1 (1.5 oz)	110	21	—	1
Hot Dog Bran'nola	1 (1.5 oz)	110	18	—	1
Hot Dog New England Style	1	110	20	—	1
Italian 8-inch Savoni	1	210	38	—	3
Kaiser Francisco	1 (2 oz)	180	34	—	—
Onion Premium	1 (2.6 oz)	180	38	—	2
Onion Soft	1	140	28	—	2
Party Petite	2	70	10	—	1
Potato	1	140	25	—	2
Sandwich Soft Sesame	1	130	23	—	2
Sourdough Brown N' Serve	1 (1 oz)	100	19	—	—
Sourdough Francisco	1 (1 oz)	100	19	—	—
Wheat Old Fashioned	2	80	11	—	—

FOOD	PORTION	CALS.	CARB.	SUG.	FIB.
August Bros.					
Dinner	1	90	18	—	—
Kaiser	1	170	35	—	2
Onion	1	160	33	—	2
Sesame Cubano	1	170	35	—	2
Bread Du Jour					
Bavarian Cracked Wheat	1 (1.2 oz)	90	17	2	1
Crusty Italian	1 (1.2 oz)	80	16	1	tr
French Petite	1 (3.5 oz)	230	47	4	2
Rye	1 (1.2 oz)	90	16	0	1
Sourdough	1 (2.2 oz)	140	29	tr	2
Dicarlo's					
Extra Sourdough	1 (1.6 oz)	100	20	0	1
French	1 (1 oz)	70	14	tr	tr
Home Pride					
Dinner Wheat	1 (1.9 oz)	160	26	2	2
Hamburger Potato Bun	1 (1.9 oz)	130	27	3	2
Hot Dog Potato Bun	1 (1.9 oz)	130	27	3	2
Sandwich Roll Wheat	1 (1.9 oz)	160	26	2	2
White	2 (1.6 oz)	130	22	1	1
Levy					
Sub Old Country	1	180	34	—	—
Martin's					
Big Marty Poppy	1	170	31	—	3
Big Marty Sesame	1	170	31	—	3
Hoagie	1	240	41	—	3
Hoagie Sesame	1	240	41	—	4
Potato Dinner	1	100	18	—	1
Potato Long	1	140	27	—	2
Potato Party	1	50	10	—	1
Potato Sandwich	1	140	26	—	2
Sandwich Whole Wheat 100% Stoneground	1	160	28	—	5
Matthew's					
Salad Roll	1	110	19	—	2
Sandwich	1	110	19	—	2
Pepperidge Farm					
Brown 'N Serve Club	1	100	19	—	1
Brown 'N Serve French	½ roll	180	36	—	1
Brown 'N Serve Hearth	1	50	10	—	tr
Dinner	1	60	8	—	tr
Dinner Country Style Classic	1	50	9	—	0
Finger Poppy Seed	1	50	8	—	tr

FOOD	PORTION	CALS.	CARB.	SUG.	FIB.
Pepperidge Farm (CONT.)					
Finger Sesame Seed	1	60	9	—	tr
Frankfurter Dijon	1	160	23	—	2
Frankfurter Side Sliced	1	140	24	—	1
Frankfurter Top Sliced	1	140	24	—	1
Frankfurter w/ Poppy Seeds	1	130	23	—	1
French Style	1	100	20	—	1
Hamburger	1	130	22	—	1
Hamburger	1	130	22	—	1
Heat & Serve Butter Crescent	1	110	13	—	tr
Heat & Serve Golden Twist	1	110	14	—	tr
Hoagie Soft	1	210	34	—	1
Old Fashioned	1	50	7	—	tr
Parker House	1	60	9	—	tr
Party	1	30	5	—	tr
Potato Sandwich	1	160	28	—	1
Sandwich Onion w/ Poppy Seeds	1	150	26	—	1
Sandwich Salad	1	110	16	—	—
Sandwich w/ Sesame Seeds	1	140	23	—	1
Soft Family	1	100	18	—	1
Sourdough French	1	100	19	—	1
Roman Meal					
Brown & Serve	2 (2 oz)	140	24	4	2
Dinner	2 (2 oz)	136	24	4	2
Hamburger	1 (1.6 oz)	111	19	3	2
Hotdog	1 (1.5 oz)	103	18	3	2
Sandwich	1 (2.7 oz)	181	31	3	3
Sandwich	1 (2.7 oz)	181	31	3	3
San Francisco					
Sourdough	1 (1.8 oz)	180	37	tr	3
The Baker					
Honey Cinnamon Raisin	1 (2 oz)	150	31	12	4
Wonder					
Brown 'N Serve Buttermilk	1 (1 oz)	70	13	1	tr
Brown 'N Serve Wheat	1 (1 oz)	70	14	tr	tr
Brown 'N Serve White	1 (1 oz)	70	14	tr	tr
Dinner White Light	1 (1 oz)	60	9	1	4
Hamburger	1 (1.5 oz)	110	21	1	tr
Hamburger Light	1 (1.5 oz)	80	13	1	5
Hamburger Wheat	1 (2.2 oz)	170	31	2	1
Hot Dog	1 (1.5 oz)	110	21	1	tr

FOOD	PORTION	CALS.	CARB.	SUG.	FIB.
Wonder (CONT.)					
Hot Dog Light	1 (1.5 oz)	80	13	1	5
Tea Dinner Rolls	1 (1.5 oz)	80	19	1	5
REFRIGERATED					
cinnamon w/ frosting	1	109	17	—	—
crescent	1 (1 oz)	98	14	—	—
Pillsbury					
Best Quick Cinnamon Rolls w/ Icing	1	110	17	—	—
Butterflake	1	140	20	—	—
Crescent	1	100	11	—	—
ROSE APPLE					
fresh	3½ oz	32	7	—	—
ROSE HIP					
fresh	3½ oz	91	19	—	—
ROSELLE					
fresh	1 cup	28	6	—	—
ROSEMARY					
dried	1 tsp	4	1	—	—
ROUGHY					
orange baked	3 oz	75	0	0	0
RUTABAGA					
CANNED					
Sunshine					
Diced	½ cup (4.2 oz)	30	7	2	3
FRESH					
cooked mashed	½ cup	41	9	—	—
raw cubed	½ cup	25	6	—	—
SABLEFISH					
baked	3 oz	213	0	0	0
fillet baked	5.3 oz	378	0	0	0
smoked	3 oz	218	0	0	0
smoked	1 oz	72	0	0	0
SAFFLOWER					
seeds dried	1 oz	147	10	—	—
SAFFRON					
saffron	1 tsp	2	tr	—	—
SAGE					
ground	1 tsp	2	tr	—	—

FOOD	PORTION	CALS.	CARB.	SUG.	FIB.
Watkins					
Sage	¼ tsp (0.5 g)	0	0	0	0

SALAD
(*see also* LETTUCE, PASTA SALAD)

MIX

Dole

Caesar Salad	⅓ pkg (3.5 oz)	170	9	2	1
Classic Blend	3.5 oz	25	4	0	1
Coleslaw Blend	3.5 oz	30	5	0	2
French Blend	3.5 oz	25	4	0	1
Italian Blend	3.5 oz	25	3	0	1
Salad-In-A- Minute Oriental	3.5 oz	110	12	4	2
Salad-In-A- Minute Spinach	3.5 oz	180	19	11	3

Fresh Express

American Salad	1½ cups (3 oz)	20	3	2	1
Caesar Salad	1½ cups (3 oz)	140	8	3	1
European Salad	1½ cups (3 oz)	20	3	2	1
Garden Salad	1½ cups (3 oz)	20	3	2	1
Italian Salad	1½ cups (3 oz)	20	3	2	1
Oriental Salad	1½ cups (3 oz)	120	11	3	1
Riviera Salad	1½ cups (3 oz)	10	2	2	1
Spinach Salad	1½ cups (3 oz)	130	23	13	3

Suddenly Salad

Caesar Low Fat Recipe as prep	¾ cup	170	30	3	1
Caesar as prep	¾ cup	220	30	3	1
Italian Pepperoni Low Fat Recipe as prep	1 cup	180	35	6	2
Italian Pepperoni as prep	1 cup	200	35	6	1
Ranch & Bacon Low Fat Recipe as prep	¾ cup	180	31	3	1
Ranch & Bacon as prep	¾ cup	320	31	3	1

Weight Watchers

Caesar Salad	1 serv (3.5 oz)	60	11	1	1
Caesar Salad w/ Cookies	1 pkg (4.3 oz)	160	29	12	3
European Salad	1 serv (3.5 oz)	60	13	9	2
European Salad w/ Cookies	1 pkg (4.3 oz)	160	31	11	2
Garden Salad	1 serv (3.5 oz)	60	12	4	1
Garden Salad w/ Cookies	1 pkg (4 oz)	120	24	10	2

SALAD DRESSING
HOME RECIPE

french	1 tbsp	88	1	—	—
vinegar & oil	1 tbsp	72	tr	—	—

FOOD	PORTION	CALS.	CARB.	SUG.	FIB.
MIX					
Good Seasons					
Cheese Garlic as prep	2 tbsp (1 oz)	140	1	1	0
Fat Free Honey Mustard as prep	2 tbsp (1.2 oz)	20	5	4	0
Fat Free Italian as prep	2 tbsp (1.1 oz)	10	2	3	0
Fat Free Ranch as prep	2 tbsp (1.2 oz)	20	5	4	0
Fat Free Zesty Herb as prep	2 tbsp (1.1 oz)	10	2	1	0
Garlic & Herbs as prep	2 tbsp (1 oz)	140	1	1	0
Gourmet Caesar as prep	2 tbsp (1.1 oz)	150	3	2	0
Gourmet Parmesan Italian as prep	2 tbsp (1.1 oz)	150	2	1	0
Honey French as prep	2 tbsp (1.2 oz)	160	5	4	0
Honey Mustard as prep	2 tbsp (1.1 oz)	150	3	2	0
Italian as prep	2 tbsp (1 oz)	140	1	1	0
Mexican Spice as prep	2 tbsp (1.1 oz)	140	2	1	0
Mild Italian as prep	2 tbsp (1.1 oz)	150	2	2	0
Oriental Sesame as prep	2 tbsp (1.1 oz)	150	3	2	0
Reduced Calorie Italian as prep	2 tbsp (1 oz)	50	2	1	0
Reduced Calorie Zesty Italian as prep	2 tbsp (1 oz)	50	2	1	0
Roasted Garlic as prep	2 tbsp (1.1 oz)	150	2	1	0
Zesty Italian as prep	2 tbsp (1 oz)	140	1	1	0
Hain					
No Oil 1000 Island	1 tbsp	12	3	—	—
No Oil Bleu Cheese	1 tbsp	14	1	—	—
No Oil Buttermilk	1 tbsp	11	1	—	—
No Oil Caesar	1 tbsp	6	1	—	—
No Oil French	1 tbsp	12	3	—	—
No Oil Garlic & Cheese	1 tbsp	6	1	—	—
No Oil Herb	1 tbsp	2	1	—	—
No Oil Italian	1 tbsp	2	1	—	—
READY-TO-EAT					
blue cheese	1 tbsp	77	1	—	—
french	1 tbsp	67	3	—	—
french reduced calorie	1 tbsp	22	4	—	—
italian	1 tbsp	69	2	—	—
italian reduced calorie	1 tbsp	16	1	—	—
russian	1 tbsp	76	2	—	—
russian reduced calorie	1 tbsp	23	5	—	—
sesame seed	1 tbsp	68	1	—	—
thousand island	1 tbsp	59	2	—	—
thousand island reduced calorie	1 tbsp	24	3	—	—

FOOD	PORTION	CALS.	CARB.	SUG.	FIB.
Estee					
Blue Cheese	2 tbsp (1 oz)	15	1	tr	—
Creamy French	2 tbsp (1 oz)	10	2	2	—
Creamy French Fat Free	1 pkg (0.5 oz)	5	1	1	—
Creamy Garlic	2 tbsp (1 oz)	60	2	2	—
Creamy Garlic Fat Free	1 pkg (0.5 oz)	5	1	1	—
Creamy Italian	2 tbsp (1 oz)	15	2	2	—
Fat Free Thousand Island	1 pkg (0.5 oz)	5	1	tr	—
Italian	2 tbsp (1 oz)	5	1	1	—
Italian Fat Free	1 pkg (0.5 oz)	0	tr	0	—
Low Fat Blue Cheese	1 pkg (0.5 oz)	5	tr	0	—
Thousand Island	2 tbsp (1 oz)	10	2	2	—
Hain					
1000 Island	1 tbsp	50	0	0	0
Canola Garden Tomato	1 tbsp	60	1	—	—
Canola Italian	1 tbsp	50	1	—	—
Canola Spicy French Mustard	1 tbsp	50	1	—	—
Canola Tangy Citrus	1 tbsp	50	1	—	—
Creamy Caesar	1 tbsp	60	1	—	—
Creamy Caesar Low Salt	1 tbsp	60	1	—	—
Creamy French	1 tbsp	60	1	—	—
Creamy Italian	1 tbsp	80	0	0	0
Creamy Italian No Salt Added	1 tbsp	80	1	—	—
Cucumber Dill	1 tbsp	80	0	0	0
Dijon Vinaigrette	1 tbsp	50	0	0	0
Garlic & Sour Cream	1 tbsp	70	0	0	0
Honey & Sesame	1 tbsp	60	2	—	—
Italian Cheese Vinaigrette	1 tbsp	55	0	0	0
Old Fashioned Buttermilk	1 tbsp	70	0	0	0
Poppyseed Rancher's	1 tbsp	60	0	0	0
Savory Herb No Salt Added	1 tbsp	90	0	0	0
Swiss Cheese Vinaigrette	1 tbsp	60	0	0	0
Traditional Italian	1 tbsp	80	0	0	0
Traditional Italian No Salt Added	1 tbsp	60	1	—	—
Hollywood					
Caesar	1 tbsp	70	2	—	0
Creamy French	1 tbsp	70	2	—	0
Creamy Italian	1 tbsp	90	2	—	0
Dijon Vinaigrette	1 tbsp	60	2	—	0
Italian	1 tbsp	90	1	—	0
Italian Cheese	1 tbsp	80	2	—	0

FOOD	PORTION	CALS.	CARB.	SUG.	FIB.
Hollywood (CONT.)					
Old Fashion Buttermilk	1 tbsp	75	1	—	0
Poppy Seed Rancher's	1 tbsp	75	1	—	0
Thousand Island	1 tbsp	60	3	—	0
Kraft					
⅓ Less Fat Catalina	2 tbsp (1.2 oz)	80	9	8	0
⅓ Less Fat Cucumber Ranch	2 tbsp (1.1 oz)	60	2	2	0
⅓ Less Fat Italian	2 tbsp (1.1 oz)	70	3	2	0
⅓ Less Fat Ranch	2 tbsp (1.1)	110	1	1	0
⅓ Less Fat Thousand Island	2 tbsp (1.2 oz)	70	7	5	0
Bacon & Tomato	2 tbsp (1.1 oz)	140	2	2	0
Buttermilk Ranch	2 tbsp (1.1 oz)	150	1	tr	0
Caesar Italian	2 tbsp (1.1 oz)	100	2	1	0
Caesar Ranch	2 tbsp (1.1 oz)	110	1	0	0
Catalina	2 tbsp (1.1 oz)	120	7	7	0
Catalina With Honey	2 tbsp (1.1 oz)	130	7	6	0
Classic Caesar	2 tbsp (1.1 oz)	110	1	0	0
Coleslaw	2 tbsp (1.1 oz)	130	7	7	0
Creamy French	2 tbsp (1.1 oz)	160	5	5	0
Creamy Garlic	2 tbsp (1.1 oz)	110	2	2	0
Creamy Italian	2 tbsp (1.1 oz)	110	2	2	0
Cucumber Ranch	2 tbsp (1.1 oz)	140	2	2	0
Free Blue Cheese	2 tbsp (1.2 oz)	45	11	2	1
Free Caesar Italian	2 tbsp (1.2 oz)	25	4	3	0
Free Catalina	2 tbsp (1.2 oz)	35	8	7	tr
Free Classic Caesar	2 tbsp (1.2 oz)	45	11	2	tr
Free Creamy Italian	2 tbsp (1.2 oz)	50	12	4	tr
Free French	2 tbsp (1.2 oz)	45	11	5	tr
Free Garlic Ranch	2 tbsp (1.2 oz)	45	11	2	1
Free Honey Dijon	2 tbsp (1.2 oz)	45	10	4	1
Free Italian	2 tbsp (1.2 oz)	20	4	2	0
Free Peppercorn Ranch	2 tbsp (1.2 oz)	45	11	2	tr
Free Ranch	1 tbsp (1.2 oz)	50	11	2	1
Free Red Wine Vinegar	2 tbsp (1.1 oz)	15	3	3	0
Free Thousand Island	2 tbsp (1.2 oz)	40	9	5	1
Garlic Ranch	2 tbsp (1.1 oz)	180	1	tr	0
Herb Vinaigrette	2 tbsp (1.1 oz)	140	tr	0	0
Honey Dijon	2 tbsp (1.1 oz)	110	6	4	0
Honey Mustard	2 tbsp (1.1 oz)	110	6	4	0
House Italian w/ Olive Oil Blend	2 tbsp (1.1 oz)	120	2	2	0
Peppercorn Ranch	2 tbsp (1 oz)	170	1	1	0

FOOD	PORTION	CALS.	CARB.	SUG.	FIB.
Kraft (CONT.)					
Pesto Italian	2 tbsp (1.1 oz)	90	2	1	0
Ranch	2 tbsp (1 oz)	170	1	1	0
Roka Blue Cheese	2 tbsp (1.1 oz)	130	2	tr	tr
Russian	2 tbsp (1.2 oz)	130	10	10	0
Sour Cream & Onion Ranch	2 tbsp (1 oz)	170	1	1	0
Thousand Island	2 tbsp (1.1 oz)	110	5	4	0
Thousand Island With Bacon	2 tbsp (1.1 oz)	130	5	5	0
Tomato & Herb Italian	2 tbsp (1.1 oz)	100	3	3	0
Zesty Italian	2 tbsp (1.1 oz)	110	2	1	0
Marzetti					
Bacon Spinach Salad	2 tbsp	80	16	0	15
Blue Cheese	2 tbsp	160	0	0	0
Buttermilk & Herb	2 tbsp	180	1	1	0
Buttermilk Bacon Ranch	2 tbsp	180	1	1	0
Buttermilk Blue Cheese	2 tbsp	160	1	1	0
Buttermilk Parmesan Pepper	2 tbsp	170	1	1	0
Buttermilk Parmesan Ranch	2 tbsp	160	1	1	0
Buttermilk Ranch	2 tbsp	180	1	1	0
Buttermilk Veggie Dip	2 tbsp	170	1	1	0
Caesar	2 tbsp	150	1	1	0
Caesar Ranch	2 tbsp	190	2	1	0
California French	2 tbsp	160	11	11	0
Celery Seed	2 tbsp	160	10	9	0
Chunky Blue Cheese	2 tbsp	150	1	1	0
Classic Caesar Ranch	2 tbsp	190	2	1	0
Country French	2 tbsp	150	7	7	0
Cracked Peppercorn	2 tbsp	140	1	0	0
Creamy Garlic Italian	2 tbsp	160	1	1	0
Creamy Italian	2 tbsp	150	1	1	0
Crispy Celery Seed	2 tbsp	160	11	10	0
Dijon Honey Mustard	2 tbsp	140	6	6	0
Dijon Ranch	2 tbsp	170	2	2	0
Dutch Sweet'N Sour	2 tbsp	160	10	10	0
Fat Free California French	2 tbsp	45	11	8	0
Fat Free Honey Dijon	2 tbsp	60	14	12	1
Fat Free Honey French	2 tbsp	45	11	8	0
Fat Free Italian	2 tbsp	15	3	2	0
Fat Free Peppercorn Ranch	2 tbsp	30	7	2	1
Fat Free Ranch	2 tbsp	30	7	2	1
Fat Free Raspberry	2 tbsp	70	18	14	0

FOOD	PORTION	CALS.	CARB.	SUG.	FIB.
Marzetti (CONT.)					
Fat Free Slaw	2 tbsp	45	11	9	0
Fat Free Sweet & Sour	2 tbsp	45	14	10	0
Fat Free Thousand Island	2 tbsp	35	9	6	0
Garden Ranch	2 tbsp	180	1	1	0
Gusto Italian	2 tbsp	120	1	1	0
Honey Dijon	2 tbsp	140	6	6	0
Honey Dijon Ranch	2 tbsp	150	2	2	0
Honey French	2 tbsp	160	11	11	0
Honey French Blue Cheese	2 tbsp	160	11	11	0
House Caesar	2 tbsp	150	1	0	0
Italian With Olive Oil	2 tbsp	120	1	1	0
Light Blue Cheese	2 tbsp	60	4	3	0
Light Buttermilk Ranch	2 tbsp	90	3	1	0
Light California French	2 tbsp	80	8	7	0
Light Chunky Blue Cheese	2 tbsp	80	4	1	0
Light French	2 tbsp	40	6	5	0
Light French	2 tbsp	40	6	5	0
Light Honey French	2 tbsp	80	12	12	0
Light Italian	2 tbsp	60	3	2	0
Light Ranch	2 tbsp	90	7	2	0
Light Red Wine Vinegar & Oil	2 tbsp	20	3	2	0
Light Slaw	2 tbsp	60	10	9	0
Light Sweet & Sour	2 tbsp	100	11	10	0
Light Thousand Island	2 tbsp	70	6	5	0
Old Fashioned Poppyseed	2 tbsp	140	10	10	0
Olde Venice Italain	2 tbsp	130	2	1	0
Olde World Caesar	2 tbsp	150	1	1	0
Parmesan Pepper	2 tbsp	160	1	1	0
Peppercorn Ranch	2 tbsp	180	1	1	0
Poppyseed	2 tbsp	160	10	7	0
Potato Salad Dressing	2 tbsp	120	7	6	0
Ranch	2 tbsp	180	1	1	0
Red Wine Vinegar & Oil	2 tbsp	130	2	2	0
Romano Cheese Caesar	2 tbsp	150	1	1	0
Romano Italian	2 tbsp	160	1	1	0
Savory Italian	2 tbsp	110	3	2	0
Slaw	2 tbsp	170	6	6	0
Southern Slaw	2 tbsp	100	14	13	0
Sweet & Saucy	2 tbsp	140	9	9	0
Sweet & Sour	2 tbsp	160	10	9	0
Thousand Island	2 tbsp	150	5	5	0
Vintage Champagne	2 tbsp	150	2	1	0

FOOD	PORTION	CALS.	CARB.	SUG.	FIB.
Marzetti (CONT.)					
Wilde Raspberry	2 tbsp	150	12	11	0
Nasoya					
Creamy Dill	2 tbsp (1 oz)	63	3	2	tr
Creamy Italian	2 tbsp (1 oz)	60	3	2	tr
Garden Herb	2 tbsp (1 oz)	61	3	2	tr
Sesame Garlic	2 tbsp (1 oz)	63	3	2	tr
Thousand Island	2 tbsp (1 oz)	62	6	5	tr
Newman's Own					
Balsamic Vinaigrette	2 tbsp (1.1 oz)	90	3	1	0
Caesar	2 tbsp (1.1 oz)	150	1	1	0
Light Italian	2 tbsp (1.1 oz)	20	3	2	0
Olive Oil & Vinegar	2 tbsp (1 oz)	150	1	1	0
Ranch	2 tbsp (1 oz)	180	2	1	0
Pfeiffer					
1000 Island	2 tbsp	140	4	4	0
California French	2 tbsp	140	9	9	0
French	2 tbsp	150	7	7	0
Honey Dijon	2 tbsp	140	6	6	0
Lite Italian	2 tbsp	50	3	2	0
Ranch	2 tbsp	180	1	1	0
Savory Italian	2 tbsp	110	3	2	0
Pritikin					
Dijon Balsamic Vinaigrette	2 tbsp (1 oz)	3	6	—	—
French	2 tbsp (1 oz)	35	8	—	—
Honey Dijon	2 tbsp (1 oz)	45	11	—	—
Honey French	2 tbsp (1 oz)	40	11	—	—
Italian	2 tbsp (1 oz)	20	5	—	—
Raspberry Vinaigrette	2 tbsp (1 oz)	45	11	—	—
Red Wing					
"K" Dressing	1 tbsp (0.5 oz)	70	4	2	0
Chunky Blue Cheese	2 tbsp (1 oz)	130	3	2	0
Creamy Ranch	2 tbsp (1 oz)	150	2	0	0
French Traditional	2 tbsp (1 oz)	130	8	4	0
Italian Traditional	2 tbsp (1 oz)	100	4	3	0
Spicy Sweet French	2 tbsp (1 oz)	130	8	6	0
Thousand Island Thick & Rich	2 tbsp (1 oz)	110	8	6	0
S&W					
Blue Cheese Low Calorie	1 tbsp	25	2	—	—
Creamy Cucumber Low Calorie	1 tbsp	25	2	—	—
Creamy Italian Low Calorie	1 tbsp	10	1	—	—
French Low Calorie	1 tbsp	18	3	—	—

FOOD	PORTION	CALS.	CARB.	SUG.	FIB.
S&W (CONT.)					
Italian No-Oil	1 tbsp	2	0	0	0
Russian Low Calorie	1 tbsp	25	4	—	—
Thousand Island Low Calorie	1 tbsp	25	2	—	—
Seven Seas					
⅓ Less Fat Creamy Italian	2 tbsp (1.1 oz)	60	2	2	0
⅓ Less Fat Italian w/ Olive Oil Blend	2 tbsp (1.1 oz)	45	2	2	0
⅓ Less Fat Ranch	2 tbsp (1.1 oz)	100	5	2	0
⅓ Less Fat Red Wine Vinegar & Oil	2 tbsp (1.1 oz)	45	3	2	0
⅓ Less Fat Viva Italian	2 tbsp (1.1 oz)	45	2	1	0
2 Cheese Italian	2 tbsp (1.1 oz)	70	3	2	0
Chunky Blue Cheese	2 tbsp (1.1 oz)	130	2	tr	tr
Classic Caesar	2 tbsp (1.1 oz)	100	2	1	0
Creamy Italian	2 tbsp (1.1 oz)	120	1	1	0
Free Ranch	2 tbsp (1.2 oz)	45	11	2	1
Free Red Wine Vinegar	2 tbsp (1.1 oz)	15	3	3	0
Free Sour Cream & Onion Ranch	2 tbsp (1.2 oz)	50	11	3	1
Free Viva Italian	2 tbsp (1.1 oz)	10	2	1	1
Green Goddess	2 tbsp (1.1 oz)	130	1	tr	0
Herbs & Spices	2 tbsp (1.1 oz)	90	1	1	0
Ranch	2 tbsp (1.1 oz)	160	2	1	0
Red Wine Vinegar & Oil	2 tbsp (1.1 oz)	90	2	2	0
Viva Italian	2 tbsp (1.1 oz)	90	2	1	0
Viva Russian	2 tbsp (1.1 oz)	150	3	2	0
Tree Of Life					
Cafe Venice	2 tbsp (1 oz)	100	2	2	0
Fat Free Blue Cheese	2 tbsp (1 oz)	15	2	—	—
Fat Free Honey French	2 tbsp (1 oz)	35	8	8	—
Fat Free Italian Garlic	2 tbsp (1 oz)	20	4	—	—
Fat Free Oriental Ginger	2 tbsp (1 oz)	15	3	—	—
Frisco's Raspberry	2 tbsp (1 oz)	120	5	3	0
Maison Caesar	2 tbsp (1 oz)	70	1	0	0
Shanghai Palace	2 tbsp (1 oz)	80	3	0	0
Ultra Slim-Fast					
French	1 tbsp	20	4	—	0
Italian	1 tbsp	6	1	—	0
W.J. Clark					
Ginger Orange Vinaigrette	1 tbsp	73	tr	1	0
Herbs & Romano	1 tbsp	67	2	1	0
Lemon Peppercorn	1 tbsp	72	tr	tr	0

FOOD	PORTION	CALS.	CARB.	SUG.	FIB.
W.J. Clark (CONT.)					
Lime Cilantro Vinaigrette	1 tbsp	73	tr	tr	0
Poppy Seed	1 tbsp	75	3	3	0
Sweet Pepper Basil	1 tbsp	69	2	2	0
Tarragon Honey Mustard	1 tbsp	66	2	2	0
Walden Farms					
Fat Free Balsamic Vinaigrette	2 tbsp (1 oz)	15	3	2	0
Fat Free Bleu Cheese	2 tbsp (1 oz)	25	4	3	0
Fat Free Caesar	2 tbsp (1 oz)	25	4	2	0
Fat Free Creamy Italian With Parmesan	1 tbsp (1 oz)	25	4	2	0
Fat Free French Style	2 tbsp (1 oz)	25	4	2	0
Fat Free Honey Dijon	2 tbsp (1 oz)	25	6	2	0
Fat Free Italian	2 tbsp (1 oz)	10	2	2	0
Fat Free Ranch	2 tbsp (1 oz)	25	4	2	0
Fat Free Raspberry Vinaigrette	2 tbsp (1 oz)	20	4	4	0
Fat Free Russian	2 tbsp (1 oz)	30	6	5	0
Fat Free Sodium Free Italian	2 tbsp (1 oz)	10	2	2	0
Fat Free Sugar Free Italian	2 tbsp (1 oz)	0	0	0	0
Fat Free Thousand Island	2 tbsp (1 oz)	35	7	5	0
Italian With Sun Dried Tomato	2 tbsp (1 oz)	15	3	2	0
Ranch With Sun Dried Tomato	2 tbsp (1 oz)	25	4	2	0
Weight Watchers					
Fat Free Caesar	1 pkg (0.75 oz)	5	1	1	0
Fat Free Caesar	2 tbsp	10	1	1	0
Fat Free Creamy Italian	2 tbsp	30	7	2	0
Fat Free French Style	2 tbsp	40	9	6	0
Fat Free Honey Dijon	2 tbsp	45	11	5	0
Fat Free Italian	2 tbsp	10	2	1	0
Fat Free Ranch	1 pkg (0.75 oz)	25	6	2	0
Fat Free Ranch	2 tbsp	35	7	3	0
Wishbone					
Caesar	2 tbsp (1 oz)	90	2	2	0
Chunky Blue Cheese	2 tbsp (1 oz)	150	3	1	0
Classic House Italian	2 tbsp (1 oz)	140	2	1	0
Classic Olive Oil Italian	2 tbsp (1 oz)	60	4	3	0
Creamy Caesar	2 tbsp (1 oz)	180	1	1	0
Creamy Italian	2 tbsp (1 oz)	110	4	1	0
Creamy Roasted Garlic	2 tbsp (1 oz)	110	3	3	0
Deluxe French	2 tbsp (1 oz)	120	5	4	0

FOOD	PORTION	CALS.	CARB.	SUG.	FIB.
Wishbone (CONT.)					
Fat Free Chunky Blue Cheese	2 tbsp (1 oz)	35	7	1	tr
Fat Free Chunky Blue Cheese	2 tbsp	35	7	1	tr
Fat Free Creamy Italian	2 tbsp (1 oz)	35	9	3	tr
Fat Free Creamy Roasted Garlic	2 tbsp (1 oz)	40	9	3	0
Fat Free Deluxe French	2 tbsp (1 oz)	30	7	6	tr
Fat Free Honey Dijon	2 tbsp (1 oz)	45	10	9	0
Fat Free Italian	2 tbsp (1 oz)	10	2	1	0
Fat Free Parmesan & Onion	2 tbsp (1 oz)	45	9	2	tr
Fat Free Ranch	2 tbsp (1 oz)	40	9	2	tr
Fat Free Red Wine Vinaigrette	2 tbsp (1 oz)	35	7	6	0
Fat Free Sweet N' Spicy French	2 tbsp (1 oz)	30	7	6	0
Fat Free Thousand Island	2 tbsp (1 oz)	35	9	6	tr
Italian	2 tbsp (1 oz)	80	3	2	0
Lite French	2 tbsp (1 oz)	50	8	7	0
Lite Italian	2 tbsp (1 oz)	15	2	1	0
Lite Ranch	2 tbsp (1 oz)	100	5	1	0
Olive Oil Vinaigrette	2 tbsp (1 oz)	60	4	3	0
Oriental	2 tbsp (1 oz)	70	5	3	0
Parmesan & Onion	2 tbsp (1 oz)	110	5	1	0
Ranch	2 tbsp (1 oz)	160	1	1	0
Red Wine Vinaigrette	2 tbsp (1 oz)	80	9	8	0
Robusto Italian	2 tbsp (1 oz)	90	4	3	0
Russian	2 tbsp (1 oz)	110	15	7	0
Sweet N' Spicy French	2 tbsp (1 oz)	140	6	5	0
Thousand Island	2 tbsp (1 oz)	140	7	6	0
SALMON					
CANNED					
chum w/ bone	1 can (13.9 oz)	521	0	0	0
chum w/ bone	3 oz	120	0	0	0
pink w/ bone	1 can (15.9 oz)	631	0	0	0
pink w/ bone	3 oz	118	0	0	0
sockeye w/ bone	1 can (12.9 oz)	566	0	0	0
sockeye w/ bone	3 oz	130	0	0	0
Bumble Bee					
Keta	3.5 oz	160	0	0	0
Pink	3.5 oz	160	0	0	0
Pink Skinless & Boneless	3.25 oz	120	0	0	0

FOOD	PORTION	CALS.	CARB.	SUG.	FIB.
Bumble Bee (CONT.)					
Red	3.5 oz	180	0	0	0
Red Skinless & Boneless	3.25 oz	130	0	0	0
Deming's					
Alaska Keta	½ cup	140	0	0	0
Alaska Pink	½ cup	140	0	0	0
Alaska Red Sockeye	½ cup	170	0	0	0
Double Q					
Alaska Pink	½ cup	140	0	0	0
Humpty Dumpty					
Alaska Chum	½ cup	140	0	0	0
S&W					
Bluepack Fancy Diet	½ cup	188	0	0	0
Red Fancy Sockeye Bluepack	½ cup	190	0	0	0
FRESH					
atlantic baked	3 oz	155	0	0	0
chinook baked	3 oz	196	0	0	0
chum baked	3 oz	131	0	0	0
coho cooked	3 oz	157	0	0	0
coho cooked	½ fillet (5.4 oz)	286	0	0	0
coho raw	3 oz	124	0	0	0
pink baked	3 oz	127	0	0	0
roe raw	3.5 oz	207	1	—	—
sockeye cooked	½ fillet (5.4 oz)	334	0	0	0
sockeye cooked	3 oz	183	0	0	0
sockeye raw	3 oz	143	0	0	0
SMOKED					
chinook	1 oz	33	0	0	0
chinook	3 oz	99	0	0	0
Nathan's					
Nova	2 oz	80	1	0	0

SALSA

(*see also* KETCHUP, SAUCE, SPANISH FOODS)

FOOD	PORTION	CALS.	CARB.	SUG.	FIB.
Casa Fiesta					
Chili Salsa	1 oz	9	2	—	—
Picante Mild	1 oz	9	2	—	—
Chi-Chi's					
Con Queso	2 tbsp (1.1 oz)	90	4	3	0
Hot	2 tbsp (1 oz)	10	2	1	0
Medium	2 tbsp (1 oz)	10	2	1	0
Mild	2 tbsp (1 oz)	10	1	1	0
Picante Hot	2 tbsp (1 oz)	10	2	2	0

FOOD	PORTION	CALS.	CARB.	SUG.	FIB.
Chi-Chi's (CONT.)					
Picante Medium	2 tbsp (1 oz)	10	2	2	0
Picante Mild	2 tbsp (1 oz)	10	2	2	0
Verde Medium	2 tbsp (1.2 oz)	15	3	2	0
Verde Mild	2 tbsp (1.2 oz)	15	3	2	0
Del Monte					
Mexicana	2 tbsp (1.1 oz)	5	2	0	1
Taquera	2 tbsp (1.1 oz)	5	2	0	1
Verde	2 tbsp (1.1 oz)	10	2	1	tr
Guiltless Gourmet					
Picante Hot	1 oz	6	1	—	tr
Picante Medium	1 oz	6	1	—	tr
Hain					
Hot	¼ cup	22	4	—	—
Mild	¼ cup	20	4	—	—
Heluva Good Cheese					
Cheese & Salsa	2 tbsp (1.1 oz)	80	3	3	0
Thick & Chunky Hot	2 tbsp (1.2 oz)	10	2	2	0
Thick & Chunky Mild	2 tbsp (1.2 oz)	10	2	2	0
Hot Cha Cha					
Medium	2 tbsp (1 oz)	5	2	0	—
Hunt's					
Alfresco Medium	2 tbsp (1.1 oz)	10	2	1	tr
Alfresco Mild	2 tbsp (1.1 oz)	10	2	1	tr
Hot	2 tbsp (1.1 oz)	27	6	1	1
Medium	2 tbsp (1.1 oz)	27	6	1	1
Mild	2 tbsp (1.1 oz)	27	6	1	1
Picante Medium	2 tbsp (1.1 oz)	11	2	1	tr
Picante Mild	2 tbsp (1.1 oz)	11	2	1	tr
Louise's					
Fat Free BBQ Black Bean	1 oz	10	2	0	0
Fat Free Black Bean	1 oz	10	2	0	0
Fat Free Medium	1 oz	10	3	1	1
Fat Free Mild	1 oz	10	3	1	1
Fat Free Nacho Queso	1 oz	15	3	1	0
Muir Glen					
Organic Fat Free Hot	2 tbsp (1.1 oz)	10	2	1	0
Organic Fat Free Medium	2 tbsp (1.1 oz)	10	2	1	0
Organic Fat Free Mild	2 tbsp (1.1 oz)	10	2	1	0
Newman's Own					
Bandito Hot	2 tbsp (1.1 oz)	10	2	1	tr
Bandito Medium	2 tbsp (1.1 oz)	10	2	1	tr
Bandito Mild	2 tbsp (1.1 oz)	10	2	1	tr
Peach	2 tbsp (1.1 oz)	25	6	5	1

FOOD	PORTION	CALS.	CARB.	SUG.	FIB.
Newman's Own (CONT.)					
Pineapple	2 tbsp (1.1 oz)	15	3	3	1
Roasted Garlic	2 tbsp (1.1 oz)	10	2	1	1
Old El Paso					
Green Chili Medium	2 tbsp (1 oz)	10	2	tr	tr
Homestyle	2 tbsp (1 oz)	5	1	1	0
Homestyle Mild	2 tbsp (1 oz)	5	1	1	0
Picante Hot	2 tbsp (1 oz)	10	2	1	0
Picante Medium	2 tbsp (1 oz)	10	2	1	0
Picante Mild	2 tbsp (1 oz)	10	2	1	0
Picante Thick'n Chunky Hot	2 tbsp (1 oz)	10	2	1	0
Picante Thick'n Chunky Medium	2 tbsp (1 oz)	10	2	1	0
Picante Thick'n Chunky Mild	2 tbsp (1 oz)	10	2	1	0
Pico De Gallo Hot	2 tbsp (1 oz)	5	2	tr	tr
Pico De Gallo Medium	1 tbsp (1 oz)	5	2	tr	tr
Salsa Verde	2 tbsp (1 oz)	10	2	tr	0
Thick'n Chunky Hot	2 tbsp (1 oz)	10	2	1	0
Thick'n Chunky Medium	2 tbsp (1 oz)	10	2	1	0
Thick'n Chunky Mild	2 tbsp (1 oz)	10	2	1	0
Ortega					
Hot Green Chili	1 tbsp	6	2	—	—
Medium Green Chili	1 tbsp	6	1	—	—
Mild Green Chili	1 tbsp	8	2	—	—
Pace					
Picante	2 tbsp (1 fl oz)	7	2	1	tr
Thick & Chunky	2 tbsp (1 fl oz)	12	2	1	1
Progresso					
Italian Hot	2 tbsp (1 oz)	30	2	1	tr
Italian Medium	2 tbsp (1 oz)	10	2	1	tr
Italian Mild	2 tbsp (1 oz)	10	2	1	tr
Rosarita					
Chunky Hot	3 tbsp (1.5 oz)	25	6	—	tr
Chunky Medium	3 tbsp (1.5 oz)	25	6	—	tr
Chunky Mild	3 tbsp (1.5 oz)	25	6	—	tr
Taco Salsa Chunky Medium	3 tbsp (1.5 oz)	25	6	—	tr
Taco Salsa Chunky Mild	3 tbsp (1.5 oz)	25	6	—	tr
Tabasco					
Picante	2 tbsp (1.5 oz)	17	3	2	1
Taco Bell					
Smooth 'N Zesty Picante Medium	2 tbsp (1.1 oz)	15	3	2	tr
Smooth 'N Zesty Picante Mild	2 tbsp (1.1 oz)	15	3	2	tr

FOOD	PORTION	CALS.	CARB.	SUG.	FIB.
Taco Bell (CONT.)					
Thick 'N Chunky Salsa Hot	2 tbsp (1.1 oz)	15	2	2	tr
Thick 'N Chunky Salsa Medium	2 tbsp (1.1 oz)	15	2	2	tr
Thick 'N Chunky Salsa Mild	2 tbsp (1.1 oz)	15	3	2	tr
Tostitos					
Hot	2 tbsp (1 oz)	12	3	1	1
Medium	2 tbsp (1 oz)	12	3	1	1
Mild	2 tbsp (1 oz)	12	3	1	1
Tree Of Life					
Hot	2 tbsp (1 oz)	10	2	1	—
Medium	2 tbsp (1 oz)	10	2	1	—
Mild	2 tbsp (1 oz)	10	2	1	—
No Salt	2 tbsp (1 oz)	10	2	1	—
Watkins					
Salsa Seasoning Blend	⅛ tsp (0.5 g)	0	0	0	0
Tropical	2 tbsp (1 oz)	60	13	13	0
Wise					
Picante	2 tbsp	12	3	—	—

SALSIFY

FOOD	PORTION	CALS.	CARB.	SUG.	FIB.
fresh sliced cooked	½ cup	46	10	—	—
raw sliced	½ cup	55	12	—	—

SALT/SEASONED SALT
(*see also* SALT SUBSTITUTES)

FOOD	PORTION	CALS.	CARB.	SUG.	FIB.
salt	1 tbsp (18 g)	0	0	0	0
salt	1 tsp (6 g)	0	0	0	0
Hain					
Sea Salt	1 tsp	0	0	0	0
Sea Salt Iodized	1 tsp	0	0	0	0
Watkins					
Bacon Cheese Salt	¼ tbsp (1 g)	0	0	0	0
Butter Salt	¼ tbsp (1 g)	0	0	0	0
Cheese Salt	¼ tbsp (1 g)	0	0	0	0
Garlic Salt	¼ tsp (1 g)	0	0	0	0
Salt & Vinegar Seasoning	¼ tsp (1 g)	0	0	0	0
Seasoning Salt	¼ tsp (1 g)	0	0	0	0
Sour Cream & Onion Salt	¼ tbsp (1 g)	0	0	0	0

SALT SUBSTITUTES
Cardia

FOOD	PORTION	CALS.	CARB.	SUG.	FIB.
Salt Alternative	1 pkg (0.6 g)	0	0	0	0
Mrs. Dash					
Onion & Herb	⅛ tsp (0.02 oz)	2	tr	—	—

FOOD	PORTION	CALS.	CARB.	SUG.	FIB.
NoSalt					
Salt Alternative	1 pkg (0.75 g)	0	0	0	0
Papa Dash					
Lite Salt	½ tsp (1 g)	0	1	—	—
SAPODILLA					
fresh	1	140	34	—	—
fresh cut up	1 cup	199	48	—	—
SAPOTES					
fresh	1	301	76	—	—
SARDINES					
CANNED					
atlantic in oil w/ bone	2	50	0	0	0
atlantic in oil w/ bone	1 can (3.2 oz)	192	0	0	0
pacific in tomato sauce w/ bone	1	68	0	0	0
pacific in tomato sauce w/ bone	1 can (13 oz)	658	0	0	0
Del Monte					
In Tomato Sauce	1 fish (1.4 oz)	50	1	0	tr
Empress					
Skinless & Boneless Olive Oil	1 can (3.8 oz)	420	2	—	—
Skinless & Boneless Soy Oil	1 can (4.4 oz)	500	2	—	—
Port Clyde					
In Louisiana Hot Sauce	1 can (3.75 oz)	170	1	0	0
In Mustard Sauce	1 can (3.75 oz)	150	1	0	1
In Soybean Oil Select Small	1 can (3.3 oz)	220	0	0	0
In Soybean Oil With Hot Chilies	1 can (3.3 oz)	155	0	0	0
In Soybean Oil drained	1 can (3.3 oz)	220	0	0	0
In Spring Water	1 can (3.3 oz)	170	0	0	0
In Tomato Sauce	1 can (3.75 oz)	150	0	0	0
S&W					
Norwegian Brisling	1.5 oz	130	0	0	0
Underwood					
Brisling In Olive Oil	3.75 oz	260	1	—	—
In Mustard Sauce	3.75 oz	220	2	—	—
In Sild Oil drained	3.75 oz	460	1	—	—
In Soya Oil drained	3 oz	230	1	—	—
In Tomato Sauce	3.75 oz	220	2	—	—

FOOD	PORTION	CALS.	CARB.	SUG.	FIB.
Underwood (CONT.)					
With Tabasco Pepper Sauce drained	3 oz	220	1	—	—
Viking's Delight					
Brisling In Olive Oil	1 can (3.75 oz)	460	1	—	—
Brisling In Olive Oil drained	1 can (3.75 oz)	260	1	—	—
FRESH					
raw	3½ oz	135	0	0	0

SAUCE

(*see also* BARBECUE SAUCE, GRAVY, PIZZA, SALSA, SPAGHETTI SAUCE, TOMATO)

FOOD	PORTION	CALS.	CARB.	SUG.	FIB.
JARRED					
teriyaki	1 tbsp	15	3	—	—
teriyaki	1 oz	30	6	—	—
Armour					
Chili Hot Dog	¼ cup (2.2 oz)	120	6	—	—
Meatless Sloppy Joe Sauce	¼ cup (2.2 oz)	30	7	—	—
Best Foods					
Tartar	1 tbsp (14 g)	70	tr	—	—
Casa Fiesta					
Taco Mild	1 oz	9	2	—	—
Cheez Whiz					
Cheese	2 tbsp (1.2 oz)	90	3	tr	0
Cheese Jalapeno Pepper	2 tbsp (1.2 oz)	90	3	2	0
Cheese Mild Salsa	2 tbsp (1.2 oz)	100	3	2	0
Chi-Chi's					
Enchilada	¼ cup (2.1 oz)	30	3	0	0
Taco	1 tbsp (0.5 oz)	10	1	1	0
Contadina					
Sweet 'n Sour	2 tbsp	40	8	7	—
Del Monte					
Cocktail	¼ cup (2.7 oz)	100	24	22	0
Sloppy Joe Hickory Flavor	¼ cup (2.4 oz)	70	18	15	0
Sloppy Joe Italian Style	¼ cup (2.4 oz)	70	16	12	0
Sloppy Joe Original	¼ cup (2.4 oz)	70	16	13	0
El Molino					
Taco Red Mild	2 tbsp	10	2	—	—
Escoffier					
Diable	1 tbsp	20	4	—	—
Gebhardt					
Enchilada Sauce	3 tbsp (1.5 oz)	25	2	—	tr
Hot Dog Chili Sauce	2 tbsp	30	4	—	tr
Hot Sauce	½ tsp	tr	tr	—	tr

FOOD	PORTION	CALS.	CARB.	SUG.	FIB.
Gold's					
Rib	1 oz	60	14	—	—
Golden Dipt					
Cajun Style	1 oz	90	5	—	—
Creole	1 oz	20	2	—	—
Dijonaisse	1 oz	52	2	—	—
French White	1 oz	55	3	—	—
Ginger Teriyaki Marinade	1 oz	120	12	—	—
Lemon Butter Dill	1 oz	100	4	—	—
Lemon Herb Marinade	1 oz	130	2	—	—
Seafood Cocktail	1 tbsp	20	5	—	—
Seafood Cocktail Extra Hot	1 tbsp	20	5	—	—
Tartar	1 tbsp	70	2	—	—
Tartar Lite	1 tbsp	50	4	—	—
Green Giant					
Sloppy Joe	¼ cup (2.6 oz)	50	11	8	2
Sloppy Joe as prep w/ meat	1 serv (4.4 oz)	200	11	8	2
Heinz					
Worcestershire	1 tbsp	6	1	—	—
Hellman's					
Tartar	1 tbsp (14 g)	70	tr	—	—
Heluva Good Cheese					
Cocktail	¼ cup (1.6 oz)	40	10	—	—
Hormel					
Not-So-Sloppy- Joe Sauce	¼ cup (2.2 oz)	70	15	3	1
House Of Tsang					
Bangkok Padang	1 tbsp (0.6 oz)	45	4	3	0
Hoisin	1 tsp (6 g)	15	4	3	0
Mandarin Marinade	1 tbsp (0.6 oz)	25	6	5	0
Saigon Sizzle	1 tbsp (0.6 oz)	40	8	6	0
Spicy Brown Bean	1 tsp (6 g)	15	3	3	0
Stir Fry Classic	1 tbsp (0.6 oz)	25	4	3	0
Stir Fry Sweet & Sour	1 tbsp (0.6 oz)	30	7	6	0
Stir Fry Szechuan Spicy	1 tbsp (0.6 oz)	20	4	3	0
Sweet & Sour Concentrate	1 tsp (6 g)	10	3	2	0
Teriyaki Korean	1 tbsp (0.6 oz)	30	6	4	0
Hunt's					
Chicken Sensations Barbecue Flavor	1 tbsp (0.5 oz)	35	3	2	tr
Chicken Sensations Italian Garlic	1 tbsp (0.5 oz)	30	1	1	1
Chicken Sensations Lemon Herb	1 tbsp (0.5 oz)	31	2	1	tr
Chicken Sensations South Western	1 tbsp (0.5 oz)	27	1	1	tr

FOOD	PORTION	CALS.	CARB.	SUG.	FIB.
Hunt's (CONT.)					
Pepper Sauce Original	1 tsp (5.2 g)	1	tr	0	0
Steak	1 tbsp (0.6 oz)	10	2	2	tr
Just Rite					
Hot Dog	2 oz	60	6	—	tr
Ka-Me					
Black Bean Sauce	1 tbsp (0.5 oz)	10	2	1	1
Chili Sauce Hot Garlic	1 tbsp (0.5 oz)	15	4	2	1
Duck Sauce	2 tbsp (1 oz)	80	20	16	0
Fish Sauce	1 tbsp (0.5 fl oz)	10	1	1	0
Hoisin Sauce	2 tbsp (1 oz)	45	10	8	1
Hot Sauce	1 tsp (5 g)	0	1	0	0
Lemon Sauce	1 tbsp (0.5 oz)	45	11	5	0
Mandarin Orange Sauce	2 tbsp (1 oz)	80	21	3	0
Oyster Sauce	1 tbsp (0.5 fl oz)	10	3	2	0
Plum	2 tbsp (1 fl oz)	80	19	17	0
Stir Fry Sauce	1 tbsp	10	1	1	0
Sweet & Sour	2 tbsp (1 fl oz)	50	13	11	0
Szechuan	1 tbsp (0.5 oz)	20	2	1	2
Tamari	1 tbsp (0.5 fl oz)	10	1	1	0
Tempura Sauce	2 tbsp (1 fl oz)	15	3	3	0
Teriyaki Sauce	1 tbsp (0.5 fl oz)	10	2	1	0
Kikkoman					
Stir-Fry	1 tbsp	16	3	—	1
Sweet & Sour	1 tbsp	19	4	—	tr
Teriyaki	1 tbsp	15	3	—	0
Knorr					
Grilling And Broiling Chardonnay	1.6 oz	50	4	—	—
Grilling And Broiling Spicy Plum	1.7 oz	60	11	—	—
Grilling And Broiling Tequilla Lime	1.6 oz	50	6	—	—
Grilling And Broiling Tuscan Herb	1.6 oz	50	5	—	—
Microwave Hollandaise	1 oz	50	1	—	—
Microwave Mandarin Ginger	1.6 oz	50	5	—	—
Microwave Parmesano	1.6 oz	50	3	—	—
Microwave Vera Cruz	3.3 oz	70	9	—	—
Kraft					
Cocktail	¼ cup (2.3 oz)	60	13	9	1
Fat Free Tartar Sauce	2 tbsp (1.1 oz)	25	5	4	0
Lemon & Herb Tartar Sauce	2 tbsp (1 oz)	150	tr	tr	0

FOOD	PORTION	CALS.	CARB.	SUG.	FIB.
Kraft (CONT.)					
Reduced Fat Sandwich Spread	1 tbsp (0.5 oz)	35	3	3	0
Sandwich Spread	1 tbsp (0.5 oz)	50	3	2	0
Sweet'n Sour	2 tbsp (1.2 oz)	60	14	12	0
Tartar	2 tbsp (1.1 oz)	90	4	0	2
La Choy					
Duck Sauce Sweet & Sour	1 tbsp	25	7	—	tr
Sweet & Sour	1 tbsp	25	7	—	tr
Lawry's					
Marinade Lemon Pepper	1 tbsp (0.5 oz)	10	1	1	—
Teriyaki Marinade	2 tbsp	72	11	—	tr
Lea & Perrins					
Steak	1 oz	40	10	—	—
Worcestershire	1 tsp	5	1	—	—
Worcestershire White Wine	1 tsp	4	1	—	—
Manwich					
Bold	¼ cup (2.2 oz)	62	13	11	1
Burrito	¼ cup (2.2 oz)	25	6	1	4
Mexican	¼ cup (2.2 oz)	27	5	5	1
Original	¼ cup (2.2 oz)	32	6	5	1
Taco	¼ cup (2.2 oz)	31	7	3	1
Thick & Chunky	¼ cup (2.3 oz)	44	9	7	1
Marzetti					
Teriyaki Stir-Fry	2 tbsp	80	14	8	0
McIlhenny					
Tabasco	1 tsp	1	tr	tr	tr
Mrs. Dash					
Steak	1 tbsp (0.4 oz)	17	4	—	—
Newman's Own					
Spicy Simmer Sauce Diavolo	½ cup (4.4 oz)	70	10	4	3
Old El Paso					
Enchilada Hot	¼ cup (2 oz)	30	4	tr	0
Enchilada Mild	¼ cup (2 oz)	25	4	tr	0
Green Chili Enchilada Sauce	¼ cup (2.1 oz)	30	3	tr	0
Taco Hot	1 tbsp (0.5 oz)	5	1	0	0
Taco Medium	1 tbsp (0.5 oz)	5	1	0	0
Taco Mild	1 tbsp (0.5 oz)	5	1	0	0
Taco Sauce	1 tbsp (0.5 oz)	5	1	0	0
Taco Sauce Extra Chunky Medium	1 tbsp (0.5 oz)	5	1	0	0
Taco Sauce Extra Chunky Mild	1 tbsp (0.5 oz)	5	1	0	0

FOOD	PORTION	CALS.	CARB.	SUG.	FIB.
Ortega					
Taco Thick & Smooth Hot	1 tbsp	8	2	—	0
Taco Thick & Smooth Mild	1 tbsp	8	2	—	0
Progresso					
Alfredo	½ cup (4.4 oz)	310	5	0	0
Red Wing					
Chili Sauce	1 tbsp (0.6 oz)	20	5	3	0
Seafood Cocktail	¼ cup (2 oz)	90	22	12	0
Sauce Arturo					
Original	¼ cup (2.2 fl oz)	50	8	4	0
Simmer Chef					
Golden Honey Mustard	½ cup (4 fl oz)	150	30	29	1
Hearty Onion & Mushroom	½ cup (4 fl oz)	50	9	2	1
Snow's					
Newburg With Sherry	⅓ cup	120	10	—	—
Welsh Rarebit Cheese	½ cup	170	10	—	—
Tabasco					
Caribbean Steak Sauce	1 tbsp (0.6 oz)	15	4	3	0
Garlic Basting Sauce	1 tbsp (0.6 oz)	20	4	4	0
Habanero Sauce	1 tsp (0.2 oz)	5	1	tr	0
Hot Sauce w/ Garlic	1 tsp (0.2 oz)	0	0	0	0
Jalapeno Pepper Sauce	1 tbsp	15	3	0	tr
New Orleans Steak Sauce	1 tbsp (0.6 oz)	15	4	3	0
Pepper Sauce	1 tsp (0.2 oz)	0	0	0	0
Taco Bell					
Taco Sauce Medium	2 tbsp (1.1 oz)	15	3	1	tr
Taco Sauce Mild	2 tbsp (1.1 oz)	15	3	1	tr
The Restaurant Hot Sauce	1 tsp (5 g)	0	0	0	0
Watkins					
Inferno Hot Pepper Sauce	2 tbsp (1 oz)	35	8	7	1
Steak Sauce	1 tbsp (0.5 oz)	20	4	2	0
Wolf Brand					
Hot Dog	1.25 oz	44	4	—	—
MIX					
bearnaise as prep w/ milk & butter	1 cup	701	18	—	—
cheese as prep w/ milk	1 cup	307	23	—	—
curry as prep w/ milk	1 cup	270	26	—	—
mushroom as prep w/ milk	1 cup	228	24	—	—
sourcream as prep w/ milk	1 cup	509	45	—	—
stroganoff as prep	1 cup	271	34	—	—
sweet & sour as prep	1 cup	294	73	—	—
teriyaki as prep	1 cup	131	28	—	—
white as prep w/ milk	1 cup	241	21	—	—

FOOD	PORTION	CALS.	CARB.	SUG.	FIB.
Cajun King					
Etoufee Seasoning Mix	3.5 oz	383	70	—	—
Jambalaya Seasoning Mix	3.5 oz	375	61	—	—
Durkee					
A La King as prep	1 cup	60	8	2	0
Cheese as prep	¼ cup	25	4	0	0
Hollandaise as prep	2 tbsp	10	2	0	0
Nacho Cheese as prep	2 tbsp	25	2	0	0
White as prep	¼ cup	20	5	0	0
French's					
Cheese as prep	¼ cup	25	4	0	0
Hollandaise as prep	2 tbsp	10	2	0	0
Knorr					
Au Jus as prep	2 oz	8	1	—	—
Bearnaise as prep	2 oz	170	5	—	—
Classic Brown Gravy as prep	2 oz	25	3	—	—
Demi-Glace as prep	2 oz	30	4	—	—
Hollandaise as prep	2 oz	170	5	—	—
Hunter as prep	2 oz	25	4	—	—
Lyonnaise as prep	2 oz	20	3	—	—
Mushroom as prep	2 oz	60	5	—	—
Napoli as prep	4 oz	100	17	—	—
Pepper as prep	2 oz	20	3	—	—
Watkins					
Beef Marinade	¼ tbsp (2 g)	5	1	0	0
Calypso Hot Pepper Sauce	1 tsp (5 g)	10	3	2	0
Caribbean Red Pepper Sauce	1 tsp (5 g)	10	3	2	0
Chicken & Pork Marinade	¼ tbsp (2 g)	5	2	0	0
Fish & Seafood Marinade	¼ tbsp (2 g)	10	1	1	0
Meat Magic	1 tsp (6 g)	10	2	1	0
SHELF-STABLE					
Cheez Whiz					
Cheese Sqeezable	2 tbsp (1.2 oz)	100	4	1	0
Fresh Gourmet					
Stir 'n Sauce Italian	1 tbsp (0.5 oz)	30	5	tr	—
SAUERKRAUT					
canned	½ cup	22	5	—	—
Del Monte					
Canned	½ cup (4.2 oz)	15	4	0	2
Hebrew National					
Gallon Kraut	½ cup	25	4	—	—

FOOD	PORTION	CALS.	CARB.	SUG.	FIB.
Hebrew National (CONT.)					
New Kraut	½ cup (3.1 oz)	50	11	—	—
Rosoff's					
Sauerkraut	½ cup (3.2 oz)	50	11	—	—
S&W					
Canned	½ cup	25	5	—	—
Schorr's					
New Kraut	½ cup (3.2 oz)	50	11	—	—
Seneca					
Canned	2 tbsp	5	0	—	1
SnowFloss					
Kraut	4 oz	28	4	—	1
Kraut Bavarian Style	4 oz	64	12	—	1
Vlasic					
Old Fashioned	1 oz	4	1	—	—

SAUERKRAUT JUICE
S&W
Juice	4 oz	14	3	—	—

SAUSAGE
(*see also* HOT DOG, SAUSAGE SUBSTITUTES)

FOOD	PORTION	CALS.	CARB.	SUG.	FIB.
bierschinken	3.5 oz	174	tr	—	—
bierwurst	3.5 oz	258	0	0	0
blutwurst uncooked	3½ oz	424	0	0	0
bockwurst	3.5 oz	276	0	0	0
bockwurst pork & veal raw	1 link (2.3 oz)	200	tr	—	—
bratwurst pork cooked	1 link (3 oz)	256	2	—	—
brotwurst pork	1 oz	92	1	—	—
brotwurst pork & beef	1 link (2.5 oz)	226	2	—	—
chipolata	3.5 oz	342	1	1	0
chorizo	3.5 oz	499	4	4	tr
country-style pork cooked	1 patty (1 oz)	100	tr	—	—
country-style pork cooked	1 link (½ oz)	48	tr	—	—
fleischwurst	3.5 oz	305	0	0	0
gelbwurst uncooked	3½ oz	363	0	0	0
italian pork cooked	1 (2.4 oz)	216	1	—	—
italian pork cooked	1 (3 oz)	268	1	—	—
jagdwurst	3.5 oz	211	0	0	0
kielbasa pork	1 oz	88	1	—	—
knockwurst pork & beef	1 oz	87	1	—	—
knockwurst pork & beef	1 (2.4 oz)	209	1	—	—
mettwurst uncooked	3½ oz	483	0	0	0
plockwurst uncooked	3½ oz	312	0	0	0
polish pork	1 (8 oz)	739	4	—	—

FOOD	PORTION	CALS.	CARB.	SUG.	FIB.
polish pork	1 oz	92	tr	—	—
pork & beef cooked	1 patty (1 oz)	107	1	—	—
pork & beef cooked	1 link (½ oz)	52	tr	—	—
pork cooked	1 link (½ oz)	48	tr	—	—
pork cooked	1 patty (1 oz)	100	tr	—	—
regensburger uncooked	3½ oz	354	0	0	0
smoked pork	1 sm link (½ oz)	62	tr	—	—
smoked pork	1 link (2.4 oz)	265	1	—	—
smoked pork & beef	1 link (2.4 oz)	229	1	—	—
smoked pork & beef	1 sm link (½ oz)	54	tr	—	—
vienna canned	1 (½ oz)	45	tr	—	—
vienna canned	7 (4 oz)	315	2	—	—
weisswurst uncooked	3½ oz	305	0	0	0
zungenwurst (tongue)	3.5 oz	285	0	0	0
Aidells					
Andouille Cajun Cooked	1 (3.5 oz)	220	1	—	—
Burmese Curry Cooked	1 (3.5 oz)	220	3	—	—
Chicken & Apple Fresh	1 (1.9 oz)	110	1	—	—
Chicken & Apple Smoked	1 (3.5 oz)	220	0	0	0
Chicken & Turkey New Mexico Smoked	1 (3.5 oz)	220	2	—	—
Chicken & Turkey Thai Fresh	1 (3.5 oz)	200	0	0	0
Chicken & Turkey Thai Smoked	1 (3.5 oz)	220	0	0	0
Chicken & Turkey With Sun-Dried Tomatoes & Basil Fresh	1 (3.5 oz)	200	1	—	—
Chicken & Turkey With Sun-Dried Tomatoes & Basil Smoked	1 (3.5 oz)	200	0	0	0
Creole Hot Cooked	1 (3.5 oz)	220	2	—	—
Duck & Turkey Smoked	1 (3.5 oz)	220	1	—	—
Hunter's Cooked	1 (3.5 oz)	240	0	0	0
Italian Hot Fresh	1 (3.5 oz)	230	0	0	0
Italian Mild Fresh	1 (3.5 oz)	230	0	0	0
Lamb & Beef With Rosemary Fresh	1 (3.5 oz)	220	2	—	—
Lemon Chicken Cooked	1 (3.5 oz)	220	1	—	—
Mexican Chorizo Beef Fresh	1 (3.5 oz)	400	3	—	—
Whiskey Fennel Cooked	1 (3.5 oz)	230	1	—	—
Armour					
Vienna Sausage 25% Less Fat	3 (1.9 oz)	130	1	—	—

FOOD	PORTION	CALS.	CARB.	SUG.	FIB.
Armour (CONT.)					
Vienna Sausage In BBQ Sauce	3 (2.1 oz)	160	4	—	—
Vienna Sausage In Beef Stock	3 (1.9 oz)	170	1	—	—
Vienna Sausage In Hot Sauce	3 (2.1 oz)	170	3	—	—
Vienna Sausage Smoked	3 (1.9 oz)	170	1	—	—
Banner					
Sausage Tripe	2 oz	90	2	—	—
Bilinski's					
Chicken & Vegetable	1 (3 oz)	80	2	1	tr
Chicken Italian With Peppers & Onions	1 (3 oz)	120	1	—	—
Golden Brown					
Beef	1	80	tr	—	—
Mild	1	100	tr	—	—
Spicy	1	100	tr	—	—
Healthy Choice					
Low Fat Smoked	2 oz	70	4	2	1
Low Fat Smoked Polska Kielbasa	2 oz	70	4	2	1
Hillshire					
Beer Bratwurst	1 (2 oz)	190	2	—	—
Bratwurst Fresh	1 (2 oz)	190	1	—	—
Bratwurst Light Fresh	1 (2 oz)	150	2	—	—
Bratwurst Spicy	1 (2 oz)	180	1	—	—
Flavorseal Kielbasa Polska	2 oz	190	2	—	—
Flavorseal Kielbasa Polska Beef	2 oz	190	2	—	—
Flavorseal Kielbasa Polska Lite	2 oz	130	1	—	—
Flavorseal Kielbasa Polska Mild	2 oz	190	2	—	—
Flavorseal Kielbasa Polska Turkey	2 oz	90	2	—	—
Flavorseal Smoked	2 oz	190	2	—	—
Flavorseal Smoked Beef	2 oz	180	2	—	—
Flavorseal Smoked Beef & Cheddar	2 oz	190	1	—	—
Flavorseal Smoked Country Recipe	2 oz	180	2	—	—
Flavorseal Smoked Hot	2 oz	180	2	—	—
Flavorseal Smoked Lite	2 oz	130	1	—	—

FOOD	PORTION	CALS.	CARB.	SUG.	FIB.
Hillshire (CONT.)					
Flavorseal Smoked Turkey	2 oz	90	2	—	—
Flavorseal Smoked w/ Italian Seasoning	2 oz	200	1	—	—
Italian Mild	1 (2 oz)	190	1	—	—
Italian Mild Light	1 (2 oz)	150	2	—	—
Italian Hot	1 (2 oz)	180	1	—	—
Italian Hot Light	1 (2 oz)	150	2	—	—
Kielbasa Fresh Polska	1 (2 oz)	190	1	—	—
Kielbasa Fresh Polska Lower Fat	1 (2 oz)	150	2	—	—
Links 80% Fat Free Cheddar Hots	2 oz	150	1	—	—
Links 80% Fat Free Kielbasa	2 oz	130	2	—	—
Links 80% Fat Free Smokies	2 oz	130	2	—	—
Links Brats Fully Cooked	2 oz	170	1	—	—
Links Bratwurst Smoked	2 oz	190	1	—	—
Links Bun Size Cheddarwurst	2 oz	200	1	—	—
Links Bun Size Kielbasa	2 oz	180	2	—	—
Links Bun Size Smoked	2 oz	180	2	—	—
Links Bun Size Smoked Beef	2 oz	180	2	—	—
Links Cheddarwurst	2 oz	190	1	—	—
Links Cheddarwurst Lite	1 link (2.7 oz)	190	2	—	—
Links Hot	2 oz	190	2	—	—
Links Hot Beef	2 oz	190	1	—	—
Links Hot Lite	1 link (2.7 oz)	190	2	—	—
Links Keilbasa Polska	2 oz	190	2	—	—
Links Keilbasa Polska Lite	1 link (2.7 oz)	190	2	—	—
Links Knockwurst Lite	2 oz	180	1	—	—
Links Lit'l Polskas	2 oz	180	2	—	—
Links Lit'l Smokies	2 oz	180	2	—	—
Links Lit'l Smokies Beef	2 oz	180	2	—	—
Links Lit'l Smokies Cheddar	2 oz	180	2	—	—
Links Lit'l Smokies Light	2 oz	120	1	—	—
Links Polish	2 oz	190	2	—	—
Links Smoked	2 oz	190	1	—	—
Mexican Style	1 (2 oz)	190	1	—	—
Mexican Style Lower Fat	1 (2 oz)	150	2	—	—

FOOD	PORTION	CALS.	CARB.	SUG.	FIB.
Hormel					
Light & Lean 97 Dinner Smoked	2 oz	60	2	2	0
Pickled Hot	6 (2 oz)	140	1	1	0
Pickled Smoked	6 (2 oz)	140	1	1	0
Smoked Summer	2 oz	200	2	2	0
Vienna	2 oz	140	0	0	0
Vienna Chicken	2 oz	110	1	0	0
Jimmy Dean					
Brick Sausage	2.5 oz	270	0	0	0
Bulk	2.5 oz	300	0	0	0
Hickory Smoked Dinner Sausage	2 oz	170	2	1	0
Pattie Pre-Cooked	1 (1.9 oz)	230	0	0	0
Polska Kielbaska	2 oz	170	1	1	0
Sage Pattie	1 (2 oz)	200	0	0	0
Sausage Pattie Raw	1 (2 oz)	200	0	0	0
Skinless Link	2 (2 oz)	200	0	0	0
Skinless Link	4 (2 oz)	200	0	0	0
Jones					
Brown & Serve Bacon	1	90	tr	—	—
Brown & Serve Beef	1	90	tr	—	—
Brown & Serve Light	1	60	1	—	—
Brown & Serve Regular	1	100	tr	—	—
Cello Beef	1 slice (1 oz)	130	tr	—	—
Cello Hot Country	1 slice (1 oz)	110	tr	—	—
Cello Original	1 slice (1 oz)	100	tr	—	—
Dinner Link	1	280	tr	—	—
Golden Brown Light Links	1	60	1	—	—
Golden Brown Mild Pattie	1	150	tr	—	—
Italian	1	160	tr	—	—
Light Link	1	70	1	—	—
Little Link	1	140	tr	—	—
Patties	1	150	tr	—	—
Scrapple	1 slice	90	5	—	—
Scrapple	1 slice (1.5 oz)	90	5	—	—
Little Sizzlers					
Brown & Serve	3 links (2.1 oz)	190	1	1	0
Brown & Serve	2 patties (1.8 oz)	190	1	1	0
Cooked	2 patties (1.8 oz)	230	0	0	0
Cooked	3 links (1.8 oz)	230	0	0	0
Heat & Serve Pork cooked	3 links (1.8 oz)	230	0	0	0
Louis Rich					
Polska Kielbasa	2 oz	90	2	tr	0

FOOD	PORTION	CALS.	CARB.	SUG.	FIB.
Louis Rich (CONT.)					
Turkey Hot	2.5 oz	120	1	0	0
Turkey Original	2.5 oz	120	1	0	0
Turkey Smoked	2 oz	90	2	1	0
Mr. Turkey					
Breakfast	2.5 oz	130	0	0	0
Hearty Blend Polish Kielbasa	1 oz	70	1	—	—
Hearty Blend Smoked	1 oz	70	1	—	—
Hot Smoked	1 oz	45	2	—	—
Italian Smoked	1 oz	45	2	—	—
Polish Kielbasa	1 oz	45	2	—	—
Smoked	1 oz	45	2	—	—
Old Smokehouse					
Summer Sausage	2 oz	200	2	2	0
Oscar Mayer					
Pork cooked	2 links (1.7 oz)	170	1	0	0
Smokies Beef	1 (1.5 oz)	120	1	tr	0
Smokies Cheese	1 (1.5 oz)	130	1	tr	0
Smokies Link	1 (1.5 oz)	130	1	tr	0
Smokies Little	6 (2 oz)	170	1	tr	0
Smokies Little Cheese	6 (2 oz)	180	1	0	0
Perdue					
Breakfast Links Turkey Cooked	2 links (2 oz)	100	0	0	0
Hot Italian Turkey Cooked	1 link (2.4 oz)	110	1	—	—
Sweet Italian Turkey Cooked	1 link (2.4 oz)	110	1	—	—
Rudy's Farm					
Italian Hot	2.5 oz	240	0	0	0
Italian Mild	2.5 oz	240	0	0	0
Italian Mild Natural Casing	1 (2 oz)	190	0	0	0
Morning Right Link	3 (2.9 oz)	150	0	0	0
Morning Right Pattie	2 (2.9 oz)	150	0	0	0
Pattie Pre-Cooked	1 (1.4 oz)	100	0	0	1
Smoked	4 (2.1 oz)	200	1	0	0
Sweet Link	1 (3.9 oz)	380	1	0	0
Shofar					
Knockwurst Beef	1 (3 oz)	260	tr	0	0
Tyson					
Country Pork	3.5 oz	320	1	—	—
Wampler Longacre					
Breakfast Links	1 (2.8 oz)	170	2	—	—
Italian Links	1 (2.8 oz)	170	2	—	—

FOOD	PORTION	CALS.	CARB.	SUG.	FIB.
Wampler Longacre (CONT.)					
Tinderlings Garlic & Pepper	1 (3.5 oz)	143	3	—	—
Turkey	1 link (1 oz)	60	1	—	—
Turkey	1 pattie (2 oz)	120	4	—	—

SAUSAGE DISHES
Jimmy Dean

Italian Sausage & Mozzarella Sandwich	1 (4.5 oz)	380	28	2	2
Ovenstuffs					
French Roll Italian Sausage	1 (4.75 oz)	390	29	—	—
French Roll Pepperoni	1 (4.75 oz)	370	30	—	—

SAUSAGE SUBSTITUTES
GardenSausage

Patty	1 (2.5 oz)	140	20	2	5
Knox Mountain Farm					
No-So-Sausage	1 serv (1/10 pkg)	120	6	—	2
Lightlife					
Lean Links Breakfast	1.25 oz	69	4	—	—
Lean Links Italian	1.5 oz	83	5	—	—
Loma Linda					
Linketts	1 (1.2 oz)	70	1	0	1
Little Links	2 (1.6 oz)	90	2	0	2
Morningstar Farms					
Breakfast Links	2 (1.6 oz)	60	2	0	2
Breakfast Patties	1 (1.3 oz)	70	2	0	2
Grillers	1 patty (2.2 oz)	140	5	tr	3
Sausage Style Recipe Crumbles	2/3 cup (1.9 oz)	90	5	tr	3
Natural Touch					
Vegan Sausage Crumbles	1/2 cup (1.9 oz)	60	4	0	2
White Wave					
Meatless Healthy Links	2 (1.6 oz)	140	5	0	3
Worthington					
Leanies	1 link (1.4 oz)	110	2	tr	1
Prosage Links	2 (1.6 oz)	60	2	0	2
Saucettes	1 link (1.3 oz)	90	1	0	1
Super Links	1 (1.7 oz)	110	2	0	1
Veja Links	1 (1.1 oz)	50	1	0	0

SAVORY

ground	1 tsp	4	1	—	—

SCALLOP
FRESH

raw	3 oz	75	2	—	—

FOOD	PORTION	CALS.	CARB.	SUG.	FIB.
FROZEN					
Mrs. Paul's					
Fried	2 oz	160	18	—	—
HOME RECIPE					
breaded & fried	2 lg	67	3	—	—
SCONE					
apricot scone	1	232	39	—	—
Finnegan's					
Cranberry	1 (2.7 oz)	90	20	1	1
Irish Raisin	1 (2.7 oz)	90	20	1	1
SCROD					
Gorton's					
Microwave Entree Baked	1 pkg	320	18	—	—
SCUP					
fresh baked	3 oz	115	0	0	0
SEA BASS					
(*see* BASS)					
SEATROUT					
(*see* TROUT)					
SEAWEED					
agar dried	1 oz	87	23	—	—
agar fresh	1 oz	tr	2	—	—
irishmoss fresh	1 oz	14	4	—	—
kelp fresh	1 oz	12	3	—	—
kombu fresh	1 oz	12	3	—	—
laver fresh	1 oz	10	1	—	—
nori fresh	1 oz	10	1	—	—
spirulina dried	1 oz	83	7	—	—
spirulina fresh	1 oz	7	1	—	—
tangle fresh	1 oz	12	3	—	—
wakame fresh	1 oz	13	3	—	—
Eden					
Agar Agar Bars	1 tbsp (2.5 oz)	10	2	0	2
Agar Agar Flakes	1 tbsp (2.5 oz)	10	2	0	2
Arame	½ cup (0.3 oz)	30	7	0	7
Hiziki	½ cup (0.3 oz)	30	6	0	6
Kombu	3.5 in piece (3.3 g)	10	2	0	1
Nori	1 sheet (2.5 g)	10	1	0	1
Sushi Nori	1 sheet (2.5 g)	10	1	0	1
Wakame	½ cup (0.3 oz)	25	4	0	4
Wakame Flakes	½ cup (0.3 oz)	25	4	0	4

FOOD	PORTION	CALS.	CARB.	SUG.	FIB.
Maine Coast					
Alaria	⅓ cup (7 g)	18	3	0	2
Dulse	⅓ cup (7 g)	18	3	0	2
Dulse Flakes	1 oz	75	13	—	9
Kelp	⅓ cup (7 g)	17	3	0	3
Kelp Crunch	1 bar (1 oz)	129	14	4	2
Kelp Crunch Peanut-Raisin	1 bar (1 oz)	129	14	4	2
Laver	⅓ cup (7 g)	22	3	0	3
Sea Seasoning Dulse	1 g	3	1	—	—
Sea Seasoning Dulse With Celery	1 g	3	1	—	—
Sea Seasoning Dulse With Garlic	1 g	3	1	—	—
Sea Seasoning Dulse With Sesame	1 g	3	1	—	—
Sea Seasoning Kelp	1 g	3	1	—	—
Sea Seasoning Kelp With Cayenne	1 g	3	1	—	—
Sea Seasoning Nori	1 g	3	1	—	—
Sea Seasoning Nori With Ginger	1 g	3	1	—	—

SEITAN
(*see* WHEAT)

SEMOLINA

FOOD	PORTION	CALS.	CARB.	SUG.	FIB.
dry	1 cup (5.9 oz)	601	122	—	7

SESAME

FOOD	PORTION	CALS.	CARB.	SUG.	FIB.
seeds	1 tsp	16	tr	—	—
seeds dried	1 tbsp	52	2	—	—
seeds dried	1 cup	825	34	—	—
seeds roasted & toasted	1 oz	161	7	—	—
sesame butter	1 tbsp	95	4	—	1
sesame crunch candy	20 pieces (1.2 oz)	181	18	—	—
sesame crunch candy	1 oz	146	14	—	—
sesame sticks	1 oz	153	13	—	—
sesame sticks unsalted	1 oz	153	13	—	—
tahini from roasted & toasted kernels	1 tbsp	89	3	—	—
tahini from stone ground kernels	1 tbsp	86	4	—	—
tahini from unroasted kernels	1 tbsp	85	3	—	—
Arrowhead					
Sesame Tahini	1 oz	170	4	—	—

FOOD	PORTION	CALS.	CARB.	SUG.	FIB.
Casbah					
Tahini Sauce Mix as prep	¼ cup	160	10	5	tr
Eden					
Sesame Shake	½ tsp (1.5 g)	10	0	0	tr
Sesame Shake Garlic	½ tsp (1.5 g)	10	0	0	tr
Sesame Shake Organic Seaweed	½ tsp (1.5 g)	10	0	0	tr
Erewhon					
Sesame Butter	2 tbsp (32 g)	190	3	—	—
Sesame Tahini	2 tbsp (32 g)	200	3	—	—
Joyva					
Tahini	2 tbsp (1 oz)	200	3	0	1
Planters					
Nut Mix	1 oz	150	9	tr	2
Stone-Buhr					
Seeds Raw	4 tsp (1 oz)	180	3	0	1
SESBANIA					
flower	1	1	tr	—	—
flowers	1 cup	5	1	—	—
flowers cooked	1 cup	23	5	—	—
SHAD					
american baked	3 oz	214	0	0	0
roe baked w/ butter & lemon	3.5 oz	126	2	—	—
roe raw	3.5 oz	130	2	—	—
SHALLOTS					
dried	1 tbsp	3	1	—	—
raw chopped	1 tbsp	7	2	—	—
SHARK					
batter-dipped & fried	3 oz	194	5	—	—
raw	3 oz	111	0	0	0
SHEEPSHEAD FISH					
cooked	3 oz	107	0	0	0
cooked	1 fillet (6.5 oz)	234	0	0	0
raw	3 oz	92	0	0	0
SHELLFISH					
(*see individual names,* SHELLFISH SUBSTITUTES)					
SHELLFISH SUBSTITUTES					
crab imitation	3 oz	87	1	—	—
scallop imitation	3 oz	84	9	—	—
shrimp imitation	3 oz	86	8	—	—
surimi	3 oz	84	6	—	—
surimi	1 oz	28	2	—	—

FOOD	PORTION	CALS.	CARB.	SUG.	FIB.
Louis Kemp					
Crab Delights Chunk Style	2 oz	54	5	—	—
Lobster Delights	2 oz	60	6	—	—
Maryland Style Cakes	2.5 oz	154	10	—	—
Ocean Magic					
Imitation King Crab	3 oz	80	11	—	—

SHELLIE BEANS

canned	½ cup	37	8	—	—

SHERBET
(*see also* ICES AND ICE POPS)

orange	½ cup (4 fl oz)	132	29	—	—
orange	½ gal	2158	469	—	—
orange	1 bar (2.75 fl oz)	91	20	—	—
orange home recipe	½ cup	120	24	—	—
Borden					
Orange	½ cup	110	25	—	—
Bresler's					
All Flavors	3.5 oz	140	30	—	—
Breyers					
Fat Free Orange	½ cup (3 oz)	110	27	21	0
Fat Free Rainbow	½ cup (3 oz)	110	28	21	0
Fat Free Raspberry	½ cup (3 oz)	120	28	22	0
Fat Free Tropical	½ cup (3 oz)	110	27	21	0
Orange	½ cup (3 oz)	120	26	19	0
Rainbow	½ cup (3 oz)	120	27	21	0
Raspberry	½ cup (3 oz)	120	28	21	0
Tropical	½ cup (3 oz)	120	27	21	0
Hood					
Lime Orange Lemon	½ cup (3.1 oz)	120	26	26	0
Orange	½ cup (3.1 oz)	120	26	26	0
Rainbow Swirl	½ cup (3.1 oz)	120	26	26	0
Raspberry Orange Lime	½ cup (3.1 oz)	120	26	26	0
Sealtest					
Lime	½ cup (3 oz)	130	28	20	0
Orange	½ cup (3 oz)	130	28	20	0
Rainbow Orange Red Raspberry Lime	½ cup (3 oz)	130	28	21	0
Red Raspberry	½ cup (3 oz)	130	28	21	0

SHRIMP
CANNED

canned	3 oz	102	1	—	—
canned	1 cup	154	1	—	—

FOOD	PORTION	CALS.	CARB.	SUG.	FIB.
S&W					
Deveined Medium Whole Shrimp	2 oz	65	1	—	—
FRESH					
cooked	4 large	22	0	0	0
cooked	3 oz	84	0	0	0
raw	3 oz	90	1	—	—
raw	4 large	30	tr	—	—
FROZEN					
Cajun Cookin'					
Shrimp Creole	12 oz	390	55	—	—
Shrimp Etouffee	17 oz	360	52	—	—
Shrimp Jambalaya	12 oz	450	43	—	—
Gorton's					
Butterfly Shrimp	4 oz	160	16	—	—
Microwave Crunchy Shrimp	5 oz	380	35	—	—
Microwave Entree Shrimp Scampi	1 pkg	390	21	—	—
Shrimp Crisps	4 oz	280	26	—	—
Mrs. Paul's					
Entrees Light Seafood & Clams With Linguini	10 oz	240	36	—	—
Van De Kamp's					
Breaded Butterfly	7 (4 oz)	280	28	1	2
Breaded Popcorn	20 (4 oz)	270	28	2	1
Breaded Whole	7 (4 oz)	240	26	2	2
SMELT					
rainbow cooked	3 oz	106	0	0	0
rainbow raw	3 oz	83	0	0	0
SNACKS					
(*see also* CHIPS, FRUIT SNACKS, NUTS MIXED, POPCORN, PRETZELS)					
oriental mix	1 oz	155	9	—	—
pork skins	1 oz	154	0	0	0
pork skins barbecue	1 oz	152	1	—	—
trail mix	1 oz	131	13	—	—
trail mix	1 cup (5.3 oz)	693	67	—	—
trail mix tropical	1 oz	115	19	—	—
trail mix w/ chocolate chips	1 oz	137	13	—	—
trail mix w/ chocolate chips	1 cup (5.1 oz)	707	66	—	—
Bakem-ets					
Hot'N Spicy	21 pieces (1 oz)	150	1	—	—
Snacks	21 pieces (1 oz)	160	2	—	—

FOOD	PORTION	CALS.	CARB.	SUG.	FIB.
Barbara's					
Cheese Puffs Bakes	1½ cups (1 oz)	160	13	1	0
Cheese Puffs Jalapeno	¾ cup (1 oz)	150	15	1	0
Cheese Puffs Original	¾ cup (1 oz)	150	16	0	0
Big Dipper					
Bagel Chips Lowfat Barbeque	12 (1 oz)	110	21	1	1
Bagel Chips Lowfat Garlic	12 (1 oz)	120	21	1	1
Bagel Chips Lowfat Original	12 (1 oz)	110	21	1	1
Bugles					
Baked Cheddar Cheese	1½ cups (1 oz)	130	22	—	tr
Baked Original	1½ cups (1 oz)	130	23	—	tr
Cheetos					
Cheddar Valley	26 pieces (1 oz)	160	16	—	1
Crunchy	26 pieces (1 oz)	150	17	—	1
Curls	15 pieces (1 oz)	150	17	—	1
Flamin' Hot	26 pieces (1 oz)	150	16	—	1
Light	38 pieces (1 oz)	140	19	—	1
Paws	16 pieces (1 oz)	160	15	—	1
Puffed Ball	38 pieces (1 oz)	160	16	—	1
Puffs	33 pieces (1 oz)	160	16	—	1
Cheez Doodles					
Crunchy	1 oz	160	16	—	—
Puffed	1 oz	150	16	—	—
Cheez Waffies					
Snacks	1 oz	140	14	—	—
Chex Mix					
Bold 'n Zesty	½ cup (1 oz)	140	20	—	2
Cheddar Cheese	½ cup (1 oz)	130	20	—	1
Hot'n Spicy	⅔ cup (1 oz)	130	21	—	2
Traditional	⅔ cup (1 oz)	130	21	—	1
Combos					
Cheddar Cheese Cracker	1 pkg (1.7 oz)	250	28	3	1
Cheddar Cheese Cracker	1 oz	140	16	2	0
Cheddar Cheese Pretzel	1 oz	130	18	4	0
Cheddar Cheese Pretzel	1 pkg (1.8 oz)	240	33	7	1
Chili Cheese w/ Corn Shell	1 oz	140	17	2	1
Chili Cheese w/ Corn Shell	1 pkg (1.7 oz)	230	29	4	2
Mustard Pretzel	1 pkg (1.8 oz)	230	35	4	1
Mustard Pretzel	1 oz	130	19	2	1
Nacho Cheese Pretzel	1 pkg (1.7 oz)	230	34	8	1
Nacho Cheese Pretzel	1 oz	130	19	5	1
Nacho Cheese w/ Tortilla Shell	1 oz	140	17	2	1

FOOD	PORTION	CALS.	CARB.	SUG.	FIB.
Combos (CONT.)					
Nacho Cheese w/ Tortilla Shell	1 pkg (1.7 oz)	230	30	4	1
Peanut Butter Cracker	1 oz	140	15	0	1
Pepperoni & Cheese Pizza	1 oz	140	17	3	0
Pepperoni & Cheese Pizza	1 pkg (1.7 oz)	240	30	6	1
Pizzeria Pretzel	1 pkg (1.8 oz)	230	35	6	1
Pizzeria Pretzel	1 oz	130	19	3	1
Tortilla Ranch	1 bag (1.7 oz)	240	29	3	1
Tortilla Ranch	1 oz	140	17	2	1
Cornnuts					
Barbecue	1 oz	120	22	5	2
Nacho Cheese	1 oz	120	22	1	2
Original	1 oz	120	22	tr	2
Original	1 pkg (2 oz)	260	40	0	4
Picante	1 oz	120	22	1	2
Ranch	1 oz	120	20	1	2
Doo Dads					
Snacks	1 oz	130	17	—	—
Energy Food Factory					
Poprice Cheddar Cheese	½ oz	60	8	—	—
Poprice Herb & Garlic	½ oz	50	10	—	—
Poprice Lite	½ oz	50	9	—	—
Poprice Original No Salt	½ oz	45	11	—	—
Estee					
Snack Crisps Apple Cinnamon	1 pkg (0.66 oz)	90	16	5	tr
Snack Crisps Apple Cinnamon	27 crisps (1 oz)	130	24	8	1
Snack Crisps Chocolate	1 pkg (0.66 oz)	90	15	5	1
Snack Crisps Chocolate	30 crisps (1 oz)	130	23	8	2
Snack Crisps Lemon	30 (1 oz)	130	23	9	tr
Snack Crisps Lemon	1 pkg (0.66 oz)	90	16	6	tr
Snack Crisps Ranch	1 pkg (0.6 oz)	90	15	4	0
Snack Crisps Ranch	30 (1 oz)	130	22	6	tr
Snack Crisps White Cheddar	1 pkg (0.6 oz)	90	14	3	tr
Snack Crisps With Cheddar	27 crisps (1 oz)	130	22	5	tr
Frito Lay					
Corn Nuggets Toasted	1.38 oz	170	29	—	—
Funyums					
Onion Rings	11 pieces (1 oz)	140	18	—	1
Hapi					
Chili Bits	½ cup (1 oz)	110	25	1	1

FOOD	PORTION	CALS.	CARB.	SUG.	FIB.
Health Valley					
Cheddar Lites	0.75 oz	40	4	—	tr
Cheddar Lites With Green Onion	0.75 oz	40	4	—	tr
Innovative Foods					
Roasted Sweet Corn	1 pkg (0.8 oz)	76	17	2	2
Lance					
Cheese Balls	1 pkg (32 g)	190	16	—	—
Crunchy Cheese Twists	1 pkg (42 g)	260	25	—	—
Gold-N-Chees	1 pkg (39 g)	180	23	—	—
Pork Skins	1 pkg (14 g)	80	0	0	0
Pork Skins BBQ	1 pkg (14 g)	80	0	0	0
Mr. Peanut					
Peanut Butter Crisps Graham	12 pieces (1.1 oz)	150	18	9	2
Munchos					
Snack	16 pieces (1 oz)	160	15	—	—
Pita Puffs					
Barbeque	35 (1 oz)	120	20	1	1
Lowfat Garlic	35 (1 oz)	110	22	1	1
Lowfat Original	35 (1 oz)	110	22	1	1
Lowfat Salsa	35 (1 oz)	110	21	1	1
Pizza	35 (1 oz)	120	21	1	1
Ranch	35 (1 oz)	120	21	1	1
Planters					
Cheez Balls	1 oz	150	15	tr	1
Cheez Balls	1 pkg (1 oz)	150	15	tr	1
Cheez Curls	1 pkg (1.2 oz)	190	19	1	1
Cheez Curls	1 oz	150	15	tr	1
Heat Snack Mix	1 oz	140	13	1	2
Snyder's					
Cheddar Cheese Twists	1 oz	150	17	—	—
Kruncheez	1 oz	160	15	—	—
Onion Toasters	1 oz	150	17	—	3
Snack Mix	1 oz	170	11	—	tr
Sopaipillas Apple & Cinnamon	1 oz	150	18	—	1
Splurge					
Snack Mix Fat Free Original	⅔ cup (1 oz)	100	25	2	tr
Ultra Slim-Fast					
Lite N' Tasty Cheese Curls	1 oz	110	20	—	3
Weight Watchers					
Cheese Curls	1 pkg (0.5 oz)	70	10	0	0

FOOD	PORTION	CALS.	CARB.	SUG.	FIB.
SNAIL					
cooked	3 oz	233	13	—	—
raw	3 oz	117	7	—	—
SNAPPER					
cooked	3 oz	109	0	0	0
cooked	1 fillet (6 oz)	217	0	0	0
raw	3 oz	85	0	0	0
SODA					
(see also DRINK MIXERS, MINERAL/BOTTLED WATER, SPORTS DRINKS)					
club	12 oz	0	0	0	0
cola	12 oz	151	39	—	—
cream	12 oz	191	49	—	—
diet cola	12 oz	2	tr	—	—
diet cola w/ equal	12 oz	2	tr	—	—
diet cola w/ saccharin	12 oz	2	tr	—	—
ginger ale	12 oz can	124	32	—	—
grape	12 oz	161	42	—	—
lemon lime	12 oz	149	38	—	—
orange	12 oz	177	46	—	—
pepper type	12 oz	151	38	—	—
quinine	12 oz	125	32	—	—
root beer	12 oz	152	39	—	—
tonic water	12 oz	125	32	—	—
After The Fall					
Raspberry Ginger Ale	1 can (12 oz)	150	36	30	0
Barrelhead					
Root Beer	8 fl oz	110	27	27	0
Burst					
Cola Strawberry	8 fl oz	117	31	31	—
Canada Dry					
Birch Beer Brown	8 fl oz	110	27	27	0
Birch Beer Clear	8 fl oz	110	27	27	0
Black Cherry Wishniak	8 fl oz	130	32	32	0
Cactus Cooler	8 fl oz	110	27	27	0
California Strawberry	8 fl oz	110	27	27	0
Club	8 fl oz	0	0	0	0
Club Sodium Free	8 fl oz	0	0	0	0
Concord Grape	8 fl oz	120	29	29	0
Diet Ginger Ale	8 fl oz	0	0	0	0
Diet Ginger Ale Cherry	8 fl oz	0	0	0	0
Diet Ginger Ale Cranberry	8 fl oz	0	tr	tr	0
Diet Ginger Ale Lemon	8 fl oz	5	0	0	0
Diet Tonic Water	8 fl oz	0	0	0	0

FOOD	PORTION	CALS.	CARB.	SUG.	FIB.
Canada Dry (CONT.)					
Diet Tonic Water Twist Of Lime	8 fl oz	0	0	0	0
Ginger Ale	8 fl oz	100	25	25	0
Ginger Ale Cherry	8 fl oz	110	27	27	0
Ginger Ale Cranberry	8 fl oz	100	25	25	0
Ginger Ale Golden	8 fl oz	100	24	24	0
Ginger Ale Lemon	8 fl oz	100	25	25	0
Half & Half	8 fl oz	110	27	27	0
Hi-Spot	8 fl oz	110	28	28	0
Island Lime	8 fl oz	140	33	33	0
Jamaica Cola	8 fl oz	110	27	27	0
Lemon Sour	8 fl oz	100	21	21	0
Peach	8 fl oz	120	30	30	0
Pina Pineapple	8 fl oz	110	26	26	0
Seltzer	8 fl oz	0	0	0	0
Seltzer Cherry	8 fl oz	0	0	0	0
Seltzer Cranberry Lime	8 fl oz	0	0	0	0
Seltzer Grapefruit	8 fl oz	0	0	0	0
Seltzer Lemon Lime	8 fl oz	0	0	0	0
Seltzer Mandarin Orange	8 fl oz	0	0	0	0
Seltzer Peach	8 fl oz	0	0	0	0
Seltzer Raspberry	8 fl oz	0	0	0	0
Seltzer Strawberry	8 fl oz	0	0	0	0
Seltzer Tropical	8 fl oz	0	0	0	0
Sunripe Orange	8 fl oz	140	35	35	0
Tahitian Treat	8 fl oz	150	36	36	0
Tonic Water	8 fl oz	100	24	24	0
Tonic Water Twist Of Lime	8 fl oz	100	24	24	0
Vanilla Cream	8 fl oz	120	30	30	0
Vichy Water	8 fl oz	0	0	0	0
Wild Cherry	8 fl oz	110	28	28	0
Clearly 2					
Black Cherry	8 fl oz	2	0	0	0
Key Lime	8 fl oz	2	0	0	0
Clearly Canadian					
Alpine Fruit & Berries	8 fl oz	90	23	—	—
Boysenberry Mist	8 fl oz	2	0	0	0
Coastal Cranberry	8 fl oz	90	22	—	—
Country Raspberry	8 fl oz	80	19	—	—
Green Apple	8 fl oz	80	19	—	—
Mountain Blackberry	8 fl oz	100	24	—	—
Orchard Peach Strawberry	8 fl oz	90	22	—	—
Soda	8 fl oz	0	0	0	0

FOOD	PORTION	CALS.	CARB.	SUG.	FIB.
Clearly Canadian (CONT.)					
Summer Strawberry	8 fl oz	80	19	—	—
Western Longanberry	8 fl oz	80	19	—	—
Wild Cherry	8 fl oz	90	23	—	—
Coca-Cola					
Cherry	8 fl oz	104	28	28	—
Classic	8 fl oz	97	27	27	—
Classic Caffeine-Free	8 fl oz	97	27	27	—
Coke II	8 fl oz	105	29	29	—
Diet	8 fl oz	1	tr	—	—
Diet Cherry	8 fl oz	1	tr	—	—
Diet Coke Caffeine-free	8 fl oz	1	tr	—	—
Cott					
Cola	8 fl oz	110	27	27	0
Ginger Ale	8 fl oz	90	20	20	0
Grape	8 fl oz	130	30	30	0
Orange	8 fl oz	140	33	33	0
Pineapple	8 fl oz	130	32	32	0
Punch	8 fl oz	130	32	32	0
Seltzer	8 fl oz	0	0	0	0
Crush					
Cherry	8 fl oz	140	35	35	0
Orange Diet	8 fl oz	0	0	0	0
Pineapple	8 fl oz	140	35	35	0
Tropical Fruit Punch	1 bottle (10 fl oz)	180	44	37	0
Diet Rite					
Black Cherry Salt/Sodium Free	8 fl oz	2	1	—	—
Cola	8 fl oz	1	tr	—	—
Cola Caffeine/Sugar Free	8 fl oz	1	tr	—	—
Cola Salt/Sodium Free	8 fl oz	1	tr	—	—
Fruit Punch Salt/Sodium Free	8 fl oz	2	tr	—	—
Golden Peach Salt/Sodium Free	8 fl oz	2	tr	—	—
Key Lime Salt/Sodium Free	8 fl oz	7	2	—	—
Pink Grapefruit Salt/ Sodium Free	8 fl oz	2	1	—	—
Red Raspberry Salt/ Sodium Free	8 fl oz	3	1	—	—
Tangerine Salt/Sodium Free	8 fl oz	2	tr	—	—
White Grape Salt/Sodium Free	8 fl oz	1	tr	—	—

FOOD	PORTION	CALS.	CARB.	SUG.	FIB.
Dr. Nehi					
Soda	8 fl oz	100	26	—	—
Fanta					
Ginger Ale	8 fl oz	86	23	23	—
Grape	8 fl oz	117	31	31	—
Orange	8 fl oz	118	32	32	—
Root Beer	8 fl oz	111	29	29	—
Fresca					
Soda	8 fl oz	3	tr	—	—
Health Valley					
Ginger Ale	12 oz	153	35	—	0
Rootbeer Old Fashioned	12 oz	120	26	—	—
Sarsaparilla Rootbeer	12 oz	153	35	—	—
Wild Berry	12 oz	142	33	—	—
Hires					
Cream	8 fl oz	130	0	0	0
Cream Soda Diet	8 fl oz	0	0	0	0
Original Mocha	8 fl oz	100	24	24	0
Original Mocha Diet	8 fl oz	5	0	0	0
Root Beer	8 fl oz	130	31	31	0
Root Beer Diet	8 fl oz	0	0	0	0
IBC					
Root Beer	8 oz	110	29	29	—
Kick					
Soda	8 fl oz	120	32	—	—
Lucozade					
Soda	7 oz	136	36	—	0
Manischewitz					
Seltzer No Salt Added No Calories	8 fl oz	0	0	0	0
Mello Yellow					
Diet	8 fl oz	4	tr	—	—
Soda	8 fl oz	119	32	32	—
Minute Maid					
Berry	8 fl oz	111	30	30	—
Diet Orange	8 fl oz	2	0	0	0
Fruit Punch	8 fl oz	117	32	32	—
Grape	8 fl oz	121	32	32	—
Grapefruit	8 fl oz	108	29	29	—
Orange	8 fl oz	118	32	32	—
Peach	8 fl oz	110	29	29	—
Pineapple	8 fl oz	109	30	30	—
Raspberry	8 fl oz	111	30	30	—
Soda	8 fl oz	110	29	29	—

FOOD	PORTION	CALS.	CARB.	SUG.	FIB.
Minute Maid (CONT.)					
Strawberry	8 fl oz	122	33	33	—
Mountain Dew					
Diet	8 fl oz	2	tr	tr	—
Soda	8 fl oz	118	30	30	—
Mr. PiBB					
Diet	8 fl oz	1	tr	—	—
Soda	6 oz	97	26	26	—
Mug					
Cream	8 fl oz	122	32	32	—
Diet Cream	8 fl oz	2	0	0	0
Diet Root Beer	8 fl oz	1	tr	tr	—
Root Beer	8 fl oz	141	29	29	—
Nehi					
Cream	8 fl oz	120	32	—	—
Fruit Punch	8 fl oz	120	34	—	—
Ginger Ale	8 fl oz	90	24	—	—
Grape	8 fl oz	120	32	—	—
Orange	8 fl oz	130	35	—	—
Peach	8 fl oz	130	34	—	—
Pineapple	8 fl oz	130	36	—	—
Quinine Water	8 fl oz	90	23	—	—
Root Beer	8 fl oz	120	32	—	—
Strawberry	8 fl oz	120	32	—	—
Wild Red	8 fl oz	120	32	—	—
Old Colony					
Grape	8 fl oz	140	32	32	0
Orangina					
Sparkling Citrus	6 oz	80	19	—	—
Pepsi					
Caffeine Free	8 fl oz	105	27	27	—
Diet	8 fl oz	1	tr	tr	—
Diet Caffeine Free	8 fl oz	1	tr	tr	—
Regular	8 fl oz	105	27	27	—
Ramblin' Root Beer					
Ramblin' Root Beer	8 fl oz	120	33	33	—
Razing Razberry					
Cola	8 fl oz	117	31	31	—
Royal Crown					
Caffeine Free Cola	8 fl oz	110	29	—	—
Cherry	8 fl oz	110	29	—	—
Cola	8 fl oz	100	28	—	—
Diet	8 fl oz	1	tr	—	—
Diet Caffeine Free	8 fl oz	1	tr	—	—

FOOD	PORTION	CALS.	CARB.	SUG.	FIB.
Royal Crown (CONT.)					
Diet Cranberry Apple Salt/ Sodium Free	8 fl oz	2	tr	—	—
Diet Cranberry Salt/Sodium Free	8 fl oz	2	tr	—	—
Royal Mistic					
'N Juice Black Cherry	12 fl oz	146	36	—	—
'N Juice Peach Vanilla	12 fl oz	146	36	—	—
'N Juice Tangerine Orange	12 fl oz	146	36	—	—
'N Juice Tropical Supreme	12 fl oz	152	38	—	—
'N Juice Wild Berry	12 fl oz	156	38	—	—
Caribbean Fruit Punch	16 fl oz	230	57	—	—
Grape Strawberry	16 fl oz	230	57	—	—
Sparkling Diet With Lime Kiwi	11.1 fl oz	0	0	0	0
Sparkling Diet With Raspberry Boysenberry	11.1 fl oz	0	0	0	0
Sparkling Diet With Royal Peach	11.1 fl oz	0	0	0	0
Sparkling Diet With Wild Cherry	11.1 fl oz	0	0	0	0
Sparkling With Lime Kiwi	11.1 fl oz	112	28	—	—
Sparkling With Mandarin Orange Pineappple	11.1 fl oz	120	30	—	—
Sparkling With Mango Passion	11.1 fl oz	112	28	—	—
Sparkling With Raspberry Boysenberry	11.1 fl oz	112	28	—	—
Sparkling With Royal Peach	11.1 fl oz	112	28	—	—
Sparkling With Wild Cherry	11.1 fl oz	112	28	—	—
Schweppes					
Bitter Lemon	8 fl oz	110	28	28	0
Club	8 fl oz	0	0	0	0
Club Sodium Free	8 fl oz	0	0	0	0
Diet Ginger Ale	8 fl oz	0	0	0	0
Diet Ginger Ale Dry Grape	8 fl oz	2	0	0	0
Diet Ginger Ale Raspberry	8 fl oz	0	0	0	0
Ginger Ale	8 fl oz	90	22	22	0
Ginger Ale Dry Grape	8 fl oz	100	26	26	0
Ginger Ale Raspberry	8 fl oz	100	26	26	0
Ginger Beer	8 fl oz	100	25	25	0
Grape	8 fl oz	130	33	33	0
Grapefruit	8 fl oz	110	27	27	0
Lemon Sour	8 fl oz	110	26	26	0

FOOD	PORTION	CALS.	CARB.	SUG.	FIB.
Schweppes (CONT.)					
Lemon-Lime	8 fl oz	100	25	25	0
Seltzer Black Berry	8 fl oz	0	0	0	0
Seltzer Lemon	8 fl oz	0	0	0	0
Seltzer Lemon Lime	8 fl oz	0	0	0	0
Seltzer Lime	8 fl oz	0	0	0	0
Seltzer Orange	8 fl oz	0	0	0	0
Seltzer Peaches & Cream	8 fl oz	0	0	0	0
Seltzer Raspberry	8 fl oz	0	0	0	0
Tonic Citrus	8 fl oz	90	20	20	0
Tonic Cranberry	8 fl oz	90	20	20	0
Tonic Raspberry	8 fl oz	90	20	20	0
Tonic Water Diet	8 fl oz	0	0	0	0
Shasta					
Black Cherry	1 can (12 oz)	170	41	41	0
Caffeine Free Cola	1 can (12 oz)	160	41	41	—
Cherry Cola	1 can (12 oz)	160	39	39	—
Club Soda	1 can (12 oz)	0	0	0	0
Cola	1 can (12 oz)	170	42	42	0
Creme	1 can (12 oz)	190	47	47	0
Diet Black Cherry	1 can (12 oz)	0	0	0	0
Diet Caffeine Free Cola	1 can (12 oz)	0	0	0	0
Diet Cherry Cola	1 can (12 oz)	0	0	0	0
Diet Cola	1 can (12 oz)	0	0	0	0
Diet Creme	1 can (12 oz)	0	0	0	0
Diet Doc Shasta	1 can (12 oz)	0	0	0	0
Diet Ginger Ale	1 can (12 oz)	0	0	0	0
Diet Grape	1 can (12 oz)	0	0	0	0
Diet Grapefruit	1 can (12 oz)	0	0	0	0
Diet Grapefruit	1 can (12 oz)	0	0	0	0
Diet Kiwi-Strawberry	1 can (12 oz)	0	0	0	0
Diet Lemon-Lime Twist	1 can (12 oz)	0	0	0	0
Diet Orange	1 can (12 oz)	0	0	0	0
Diet Pineapple-Orange	1 can (12 oz)	0	0	0	0
Diet Raspberry Creme	1 can (12 oz)	0	0	0	0
Diet Red Pop	1 can (12 oz)	0	0	0	0
Diet Root Beer	1 can (12 oz)	0	0	0	0
Diet Strawberry	1 can (12 oz)	0	0	0	0
Diet Strawberry-Peach	1 can (12 oz)	0	0	0	0
Doc Shasta	1 can (12 oz)	160	39	39	0
Fruit Punch	1 can (12 oz)	200	50	50	0
Ginger Ale	1 can (12 oz)	130	32	32	0
Grape	1 can (12 oz)	190	48	48	0
Kiwi-Strawberry	1 can (12 oz)	170	43	43	0

FOOD	PORTION	CALS.	CARB.	SUG.	FIB.
Shasta (CONT.)					
Lemon-Lime Twist	1 can (12 oz)	150	38	38	0
Moon Mist	1 can (12 oz)	180	46	46	0
Orange	1 can (12 oz)	200	49	49	0
Peach	1 can (12 oz)	170	43	43	0
Pineapple	1 can (12 oz)	200	51	51	0
Pineapple-Orange	1 can (12 oz)	180	46	46	0
Quinine/Tonic	1 can (12 oz)	130	32	32	0
Raspberry Creme	1 can (12 oz)	170	44	44	0
Red Pop	1 can (12 oz)	170	43	43	0
Root Beer	1 can (12 oz)	170	42	42	0
Strawberry	1 can (12 oz)	190	46	46	0
Strawberry-Peach	1 can (12 oz)	170	42	42	0
Slice					
Diet Lemon Lime	8 fl oz	5	tr	tr	—
Diet Mandarin	8 fl oz	5	tr	tr	—
Lemon Lime	8 fl oz	100	26	26	—
Mandarin Orange	8 fl oz	128	33	33	—
Red	8 fl oz	128	33	33	—
Snapple					
Amazin' Grape	8 fl oz	120	28	—	—
Cherry Lime Ricky	8 fl oz	110	27	—	—
Creme D'Vanilla	8 fl oz	130	33	—	—
French Cherry	8 fl oz	120	29	—	—
Kiwi Peach	8 fl oz	120	29	—	—
Kiwi Strawberry	8 fl oz	130	33	—	—
Mango Madness	8 fl oz	130	33	—	—
Passion Supreme	8 fl oz	120	29	—	—
Peach Melba	8 fl oz	120	31	—	—
Raspberry	8 fl oz	120	31	—	—
Seltzer Black Cherry	8 fl oz	0	0	0	0
Seltzer Lemon Lime	8 fl oz	0	0	0	0
Seltzer Original	8 fl oz	0	0	0	0
Seltzer Tangerine	8 fl oz	0	0	0	0
Tru Root Beer	8 fl oz	110	29	—	—
Sprite					
Diet	8 fl oz	3	0	0	0
Soda	8 fl oz	100	26	26	—
Sundrop					
Cherry	8 fl oz	130	21	21	0
Diet	8 fl oz	5	0	0	0
Soda	8 fl oz	140	34	34	0
Sunkist					
Cactus Cooler	8 fl oz	110	27	27	0

FOOD	PORTION	CALS.	CARB.	SUG.	FIB.
Sunkist (CONT.)					
Cherry	8 fl oz	140	35	35	0
Diet Citrus	8 fl oz	0	0	0	0
Diet Orange	8 fl oz	5	0	0	0
Fruit Punch	8 fl oz	130	33	33	0
Orange	8 fl oz	140	35	35	0
Peach	8 fl oz	120	30	30	0
Pineapple	8 fl oz	140	35	35	0
Strawberry	8 fl oz	140	34	34	0
TAB					
Soda	8 fl oz	1	tr	—	—
Tropical Chill					
Cola	8 fl oz	117	31	31	—
Diet	8 fl oz	1	tr	tr	—
Upper 10					
Diet	8 fl oz	3	1	—	—
Diet Salt/Sodium Free	8 fl oz	3	1	—	—
Salt Free	8 fl oz	100	29	—	—
Soda	8 fl oz	100	28	—	—
Wink					
Diet	8 fl oz	5	1	1	0
Soda	8 fl oz	130	31	31	0
Yoo-Hoo					
Original	9 fl oz	150	31	—	tr
SOLE					
FRESH					
cooked	1 fillet (4.5 oz)	148	0	0	0
cooked	3 oz	99	0	0	0
lemon raw	3½ oz	85	0	0	0
raw	3½ oz	90	0	0	0
FROZEN					
Gorton's					
Fishmarket Fresh	5 oz	110	1	—	—
Microwave Entree In Lemon Butter	1 pkg	380	17	—	—
Microwave Entree In Wine Sauce	1 pkg	180	3	—	—
Mrs. Paul's					
Light Fillets	1 fillet	240	20	—	—
Van De Kamp's					
Lightly Breaded Fillets	1 (4 oz)	220	17	3	0

FOOD	PORTION	CALS.	CARB.	SUG.	FIB.
Van De Kamp's (CONT.)					
Natural Fillets	1 (4 oz)	110	0	0	0

SORBET
(*see* ICES AND ICE POPS)

SORGHUM
| sorghum | 1 cup (6.7 oz) | 651 | 143 | — | — |

SOUFFLE
grand marnier	1 cup	109	14	—	—
lemon chilled	1 cup	176	34	—	—
raspberry chilled	1 cup	173	34	—	—
spinach	1 cup	218	3	—	—

SOUP
CANNED
asparagus cream of as prep w/ milk	1 cup	161	16	—	—
asparagus cream of as prep w/ water	1 cup	87	11	—	—
beef broth ready-to-serve	1 can (14 oz)	27	tr	—	—
beef broth ready-to-serve	1 cup	16	tr	—	—
beef noodle as prep w/water	1 cup	84	9	—	—
black bean turtle soup	1 cup	218	40	—	—
black bean as prep w/water	1 cup	116	20	—	—
celery cream of as prep w/ milk	1 cup	165	15	—	—
celery cream of as prep w/ water	1 cup	90	9	—	—
celery cream of not prep	1 can (10.75 oz)	219	21	—	—
cheese as prep w/ milk	1 cup	230	16	—	—
cheese as prep w/ water	1 cup	155	11	—	—
cheese not prep	1 can (11 oz)	377	26	—	—
chicken broth as prep w/ water	1 cup	39	1	—	—
chicken cream of as prep w/ milk	1 cup	191	15	—	—
chicken cream of as prep w/ water	1 cup	116	9	—	—
chicken gumbo as prep w/ water	1 cup	56	8	—	—
chicken noodle as prep w/ water	1 cup	75	9	—	—
chicken rice as prep w/ water	1 cup	251	7	—	—

FOOD	PORTION	CALS.	CARB.	SUG.	FIB.
clam chowder manhattan as prep w/ water	1 cup	77	12	—	—
clam chowder new england as prep w/ water	1 cup	95	12	—	—
clam chowder new england as prep w/ milk	1 cup	163	17	—	—
consomme w/ gelatin not prep	1 can (10.5 oz)	71	4	—	—
consomme w/ gelatin as prep w/ water	1 cup	29	2	—	—
escarole ready-to-serve	1 cup	27	2	—	—
french onion as prep w/ water	1 cup	57	8	—	—
gazpacho ready-to-serve	1 cup	57	1	—	—
minestrone as prep w/water	1 cup	83	11	—	—
mushroom cream of as prep w/ milk	1 cup	203	15	—	—
mushroom cream of as prep w/ water	1 cup	129	9	—	—
oyster stew as prep w/ milk	1 cup	134	10	—	—
oyster stew as prep w/ water	1 cup	59	4	—	—
pepperpot as prep w/ water	1 cup	103	9	—	—
potato cream of as prep w/ milk	1 cup	148	17	—	—
potato cream of as prep w/ water	1 cup	73	11	—	—
scotch broth as prep w/ water	1 cup	80	9	—	—
split pea w/ ham as prep w/ water	1 cup	189	28	—	—
tomato as prep w/ milk	1 cup	160	22	—	—
tomato as prep w/water	1 cup	86	17	—	—
vegetarian vegetable as prep w/ water	1 cup	72	12	—	—
vichyssoise	1 cup	148	17	—	—
Campbell					
Asparagus Cream Of as prep	8 oz	80	10	—	—
Bean Homestyle as prep	8 oz	130	25	—	—
Bean With Bacon as prep	8 oz	140	21	—	—
Beef as prep	8 oz	80	10	—	—
Beef Broth as prep	8 oz	16	1	—	—
Beef Noodle Homestyle as prep	8 oz	80	7	—	—
Beef Noodle as prep	8 oz	70	7	—	—
Beefy Mushroom as prep	8 oz	60	5	—	—

FOOD	PORTION	CALS.	CARB.	SUG.	FIB.
Campbell (CONT.)					
Broccoli Cream Of as prep	8 oz	80	8	—	—
Broccoli Cream Of as prep w/ 2% milk	8 oz	140	14	—	—
Celery Cream Of as prep	8 oz	100	8	—	—
Cheddar Cheese as prep	8 oz	110	10	—	—
Chicken Alphabet as prep	8 oz	80	10	—	—
Chicken Noodle-O's as prep	8 oz	70	9	—	—
Chicken Vegetable as prep	8 oz	70	8	—	—
Chicken & Pasta With Garden Vegetables	1 cup (8.4 oz)	90	14	2	1
Chicken & Stars as prep	8 oz	60	7	—	—
Chicken 'n Dumplings as prep	8 oz	80	9	—	—
Chicken Barley as prep	8 oz	70	10	—	—
Chicken Broth as prep	8 oz	30	2	—	—
Chicken Broth & Noodles as prep	8 oz	45	8	—	—
Chicken Cream Of as prep	8 oz	110	9	—	—
Chicken Gumbo as prep	8 oz	60	8	—	—
Chicken Mushroom Creamy as prep	8 oz	120	8	—	—
Chicken Noodle Homestyle as prep	8 oz	70	8	—	—
Chicken Noodle as prep	8 oz	60	8	—	—
Chicken With Rice as prep	8 oz	60	7	—	—
Chili Beef as prep	8 oz	140	20	—	—
Chunky Chicken Nuggets w/ Vegetables & Noodles	10.75 oz	190	24	—	—
Clam Chowder Manhattan Style as prep	8 oz	70	10	—	—
Clam Chowder New England as prep	8 oz	80	12	—	—
Clam Chowder New England as prep w/ whole milk	8 oz	150	17	—	—
Consomme as prep	8 oz	25	2	—	—
Curly Noodle With Chicken as prep	8 oz	80	11	—	—
French Onion as prep	8 oz	60	9	—	—
Green Pea as prep	8 oz	160	25	—	—
Healthy Request Bean With Bacon as prep	8 oz	140	22	—	—
Healthy Request Chicken Noodle as prep	8 oz	60	8	—	—

FOOD	PORTION	CALS.	CARB.	SUG.	FIB.
Campbell (CONT.)					
Healthy Request Chicken With Rice as prep	8 oz	60	7	—	—
Healthy Request Cream Of Mushroom as prep	8 oz	60	9	—	—
Healthy Request Cream Of Chicken	8 oz	70	11	—	—
Healthy Request Hearty Chicken Vegetable	8 oz	120	16	—	—
Healthy Request Ready-To-Serve Chicken Broth	8 oz	10	1	—	—
Healthy Request Ready-To-Serve Hearty Minestrone	8 oz	90	13	—	—
Healthy Request Ready-To-Serve Hearty Chicken Noodle	8 oz	80	7	—	—
Healthy Request Ready-To-Serve Hearty Chicken Rice	8 oz	110	15	—	—
Healthy Request Ready-To-Serve Hearty Vegetable	8 oz	110	17	—	—
Healthy Request Ready-To-Serve Hearty Vegetable Beef	8 oz	120	15	—	—
Healthy Request Tomato as prep	8 oz	90	17	—	—
Healthy Request Tomato as prep w/ skim milk	8 oz	130	22	—	—
Healthy Request Vegetable as prep	8 oz	90	14	—	—
Healthy Request Vegetable Beef as prep	8 oz	70	9	—	—
Home Cookin' Bean & Ham	10.75 oz	210	29	—	—
Home Cookin' Beef With Vegetables & Pasta	10.75 oz	140	18	—	—
Home Cookin' Chicken Minestrone	10.75 oz	180	17	—	—
Home Cookin' Chicken Gumbo With Sausages	10.75 oz	140	15	—	—
Home Cookin' Chicken Rice	10.75 oz	150	10	—	—
Home Cookin' Chicken With Noodles	10.75 oz	140	12	—	—
Home Cookin' Country Vegetable	10.75 oz	120	20	—	—

FOOD	PORTION	CALS.	CARB.	SUG.	FIB.
Campbell (cont.)					
Home Cookin' Garden Tomato	10.75 oz	150	29	—	—
Home Cookin' Hearty Lentil	10.75 oz	170	28	—	—
Home Cookin' Minestrone	10.75 oz	140	22	—	—
Home Cookin' Split Pea With Ham	10.75 oz	230	38	—	—
Home Cookin' Vegetable Beef	10.75 oz	140	17	—	—
Minestrone as prep	8 oz	80	13	—	—
Mushroom Cream Of as prep	8 oz	100	8	—	—
Mushroom Golden as prep	8 oz	70	9	—	—
Nacho Cheese as prep	8 oz	110	8	—	—
Nacho Cheese as prep w/ milk	8 oz	180	13	—	—
Noodles & Ground Beef as prep	8 oz	90	10	—	—
Onion Cream Of as prep	8 oz	100	12	—	—
Onion Cream Of as prep w/ whole milk & water	8 oz	140	15	—	—
Oyster Stew as prep	8 oz	70	5	—	—
Oyster Stew as prep w/ whole milk	8 oz	140	10	—	—
Pepper Pot as prep	8 oz	90	9	—	—
Potato Cream Of as prep	8 oz	80	12	—	—
Potato Cream Of as prep w/ whole milk & water	8 oz	120	15	—	—
Ready-To-Serve Chunky Chili Beef	11 oz	290	37	—	—
Ready-To-Serve Chunky Mediterranean Vegetable	9.5 oz	170	24	—	—
Ready-To-Serve Chunky Minestrone	9.5 oz	160	24	—	—
Ready-To-Serve Chunky Beef	10.75 oz	200	24	—	—
Ready-To-Serve Chunky Beef Stroganoff	10.75 oz	320	28	—	—
Ready-To-Serve Chunky Chicken Corn Chowder	10.75 oz	340	23	—	—
Ready-To-Serve Chunky Chicken Noodle	10.75 oz	200	20	—	—
Ready-To-Serve Chunky Chicken Vegetable	9.5 oz	170	19	—	—

FOOD	PORTION	CALS.	CARB.	SUG.	FIB.
Campbell (CONT.)					
Ready-To-Serve Chunky Chicken With Rice	9.5 oz	140	16	—	—
Ready-To-Serve Chunky Creamy Chicken Mushroom	10.5 oz	270	13	—	—
Ready-To-Serve Chunky Creole Style	10.75 oz	240	31	—	—
Ready-To-Serve Chunky Ham 'n Butter Bean	10.75 oz	280	34	—	—
Ready-To-Serve Chunky Manhattan Style Clam Chowder	10.75 oz	160	24	—	—
Ready-To-Serve Chunky New England Clam Chowder	10.75 oz	290	26	—	—
Ready-To-Serve Chunky Old Fashioned Chicken	10.75 oz	180	21	—	—
Ready-To-Serve Chunky Old Fashioned Vegetable Beef	10.75 oz	190	20	—	—
Ready-To-Serve Chunky Old Fashioned Bean w/ Ham	11 oz	290	38	—	—
Ready-To-Serve Chunky Pepper Steak	10.75 oz	180	24	—	—
Ready-To-Serve Chunky Sirloin Burger	10.75 oz	220	23	—	—
Ready-To-Serve Chunky Split Pea w/ Ham	10.75 oz	230	33	—	—
Ready-To-Serve Chunky Steak & Potato	10.75 oz	200	24	—	—
Ready-To-Serve Chunky Turkey Vegetable	9.5 oz	150	16	—	—
Ready-To-Serve Low Sodium Chicken Vegetable Beef	10.75 oz	180	19	—	—
Ready-To-Serve Low Sodium Chicken Broth	10.5 oz	30	2	—	—
Ready-To-Serve Low Sodium Chicken With Noodles	10.75 oz	170	17	—	—
Ready-To-Serve Low Sodium Mushroom Cream Of	10.5 oz	210	18	—	—

FOOD	PORTION	CALS.	CARB.	SUG.	FIB.
Campbell (CONT.)					
Ready-To-Serve Low Sodium Split Pea	10.75 oz	230	37	—	—
Ready-To-Serve Low Sodium Tomato With Tomato Pieces	10.5 oz	190	30	—	—
Scotch Broth as prep	8 oz	80	9	—	—
Shrimp Cream Of as prep	8 oz	90	8	—	—
Shrimp Cream Of as prep w/ whole milk	8 oz	160	13	—	—
Split Pea With Bacon as prep	8 oz	160	24	—	—
Teddy Bear as prep	8 oz	70	11	—	—
Tomato as prep	8 oz	90	17	—	—
Tomato as prep w/ 2% milk	8 oz	150	22	—	—
Tomato Bisque as prep	8 oz	120	22	—	—
Tomato Homestyle Cream Of as prep	8 oz	110	20	—	—
Tomato Homestyle Cream Of as prep w/ whole milk	8 oz	180	25	—	—
Tomato Rice Old Fashioned as prep	8 oz	110	22	—	—
Tomato Zesty as prep	8 oz	100	20	—	—
Turkey Vegetable as prep	8 oz	70	8	—	—
Turkey Noodle as prep	8 oz	70	9	—	—
Vegetable Homestyle as prep	8 oz	60	9	—	—
Vegetable as prep	8 oz	90	14	—	—
Vegetable Beef as prep	8 oz	70	10	—	—
Vegetable Old Fashioned as prep	8 oz	60	9	—	—
Vegetarian Vegetable as prep	8 oz	80	13	—	—
Won Ton as prep	8 oz	40	5	—	—
College Inn					
Beef Broth	½ can (7 oz)	16	1	—	—
Chicken Broth	½ can (7 oz)	35	0	0	0
Chicken Broth Lower Salt	½ can (7 oz)	20	0	0	0
Gold's					
Borscht	8 oz	100	21	—	—
Borscht Lo-Cal	8 oz	20	5	—	—
Schav	8 oz	25	4	—	—
Gorton's					
New England Clam Chowder as prep w/ whole milk	¼ can	140	17	—	—

FOOD	PORTION	CALS.	CARB.	SUG.	FIB.
Goya					
Black Bean	7.5 oz	160	29	—	9
Hain					
Chicken Broth	8.75 fl oz	70	0	0	0
Chicken Broth No Salt Added	8.75 fl oz	60	0	0	0
Chicken Noodle	9.5 fl oz	120	11	—	—
Chicken Noodle No Salt Added	9.5 fl oz	120	12	—	—
Creamy Mushroom	9.25 fl oz	110	16	—	—
Italian Vegetable Pasta	9.5 fl oz	160	25	—	—
Italian Vegetable Pasta Low Sodium	9.5 fl oz	140	22	—	—
Minestrone	9.5 fl oz	170	27	—	—
Minestrone No Salt Added	9.5 fl oz	160	28	—	—
Mushroom Barley	9.5 fl oz	100	17	—	—
New England Clam Chowder	9.5 fl oz	180	26	—	—
Split Pea	9.5 fl oz	170	28	—	—
Split Pea No Salt Added	9.5 fl oz	170	29	—	—
Turkey Rice	9.5 fl oz	100	10	—	—
Turkey Rice No Salt Added	9.5 fl oz	120	13	—	—
Vegetable Chicken	9.5 fl oz	120	14	—	—
Vegetable Chicken No Salt Added	9.5 fl oz	130	14	—	—
Vegetable Broth	9.5 fl oz	45	10	—	—
Vegetable Broth Low Sodium	9.5 fl oz	40	8	—	—
Vegetable Split Pea	9.5 fl oz	170	28	—	—
Vegetable Split Pea No Salt Added	9.5 fl oz	170	27	—	—
Vegetarian Lentil	9.5 fl oz	160	25	—	—
Vegetarian Lentil No Salt Added	9.5 fl oz	160	24	—	—
Vegetarian Vegetable	9.5 fl oz	140	22	—	—
Vegetarian Vegetable No Salt Added	9.5 fl oz	150	23	—	—
Health Valley					
Beef Broth	7.5 oz	10	2	—	0
Beef Broth No Salt Added	7.5 oz	10	2	—	0
Black Bean	7.5 oz	150	24	—	16
Black Bean No Salt Added	7.5 oz	150	24	—	16
Chicken Broth	7.5 oz	35	1	—	0
Chicken Broth No Salt Added	7.5 oz	35	1	—	0

FOOD	PORTION	CALS.	CARB.	SUG.	FIB.
Health Valley (CONT.)					
Chunky Chicken Vegetable	7.5 oz	125	20	—	4
Chunky Five Bean Vegetable	7.5 oz	110	21	—	11
Chunky Five Bean Vegetable No Salt Added	7.5 oz	110	21	—	11
Chunky Vegetable Chicken No Salt Added	7.5 oz	125	20	—	4
Green Split Pea	7.5 oz	180	34	—	15
Green Split Pea No Salt Added	7.5 oz	180	34	—	15
Lentil	7.5 oz	220	33	—	10
Lentil No Salt Added	7.5 oz	220	4	—	10
Manhattan Clam Chowder	7.5 oz	110	15	—	2
Manhattan Clam Chowder No Salt Added	7.5 oz	110	15	—	2
Minestrone	7.5 oz	130	19	—	13
Minestrone No Salt Added	7.5 oz	130	19	—	13
Mushroom Barley	7.5 oz	100	2	—	9
Mushroom Barley No Salt Added	7.5 oz	100	16	—	9
Potato Leek	7.5 oz	130	23	—	7
Potato Leek No Salt Added	7.5 oz	130	23	—	7
Tomato	7.5 oz	130	21	—	1
Tomato No Salt Added	7.5 oz	130	21	—	1
Vegetable	7.5 oz	110	20	—	8
Vegetable No Salt Added	7.5 oz	110	20	—	8
Healthy Choice					
Bean & Ham	1 cup (8.7 oz)	184	34	0	10
Beef & Potato	1 cup (8.5 oz)	119	18	—	3
Chicken Corn Chowder	1 cup (8.8 oz)	176	30	2	2
Chicken Pasta	1 cup (8.6 oz)	118	18	0	1
Chicken With Rice	1 cup (8.4 oz)	108	15	0	1
Chili Beef	1 cup (9.1 oz)	166	30	5	5
Clam Chowder	1 cup (8.8 oz)	123	23	3	2
Country Vegetable	1 cup (8.6 oz)	104	23	1	2
Cream Of Mushroom	1 cup (8.8 oz)	77	14	0	1
Cream Of Chicken With Mushrooms	1 cup (8.9 oz)	127	20	0	1
Cream Of Chicken With Vegetables	1 cup (8.9 oz)	127	21	0	1
Garden Vegetable	1 cup (8.6 oz)	118	26	0	3
Hearty Chicken	1 cup (8.7 oz)	132	20	0	1
Lentil	1 cup (8.7 oz)	146	28	1	5

FOOD	PORTION	CALS.	CARB.	SUG.	FIB.
Healthy Choice (CONT.)					
Minestrone	1 cup (8.6 oz)	112	23	3	3
Old Fashion Chicken Noodle	1 cup (8.8 oz)	137	19	0	1
Split Pea & Ham	1 cup (8.8 oz)	155	26	3	2
Tomato Garden	1 cup (8.6 oz)	106	21	7	3
Turkey With Wild Rice	1 cup (8.4 oz)	92	13	0	1
Vegetable Beef	1 cup (8.8 oz)	130	22	0	2
Herb-Ox					
Beef Liquid	2 tsp (0.4 oz)	20	2	1	0
Chicken Liquid	2 tsp (0.4 oz)	15	1	0	0
Manischewitz					
Borscht Low Calorie	8 fl oz	20	4	—	—
Borscht With Beets	8 fl oz	80	20	—	—
Old El Paso					
Black Bean With Bacon	1 cup (8.6 oz)	160	26	2	7
Chicken Vegetable	1 cup (8.4 oz)	110	13	4	0
Chicken With Rice	1 cup (8.4 oz)	90	10	1	0
Garden Vegetable	1 cup (8.4 oz)	110	17	0	0
Hearty Beef	1 cup (8.4 oz)	120	14	2	0
Hearty Chicken Noodle	1 cup (8.4 oz)	110	10	0	0
Pritikin					
Chicken & Rice	1 cup (8.8 oz)	80	13	—	—
Chicken Broth	1 cup (8.5 oz)	15	1	—	—
Chicken Pasta	1 cup (8.6 oz)	100	18	—	—
Hearty Vegetable	1 cup (8.8 oz)	90	20	—	—
Lentil	1 cup (8.4 oz)	130	24	—	—
Minestrone	1 cup (8.8 oz)	90	19	—	—
Split Pea	1 cup (9.2 oz)	140	29	—	—
Three Bean Chili	½ cup (4.5 oz)	90	19	—	—
Vegetable Broth	1 cup (8.3 oz)	20	3	—	—
Vegetarian Vegetables	1 cup (9 oz)	100	23	—	—
Progresso					
Bean And Ham	1 cup (8.4 oz)	160	25	2	8
Beef	1 can (10.5 fl oz)	180	17	—	—
Beef Barley	1 cup (8.5 oz)	130	13	0	3
Beef Minestrone	1 cup (8.5 oz)	140	14	0	3
Beef Noodle	1 cup (8.5 oz)	140	15	2	1
Beef Vegetable & Rotini	1 cup (8 oz)	120	10	tr	3
Broccoli & Shells	1 cup (8.5 oz)	70	14	2	3
Chickarina	1 cup (8.3 oz)	120	10	0	1
Chicken Minestrone	1 cup (8.4 oz)	120	12	0	2
Chicken Vegetables & Penne	1 cup (8.4 oz)	100	11	2	3

FOOD	PORTION	CALS.	CARB.	SUG.	FIB.
Progresso (CONT.)					
Chicken & Wild Rice	1 cup (8.4 oz)	100	15	0	2
Chicken Barley	1 cup (8.5 oz)	110	14	0	3
Chicken Broth	1 cup ((8.2 oz)	20	1	—	0
Chicken Noodle	1 cup (8.4 oz)	80	8	0	1
Chicken Noodle	1 can (10.5 oz)	110	10	0	1
Chicken Rice Vegetable	1 cup (8.4 oz)	110	12	0	tr
Chicken Rice Vegetable	1 can (10.5 oz)	130	15	0	tr
Clam & Rotini Chowder	1 cup (8.8 oz)	200	21	3	0
Corn Chowder	1 cup (8.6 oz)	180	20	4	2
Cream Of Chicken	1 cup (8.4 oz)	170	11	0	0
Cream Of Mushroom	1 cup (8.4 oz)	140	12	0	1
Creamy Tortellini	1 cup (8.4 oz)	210	15	0	0
Escarole In Chicken Broth	1 cup (8.1 oz)	25	2	0	0
Green Split Pea	1 cup (8.6 oz)	170	25	4	5
Healthy Classics Beef Barley	1 cup (8.5 oz)	140	20	1	3
Healthy Classics Beef Vegetable	1 cup (8.5 oz)	150	25	3	6
Healthy Classics Chicken Noodle	1 cup (8.3 oz)	80	10	1	1
Healthy Classics Chicken Rice With Vegetables	1 cup (8.4 oz)	90	12	0	1
Healthy Classics Cream Of Broccoli	1 cup (8.6 oz)	90	13	tr	2
Healthy Classics Garlic & Pasta	1 cup (8.5 oz)	100	18	3	3
Healthy Classics Lentil	1 cup (8.5 oz)	120	20	0	1
Healthy Classics Minestrone	1 cup (8.5 oz)	120	20	0	1
Healthy Classics New England Clam Chowder	1 cup (8.6 oz)	120	20	1	1
Healthy Classics Split Pea	1 cup (8.9 oz)	180	30	2	5
Healthy Classics Tomato Garden Vegetable	1 cup (8.6 oz)	100	19	8	4
Healthy Classics Vegetable	1 cup (8.4 oz)	80	13	2	1
Hearty Minestrone With Shells	1 cup (8.4 oz)	120	20	2	4
Hearty Black Bean	1 cup (8.5 oz)	170	30	0	10
Hearty Chicken	1 can (10.5 fl oz)	120	10	0	0
Hearty Chicken & Rotini	1 cup (8.4 oz)	90	8	0	0
Hearty Penne In Chicken Broth	1 cup (8.4 oz)	70	12	0	0
Hearty Tomato & Rotini	1 cup (8.4 oz)	90	16	5	3

FOOD	PORTION	CALS.	CARB.	SUG.	FIB.
Progresso (CONT.)					
Hearty Vegetable With Rotini	1 cup (8.4 oz)	110	20	2	3
Homestyle Chicken Vegetable	1 cup (8.4 oz)	100	10	0	1
Lentil	1 can (10.5 fl oz)	170	27	0	8
Lentil	1 cup (8.5 oz)	140	22	0	7
Lentil & Shells	1 cup (8.5 oz)	130	22	0	4
Lentil With Sausage	1 cup (8.5 oz)	170	19	0	5
Macaroni & Bean	1 cup (8.6 oz)	160	23	1	6
Manhattan Clam Chowder	1 cup (8.4 oz)	110	11	3	3
Meatballs & Pasta Pearls	1 cup (8.3 oz)	140	13	0	0
Minestrone	1 cup (8.4 oz)	130	22	4	5
Minestrone	1 can (10.5 fl oz)	170	27	5	6
New England Clam Chowder	1 can (10.5 oz)	220	21	7	2
New England Clam Chowder	1 cup (8.4 oz)	180	17	6	2
Spicy Chicken & Penne	1 cup (8.5 oz)	120	13	2	0
Split Pea With Ham	1 cup (8.5 oz)	160	20	1	5
Tomato	1 cup (8.5 oz)	90	15	8	4
Tomato Tortellini	1 cup (8.4 oz)	120	13	5	2
Tomato Beef & Rotini	1 cup (8.5 oz)	140	15	2	2
Tortellini In Chicken Broth	1 cup (8.3 oz)	80	10	1	2
Vegetable	1 cup (8.4 oz)	90	15	4	3
Zesty Minestrone	1 cup (8.3 oz)	150	17	0	4
Snow's					
Manhattan Clam Chowder as prep w/ water	7.5 fl oz	70	9	—	—
New England Clam Chowder as prep w/ milk	7.5 fl oz	140	13	—	—
New England Corn Chowder as prep w/ milk	7.5 fl oz	150	18	—	—
New England Fish Chowder as prep w/ milk	7.5 fl oz	130	11	—	—
New England Seafood Chowder as prep w/ milk	7.5 fl oz	130	11	—	—
Swanson					
Beef Broth	7.25 oz	18	1	—	—
Chicken Broth	7.25 oz	30	2	—	—
Natural Goodness Clear Chicken Broth	7.25 oz	20	1	—	—
Vegetable Broth	7.25 fl oz	20	3	—	—
Weight Watchers					
Chicken & Rice	1 can (10.5 oz)	110	17	11	4

FOOD	PORTION	CALS.	CARB.	SUG.	FIB.
Weight Watchers (CONT.)					
Chicken Noodle	1 can (10.5 oz)	150	25	15	4
Minestrone	1 can (10.5 oz)	130	23	7	6
Vegetable	1 can (10.5 oz)	130	27	11	6
FROZEN					
Jaclyn's					
Barley & Mushroom	7.5 fl oz	90	16	—	—
Split Pea	7.5 fl oz	180	31	—	—
Vegetable	7.5 fl oz	90	18	—	—
Tabatchnick					
Barley Mushroom	1 serv (7.5 oz)	70	13	0	3
Barley Mushroom No Salt Added	1 serv (7.5 oz)	70	13	0	3
Broccoli Cream Of	1 serv (7.5 oz)	90	12	6	3
Cabbage	1 serv (7.5 oz)	60	14	9	2
Chicken With Dumplings	1 serv (7.5 oz)	70	13	2	1
Corn Chowder	1 serv (7.5 oz)	150	22	4	1
Minestrone	1 serv (7.5 oz)	150	27	3	10
New England Potato	1 serv (7.5 oz)	150	21	4	2
New York Chicken	1 serv (7.5 oz)	35	6	2	0
Old Fashion Potato	1 serv (7.5 oz)	70	16	2	2
Pea	1 serv (7.5 oz)	180	31	2	11
Pea No Salt Added	1 serv (7.5 oz)	180	31	2	11
Spinach Cream Of	1 serv (7.5 oz)	90	11	5	2
Vegetable	1 serv (7.5 oz)	110	20	3	4
Vegetable No Salt Added	1 serv (7.5 oz)	110	20	3	4
Wisconsin Cheddar Vegetable	1 serv (7.5 oz)	140	12	4	1
Yankee Bean	1 serv (7.5 oz)	160	27	1	11
MIX					
asparagus cream of as prep w/ water	1 cup	59	9	—	—
beef broth	1 pkg (0.2 oz)	14	1	—	—
beef broth as prep w/ water	1 cup	19	2	—	—
beef broth cube	1 cube (3.6 g)	6	1	—	—
beef broth cube as prep w/ water	1 cup	8	1	—	—
celery cream of as prep w/ water	1 cup	63	10	—	—
chicken broth	1 pkg (0.2 oz)	16	1	—	—
chicken broth as prep w/water	1 cup	21	1	—	—
chicken broth cube	1 cube (4.8 g)	9	1	—	—
chicken broth cube, as prep w/ water	1 cup	13	2	—	—

FOOD	PORTION	CALS.	CARB.	SUG.	FIB.
chicken cream of as prep w/ water	1 cup	107	13	—	—
chicken noodle as prep w/ water	1 cup	53	7	—	—
french onion not prep	1 pkg (1.4 oz)	115	21	—	—
leek as prep w/ water	1 cup	71	11	—	—
onion as prep w/ water	1 cup	28	5	—	—
tomato as prep w/ water	1 cup	102	19	—	—
4C					
Noodle	8 oz	50	7	—	—
Onion Reduced Salt	8 oz	30	5	—	—
Armour					
Bouillon Cubes Beef	1 (4 g)	5	1	—	—
Bouillon Cubes Chicken	1 (4 g)	5	1	—	—
Arrowhead					
Bean & Barley	¼ cup (1.9 oz)	170	35	0	7
Bean Cuisine					
Bean Bouillabaisse	1 cup (7.5 fl oz)	174	18	1	5
Island Black Bean	1 cup (8.7 fl oz)	210	33	3	10
Lots of Lentil	1 cup (7.7 oz)	166	19	0	6
Mesa Maize	1 cup (9.2 fl oz)	179	21	0	6
Rocky Mountain Red Bean	1 cup (8.6 oz)	202	24	0	8
Sante Fe Corn Chowder	1 cup (9.2 oz)	179	21	0	6
Thick As Fog Split Pea	1 cup (8.6 fl oz)	189	21	0	1
Ultima Pasta E Fagioli	1 cup (8.6 fl oz)	179	22	0	4
White Bean Provencal	1 cup (7.7 fl oz)	166	19	0	6
Campbell					
Bean With Bacon 'n Ham Microwave	7.5 oz	230	38	—	—
Chicken Noodle Microwave	7.5 oz	100	11	—	—
Chicken Noodle as prep	8 oz	100	16	—	—
Chicken With Rice Microwave	7.5 oz	100	14	—	—
Chili Beef Microwave	7.5 oz	190	32	—	—
Hearty Noodle as prep	8 oz	90	15	—	—
Noodle as prep	8 oz	110	19	—	—
Onion as prep	8 oz	30	7	—	—
Vegetable as prep	8 oz	40	8	—	—
Vegetable Beef Microwave	7.5 oz	100	16	—	—
Campbell's Cup					
Beef Noodle	1 (1.35 oz)	130	23	—	—
Chicken Noodle	1 (1.35 oz)	140	22	—	—
Chicken Noodle w/ White Meat as prep	6 oz	90	12	—	—

FOOD	PORTION	CALS.	CARB.	SUG.	FIB.
Campbell's Cup (CONT.)					
Creamy Chicken w/ White Meat as prep	6 oz	90	12	—	—
Hearty Noodles With Vegetables	1 (1.7 oz)	180	32	—	—
Noodle With Chicken Broth as prep	6 oz	90	15	—	—
Casbah					
Black Bean	1 pkg (1.7 oz)	170	30	0	9
Split Pea	1 pkg (2.3 oz)	230	40	2	10
Sweet Corn Chowder	1 pkg (1.2 oz)	125	26	4	2
Vegetarian Chili	1 pkg (1.8 oz)	170	31	5	7
Cup-A-Ramen					
Beef With Vegetables Low Fat as prep	8 oz	220	44	—	—
Beef With Vegetables as prep	8 oz	270	38	—	—
Chicken With Vegetables Low Fat as prep	8 oz	220	44	—	—
Chicken With Vegetables as prep	8 oz	270	38	—	—
Oriental With Vegetables Low Fat as prep	8 oz	220	44	—	—
Oriental With Vegetables as prep	8 oz	270	38	—	—
Shrimp With Vegetables Low Fat as prep	8 oz	230	45	—	—
Shrimp With Vegetables as prep	8 oz	280	40	—	—
Cup-a-Soup					
Broccoli & Cheese as prep	1 serv (6 oz)	70	9	2	tr
Chicken Vegetable as prep	1 serv (6 oz)	50	10	1	0
Chicken Broth as prep	1 serv (6 oz)	20	3	0	0
Chicken Broth w/ Pasta Fat Free as prep	1 serv (6 oz)	45	8	0	0
Chicken Noodle as prep	1 serv (6 oz)	50	8	0	0
Cream Of Chicken as prep	1 serv (6 oz)	70	12	2	tr
Creamy Chicken Vegetable as prep	1 serv (6 oz)	80	10	2	tr
Creamy Mushroom as prep	1 serv (6 oz)	60	10	1	0
Green Pea as prep	1 serv (6 oz)	80	12	1	3
Hearty Chicken Noodle as prep	1 serv (6 oz)	60	10	0	0
Ring Noodle as prep	1 serv (6 oz)	50	9	0	0

FOOD	PORTION	CALS.	CARB.	SUG.	FIB.
Cup-a-Soup (CONT.)					
Spring Vegetable as prep	1 serv (6 oz)	45	21	1	tr
Tomato as prep	1 serv (6 oz)	100	20	14	tr
Emes					
Beef Base	1 tsp	18	2	—	—
Chicken Base	1 tsp	18	2	—	—
Fantastic					
Cha-Cha Chili Low Fat	1 pkg	220	37	4	13
Golden Dipt					
Lobster Bisque	¼ pkg	30	5	—	—
Manhattan Clam Chowder	¼ pkg	80	13	—	—
New England Clam Chowder	¼ pkg	24	12	—	—
Seafood Chowder	¼ pkg	70	12	—	—
Shrimp Bisque	¼ pkg	30	5	—	—
Goodman's					
Cup Of Soup Beef	1 pkg (1½ cups)	180	32	5	2
Cup Of Soup Chicken Noodle	1 pkg (1½ cups)	180	31	5	2
Cup Of Soup Vegetable	1 pkg (1½ cups)	180	32	4	2
Matzo Ball & Soup	1 cup	40	9	2	1
Matzo Ball & Soup 50% Less Salt	1 serv	50	10	2	1
Noodleman	1 cup	45	9	4	0
Noodleman Low Sodium	1 cup	50	9	2	1
Onion	1 cup	30	5	2	1
Onion Low Sodium	1 cup	30	6	3	1
Hain					
Cheese & Broccoli	¾ cup	310	19	—	—
Cheese Savory	¾ cup	250	20	—	—
Savory Lentil	¾ cup	130	20	—	—
Savory Minestrone	¾ cup	110	20	—	—
Savory Mushroom	¾ cup	210	11	—	—
Savory Mushroom No Salt Added	¾ cup	250	15	—	—
Savory Onion	¾ cup	50	6	—	—
Savory Onion No Salt Added	¾ cup	50	9	—	—
Savory Potato Leek	¾ cup	260	20	—	—
Savory Split Pea	¾ cup	310	16	—	—
Savory Tomato	¾ cup	220	19	—	—
Savory Vegetable	¾ cup	80	13	—	—
Savory Vegetable No Salt Added	¾ cup	80	13	—	—

FOOD	PORTION	CALS.	CARB.	SUG.	FIB.
Herb-Ox					
Beef Bouillon	1 cube (3.5 g)	5	tr	0	0
Beef Instant Bouillon Powder	1 tsp (4 g)	5	tr	0	0
Beef Instant Broth & Seasoning Pack	1 pkg (4.5 g)	5	tr	0	0
Beef Instant Broth & Seasoning Pack Low Sodium	1 pkg (4 g)	10	2	1	0
Chicken Bouillon	1 cube (4 g)	5	tr	0	0
Chicken Instant Bouillon Powder	1 tsp (4 g)	5	tr	0	0
Chicken Instant Broth & Seasoning Pack	1 pkg (4 g)	5	tr	0	0
Chicken Instant Broth & Seasoning Pack Low Sodium	1 pkg (4 g)	10	2	1	0
Vegetable Bouillon	1 cube (4 g)	5	tr	0	0
Hodgson Mill					
13 Bean not prep	1.5 oz	100	14	0	12
Hurst					
15 Bean Soup Beef	1 serv (6 oz)	120	20	1	9
15 Bean Soup Cajun	1 serv	120	20	1	9
15 Bean Soup Chicken	1 serv (6 oz)	120	20	1	9
15 Bean Soup Chili	1 serv (6 oz)	120	20	1	9
15 Bean Soup Ham	1 serv	120	20	1	9
HamBeens Great Northern Bean	1 serv	120	22	1	11
HamBeens Navy Bean	1 serv	120	21	1	11
Pasta Fagioli	1 serv	120	23	1	9
Spanish American Pinto Bean	1 serv	120	22	1	6
Spanish-American Black Bean	1 serv	120	22	1	8
Ka-Me					
Won Ton Chicken not prep	1 pkg (1.25 oz)	180	18	0	1
Won Ton Pork not prep	1 pkg (1.25 oz)	180	18	0	1
Knorr					
Black Bean Cup-A-Soup as prep	1 pkg	200	37	1	9
Broccoli as prep	8 fl oz	160	16	—	—
Cauliflower as prep	8 fl oz	100	13	—	—
Chef's Series Wild Mushroom as prep	8 fl oz	100	14	—	—

FOOD	PORTION	CALS.	CARB.	SUG.	FIB.
Knorr (CONT.)					
Chick 'N Pasta as prep	8 fl oz	90	16	—	—
Chicken Bouillon as prep	8 fl oz	16	tr	—	—
Chicken Flavored Noodle as prep	8 fl oz	100	18	—	—
Chicken Noodle Instant as prep	6 fl oz	25	4	—	—
Fine Herb as prep	8 fl oz	130	15	—	—
Fish Bouillon as prep	8 fl oz	10	tr	—	—
French Onion as prep	8 fl oz	50	9	—	—
Hearty Minestrone Cup-A-Soup as prep	1 pkg	150	29	1	1
Lentil Cup-A-Soup as prep	1 pkg	220	40	1	6
Mushroom as prep	8 fl oz	100	12	—	—
Navy Bean Cup-A-Soup as prep	1 pkg	140	27	1	5
Oriental Hot And Sour as prep	8 fl oz	50	9	—	—
Oxtail Hearty Beef as prep	8 fl oz	70	10	—	—
Potato Leek Cup-A-Soup as prep	1 pkg	120	24	4	1
Spinach as prep	8 fl oz	100	11	—	—
Spring Vegetable With Herbs as prep	8 fl oz	30	6	—	—
Tomato Basil as prep	8 fl oz	90	14	—	—
Tortellini In Brodo as prep	8 fl oz	60	11	—	—
Vegetable Cup-A-Soup as prep	1 pkg	100	21	0	0
Vegetable as prep	8 fl oz	35	7	—	—
Vegetarian Vegetable Bouillon as prep	8 fl oz	16	1	—	—
Kojel					
Hearty Potato With Vegetables Instant	1 serv (6 fl oz)	60	15	3	2
Noodle Soup Chicken Flavor Instant	1 serv (6 fl oz)	70	11	4	2
Split Pea Instant	1 serv (6 fl oz)	60	14	5	3
Tomato Instant	1 serv (6 fl oz)	50	15	4	1
Vegetable Chicken Couscous Instant	1 serv (6 fl oz)	80	18	2	2
Lipton					
Chicken Noodle w/ White Chicken Meat as prep	1 cup	80	11	0	0
Extra Noodle w/ Chicken Broth as prep	1 cup	90	15	1	tr

FOOD	PORTION	CALS.	CARB.	SUG.	FIB.
Lipton (CONT.)					
Giggle Noodle w/ Chicken Broth as prep	1 cup	70	11	1	0
Recipe Secrets Beefy Mushroom	1½ tbsp (0.4 oz)	35	7	2	0
Recipe Secrets Beefy Onion	1 tbsp (0.3 oz)	25	5	0	0
Recipe Secrets Fiesta Herb w/ Red Pepper as prep	1 cup	30	6	tr	0
Recipe Secrets Golden Herb w/ Lemon as prep	1 cup	35	7	0	0
Recipe Secrets Golden Onion	1⅔ tbsp (0.5 oz)	50	9	2	0
Recipe Secrets Italian Herb w/ Tomato as prep	1 cup	40	9	3	0
Recipe Secrets Onion as prep	1 cup	20	4	0	tr
Recipe Secrets Onion Mushroom as prep	1 cup	30	5	0	0
Recipe Secrets Savory Herb With Garlic as prep	1 cup	30	6	0	0
Recipe Secrets Vegetable as prep	1 cup	30	7	2	1
Ring-O-Noodle w/ Chicken Broth as prep	1 cup	70	10	1	0
Soup Secrets Chicken 'N Onion as prep	1 cup	120	24	1	1
Soup Secrets Chicken w/ Pasta & Beans as prep	1 cup	110	19	1	3
Soup Secrets Country Chicken w/ Pasta & Herbs as prep	1 cup	100	18	1	1
Soup Secrets Homestyle Lentil w/ Bow Tie Pasta as prep	1 cup	130	22	1	5
Soup Secrets Minestrone as prep	1 cup	110	21	4	4
Spiral Pasta w/ Chicken Broth as prep	1 cup	60	11	1	0
Lite Line					
Beef Bouillon Instant Low Sodium	1 tsp	12	2	—	—
Chicken Bouillon Instant Low Sodium	1 tsp	12	2	—	—

FOOD	PORTION	CALS.	CARB.	SUG.	FIB.
Manischewitz					
Minestrone as prep	6 fl oz	50	9	—	—
Split Pea as prep	6 fl oz	45	9	—	—
Vegetable as prep	6 fl oz	50	9	—	—
Maruchan					
Instant Lunch Oriental Noodles Beef	1 pkg (2.25 oz)	290	37	—	—
Instant Lunch Oriental Noodles Chicken	1 pkg (2.25 oz)	290	36	2	2
Instant Lunch Oriental Noodles Chicken Mushroom	1 pkg (2.25 oz)	280	34		
Instant Lunch Oriental Noodles Mushroom	1 pkg (2.25 oz)	290	35	—	—
Instant Lunch Oriental Noodles Pork	1 pkg (2.25 oz)	290	35		
Instant Lunch Oriental Noodles Shrimp	1 pkg (2.25 oz)	290	37	—	—
Instant Lunch Oriental Noodles Toast Onion	1 pkg (2.25 oz)	270	34		
Instant Lunch Oriental Noodles Vegetable Beef	1 pkg (2.25 oz)	290	34	—	—
Instant Wonton Chicken	1 pkg (1.49 oz)	200	19	—	—
Instant Wonton Hot & Sour	1 pkg (1.49 oz)	200	21	—	—
Instant Wonton Oriental	1 pkg (1.49 oz)	190	19	—	—
Instant Wonton Pork	1 pkg (1.49 oz)	200	19	—	—
Instant Wonton Shrimp	1 pkg (1.49 oz)	200	19	—	—
Oriental Noodle Picante Style Beef	1 pkg (2.25 oz)	290	37	—	—
Oriental Noodle Picante Style Chicken	1 pkg (2.25 oz)	290	38		
Oriental Noodle Picante Style Shrimp	1 pkg (2.25 oz)	300	36		
Ramen Beef	½ pkg (1.5 oz)	190	26	—	—
Ramen Chicken	½ pkg (1.5 oz)	190	20	—	—
Ramen Chicken Mushroom	½ pkg (1.5 oz)	190	25	—	—
Ramen Chili	½ pkg (1.5 oz)	190	26	—	—
Ramen Mushroom	½ pkg (1.5 oz)	190	25	—	—
Ramen Oriental	½ pkg (1.5 oz)	190	26	—	—
Ramen Pork	½ pkg (1.5 oz)	190	25	—	—
Ramen Shrimp	½ pkg (1.5 oz)	190	26	—	—
Wonton Beef	⅓ pkg (0.68 oz)	90	8	—	—
Wonton Chicken	⅓ pkg (0.67 oz)	90	8	—	—
Wonton Pork	⅓ pkg (0.68 oz)	90	9	—	—

FOOD	PORTION	CALS.	CARB.	SUG.	FIB.
Maruchan (CONT.)					
Wonton Vegetable	⅓ pkg (0.7 oz)	90	9	—	—
Morga					
Vegetable Bouillon No Salt Added	½ cube (5 g)	25	1	tr	0
Vegetable Broth Fat Free	1 tsp (4 g)	10	2	0	0
Nile Spice					
Couscous Almondine	1 pkg	200	37	5	2
Couscous Garbanzo	1 pkg	220	39	2	2
Couscous Lentil Curry	1 pkg	200	36	5	4
Couscous Minestrone	1 pkg	180	34	7	2
Couscous Parmesan	1 pkg	200	34	0	2
Homestyle Black Bean	1 pkg	190	34	4	2
Homestyle Chicken Flavored Vegetable	1 pkg	120	20	tr	4
Homestyle Lentil	1 pkg	180	31	3	3
Homestyle Minestrone	1 pkg	160	29	3	4
Homestyle Red Beans & Rice	1 pkg	190	36	3	3
Homestyle Split Pea	1 pkg	200	35	5	6
Homestyle Sweet Corn Chowder	1 pkg	120	20	7	0
Italian Tomato	1 pkg	140	21	2	2
Potato Leek	1 pkg	150	21	3	2
Potato Romano	1 pkg	140	19	4	3
Ramen Noodle					
Beef Low Fat as prep	8 oz	160	32	—	—
Beef as prep	8 oz	190	26	—	—
Chicken Low Fat as prep	8 oz	160	32	—	—
Chicken as prep	8 oz	190	26	—	—
Oriental Low Fat as prep	8 oz	150	31	—	—
Oriental as prep	8 oz	190	26	—	—
Pork Low Fat as prep	8 oz	150	31	—	—
Pork as prep	8 oz	200	26	—	—
Ultra Slim-Fast					
Beef Noodle	6 oz	45	7	—	2
Chicken Leek	6 oz	50	7	—	2
Chicken Noodle	6 oz	45	6	—	2
Creamy Broccoli	6 oz	75	14	—	2
Creamy Tomato	6 oz	60	10	—	2
Hearty Vegetable	6 oz	50	7	—	2
Onion	6 oz	45	7	—	2
Potato Leek	6 oz	80	15	—	2

FOOD	PORTION	CALS.	CARB.	SUG.	FIB.
Weight Watchers					
Instant Beef Broth	1 pkg (0.16 oz) mix	10	2	2	0
Instant Chicken Broth	1 pkg (0.16 oz)	10	2	2	0
Wyler's					
Beef Bouillon Instant	1 tsp	6	1	—	—
Beef Bouillon Instant Cube	1	6	1	—	—
Chicken Bouillon Instant	1 tsp	8	1	—	—
Chicken Bouillon Instant Cube	1	8	1	—	—
Onion Bouillon Instant	1 tsp	10	1	—	—
Vegetable Bouillon Instant	1 tsp	6	1	—	—
SHELF-STABLE					
Hormel					
Micro Cup Bean & Ham	1 cup (7.5 oz)	190	29	2	7
Micro Cup Beef Vegetable	1 cup (7.5 oz)	90	15	3	1
Micro Cup Broccoli Cheese w/ Ham	1 cup (7.5 oz)	170	10	3	1
Micro Cup Chicken & Rice	1 cup (7.5 oz)	110	17	3	1
Micro Cup Chicken Noodle	1 cup (7.5 oz)	110	13	0	0
Micro Cup New England Clam Chowder	1 cup (7.5 oz)	130	17	0	1
Micro Cup Potato Cheese w/ Ham	1 cup (7.5 oz)	190	15	2	1
Lunch Bucket					
Chicken Noodle	1 pkg (7.25 oz)	90	13	—	—
Country Vegetable	1 pkg (7.25 oz)	70	15	—	—

SOUR CREAM

(*see also* SOUR CREAM SUBSTITUTES)

FOOD	PORTION	CALS.	CARB.	SUG.	FIB.
sour cream	1 cup (8 oz)	493	10	—	—
sour cream	1 tbsp (0.4 oz)	26	1	—	—
Breakstone's					
Free	2 tbsp (1.1 oz)	35	6	2	0
Reduced Fat	2 tbsp (1.1 oz)	45	2	2	0
Sour Cream	2 tbsp (1 oz)	60	1	1	0
Cabot					
Light	1 oz	33	2	—	—
Sour Cream	1 oz	60	1	—	—
Friendship					
Light	2 tbsp (1 oz)	35	2	2	0
Sour Cream	2 tbsp (1 oz)	60	2	2	0
Heluva Good Cheese					
Fat-Free	2 tbsp (1.1 oz)	20	3	2	0
Light	2 tbsp (1.1 oz)	40	3	2	0

FOOD	PORTION	CALS.	CARB.	SUG.	FIB.
Heluva Good Cheese (CONT.)					
Sour Cream	2 tbsp (1.1 oz)	60	2	1	0
Hood					
Fat Free	2 tbsp (1 oz)	20	3	2	0
Light	2 tbsp (1 oz)	40	2	2	0
Sour Cream	2 tbsp (1 oz)	60	2	2	0
Knudsen					
Free	2 tbsp (1.1 oz)	35	6	2	0
Hampshire	2 tbsp (1 oz)	60	1	1	0
Light	2 tbsp (1.1 oz)	50	2	2	0
Naturally Yours					
No Fat	2 tbsp (1 fl oz)	15	1	—	—
SOUR CREAM SUBSTITUTES					
nondairy	1 oz	59	2	—	—
nondairy	1 cup	479	15	—	—
Pet					
Imitation	1 tbsp	25	tr	—	—
Tofutti					
Better Than Sour Cream Sour Supreme	1 oz	50	1	—	—
SOURSOP					
fresh	1	416	105	—	—
fresh cut up	1 cup	150	38	—	—
SOY					
(*see also* CHEESE SUBSTITUTES, ICE CREAM AND FROZEN DESSERTS, MILK SUBSTITUTES, MISO, SOY SAUCE, SOYBEANS, TEMPEH, TOFU, AND YOGURT FROZEN)					
lecithin	1 tbsp	104	0	0	0
soy milk	1 cup	79	4	—	—
soya cheese	1.4 oz	128	tr	—	0
Loma Linda					
Soyagen All Purpose	¼ cup (1 oz)	130	12	7	3
Soyagen Carob	¼ cup (1 oz)	130	13	7	2
Soyagen No Sucrose	¼ cup (1 oz)	130	12	7	3
SOY SAUCE					
shoyu	1 tbsp	9	2	—	—
soy sauce	1 tbsp	7	1	—	—
tamari	1 tbsp	11	1	—	—
Eden					
Shoyu Organic	1 tbsp (0.5 oz)	15	2	0	0
Shoyu Traditional	1 tbsp (0.5 oz)	15	2	0	0
Tamari Organic Domestic	1 tbsp (0.5 oz)	15	2	0	0

FOOD	PORTION	CALS.	CARB.	SUG.	FIB.
Eden (CONT.)					
Tamari Organic Imported	1 tbsp (0.5 oz)	15	2	0	0
House Of Tsang					
Dark	1 tbsp (0.6 oz)	10	1	0	0
Ginger Flavored	1 tbsp (0.6 oz)	20	4	3	0
Light	1 tbsp (0.6 oz)	5	0	0	0
Low Sodium	1 tbsp (0.6 oz)	5	0	0	0
Low Sodium Ginger	1 tbsp (0.6 oz)	10	2	1	0
Low Sodium Mushroom	1 tbsp (0.6 oz)	10	2	1	0
Ka-Me					
Chinese Dark	1 tbsp (0.5 fl oz)	10	3	2	0
Chinese Light	1 tbsp (0.5 fl oz)	5	1	1	0
Dark	1 tbsp (0.5 fl oz)	10	3	2	0
Japanese	1 tbsp (0.5 fl oz)	5	1	0	0
Light	1 tbsp (0.5 oz)	5	1	1	0
Mild	1 tbsp (0.5 fl oz)	5	0	0	0
Kikkoman					
Lite	1 tbsp	13	2	—	—
Soy Sauce	1 tbsp	12	2	—	0
La Choy					
Lite	½ tsp	1	tr	—	tr
Soy Sauce	½ tsp	2	tr	—	tr
Trappey					
Chef Magic	1 tbsp (0.5 oz)	23	4	tr	tr
Tree Of Life					
Shoyu	1 tbsp (0.5 oz)	15	1	1	—
Tamari Reduced Sodium	1 tbsp (0.5 oz)	20	1	1	—
Tamari Wheat Free	1 tbsp (0.5 oz)	15	1	1	—

SOYBEANS
(*see also* MILK SUBSTITUTES, MISO, SOY, SOY SAUCE, TEMPEH, TOFU)

FOOD	PORTION	CALS.	CARB.	SUG.	FIB.
dried cooked	1 cup	298	17	—	—
dry-roasted	½ cup	387	28	—	—
green cooked	½ cup	127	10	—	4
honey toasted	¼ cup (1 oz)	130	19	15	0
roasted	½ cup	405	29	—	—
roasted & toasted	1 oz	129	9	—	—
roasted & toasted	1 cup	490	33	—	—
roasted & toasted salted	1 cup	490	33	—	—
roasted & toasted salted	1 oz	129	9	—	—
sprouts raw	½ cup	43	3	—	—
sprouts steamed	½ cup	38	3	—	—
sprouts stir fried	1 cup	125	9	—	—

FOOD	PORTION	CALS.	CARB.	SUG.	FIB.

SPAGHETTI
(*see* PASTA, PASTA DINNERS, PASTA SALAD, SPAGHETTI SAUCE)

SPAGHETTI SAUCE
(*see also* PIZZA, TOMATO)

JARRED

FOOD	PORTION	CALS.	CARB.	SUG.	FIB.
marinara sauce	1 cup	171	25	—	—
spaghetti sauce	1 cup	272	40	—	—
Classico					
Beef & Pork	4 fl oz	80	7	—	—
Four Cheese	4 fl oz	70	7	—	—
Ripe Olives & Mushrooms	4 fl oz	50	7	—	—
Spicy Red Pepper	4 fl oz	50	6	—	—
Sweet Peppers & Onions	4 fl oz	50	7	—	—
Tomato & Basil	4 fl oz	60	6	—	—
Contadina					
Italian	¼ cup	15	4	1	1
Sauce	¼ cup	20	4	1	tr
Thick & Zesty	¼ cup	15	4	1	1
Del Monte					
Traditional	½ cup (4.4 oz)	80	15	10	tr
Traditional No Sugar Added	½ cup (4.4 oz)	60	11	6	tr
With Garlic & Onion	½ cup (4.4 oz)	70	15	11	tr
With Green Peppers & Mushrooms	½ cup (4.4 oz)	70	13	6	tr
With Meat	½ cup (4.4 oz)	40	13	10	tr
With Mushrooms	½ cup (4.4 oz)	80	15	10	tr
Eden					
Organic No Salt Added	½ cup (4.4 oz)	80	12	6	3
Enrico's					
Fat Free Organic Basil	½ cup (4 oz)	50	8	8	4
Fat Free Organic Garlic	½ cup (4 oz)	50	9	9	5
Fat Free Organic Hot Pepper	½ cup (4 oz)	50	8	9	5
Fat Free Organic Mushroom	½ cup (4 oz)	60	10	9	7
Fat Free Organic Traditional	½ cup (4 oz)	45	4	7	6
Healthy Choice					
Extra Chunky Garlic & Onion	½ cup (4.4 oz)	43	8	7	1
Extra Chunky Italian Vegetable	½ cup (4.4 oz)	39	8	6	1
Extra Chunky Mushroom	½ cup (4.4 oz)	41	8	8	1
Garlic & Herbs	½ cup (4.4 oz)	47	10	8	2

FOOD	PORTION	CALS.	CARB.	SUG.	FIB.
Healthy Choice (CONT.)					
Super Chunky Mushroom & Sweet Peppers	½ cup (4.4 oz)	44	9	6	1
Super Chunky Tomato, Mushroom & Garlic	½ cup (4.4 oz)	46	9	6	2
Super Chunky Vegetable Primavera	½ cup (4.4 oz)	46	9	9	1
Traditional	½ cup (4.4 oz)	47	10	8	2
With Meat	½ cup (4.4 oz)	47	8	8	2
With Mushrooms	½ cup (4.4 oz)	47	10	8	3
Hunt's					
Chunky Marinara	½ cup (4.4 oz)	60	12	5	2
Chunky Tomato Garlic & Onion	½ cup (4.4 oz)	61	13	5	2
Chunky Vegetable	½ cup (4.4 oz)	63	13	5	2
Classic Garlic & Onion	½ cup (4.4 oz)	58	10	7	2
Classic Tomato & Basil	½ cup (4.4 oz)	48	8	5	4
Classic Italian With Parmesan	½ cup (4.4 oz)	50	8	5	2
Home Style With Meat	½ cup (4.4 oz)	56	7	6	2
Home Style With Mushrooms	½ cup (4.4 oz)	56	7	6	2
Homestyle Traditional	½ cup (4.4 oz)	56	7	7	2
Italian Cheese & Garlic	½ cup (4.5 oz)	65	9	6	2
Italian Sausage	½ cup (4.5 oz)	77	12	7	2
Old Country Garlic & Herbs	½ cup (4.4 oz)	63	9	7	3
Old Country Italian Style Vegetables	½ cup (4.4 oz)	64	9	7	3
Old Country Traditional	½ cup (4.4 oz)	53	7	6	3
Old Country With Meat	½ cup (4.4 oz)	56	7	6	3
Old Country With Mushrooms	½ cup (4.4 oz)	53	7	6	3
Original Traditional	½ cup (4.4 oz)	65	11	7	4
Original With Meat	½ cup (4.4 oz)	65	11	7	2
Original With Mushrooms	½ cup (4.4 oz)	65	11	7	2
Mama Rizzo's					
Mushroom Onion	½ cup (4.3 oz)	60	9	6	1
Pepper Mushroom Onion	½ cup (4.3 oz)	60	9	6	1
Pepper Primavera Vegetable	½ cup (4.2 oz)	50	8	3	2
Pepper Tomato Basil Garlic	½ cup (4.7 oz)	60	10	7	1
Primavera Vegetable	½ cup (4.2 oz)	50	8	3	2
Tomato Basil Garlic	½ cup (4.6 oz)	60	8	6	2

FOOD	PORTION	CALS.	CARB.	SUG.	FIB.
Muir Glen					
Organic Cabernet Marinara	½ cup (4.4 oz)	45	10	3	2
Organic Chunky Style	½ cup (4.5 oz)	80	13	8	3
Organic Fat Free Tomato Basil	½ cup (4.3 oz)	50	10	6	2
Organic Garlic Onion	½ cup (4.3 oz)	50	11	6	3
Organic Garlic Roasted Garlic	½ cup (4.4 oz)	45	10	3	2
Organic Green Pepper & Mushroom	½ cup (4.5 oz)	70	10	8	4
Organic Italian Herb	½ cup (4.5 oz)	60	13	10	2
Organic Romano Cheese	½ cup (4.5 oz)	90	14	7	4
Organic Sun Dried Tomato	½ cup (4.4 oz)	40	9	3	2
Organic Sweet Pepper Onion	½ cup (4.4 oz)	40	8	6	1
Organic Tomato Basil	½ cup (4.3 oz)	50	10	6	2
Newman's Own					
Marinara Ventian	½ cup (4.4 oz)	60	9	7	3
Marinara Ventian w/ Mushrooms	½ cup (4.4 oz)	60	9	7	3
Pasta Sauce Bambolina	½ cup (4.5 oz)	100	15	9	5
Pasta Sauce Roasted Garlic & Red & Green Peppers	½ cup (4.7 oz)	70	11	6	4
Pasta Sauce Say Cheese	½ cup (4.4 oz)	90	14	8	3
Sockarooni	½ cup (4.4 oz)	60	9	7	3
Prego					
Chunky Sausage & Green Peppers	4 oz	160	19	—	—
Extra Chunky Garden Combination	4 oz	80	14	—	—
Extra Chunky Mushroom & Tomato	4 oz	110	14	—	—
Extra Chunky Mushroom & Green Pepper	4 oz	100	14	—	—
Extra Chunky Mushroom & Onion	4 oz	100	13	—	—
Extra Chunky Mushroom With Extra Spice	4 oz	100	17	—	—
Extra Chunky Tomato & Onion	4 oz	110	14	—	—
Marinara	4 oz	100	10	—	—
Meat Flavored	4 oz	140	20	—	—
Mushroom	4 oz	130	20	—	—

FOOD	PORTION	CALS.	CARB.	SUG.	FIB.
Prego (CONT.)					
Onion & Garlic	4 oz	110	16	—	—
Regular	4 oz	130	20	—	—
Three Cheese	4 oz	100	17	—	—
Tomato & Basil	4 oz	100	18	—	—
Pritikin					
Chunky Garden	½ cup (4 oz)	50	12	—	—
Marinara	½ cup (4 oz)	60	13	—	—
Original	½ cup (4 oz)	60	13	—	—
Progresso					
Marinara	½ cup (4.3 oz)	90	8	5	2
Meat Flavored	½ cup (4.4 oz)	100	12	9	3
Mushroom	½ cup (4.4 oz)	100	12	7	4
Sauce	½ cup (4.4 oz)	100	12	8	2
Ragu					
Fino Italian Garden Medley	½ cup (4.5 oz)	90	14	10	2
Fino Italian Garlic & Basil	½ cup (4.5 oz)	90	15	9	2
Fino Italian Parmesan	½ cup (4.5 oz)	100	15	9	2
Fino Italian Sliced Mushroom	½ cup (4.5 oz)	90	14	10	2
Fino Italian Tomato & Herb	½ cup (4.5 oz)	90	15	10	2
Fino Italian Zesty Tomato	½ cup (4.5 oz)	90	14	8	2
Gardenstyle Chunky Garden Combination	½ cup (4.5 oz)	120	18	12	3
Gardenstyle Chunky Green & Red Pepper	½ cup (4.5 oz)	120	19	13	2
Gardenstyle Chunky Mushroom & Green Pepper	½ cup (4.5 oz)	120	18	12	3
Gardenstyle Chunky Mushroom & Onion	½ cup (4.5 oz)	120	19	13	3
Gardenstyle Chunky Tomato Garlic & Onion	½ cup (4.5 oz)	120	19	13	3
Gardenstyle Super Mushroom	½ cup (4.5 oz)	120	19	14	3
Gardenstyle Super Vegetable Primavera	½ cup (4.5 oz)	110	17	10	4
Homestyle Mushroom	½ cup (4.5 oz)	120	18	12	3
Homestyle Tomato & Herb	½ cup (4.5 oz)	120	18	12	3
Homestyle With Meat	½ cup (4.5 oz)	130	18	12	3
Light Chunky Mushroom	½ cup (4.4 oz)	50	10	8	2
Light Garden Harvest	½ cup (4.4 oz)	50	11	9	2
Light No Sugar Added	½ cup (4.4 oz)	60	9	5	3
Light Tomato & Herb	½ cup (4.4 oz)	50	10	9	2

FOOD	PORTION	CALS.	CARB.	SUG.	FIB.
Ragu (CONT.)					
Old World Style Marinara	½ cup (4.4 oz)	90	9	7	3
Old World Style Mushrooms	½ cup (4.4 oz)	80	10	7	3
Old World Style Traditional	½ cup (4.4 oz)	80	10	7	3
Old World Style With Meat	½ cup (4.4 oz)	90	9	7	3
Sauce	4 fl oz	80	9	—	—
Thick & Hearty Mushroom	½ cup (4.5 oz)	120	19	11	3
Thick & Hearty Spaghetti Sauce	4 oz	100	15	—	—
Thick & Hearty Tomato & Herb	½ cup (4.5 oz)	120	19	12	3
Thick & Hearty With Meat	1.2 cup (4.5 oz)	130	19	11	3
Tree Of Life					
Pasta Sauce	½ cup (4 oz)	50	9	8	—
Pasta Sauce Calabrese	½ cup (3.9 oz)	60	9	2	—
Pasta Sauce Fat Free Classic	½ cup (3.9 oz)	40	8	6	0
Pasta Sauce Fat Free Mushroom & Basil	½ cup (3.9 oz)	30	7	6	0
Pasta Sauce Fat Free Onion & Garlic	½ cup (3.9 oz)	30	7	6	0
Pasta Sauce Fat Free Sweet Pepper	½ cup (3.9 oz)	30	7	6	0
Pasta Sauce No Salt	½ cup (3.9 oz)	50	9	8	—
MIX					
Durkee					
American Style as prep	½ cup	15	6	1	0
Family Style as prep	½ cup	20	4	2	0
Spaghetti Sauce as prep	½ cup	15	5	1	0
With Mushrooms as prep	½ cup	15	4	2	0
Zesty as prep	½ cup	20	5	1	0
French's					
All American as prep	½ cup	20	7	1	0
Italian as prep	½ cup	16	5	1	0
Mushroom as prep	½ cup	20	4	1	0
Thick as prep	½ cup	10	4	1	0
Zesty Pasta as prep	½ cup	20	5	1	0
REFRIGERATED					
Contadina					
Alfredo	½ cup (4.2 fl oz)	400	8	3	0
Four Cheese Sauce With White Wine & Shallots	½ cup (4.2 fl oz)	320	8	3	0
Light Alfredo	½ cup (4.2 fl oz)	190	10	5	0

FOOD	PORTION	CALS.	CARB.	SUG.	FIB.
Contadina (CONT.)					
Light Chunky Tomato	½ cup (4.4 fl oz)	45	8	6	3
Light Garden Vegetable	½ cup (4.4 fl oz)	45	8	6	3
Marinara	½ cup (4.4 fl oz)	80	8	7	2
Pesto With Basil	¼ cup (2 oz)	310	5	3	0
Pesto With Sun Dried Tomatoes	¼ cup (2 oz)	250	6	2	3
Plum Tomato With Basil	½ cup (4.4 fl oz)	70	8	7	3
Spicy Italian Sausage & Bell Pepper	½ cup (4.4 fl oz)	100	9	6	3
Di Giorno					
Alfredo	¼ cup (2.2 oz)	180	3	2	0
Basil Pesto	¼ cup (2.2 oz)	320	2	tr	tr
Four Cheese	¼ cup (2.2 oz)	160	3	2	0
Garlic Pesto	¼ cup (2.1 oz)	340	3	tr	tr
Light Alfredo Sauce	¼ cup (2.4 oz)	140	9	3	0
Marinara	½ cup (4.5 oz)	70	15	10	2
Plum Tomato Cream Sauce	½ cup (4.4 oz)	160	8	6	2
Plum Tomato & Mushroom	½ cup (4.4 oz)	60	13	10	2
Roasted Red Bell Pepper Cream Sauce	¼ cup (2.3 oz)	140	8	3	0

SPANISH FOOD

(*see also* BEANS, CHIPS, CHILI, DINNER, PEPPERS, SALSA, SNACKS, SAUCE, TORTILLA)

CANNED

FOOD	PORTION	CALS.	CARB.	SUG.	FIB.
Chi-Chi's					
Pico De Gallo	2 tbsp (1.2 oz)	10	2	2	0
Derby					
Tamales	2	160	15	—	1
El Molino					
Enchilada Sauce Hot	2 tbsp	16	2	—	—
Green Chili Sauce Mild	2 tbsp	10	2	—	—
Gebhardt					
Enchiladas	2	310	20	—	2
Tamales	2	290	19	—	2
Tamales Jumbo	2	400	26	—	3
Guiltless Gourmet					
Picante Mild	1 oz	6	1	—	tr
Queso Mild Cheddar	1 oz	22	5	—	tr
Hormel					
Tamales Beef	3 (7.5 oz)	280	20	1	3
Tamales Chicken	3 (7.5 oz)	210	22	2	2
Tamales Hot Spicy Beef	3 (7.5 oz)	280	20	1	3

FOOD	PORTION	CALS.	CARB.	SUG.	FIB.
Hormel (CONT.)					
Tamales Jumbo Beef	2 (6.9 oz)	270	18	1	3
Old El Paso					
Tamales	3 (7.2 oz)	330	31	0	5
Rosarita					
Enchilada Sauce Mild	2.5 oz	25	3	—	tr
Picante Chunky Hot	3 tbsp (2 fl oz)	18	4	—	tr
Picante Chunky Medium	3 tbsp (2 fl oz)	16	4	—	tr
Picante Chunky Mild	3 tbsp (2 oz)	25	5	—	tr
Van Camp's					
Tamales	2 (5.1 oz)	210	20	—	3
Wolf Brand					
Tamales	7.5 oz	328	25	—	—
FROZEN					
Amy's Organic					
Black Bean Vegetable Enchilada	1 (4.75 oz)	130	20	1	2
Burritos Bean & Cheese	1 (6 oz)	280	43	1	6
Burritos Bean & Rice Non-Dairy	1 (6 oz)	250	44	1	6
Burritos Black Bean Vegetable	1 (6 oz)	320	54	4	4
Burritos Breakfast	1 (6 oz)	230	38	4	5
Cheese Enchilada	1 (4.7 oz)	210	16	0	2
Mexican Tamale Pie	1 (8 oz)	220	41	4	11
Pocket Sandwich Tamale	1 (4.5 oz)	250	39	4	3
Whole Meals Cheese Enchilada	1 pkg (9 oz)	330	38	6	6
Whole Meals Enchilada	1 pkg (10 oz)	250	41	4	5
Banquet					
Beef Enchilada	1 pkg (11 oz)	320	54	7	10
Chimichanga Meal	1 pkg (9.5 oz)	470	56	9	9
Enchilada Cheese	1 pkg (11 oz)	350	56	7	9
Enchilada Chicken	1 pkg (11 oz)	360	54	7	9
Family Entree Beef Enchilada w/ Cheese	1 serv (4.67 oz)	130	19	4	3
Chi-Chi's					
Burro Beef	1 pkg (15.9 oz)	590	76	7	11
Burro Chicken	1 pkg (15.9 oz)	540	77	8	10
Chimichanga Beef	1 pkg (15.9 oz)	630	75	8	10
Chimichanga Chicken	1 pkg (15.9 oz)	580	78	8	10
Enchilada Chicken Suprema	1 pkg (15.9 oz)	600	80	9	11
Enchilida Baja	1 pkg (15.9 oz)	590	75	7	15

FOOD	PORTION	CALS.	CARB.	SUG.	FIB.
Healthy Choice					
Beef Burrito Ranchero Medium	1 (5.4 oz)	290	44	6	6
Beef Burrito Ranchero Mild	1 (5.4 oz)	300	45	6	7
Beef Enchilada Rio Grande	1 meal (13.4 oz)	410	70	24	9
Burrito Chicken Con Queso	1 (5.4 oz)	280	43	6	5
Chicken Enchilada Supreme	1 meal (13.4 oz)	390	60	22	8
Enchiladas Suiza Chicken	1 meal (10 oz)	270	43	4	5
Fiesta Chicken Fajitas	1 meal (7 oz)	260	36	6	5
Jimmy Dean					
Burrito Breakfast Bacon	1 (4 oz)	260	37	3	1
Burrito Breakfast Sausage	1 (4 oz)	250	36	4	2
Le Menu					
Entree LightStyle Enchiladas Chicken	8 oz	280	32	—	—
Lean Cuisine					
Chicken Enchilada Suiza w/ Mexican Style Rice	1 pkg (9 oz)	280	48	7	3
Life Choice					
Burrito Black Bean	1 meal (13.2 oz)	410	86	12	13
Vegetable Enchilada Sonora	1 meal (14 oz)	420	89	23	11
Lightlife					
Vegetarian Taco	2 oz	51	4	—	—
Old El Paso					
Burrito Bean & Cheese	1 (4.9 oz)	290	44	3	3
Burrito Beef & Bean Hot	1 (5 oz)	320	45	4	3
Burrito Beef & Bean Medium	1 (5 oz)	320	46	4	3
Burrito Beef & Bean Mild	1 (5 oz)	330	48	4	4
Chimichanga Beef	1 (4.5 oz)	370	37	0	3
Chimichanga Chicken	1 (4.5 oz)	350	39	0	2
Patio					
Burrito Bean & Cheese	1 (5 oz)	270	46	2	7
Burrito Chicken	1 (5 oz)	260	44	5	3
Burrito Red Chili	1 (5 oz)	270	42	4	6
Burritos Beef & Bean	1 (5 oz)	280	45	5	7
Burritos Beef & Bean Green Chili	1 (5 oz)	260	44	3	7
Burritos Beef & Bean Red Chili	1 (5 oz)	260	42	3	7
Enchilada Beef Dinner	1 meal (12 oz)	320	52	2	9
Enchilada Cheese Dinner	1 meal (12 oz)	330	52	7	10
Enchilada Chicken	1 pkg (12 oz)	380	58	8	9

FOOD	PORTION	CALS.	CARB.	SUG.	FIB.
Patio (CONT.)					
Family Entree Beef Enchilada	2 (5.7 oz)	170	27	tr	5
Family Entree Enchilada Beef	2 (5.3 oz)	250	35	2	8
Family Entree Enchilada Beef & Cheese	2 (5.3 oz)	250	35	2	9
Family Entree Enchilada Cheese	2 (5.7 oz)	170	26	3	4
Fiesta Dinner	1 meal (12 oz)	340	51	5	11
Mexican Dinner	1 meal (13.25 oz,	440	59	3	13
Salis Con Queso	1 pkg (11 oz)	390	33	7	10
Patio Britos					
Beef & Bean	10 (6 oz)	420	51	2	7
Nacho Beef	10 (6 oz)	410	48	3	5
Nacho Cheese	10 (6 oz)	360	52	8	3
Spicy Chicken	10 (6 oz)	400	52	2	3
Rudy's Farm					
Burrito Beef/Bean	1 (5 oz)	326	43	1	5
Burrito Hot Beef/Bean	1 (5 oz)	305	44	1	5
Senor Felix's					
Burrito Black Bean	1 (10 oz)	540	70	18	7
Burrito Black Bean Soy	1 (5 oz)	240	36	6	3
Burrito Chicken	1 (10 oz)	520	51	9	3
Burrito Hot Potato	1 (10 oz)	560	67	10	5
Burrito Soy Hot	1 (10 oz)	520	70	10	5
Burritos Charbroiled Chicken	1 + 4 tsp sauce (6.7 oz)	320	40	9	7
Burritos Sonora Style	1 + 4 tsp sauce (6.7 oz)	280	45	4	3
Burritos Yucatan Style	1 + 4 tsp sauce (6.7 oz)	310	46	2	5
Empanadas Chicken	1 (4.7 oz)	340	41	9	13
Empanadas Corn & Rice	1 (4.7 oz)	280	37	2	6
Empanadas Pumpkin & Mushroom	1 (4.7 oz)	260	32	3	6
Empanadas Spinach & Ricotta	1 (4.7 oz)	260	32	2	6
Enchilada Red Pepper	1 (10 oz)	420	51	12	8
Enchilada Soy Verda	1 (10 oz)	430	41	5	6
Enchilada Supreme Soy Cheese	1 (10 oz)	460	48	11	6
Enchilada Verde	1 (5 oz)	423	41	6	6
Tamales Blue Corn & Soy Cheese	2 + 4 tsp sauce (5.7 oz)	240	28	4	3

FOOD	PORTION	CALS.	CARB.	SUG.	FIB.
Senor Felix's (CONT.)					
Tamales Chicken	2 + 4 tsp sauce (5.7 oz)	240	30	0	8
Tamales Gourmet Vegetarian	2 + 4 tsp sauce	240	30	0	8
Taquitos Blue Corn Soy	3 + 4 tsp sauce (5.2 oz)	230	27	2	3
Taquitos Chicken	2 + 4 tsp sauce (5.7 oz)	240	28	4	3
Stouffer's					
Chicken Enchilada	1 serv (4.8 oz)	230	25	4	3
Swanson					
Enchiladas Beef	13.75 oz	480	55	—	—
Mexican Style Combination	14.25 oz	490	62	—	—
Mexican Style Hungry Man	20.25 oz	820	88	—	—
Today's Tamales					
Cheese & Chili	1 pkg (7 oz)	390	38	0	6
Del Sol	1 pkg (6.5 oz)	310	40	2	15
Original Bean	1 pkg (7 oz)	330	49	0	10
Spicy Taco	1 pkg (7 oz)	310	41	0	10
Tyson					
Fajita Kit Beef	3.84 oz	160	21	—	—
Fajita Kit Chicken	4 oz	80	2	—	—
Weight Watchers					
Smart Ones Chicken Enchiladas Suiza	1 pkg (9 oz)	270	33	8	4
Smart Ones Santa Fe Style Rice & Beans	1 pkg (10 oz)	290	41	11	10
MIX					
Gebhardt					
Menudo Mix	1 tsp	5	1	—	tr
Hain					
Taco Seasoning Mix	1/10 pkg	10	2	—	—
Old El Paso					
Burrito Seasoning Mix	2 tsp (6 g)	20	3	0	1
Dinner Kit Burrito as prep	1	280	35	—	3
Dinner Kit Soft Taco as prep	2	380	45	—	3
Dinner Kit Taco as prep	2	270	21	—	4
Enchilada Sauce Mix	2 tsp (4 g)	10	2	0	tr
Taco Mix 40% Less Sodium	2 tsp (6 g)	20	4	2	0
Taco Seasoning Mix	2 tsp (6 g)	20	5	2	0
Ortega					
Taco Meat Seasoning Mix Mild	1 filled taco	90	18	—	—

FOOD	PORTION	CALS.	CARB.	SUG.	FIB.
Quaker					
Masa Harina De Maiz	2 tortillas	137	28	—	3
Masa Trigo	2 tortillas	149	25	—	1
Taco Bell					
Home Originals Chicken Fajita Dinner as prep	2 (6.9 oz)	340	45	7	3
Home Originals Chicken Fajita Seasoning Mix	1 tbsp (8 g)	25	5	1	2
Home Originals Soft Taco Dinner as prep	2 (6.3 oz)	410	41	5	2
Home Originals Taco Dinner as prep	2 (4.4 oz)	280	19	2	2
Home Originals Taco Seasoning Mix	2 tsp (6 g)	20	3	0	tr
Home Originals Ultimate Bean Burrito Dinner as prep	1 (4.4 oz)	200	34	4	3
Home Originals Ultimate Nachos as prep	12 pieces (4.6 oz)	240	31	2	4
READY-TO-EAT					
taco shell baked	1 med (0.5 oz)	61	8	—	tr
taco shell baked w/o salt	1 med (½ oz)	61	8	—	tr
Casa Fiesta					
Taco Shells	3.5 oz	480	60	—	—
Chi-Chi's					
Taco Shells White Corn	2 (1.2 oz)	170	22	0	2
Taco Shells Yellow Corn	2 shells (1.2 oz)	170	22	0	2
Gebhardt					
Taco Shells	1	50	7	—	tr
Old El Paso					
Taco Shells Mini	7 (1.1 oz)	160	18	0	2
Taco Shells Regular	3 (1.1 oz)	170	18	0	2
Taco Shells Super	2 (1.3 oz)	190	21	0	2
Taco Shells White Corn	3 (1.1 oz)	170	18	0	2
Tostaco Shells	1 (0.8 oz)	130	14	0	1
Tostada Shells	3 (1.1 oz)	160	19	0	2
Rosarita					
Taco Shells	1 shell (11 g)	50	7	—	tr
Tostada Shells	1 shell (14 g)	60	8	—	tr
Taco Bell					
Home Originals Taco Shells	3 (1.1 oz)	150	21	0	2

SPARE RIBS
(*see* PORK)

FOOD	PORTION	CALS.	CARB.	SUG.	FIB.
SPELT					
Arrowhead					
Spelt	1 oz	83	20	tr	4
SPICES					
(*see* HERBS/SPICES, *individual names*)					
SPINACH					
CANNED					
spinach	½ cup	25	4	—	—
Del Monte					
50% Less Salt	½ cup (4 oz)	30	4	0	2
Chopped	½ cup (4 oz)	30	4	0	2
No Salt Added	½ cup (4 oz)	30	4	0	2
Whole Leaf	½ cup (4 oz)	30	4	0	2
Popeye					
Chopped	½ cup (4.1 oz)	40	6	1	4
Leaf	½ cup (4.2 oz)	45	7	1	4
Low Sodium	½ cup (4.2 oz)	35	4	tr	3
S&W					
Northwest Premium	½ cup	25	3	—	—
Sunshine					
Chopped	½ cup (4.1 oz)	40	6	1	4
FRESH					
cooked	½ cup	21	3	—	2
malabar cooked	1 cup (1.5 oz)	10	1	—	1
mustard chopped cooked	½ cup	14	3	—	—
mustard raw chopped	½ cup	17	3	—	—
new zealand chopped cooked	½ cup	11	2	—	—
new zealand raw	½ cup	4	1	—	—
raw chopped	½ cup	6	1	—	1
raw chopped	1 pkg (10 oz)	46	7	—	—
Dole					
Spinach	3 oz	9	tr	—	8
Fresh Express					
Spinach	1½ cups (3 oz)	40	10	0	5
FROZEN					
cooked	½ cup	27	5	—	—
Amy's Organic					
Pocket Sandwich Spinach Feta	1 (4.5 oz)	200	27	4	2
Birds Eye					
Creamed	½ cup (4.3 oz)	100	7	3	1
Whole Leaf	1 cup (2.8 oz)	20	2	1	2

FOOD	PORTION	CALS.	CARB.	SUG.	FIB.
Budget Gourmet					
Au Gratin	1 pkg (5.5 oz)	160	9	—	—
Fresh Like					
Cut Leaf	3.5 oz	21	4	—	1
Green Giant					
Butter Sauce	½ cup (3.4 oz)	40	5	tr	2
Creamed	½ cup (3.8 oz)	80	10	4	2
Cut Leaf	¾ cup (2.6 oz)	25	3	0	3
Harvest Fresh	½ cup (3.5 oz)	25	3	0	2
Stouffer's					
Creamed	1 serv (4.5 oz)	160	8	2	2
Souffle	1 serv (4 oz)	150	9	4	0
Tabatchnick					
Creamed	7.5 oz	60	8	4	2

SPINACH JUICE

FOOD	PORTION	CALS.	CARB.	SUG.	FIB.
juice	3.5 oz	7	1	—	—

SPORTS DRINKS

(*see also* NUTRITIONAL SUPPLEMENTS)

FOOD	PORTION	CALS.	CARB.	SUG.	FIB.
Gatorade					
Citrus Cooler	1 cup (8 oz)	50	14	—	—
Fruit Punch	1 cup (8 oz)	50	14	—	—
Grape	1 cup (8 oz)	50	14	—	—
Iced Tea Cooler	1 cup (8 oz)	50	14	—	—
Lemon-Lime	1 cup (8 oz)	50	14	—	—
Lemonade	1 cup (8 oz)	50	14	—	—
Orange	1 cup (8 fl oz)	50	14	14	—
Tropical Fruit	1 cup (8 oz)	50	14	—	—
Powerade					
Fruit Punch	8 fl oz	72	19	15	—
Grape	8 fl oz	73	19	15	—
Lemon-Lime	8 fl oz	70	19	15	—
Orange	8 fl oz	72	19	15	—
Slice					
All Sport Diet Lemon Lime	8 fl oz	1	0	0	0
All Sport Lemon Lime	8 fl oz	72	19	19	—
All Sport Orange	8 fl oz	74	19	19	—
All Sport Punch	8 fl oz	81	22	22	—
Snapple					
Sport Fruit	1 bottle	80	20	—	—
Sport Lemon	1 bottle	80	20	—	—
Sport Lemon Lime	1 bottle	80	20	—	—
Sport Orange	1 bottle	80	20	—	—

FOOD	PORTION	CALS.	CARB.	SUG.	FIB.
Ultra Fuel					
Lemon Lime	16 fl oz	400	100	30	—
SPOT					
baked	3 oz	134	0	0	0
SQUAB					
breast w/o skin raw	1 (3.5 oz)	135	0	0	0
w/ skin raw	1 squab (6.9 oz)	584	0	0	0
w/o skin raw	1 squab (5.9 oz)	239	0	0	0
SQUASH					
(*see also* ZUCCHINI)					
CANNED					
crookneck sliced	½ cup	14	3	—	—
Allen					
Yellow	½ cup (4.2 oz)	25	5	3	2
Sunshine					
Yellow	½ cup (4.2 oz)	25	5	3	2
FRESH					
acorn cooked mashed	½ cup	41	11	—	3
acorn cubed baked	½ cup	57	15	—	2
butternut baked	½ cup	41	11	—	2
crookneck raw sliced	½ cup	12	3	—	1
crookneck sliced cooked	½ cup	18	4	—	1
hubbard baked	½ cup	51	11	—	3
hubbard cooked mashed	½ cup	35	8	—	3
scallop raw sliced	½ cup	12	3	—	1
scallop sliced cooked	½ cup	14	3	—	1
spaghetti cooked	½ cup	23	5	—	2
Nature's Pasta					
Spaghetti Squash	1 cup (5.5 oz)	20	4	0	2
FROZEN					
butternut cooked mashed	½ cup	47	12	—	3
crookneck sliced cooked	½ cup	24	5	—	—
SEEDS					
dried	1 oz	154	5	—	—
dried	1 cup	747	25	—	—
roasted	1 cup	1184	31	—	—
roasted	1 oz	148	4	—	—
salted & roasted	1 cup	1184	31	—	—
salted & roasted	1 oz	148	4	—	—
whole roasted	1 oz	127	15	—	—
whole roasted	1 cup	285	34	—	—
whole salted roasted	1 cup	285	34	—	—
whole salted roasted	1 oz	127	15	—	—

FOOD	PORTION	CALS.	CARB.	SUG.	FIB.
SQUID					
fried	3 oz	149	7	—	—
raw	3 oz	78	3	—	—
SQUIRREL					
roasted	3 oz	147	0	0	0
STAR FRUIT					
fresh	1	42	10	—	—
Sonoma					
Dried	7-9 pieces (1.4 oz)	140	34	—	0
STRAWBERRIES					
CANNED					
in heavy syrup	½ cup	117	30	—	—
FRESH					
strawberries	1 cup	45	10	—	4
strawberries	1 pint	97	22	—	—
Dole					
Strawberries	8	50	13	—	3
FROZEN					
sweetened sliced	1 cup	245	66	—	—
sweetened sliced	1 pkg (10 oz)	273	74	—	—
unsweetened	1 cup	52	14	—	—
whole sweetened	1 cup	200	54	—	—
whole sweetened	1 pkg (10 oz)	223	60	—	—
Big Valley					
Strawberries	⅔ cup (4.9 oz)	50	12	8	2
Birds Eye					
Halves	½ cup (4.7 oz)	120	31	28	1
Halves In Lite Syrup	½ cup (4.6 oz)	70	17	15	1
Whole	½ cup (4.5 oz)	100	25	23	1
STRAWBERRY JUICE					
Capri Sun					
Strawberry Cooler Drink	1 pkg (7 oz)	90	25	25	0
Kern's					
Nectar	6 fl oz	110	28	—	—
Kool-Aid					
Drink as prep w/ sugar	1 serv (8 oz)	100	25	25	0
Drink Mix as prep	1 serv (8 oz)	60	16	16	0
Libby					
Nectar	1 can (11.5 fl oz)	210	52	46	—
Smucker's					
Juice	8 oz	130	31	—	—

FOOD	PORTION	CALS.	CARB.	SUG.	FIB.
Veryfine					
Juice-Ups	8 fl oz	140	36	36	0
STUFFING/DRESSING					
HOME RECIPE					
bread as prep w/ water & fat	½ cup	251	25	—	—
bread as prep w/ water egg & fat	½ cup	107	9	—	—
MIX					
bread dry as prep	½ cup	178	22	—	3
cornbread as prep	½ cup	179	22	—	—
Arnold					
All Purpose Seasoned	½ oz	50	9	—	1
Corn	½ oz	50	9	—	1
Herb Seasoned	½ oz	50	2	—	1
Sage & Onion	½ oz	50	9	—	1
Brownberry					
Corn	1 oz	103	19	—	2
Herb	1 oz	100	19	—	2
Sage & Onion	1 oz	97	18	—	2
Golden Grain					
Bread Stuffing Chicken	½ cup	180	20	—	—
Bread Stuffing Corn Bread	½ cup	180	21	—	—
Bread Stuffing Herb & Butter	½ cup	180	20	—	—
Bread Stuffing With Wild Rice	½ cup	180	21	—	—
Kellogg's					
Croutettes Mix	1 cup (1.2 oz)	120	25	0	0
Pepperidge Farm					
Corn Bread	1 oz	110	22	—	—
Country Style	1 oz	100	21	—	—
Cube	1 oz	110	22	—	—
Distinctive Apple Raisin	1 oz	110	21	—	—
Distinctive Classic Chicken	1 oz	110	20	—	—
Distinctive Country Garden Herb	1 oz	120	18	—	—
Distinctive Vegetable & Almond	1 oz	110	19	—	—
Distinctive Wild Rice & Mushroom	1 oz	130	17	—	—
Herb Seasoned	1 oz	110	22	—	—
Stove Top					
Chicken as prep w/ margarine	½ cup (3.6 oz)	170	20	3	tr

FOOD	PORTION	CALS.	CARB.	SUG.	FIB.
Stove Top (CONT.)					
Cornbread as prep w/ margarine	½ cup (3.6 oz)	170	21	3	1
Flexible Serve Chicken as prep w/ margarine	½ cup (3.3 oz)	170	19	3	tr
Flexible Serve Cornbread as prep w/ margarine	½ cup (3.3 oz)	160	19	3	1
Flexible Serve Homestyle Herb as prep w/ margarine	½ cup (3.3 oz)	170	19	3	1
For Beef as prep w/ margarine	½ cup (3.7 oz)	180	22	4	1
For Pork as prep w/ margarine	½ cup (3.6 oz)	170	20	3	1
For Turkey as prep w/ margarine	½ cup (3.6 oz)	170	20	3	tr
Long Grain & Wild Rice as prep w/ margarine	½ cup (3.7 oz)	180	22	3	tr
Lower Sodium Chicken as prep w/ margarine	½ cup (3.6 oz)	180	21	3	tr
Microwave Chicken as prep w/ margarine	½ cup (3.5 oz)	160	20	3	tr
Microwave Homestyle Cornbread as prep w/ margarine	½ cup (3 oz)	160	20	3	tr
Mushroom & Onion as prep w/ margarine	½ cup (3.6 oz)	180	20	3	tr
San Francisco Style as prep w/ margarine	½ cup (3.6 oz)	170	20	3	1
Savory Herb as prep w/ margarine	½ cup (3.6 oz)	170	20	3	1
Traditional Sage as prep w/ margarine	½ cup (3.6 oz)	180	21	3	1
Wonder					
Seasoned Stuffing	1 cup (0.9 oz)	60	12	tr	tr
STURGEON					
cooked	3 oz	115	0	0	0
raw	3 oz	90	0	0	0
roe raw	3.5 oz	207	1	—	—
smoked	1 oz	48	0	0	0
smoked	3 oz	147	0	0	0
SUCKER					
white baked	3 oz	101	0	0	0

FOOD	PORTION	CALS.	CARB.	SUG.	FIB.
SUGAR					
(*see also* FRUCTOSE, SUGAR SUBSTITUTES, SYRUP)					
brown packed	1 cup (7.7 oz)	828	214	214	—
brown unpacked	1 cup (5.1 oz)	546	141	—	—
maple	1 piece (1 oz)	100	26	—	—
powdered	1 tbsp (0.3 oz)	31	8	8	—
powdered unsifted	1 cup (4.2 oz)	467	119	115	—
white	1 cup (7 oz)	773	200	200	—
white	1 packet (6 g)	25	6	—	—
white	1 tbsp	45	12	—	—
white	1 tsp (4 g)	15	4	4	—
C&H					
White	1 tsp	16	4	—	—
Domino					
White	1 tsp	16	4	—	—
Hain					
Turbinado	1 tbsp	50	12	—	—
Hollywood					
Turbinado	1 tbsp	50	12	—	—
SUGAR SUBSTITUTES					
(*see also* FRUCTOSE)					
Equal					
Packet	1 pkg	4	tr	—	—
Mrs. Bateman's					
Sugarlike	1 tsp (4 g)	4	4	0	0
NatraTaste					
Packet	1 pkg (1 g)	0	1	—	—
S&W					
Liquid Table Sweetener	⅛ tsp	0	0	0	0
Sprinkle Sweet					
Sugar Substitute	1 tsp	2	tr	—	—
Sweet One					
Packet	1 pkg (1 g)	4	1	—	—
*Sweet*10*					
Granular	⅛ tsp	0	0	0	0
Weight Watchers					
Sweetner	1 serv (1 g)	5	1	1	0
SUGAR-APPLE					
fresh	1	146	37	—	—
fresh cut up	1 cup	236	59	—	—
SUNCHOKE					
fresh raw sliced	½ cup	57	13	—	—

FOOD	PORTION	CALS.	CARB.	SUG.	FIB.
SUNDAE TOPPINGS					
(*see* ICE CREAM TOPPINGS)					
SUNFISH					
pumpkinseed baked	3 oz	97	0	0	0
SUNFLOWER					
seeds dried	1 oz	162	5	—	—
seeds dried	1 cup	821	27	—	—
seeds dry roasted	1 oz	165	7	—	—
seeds dry roasted	1 cup	745	31	—	—
seeds dry roasted salted	1 cup	745	31	—	—
seeds dry roasted salted	1 oz	165	7	—	—
seeds oil roasted	1 cup	830	20	—	—
seeds oil roasted salted	1 cup	830	20	—	—
seeds oil roasted salted	1 oz	175	4	—	—
seeds toasted	1 oz	176	6	—	—
seeds toasted	1 cup	826	28	—	—
seeds toasted salted	1 oz	176	6	—	—
seeds toasted salted	1 cup	826	28	—	—
sunflower butter	1 tbsp	93	4	—	—
sunflower butter w/o salt	1 tbsp	93	4	—	—
Erewhon					
Sunflower Seed Butter	2 tbsp (32 g)	200	3	—	—
Fisher					
Seeds Oil Roasted	1 oz	170	6	—	—
Seeds Salted In Shell shelled	1 oz	160	6	—	—
Seeds Salted In Shell unshelled	1 oz	170	6	—	—
Frito Lay					
Seeds	1 oz	160	6	—	—
Planters					
Kernels	1 pkg (1.7 oz)	290	9	0	7
Kernels	1 pkg (2 oz)	340	11	0	8
Kernels Barbecue	1 pkg (1.7 oz)	290	10	1	6
Kernels Honey Roasted	1 pkg (1.7 oz)	280	15	6	6
Kernels Salted	1 oz	170	4	0	4
Munch'N Go Singles Dry Roasted	1 pkg	120	4	0	1
Nuts Dry Roasted	¼ cup (1.1 oz)	190	6	0	4
Original With Shell Dry Roasted	¾ cup	160	5	0	2
Stone-Buhr					
Seeds Raw	4 tsp (1 oz)	170	6	0	6

FOOD	PORTION	CALS.	CARB.	SUG.	FIB.
SWAMP CABBAGE					
chopped cooked	½ cup	10	2	—	—
raw chopped	1 cup	11	2	—	—
SWEET POTATO					
(*see also* YAM)					
CANNED					
in syrup	½ cup	106	25	—	—
pieces	1 cup	183	42	—	—
Princella					
Mashed	⅔ cup (5.1 oz)	120	28	15	3
Royal Prince					
Candied	½ cup (4.9 oz)	210	50	35	2
Halves	3 pieces (5.7 oz)	190	46	16	4
Orange Pineapple	½ cup (4.8 oz)	210	43	36	3
Sugary Sam					
Mashed	⅔ cup (5.1 oz)	120	28	15	3
FRESH					
baked w/ skin	1 (3.5 oz)	118	28	—	3
leaves cooked	½ cup	11	2	—	—
mashed	½ cup	172	40	—	3
FROZEN					
cooked	½ cup	88	21	—	—
Mrs. Paul's					
Candied Sweet Potatoes	4 oz	170	42	—	—
Candied Sweets 'N Apples	4 oz	160	38	—	—
SWEETBREADS					
beef braised	3 oz	230	0	0	0
lamb braised	3 oz	199	0	0	0
veal braised	3 oz	218	0	0	0
SWISS CHARD					
cooked	½ cup	18	4	—	—
raw chopped	½ cup	3	1	—	—
SWORDFISH					
cooked	3 oz	132	0	0	0
raw	3 oz	103	0	0	0
SYRUP					
(*see also* ICE CREAM TOPPINGS, PANCAKE/WAFFLE SYRUP)					
corn	2 tbsp	122	32	—	—
corn dark	1 tbsp (0.7 oz)	56	15	—	—
corn dark	1 cup (11.5 oz)	925	251	—	—
corn light	1 cup (11.5 oz)	925	251	168	—

FOOD	PORTION	CALS.	CARB.	SUG.	FIB.
corn light	1 tbsp (0.7 oz)	56	15	10	—
malt	1 tbsp (0.8 oz)	76	17	—	—
malt	1 cup (13 oz)	1222	274	—	—
maple	1 tbsp (0.8 oz)	52	13	12	—
maple	1 cup (11.1 oz)	824	212	191	—
raspberry	3.5 oz	267	66	—	—
rose hip	3.5 oz	33	8	8	0
sorghum	1 cup (11.6 oz)	957	247	247	—
sorghum	1 tbsp (0.7 oz)	61	16	16	—
Estee					
Blueberry Lite	¼ cup (2.4 oz)	80	20	20	—
Karo					
Corn Syrup Dark	1 cup (331 g)	975	243	—	—
Corn Syrup Dark	1 tbsp (21 g)	60	15	—	—
Corn Syrup Light	1 tbsp (21 g)	60	15	—	—
Corn Syrup Light	1 cup (331 g)	960	241	—	—
McIlhenny					
Cane	2 tbsp (1.4 oz)	130	32	22	tr
Quik					
Strawberry	2 tbsp (1.5 oz)	110	27	26	0
Red Wing					
Strawberry	2 tbsp (1.4 oz)	110	28	20	0
S&W					
Blueberry Diet	1 tbsp	4	1	—	—
Maple Flavored Diet	1 tbsp	4	1	—	—
Strawberry Diet	1 tbsp	4	1	—	—
Smucker's					
All Flavors Fruit Syrup	2 tbsp	100	26		
Tree Of Life					
Maple	¼ cup (2.1 oz)	200	53	53	—
Rice Syrup	2 tbsp (1 oz)	120	29	29	—
Whistling Wings					
Blueberry	1 oz	45	10	—	tr
Raspberry	1 oz	60	14	—	0

TACO
(*see* SPANISH FOOD)

TAHINI
(*see* SESAME)

TAMARIND

fresh	1	5	1	—	—
fresh cut up	1 cup	287	75	—	—

FOOD	PORTION	CALS.	CARB.	SUG.	FIB.
TANGERINE					
CANNED					
in light syrup	½ cup	76	20	—	—
juice pack	½ cup	46	12	—	—
FRESH					
sections	1 cup	86	22	—	—
tangerine	1	37	9	—	—
Dole					
Tangerine	2	70	19	—	2
TANGERINE JUICE					
canned sweetened	1 cup	125	30	—	—
fresh	1 cup	106	25	—	—
frzn sweetened as prep	1 cup	110	27	—	—
frzn sweetened not prep	6 oz	344	83	—	—
After The Fall					
Juice	1 can (12 oz)	170	40	35	0
Dole					
Mandarin frzn as prep	8 fl oz	140	35	29	0
Fresh Samantha					
Fresh Juice	1 cup (8 oz)	106	24	—	1
Minute Maid					
Frozen	8 fl oz	120	29	29	—
TAPIOCA					
pearl dry	½ cup (2.7 oz)	272	67	—	1
starch	3½ oz	344	85	—	—
Minute					
Minute Tapioca	1½ tsp (6 g)	20	5	0	0
TARO					
chips	10 (0.8 oz)	115	16	—	—
chips	1 oz	141	19	—	—
leaves cooked	½ cup	18	3	—	—
raw sliced	½ cup	56	14	—	—
shoots sliced cooked	½ cup	10	2	—	—
sliced cooked	½ cup (2.3 oz)	94	23	—	—
tahitian sliced cooked	½ cup	30	5	—	—
TARRAGON					
ground	1 tsp	5	1	—	—
TEA/HERBAL TEA					
(*see also* ICED TEA)					
HERBAL					
Bigelow					
Almond Orange	5 fl oz	tr	tr	—	—

FOOD	PORTION	CALS.	CARB.	SUG.	FIB.
Bigelow (CONT.)					
Apple Orchard	5 fl oz	5	1	—	—
Apple Spice	5 fl oz	tr	tr	—	—
Chamomile Mint	5 fl oz	tr	tr	—	—
Cinnamon Orange	5 fl oz	tr	tr	—	—
Early Riser	5 fl oz	3	1	—	—
Feeling Free	5 fl oz	1	tr	—	—
Fruit & Almond	5 fl oz	1	tr	—	—
Hibiscus & Rose Hips	5 fl oz	1	tr	—	—
I Love Lemon	5 fl oz	1	tr	—	—
Lemon & C	5 fl oz	tr	tr	—	—
Looking Good	5 fl oz	1	1	—	—
Mint Blend	5 fl oz	tr	tr	—	—
Mint Medley	5 fl oz	1	tr	—	—
Orange & C	5 fl oz	tr	tr	—	—
Orange & Spice	5 fl oz	1	tr	—	—
Peppermint	5 fl oz	tr	tr	—	—
Roasted Grains & Carob	5 fl oz	3	1	—	—
Spearmint	5 fl oz	tr	tr	—	—
Sweet Dreams	5 fl oz	1	tr	—	—
Take-A-Break	5 fl oz	3	1	—	—
Celestial Seasonings					
Almond Sunset	8 fl oz	3	1	—	—
Bengal Spice	8 fl oz	5	tr	—	—
Caffeine Free	8 fl oz	2	1	—	—
Chamomile	8 fl oz	2	1	—	—
Cinnamon Apple Spice	8 fl oz	<3	tr	—	—
Cinnamon Rose	8 fl oz	<4	1	—	—
Country Peach Spice	8 fl oz	3	1	—	—
Cranberry Cove	8 fl oz	2	1	—	—
Emperor's Choice	8 fl oz	4	1	—	—
Ginseng Plus	8 fl oz	3	1	—	—
Grandma's Tummy Mint	8 fl oz	2	tr	—	—
Lemon Mist	8 fl oz	3	tr	—	—
Lemon Zinger	8 fl oz	4	1	—	—
Mama Bear's Cold Care	8 fl oz	6	tr	—	—
Mandarin Orange Spice	8 fl oz	5	1	—	—
Mellow Mint	8 fl oz	2	tr	—	—
Mint Magic	8 fl oz	1	tr	—	—
Orange Zinger	8 fl oz	6	1	—	—
Peppermint	8 fl oz	2	1	—	—
Raspberry Patch	8 fl oz	4	1	—	—
Red Zinger	8 fl oz	4	1	—	—
Roastaroma	8 fl oz	10	2	—	—

FOOD	PORTION	CALS.	CARB.	SUG.	FIB.
Celestial Seasonings (CONT.)					
Sleepytime	8 fl oz	4	1	—	—
Spearmint	8 fl oz	5	tr	—	—
Strawberry Fields	8 fl oz	4	1	—	—
Sunburst C	8 fl oz	3	1	—	—
Tropical Escape	8 fl oz	1	tr	—	—
Wild Forest Blackberry	8 fl oz	2	1	—	—
Lipton					
Bedtime Story	1 tea bag	0	0	0	0
Cinnamon Apple	1 tea bag	0	0	0	0
Country Cranberry	1 tea bag	0	0	0	0
Gentle Orange	1 tea bag	0	0	0	0
Ginger Twist	1 tea bag	0	0	0	0
Golden Lemon Honey	1 tea bag	0	tr	0	—
Lemon Soother	1 tea bag	0	tr	0	—
Peppermint Breeze	1 tea bag	0	0	0	0
REGULAR					
brewed tea	6 oz	2	tr	—	—
instant unsweetened as prep w/ water	8 oz	2	tr	—	—
Bigelow					
Chinese Fortune	5 fl oz	1	tr	—	—
Cinnamon Stick	5 fl oz	1	tr	—	—
Constant Comment	5 fl oz	1	tr	—	—
Darjeeling Blend	5 fl oz	1	tr	—	—
Earl Gray	5 fl oz	1	tr	—	—
English Teatime	5 fl oz	1	tr	—	—
Lemon Lift	5 fl oz	1	tr	—	—
Orange Pekoe	5 fl oz	1	tr	—	—
Peppermint Stick	5 fl oz	1	tr	—	—
Plantation Mint	5 fl oz	1	tr	—	—
Raspberry Royale	5 fl oz	1	tr	—	—
Celestial Seasonings					
Cinnamon Vienna	8 fl oz	2	1	—	—
Earl Grey Extraordinary	8 fl oz	3	1	—	—
English Breakfast Classic	8 fl oz	3	tr	—	—
Lemon	8 fl oz	7	1	—	—
Mint	8 fl oz	4	tr	—	—
Morning Thunder	8 fl oz	3	tr	—	—
Naturally Decaffeinated	8 fl oz	10	tr	—	—
Orange Spice	8 fl oz	7	1	—	—
Orange Spice Decaff	8 fl oz	7	1	—	—
Organically Grown	8 fl oz	12	1	—	—
Raspberry	8 fl oz	7	1	—	—

FOOD	PORTION	CALS.	CARB.	SUG.	FIB.
General Foods					
International Instant Tea Decaffeinated English Breakfast Creme	1 serv (8 oz)	70	13	10	0
International Instant Tea Decaffeinated Viennese Cinnamon Creme	1 serv (8 oz)	70	13	10	0
International Instant Tea English Breakfast Creme as prep	1 serv (8 oz)	70	13	10	0
International Instant Tea English Raspberry Creme as prep	1 serv (8 oz)	70	13	11	0
International Instant Tea Island Orange Creme as prep	1 serv (8 oz)	70	13	11	0
International Instant Tea Viennese Cinnamon Creme as prep	1 serv (8 oz)	70	13	11	0
Lipton					
Brisk Tea as prep	1 serv	0	0	0	0
Decaffeinated Brisk Tea as prep	1 serv	0	0	0	0
English Blend as prep	1 cup	0	0	0	0
Flavored Blackberry	1 tea bag	0	0	0	0
Flavored Decaffeinated Orange & Spice	1 tea bag	0	0	0	0
Flavored Honey & Lemon	1 tea bag	0	0	0	0
Flavored Mint	1 tea bag	0	0	0	0
Flavored Orange & Spice	1 tea bag	0	0	0	0
Flavored Raspberry	1 tea bag	0	0	0	0
Green Tea	1 tea bag	0	0	0	0
Green Tea Orange, Passionfruit & Jasmine	1 tea bag	0	0	0	0
Loose Tea	1 tsp (2 g)	0	0	0	0
Nestea					
Tea Bag as prep	6 oz	0	0	0	0
Tetley					
Tea Bag as prep	1	0	0	0	0
TEFF					
Arrowhead					
Whole Grain	¼ cup (1.6 oz)	160	32	0	6
TEMPEH					
tempeh	½ cup	165	14	—	—

FOOD	PORTION	CALS.	CARB.	SUG.	FIB.
Lightlife					
Garden Vege	4 oz	142	9	0	2
Tempeh	4 oz	182	9	—	—
White Wave					
Burger	1 patty (3 oz)	110	10	0	6
Lemon Broil	1 patty (2 oz)	130	11	2	4
Organic Wild Rice	⅓ block (2.7 oz)	140	12	0	6
Teriyaki Burger	1 patty (3 oz)	110	11	3	6
THYME					
ground	1 tsp	4	1	—	—
Watkins					
Thyme	¼ tsp (0.5 oz)	0	0	0	0
TILEFISH					
cooked	3 oz	125	0	0	0
cooked	½ fillet (5.3 oz)	220	0	0	0
raw	3 oz	81	0	0	0
TOFU					
firm	¼ block (3 oz)	118	3	—	1
firm	½ cup	183	5	—	2
fresh fried	1 piece (0.5 oz)	35	1	—	tr
fuyu salted & fermented	1 block (⅓ oz)	13	1	—	tr
koyadofu dried frozen	1 piece (½ oz)	82	2	—	tr
okara	½ cup	47	8	—	1
regular	¼ block (4 oz)	88	2	—	1
regular	½ cup	94	2	—	1
Azumaya					
Blue Label	3.5 oz	46	4	—	—
Green Label	3.5 oz	68	4	—	—
Name Age Fried	3.5 oz	144	9	—	—
Red Label	3.5 oz	68	5	—	—
Casbah					
Gyro as prep w/ tofu	1 patty (2 oz)	105	15	0	tr
Jaclyn's					
Grilled In Black Bean Sauce	10.75 oz	270	45	—	—
Grilled In Peanut Sauce	10.75 oz	260	44	—	—
Long Life					
Tofu	3 oz	60	2	0	1
Mori-Nu					
Extra Firm	1 in slice (3 oz)	55	2	—	—
Firm	1 in slice (3 oz)	50	2	—	—
Lite Extra Firm	1 in slice (3 oz)	35	1	—	—
Lite Firm	1 in slice (3 oz)	35	1	—	—

FOOD	PORTION	CALS.	CARB.	SUG.	FIB.
Mori-Nu (CONT.)					
Soft	1 in slice (3 oz)	45	2	—	—
Nasoya					
Chinise 5 Spice	¼ block (3 oz)	68	1	1	1
Extra Firm	⅕ block (3.2 oz)	92	1	tr	tr
Firm	⅕ block (3.2 oz)	76	2	1	tr
French Country	⅕ block (3 oz)	68	1	1	1
Silken	⅕ block (3.2 oz)	48	2	1	tr
Soft	⅕ block (3.2 oz)	63	2	1	tr
Spring Creek					
Baked Barbeque	2 oz	88	7	—	—
Baked Cajun	2 oz	87	5	—	—
Baked Teriyaki	2 oz	84	3	—	—
Great Balls Of Tofu!	2 (3 oz)	107	5	—	—
Nigari Firm	4 oz	140	tr	—	3
Tofu Salads !Onion Dip	2 oz	46	6	—	—
Tofu Salads !Taco Dip	2 oz	46	6	—	—
Tofu Salads Missing Egg	2 oz	49	6	—	—
Tree Of Life					
Baked	⅕ block (3.2 oz)	150	5	0	0
Firm	⅕ block (3.2 oz)	100	2	0	0
Raw Firm	⅕ block (3.2 oz)	100	2	0	0
Ready Ground Hot & Spicy	⅓ pkg (3 oz)	60	2	0	0
Ready Ground Original	⅓ pkg (3 oz)	60	2	0	0
Ready Ground Savory Garlic	⅓ pkg (3 oz)	60	2	0	0
Reduced Fat	⅕ block (3.2 oz)	90	4	0	2
Savory Baked	⅕ block (3.2 oz)	140	4	0	0
Smoked Hot'N Spicy	½ block (3 oz)	120	3	0	0
Smoked Original	½ block (3 oz)	120	3	0	0
White Wave					
Baked Tofus Teriyaki Oriental Style	¼ block (2 oz)	120	3	—	1
Hard	4 oz	120	1	—	—
International Baked Italian Garlic Herb	¼ pkg (2 oz)	120	3	0	1
International Baked Mexican Jalapeno	¼ pkg (2 oz)	120	3	0	1
International Baked Oriental Teriyaki	¼ pkg (2 oz)	120	3	0	1
International Baked Thai Sesame Peanut	¼ pkg (2 oz)	120	3	0	1
Soft	4 oz	120	1	—	—
YOGURT					
Stir Fruity					
Black Cherry	6 oz	141	25	—	—

FOOD	PORTION	CALS.	CARB.	SUG.	FIB.
Stir Fruity (CONT.)					
Blueberry	6 oz	140	26	—	—
Lemon Chiffon	6 oz	152	26	—	—
Mixed Berry	6 oz	149	26	—	—
Orange	6 oz	143	26	—	—
Peach	6 oz	160	27	—	—
Pina Colada	6 oz	162	28	—	—
Raspberry	6 oz	155	29	—	—
Spiced Apple	6 oz	167	31	—	—
Strawberry	6 oz	140	25	—	—
Tropical Fruit	6 oz	170	32	—	—
TOMATILLO					
fresh	1 (1.2 oz)	11	2	—	—
fresh chopped	½ cup	21	4	—	—
TOMATO					
(*see also* PIZZA, SPAGHETTI SAUCE)					
CANNED					
paste	½ cup	110	25	—	6
puree	1 cup	102	25	—	6
puree w/o salt	1 cup	102	25	—	6
red whole	½ cup	24	5	—	—
sauce	½ cup	37	9	—	2
sauce spanish style	½ cup	40	9	—	2
sauce w/ mushrooms	½ cup	42	10	—	—
sauce w/ onion	½ cup	52	12	—	—
stewed	½ cup	34	8	—	—
w/ green chiles	½ cup	18	4	—	—
wedges in tomato juice	½ cup	34	8	—	—
Amore					
Sun-Dried Tomato Paste	1 tsp (6 g)	15	tr	0	0
Contadina					
Crushed	¼ cup	20	4	3	1
Italian Paste	2 tbsp	40	7	2	1
Italian Style Pear	½ cup	25	4	3	1
Italian Style Stewed	½ cup	40	8	5	1
Mexican Style Stewed	½ cup	40	9	4	1
Pasta Ready Primavera	½ cup	50	8	5	1
Pasta Ready Tomatoes	½ cup	50	7	4	1
Pasta Ready With Crushed Red Pepper	½ cup	60	8	4	1
Pasta Ready With Mushrooms	½ cup	50	9	5	1
Pasta Ready With Olives	½ cup	60	8	5	1

FOOD	PORTION	CALS.	CARB.	SUG.	FIB.
Contadina (CONT.)					
Pasta Ready With Three Cheeses	½ cup	70	8	5	tr
Paste	2 tbsp	30	6	3	1
Peeled Whole	½ cup	25	4	3	1
Puree	¼ cup	20	4	1	tr
Recipe Ready	½ cup	25	5	1	3
Stewed	½ cup	40	9	5	1
Del Monte					
Paste	2 tbsp (1.2 oz)	30	7	5	2
Peeled Diced	½ cup (4.4 oz)	25	6	4	2
Puree	¼ cup (2.2 oz)	30	7	5	1
Sauce	¼ cup (2.1 oz)	20	4	4	tr
Sauce No Salt Added	¼ cup (2.1 oz)	20	4	4	tr
Stewed Cajun Style	½ cup (4.4 oz)	35	9	7	2
Stewed Chunky Chili	½ cup (4.5 oz)	30	8	6	2
Stewed Chunky Pasta	½ cup (4.5 oz)	45	11	8	2
Stewed Chunky Pizza	½ cup (4.5 oz)	35	9	7	2
Stewed Chunky Salsa	½ cup (4.5 oz)	35	8	6	2
Stewed Italian Style	½ cup (4.4 oz)	30	8	6	2
Stewed Mexican Style	½ cup (4.4 oz)	35	9	7	2
Stewed Original	½ cup (4.4 oz)	35	9	7	2
Stewed Original No Salt Added	½ cup (4.4 oz)	35	9	7	2
Wedges	½ cup (4.4 oz)	35	9	7	2
Whole Peeled	½ cup (4.4 oz)	25	6	4	2
Eden					
Crushed Organic	¼ cup (2.1 oz)	20	3	2	1
Sauce Lightly Seasoned	¼ cup (2.1 oz)	25	5	3	1
Health Valley					
Sauce	1 cup	70	13	—	tr
Sauce Low Sodium	1 cup	70	13	—	1
Hebrew National					
Pickled	⅓ tomato (1 oz)	4	1	—	—
Hunt's					
Choice Cut	½ cup (4.2 oz)	22	5	5	1
Choice Cut Diced Tomatoes & Green Chiles	2 tbsp (0.4 oz)	1	tr	tr	tr
Choice Cut Diced Tomatoes & Italian Herb	½ cup (4.2 oz)	24	5	5	1
Choice Cut Diced Tomatoes & Roasted Garlic	½ cup (4.2 oz)	24	5	5	1
Crushed	½ cup (4.2 oz)	29	7	6	2

FOOD	PORTION	CALS.	CARB.	SUG.	FIB.
Hunt's (CONT.)					
Crushed Angela Mia	½ cup (4.2 oz)	27	6	4	2
Paste	2 tbsp (1.2 oz)	30	6	4	2
Paste Italian	2 tbsp (1.2 oz)	27	6	4	2
Paste No Salt Added	2 tbsp (1.2 oz)	30	6	4	2
Paste With Garlic	2 tbsp (1.2 oz)	28	6	4	2
Pear Shaped	½ cup (4.6 oz)	20	4	4	1
Puree	¼ cup (2.2 oz)	24	5	3	2
Ready Sauce Chunky Chili	¼ cup (2.2 oz)	22	4	3	1
Ready Sauce Chunky Italian	¼ cup (2.2 oz)	26	5	4	1
Ready Sauce Chunky Mexican	¼ cup (2.2 oz)	21	4	3	1
Ready Sauce Chunky Special	¼ cup (2.2 oz)	21	4	3	1
Ready Sauce Chunky Tomato	¼ cup (2.2 oz)	15	3	2	1
Ready Sauce Country Herb	¼ cup (2.2 oz)	33	5	5	1
Ready Sauce Garlic	¼ cup (2.2 oz)	29	5	2	2
Ready Sauce Garlic & Herb	¼ cup (2.2 oz)	26	5	3	1
Ready Sauce Meatloaf Fixins	¼ cup (2.2 oz)	23	4	5	1
Ready Sauce Original	¼ cup (2.2 oz)	30	4	4	1
Ready Sauce Salsa	¼ cup (2.2 oz)	18	3	3	1
Sauce	¼ cup (2.2 oz)	16	3	3	1
Sauce Italian	¼ cup (2.2 oz)	32	5	5	1
Sauce No Salt Added	¼ cup (2.2 oz)	16	3	3	1
Sauce With Herb	¼ cup (2.2 oz)	32	5	5	1
Stewed	½ cup (4.2 oz)	33	7	6	2
Stewed Italian	4 oz	40	9	—	tr
Tomatoes	½ cup (4.2 oz)	33	7	6	2
Whole	2 (5.2 oz)	22	4	5	1
Muir Glen					
Organic Chunky Sauce	¼ cup (2.3 oz)	20	4	2	1
Organic Crushed With Basil	¼ cup (2.3 oz)	25	4	4	1
Organic Diced	½ cup (4.5 oz)	25	4	4	1
Organic Diced No Salt Added	½ cup (4.5 oz)	25	4	4	1
Organic Ground Peeled	¼ cup (2.3 oz)	10	2	2	1
Organic Italian Style Diced	½ cup (4.4 oz)	25	4	4	1
Organic Paste	2 tbsp (1.2 oz)	30	6	3	1
Organic Puree	¼ cup (2.2 oz)	20	5	3	1
Organic Sauce	¼ cup (2.2 oz)	20	5	3	1
Organic Sauce No Salt Added	¼ cup (2.2 oz)	20	5	1	1

FOOD	PORTION	CALS.	CARB.	SUG.	FIB.
Muir Glen (CONT.)					
Organic Stewed	½ cup (4.5 oz)	30	7	3	tr
Organic Stewed Italian Style	½ cup (4.4 oz)	30	7	3	tr
Organic Stewed Mexican Style	½ cup (4.4 oz)	30	7	3	tr
Organic Whole Peeled	½ cup (4.6 oz)	30	5	4	1
Old El Paso					
Tomatoes & Jalapenos	¼ cup (2 oz)	15	3	2	1
Tomatoes & Green Chilies	¼ cup (2 oz)	10	2	1	0
Progresso					
Crushed	¼ cup (2.1 oz)	20	4	2	1
Paste	2 tbsp (1.2 oz)	30	6	3	1
Peeled Whole	½ cup (4.2 oz)	25	4	3	1
Peeled w/ Basil	½ cup (4.2 oz)	25	4	3	1
Puree	¼ cup (2.2 oz)	25	5	3	1
Puree Thick Style	¼ cup (2.2 oz)	30	5	3	1
Sauce	¼ cup (2.1 oz)	20	4	2	1
Ro-Tel					
Diced Tomatoes & Green Chilies	½ cup (4.4 oz)	20	4	3	1
Rosoff's					
Pickled	⅓ tomato (1 oz)	5	1	—	—
S&W					
Aspic Supreme	½ cup	60	16	—	—
Diced In Rich Puree	½ cup	35	8	—	—
Italian Stewed Sliced	½ cup	35	9	—	—
Italian Style w/ Basil	½ cup	25	5	—	—
Paste	6 oz	150	35	—	—
Peeled Ready Cut	½ cup	25	6	—	—
Puree	½ cup	60	14	—	—
Sauce	½ cup	40	9	—	—
Sauce Chunky	½ cup	45	10	—	—
Stewed 50% Salt Reduced	½ cup	35	9	—	—
Stewed Mexican Style	½ cup	40	8	—	—
Stewed Sliced	½ cup	35	9	—	—
Whole Diet	½ cup	25	5	—	—
Whole Peeled	½ cup	25	6	—	—
Schorr's					
Pickled	⅓ tomato (1 oz)	4	1	—	—
Sonoma					
Dried Spice Medley oil drained	1 tbsp (0.5 oz)	50	3	1	1
Pesto	¼ cup (2 oz)	110	6	2	1

FOOD	PORTION	CALS.	CARB.	SUG.	FIB.
Sonoma (CONT.)					
Tapenade	1 tbsp (0.7 oz)	70	4	1	1
Tree Of Life					
Sauce	¼ cup (2 oz)	20	4	4	—
DRIED					
sun dried	1 cup	140	30	—	—
sun dried	1 piece	5	1	—	—
sun dried in oil	1 piece (3 g)	6	1	—	—
sun dried in oil	1 cup (4 oz)	235	26	—	—
Sonoma					
Bits	2-3 tsp (5 g)	15	3	1	1
Dried	2-3 halves (5 g)	15	3	1	1
Halves	2-3 halves (5 g)	15	3	1	1
Julienne	7-9 pieces (5 g)	15	3	1	1
Pasta Toss	½ cup (0.7 oz)	70	13	4	3
Season It	2-3 tsp (5 g)	20	3	1	1
FRESH					
cooked	½ cup	32	7	—	—
green	1	30	6	—	—
red	1 (4.5 oz)	26	6	—	2
red chopped	1 cup	35	8	—	2
TOMATO JUICE					
beef broth & tomato	5½ oz	61	14	—	—
clam & tomato	1 can (5½ oz)	77	18	—	—
tomato juice	6 oz	32	8	—	—
tomato juice	½ cup	21	5	—	—
Campbell					
Juice	6 oz	40	8	—	—
Del Monte					
Snap-E-Tom	6 fl oz	40	8	4	1
Snap-E-Tom	8 fl oz	50	11	6	2
Snap-E-Tom	10 fl oz	60	13	7	2
Hunt's					
Juice	8 fl oz	22	5	4	1
No Salt Added	8 fl oz	34	8	7	2
Libby					
Juice	6 oz	35	35	—	—
Mott's					
Beefamato	8 fl oz	80	20	7	1
Clamato	8 fl oz	100	24	8	2
Clamato Caesar	8 fl oz	100	24	8	0
Muir Glen					
Organic	8 oz	40	7	7	tr

FOOD	PORTION	CALS.	CARB.	SUG.	FIB.
S&W					
California	6 oz	35	8	—	—
Diet	½ cup	35	8	—	—
TONGUE					
beef simmered	3 oz	241	tr	—	—
lamb braised	3 oz	234	0	0	0
pork braised	3 oz	230	0	0	0

TOPPINGS
(*see* ICE CREAM TOPPINGS)

TORTILLA
(*see also* CHIPS TORTILLA, SPANISH FOOD)

FOOD	PORTION	CALS.	CARB.	SUG.	FIB.
corn	1 (6 in diam)	56	12	—	1
corn w/o salt	1-6 in diam (.9 oz)	56	12	—	1
flour w/o salt	1-8 in diam (1.2 oz)	114	20	—	1
Alvarado St. Bakery					
Burrito Size	1 (2.2 oz)	170	30	0	1
Fajita Size	1 (1.6 oz)	130	23	0	1
Mariachi					
Tortilla	1	112	20	—	—
Old El Paso					
Flour	1 (1.4 oz)	150	27	tr	0
Soft Taco Tortilla	2 (1.8 oz)	180	33	tr	0
Tyson					
Burrito Style Flour	1	170	29	—	—
Burrito Style Hand Stretched Small Flour	1	106	19	—	—
Burrito Style Heat Pressed Large Flour	1	182	33	—	—
Enchilada Style Corn	1	54	11	—	—
Fajito Style Flour	1	89	15	—	—
Soft Taco Flour	1	121	20	—	—
Whole Wheat	1	120	20	—	—
Wonder					
Low Fat Wheat	1 (1.4 oz)	120	24	3	1
Low Fat White	1 (1.4 oz)	110	22	1	1
Zapata					
Tortilla	1 (1.2 oz)	100	18	1	tr

TORTILLA CHIPS
(*see* CHIPS)

TREE FERN

FOOD	PORTION	CALS.	CARB.	SUG.	FIB.
chopped cooked	½ cup	28	8	—	—

FOOD	PORTION	CALS.	CARB.	SUG.	FIB.
TRITICALE					
dry	1 cup (6.7 oz)	645	138	—	—
triticale not prep	3.5 oz	329	64	—	7
TROUT					
baked	3 oz	162	0	0	0
rainbow cooked	3 oz	129	0	0	0
seatrout baked	3 oz	113	0	0	0
Clear Springs					
Rainbow	3.5 oz	140	tr	—	—
TRUFFLES					
fresh	3½ oz	25	17	—	—
TUMERIC					
ground	1 tsp	8	1	—	—
TUNA					
(*see also* TUNA DISHES)					
CANNED					
light in oil	3 oz	169	0	0	0
light in oil	1 can (6 oz)	399	0	0	0
light in water	3 oz	99	0	0	0
light in water	1 can (5.8 oz)	192	0	0	0
white in oil	3 oz	158	0	0	0
white in oil	1 can (6.2 oz)	331	0	0	0
white in water	3 oz	116	0	0	0
white in water	1 can (6 oz)	234	0	0	0
Bumble Bee					
Chunk Light In Oil	2 oz	160	0	0	0
Chunk Light In Water	2 oz	60	0	0	0
Chunk White In Oil	2 oz	160	0	0	0
Chunk White In Water	2 oz	70	0	0	0
Chunk White In Water Diet	2 oz	60	0	0	0
Solid White In Oil	2 oz	130	0	0	0
Solid White In Water	2 oz	70	0	0	0
Empress					
Chunk Light	2 oz	60	0	0	0
Chunk Light Tongol	2 oz	50	0	0	0
Solid White	2 oz	70	0	0	0
Progresso					
In Olive Oil	¼ cup (2 oz)	160	0	0	0
S&W					
Chunk Light Fancy In Oil	2 oz	140	0	0	0
Chunk Light Fancy In Water	2 oz	60	0	0	0
Fancy White Albacore in Oil	2 oz	160	0	0	0

FOOD	PORTION	CALS.	CARB.	SUG.	FIB.
Tree Of Life					
Tongol In Spring Water	2 oz	60	0	0	0
Tongol In Spring Water No Salt Water	2 oz	70	0	0	0
FRESH					
bluefin cooked	3 oz	157	0	0	0
bluefin raw	3 oz	122	0	0	0
skipjack baked	3 oz	112	0	0	0
yellowfin baked	3 oz	118	0	0	0

TUNA DISHES
FROZEN

FOOD	PORTION	CALS.	CARB.	SUG.	FIB.
Mrs. Paul's					
Microwave Tuna Sandwich	1	200	23	—	—
MIX					
Bumble Bee					
Tuna Mix-ins Classic Italian	⅓ pkg (0.17 oz)	25	5	—	—
Tuna Mix-ins Garden & Herb	⅓ pkg (0.17 oz)	25	5	—	—
Tuna Mix-ins Lemon Herb	⅓ pkg (0.17 oz)	25	6	—	—
Tuna Mix-ins Zesty Tomato	⅓ pkg (0.17 oz)	25	5	—	—
Tuna Helper					
AuGratin 50% Less Fat Recipe as prep	1 cup	250	36	5	1
AuGratin as prep	1 cup	310	36	5	1
Cheesy Pasta 50% Less Fat Recipe as prep	1 cup	230	32	5	tr
Cheesy Pasta as prep	1 cup	280	32	5	tr
Creamy Broccoli 50% Less Fat Recipe as prep	1 cup	240	35	6	1
Creamy Broccoli as prep	1 cup	280	35	6	1
Creamy Pasta 50% Less Fat Recipe as prep	1 cup	230	31	4	1
Creamy Pasta as prep	1 cup	300	31	4	1
Fettuccine Alfredo 50% Less Fat Recipe as prep	1 cup	240	32	6	1
Fettuccine Alfredo as prep	1 cup	310	32	6	1
Garden Cheddar 50% Less Fat Recipe as prep	1 cup	250	35	5	1
Garden Cheddar as prep	1 cup	310	35	5	1
Pasta Salad Low Fat Recipe as prep	⅔ cup	230	26	4	1
Pasta Salad as prep	⅔ cup	380	26	4	1
Tetrazzini 50% Less Fat Recipe as prep	1 cup	240	33	3	1

FOOD	PORTION	CALS.	CARB.	SUG.	FIB.
Tuna Helper (CONT.)					
Tetrazzini as prep	1 cup	310	33	3	1
Tuna Melt Reduced Fat Recipe as prep	1 cup	240	34	6	0
Tuna Melt as prep	1 cup	300	34	6	0
Tuna Pot Pie as prep	1 cup	440	40	9	1
Tuna Romanoff 50% Less Fat Recipe as prep	1 cup	240	38	3	1
Tuna Romanoff as prep	1 cup	280	38	3	1

TURBOT

FOOD	PORTION	CALS.	CARB.	SUG.	FIB.
european baked	3 oz	104	0	0	0

TURKEY

(*see also* DINNER, HOT DOG, TURKEY DISHES, TURKEY SUBSTITUTES)

FOOD	PORTION	CALS.	CARB.	SUG.	FIB.
CANNED					
w/ broth	1 can (5 oz)	231	0	0	0
w/ broth	½ can (2.5 oz)	116	0	0	0
Armour					
Turkey Loaf	2 oz	110	1	—	—
Hormel					
Chunk Turkey Ham	2 oz	70	0	0	0
Swanson					
White	2½ oz	80	1	—	—
Underwood					
Chunky Light	2.08 oz	75	2	—	—
FRESH					
back w/ skin roasted	½ back (9 oz)	637	0	0	0
breast w/ skin roasted	4 oz	212	0	0	0
dark meat w/ skin roasted	3.6 oz	230	0	0	0
dark meat w/o skin roasted	1 cup (5 oz)	262	0	0	0
dark meat w/o skin roasted	3 oz	170	0	0	0
ground cooked	3 oz	188	0	0	0
leg w/ skin roasted	1 (1.2 lbs)	1133	0	0	0
leg w/ skin roasted	2.5 oz	147	0	0	0
light meat w/ skin roasted	4.7 oz	268	0	0	0
light meat w/ skin roasted	from ½ turkey (2.3 lbs)	2069	0	0	0
light meat w/o skin roasted	4 oz	183	0	0	0
neck simmered	1 (5.3 oz)	274	0	0	0
skin roasted	from ½ turkey (9 oz)	1096	0	0	0
skin roasted	1 oz	141	0	0	0
w/ skin roasted	½ turkey (4 lbs)	3857	0	0	0
w/ skin roasted	8.4 oz	498	0	0	0

FOOD	PORTION	CALS.	CARB.	SUG.	FIB.
w/ skin neck & giblets roasted	½ turkey (8.8 lbs)	4123	1	—	—
w/o skin roasted	1 cup (5 oz)	238	0	0	0
w/o skin roasted	7.3 oz	354	0	0	0
wing w/ skin roasted	1 (6.5 oz)	426	0	0	0
Butterball					
Ground All White Meat	3 oz	100	tr	—	—
Louis Rich					
Ground	4 oz	190	0	0	0
Patties White	1 (4 oz)	170	0	0	0
Mr. Turkey					
Ground 85% Fat Free	3.5 oz	210	0	0	0
Ground 91% Fat Free	3.5 oz	170	1	—	—
Perdue					
Breast Tenderloins Cooked	3 oz	110	0	0	0
Breast Boneless Cooked	3 oz	110	0	0	0
Breast Cutlets Thin Sliced Cooked	1 (2.5 oz)	90	0	0	0
Breast Fillets Cooked	3 oz	110	0	0	0
Burger Cooked	1 (3 oz)	170	0	0	0
Cubed Steak Cooked	3 oz	120	0	0	0
Dark Cooked	3 oz	200	0	0	0
Drumsticks Roasted	3 oz	150	0	0	0
Drumsticks Cooked	3 oz	150	0	0	0
Ground Cooked	3 oz	170	0	0	0
Ground Breast Cooked	3 oz	110	0	0	0
Half Breast Cooked	3 oz	170	0	0	0
Thighs Cooked	3 oz	180	0	0	0
Tom Wings Cooked	3 oz	160	0	0	0
White Cooked	3 oz	170	0	0	0
Whole Breast Cooked	3 oz	170	0	0	0
Wings Roasted	1 (3 oz)	180	0	0	0
Wings Drummettes Roasted	1 (3.5 oz)	180	0	0	0
Swift-Eckrich					
Ground All White	3 oz	100	tr	—	—
The Turkey Store					
Seasoned Cuts Turkey Breast Roast	4 oz	110	4	—	—
Wampler Longacre					
Ground raw	1 oz	60	0	0	0
FROZEN					
roast boneless seasoned light & dark meat roasted	1 pkg (1.7 lbs)	1213	24	—	—

FOOD	PORTION	CALS.	CARB.	SUG.	FIB.
Empire					
Patties	1 (3.1 oz)	200	14	1	1
READY-TO-EAT					
bologna	1 oz	57	tr	—	—
breast	1 slice (0.75 oz)	23	0	0	0
diced light & dark seasoned	½ lb	313	2	—	—
diced light & dark seasoned	1 oz	39	tr	—	—
ham thigh meat	2 oz	73	tr	—	—
ham thigh meat	1 pkg (8 oz)	291	1	—	—
pastrami	2 oz	80	1	—	—
pastrami	1 pkg (8 oz)	320	4	—	—
patties battered & fried	1 (3.3 oz)	266	15	—	—
patties battered & fried	1 (2.3 oz)	181	10	—	—
patties breaded & fried	1 (3.3 oz)	266	15	—	—
patties breaded & fried	1 (2.3 oz)	181	10	—	—
poultry salad sandwich spread	1 tbsp	109	1	—	—
poultry salad sandwich spread	1 oz	238	2	—	—
prebasted breast w/ skin roasted	1 breast (3.8 lbs)	2175	0	0	0
prebasted breast w/ skin roasted	½ breast (1.9 lbs)	1087	0	0	0
prebasted thigh w/ skin roasted	1 thigh (11 oz)	494	0	0	0
roll light & dark meat	1 oz	42	1	—	—
roll light meat	1 oz	42	2	—	—
salami cooked	2 oz	111	tr	—	—
salami cooked	1 pkg (8 oz)	446	1	—	—
turkey loaf breast meat	1 pkg (6 oz)	187	0	0	0
turkey loaf breast meat	2 slices (1.5 oz)	47	0	0	0
turkey sticks battered & fried	1 stick (2.3 oz)	178	11	—	—
turkey sticks breaded & fried	1 stick (2.3 oz)	178	11	—	—
Alpine Lace					
Breast Fat Free	2 oz	50	0	0	0
Carl Buddig					
Honey Turkey	1 oz	40	1	—	—
Turkey	1 oz	50	1	—	0
Turkey Ham	1 oz	40	1	—	0
Empire					
Barbecue Whole	5 oz	250	0	tr	0
Bologna	3 slices (1.8 oz)	90	3	0	0
Oven Prepared Breast Slices	3 slices (1.8 oz)	50	1	0	0

FOOD	PORTION	CALS.	CARB.	SUG.	FIB.
Empire (cont.)					
Pastrami	3 slices (1.8 oz)	60	0	1	1
Salami	3 slices (1.8 oz)	70	1	0	0
Smoked Breast Slices	3 slices (1.8 oz)	40	0	1	0
Hansel n'Gretel					
Breast Gourmet	1 oz	28	1	—	—
Breast Gourmet Smoked	1 oz	31	tr	—	—
Breast Honey	1 oz	28	1	—	—
Breast Lessalt Cooked	1 oz	25	tr	—	—
Breast Oven Cooked	1 oz	26	tr	—	—
Doubledecker Turkey Corned Beef	1 oz	30	1	—	—
Doubledecker Turkey Ham	1 oz	30	1	—	—
Healthy Choice					
Deli-Thin Honey Roast & Smoked	6 slices (2 oz)	70	2	2	0
Deli-Thin Roasted Breast	6 slices (2 oz)	60	1	0	0
Deli-Thin Smoked Breast	6 slices (2 oz)	60	1	0	0
Deli-Thin Turkey Ham	6 slices (2 oz)	60	1	1	0
Fresh-Trak Honey Roast & Smoked Breast	1 slice (1 oz)	35	1	1	0
Fresh-Trak Oven Roasted Breast	1 slice (1 oz)	35	1	0	0
Honey Roasted & Smoked	1 slice (1 oz)	35	1	0	0
Oven Roasted Breast	1 slice (1 oz)	35	1	0	0
Smoked Breast	1 slice (1 oz)	30	0	0	0
Variety Pack Regular	3 slices (2.2 oz)	70	2	1	0
Hillshire					
Deli Select Honey Roasted Breast	1 slice	10	tr	—	—
Deli Select Oven Roasted Breast	1 slice	10	tr	—	—
Deli Select Smoked Breast	1 slice	10	tr	—	—
Deli Select Turkey Ham	1 slice	10	tr	—	—
Flavor Pack 90-99% Fat Free Honey Roasted Breast	1 slice (0.75 oz)	20	1	—	—
Flavor Pack 90-99% Fat Free Smoked Breast	1 slice (0.75 oz)	20	tr	—	—
Honey Cured Breast	1 oz	35	2	—	—
Lunch 'N Munch Smoked Turkey/ Cheddar	1 pkg (4.5 oz)	350	20	—	—
Lunch 'N Munch Smoked Turkey/ Cheddar/ Brownie	1 pkg (4.5 oz)	400	34	—	—

FOOD	PORTION	CALS.	CARB.	SUG.	FIB.
Hillshire (CONT.)					
Lunch 'N Munch Turkey/ Cheddar/ Brownie/Hi-C	1 pkg (4.5 oz + 6 fl oz)	500	58	—	—
Smoked Breast	1 oz	35	1	—	—
Hormel					
Light & Lean 97 Breast Sliced	1 slice (1 oz)	30	0	0	0
Light & Lean 97 Mesquite Smoked Breast	1 slice (1 oz)	30	0	0	0
turkey pepperoni	17 slices (1 oz)	80	0	0	0
Jordan's					
Healthy Trim Fat Free Oven Roasted Breast	1 slice (1 oz)	20	0	0	0
Healthy Trim Fat Free Oven Roasted Smoked Breast	1 slice (1 oz)	20	0	0	0
Louis Rich					
Bologna	1 slice (28 g)	50	1	0	0
Breaded Nuggets	4 (3.2 oz)	260	15	0	0
Breaded Patties	1 (3 oz)	220	13	0	0
Breaded Sticks	3 (3 oz)	230	12	0	0
Breast Skinless Hickory Smoked	2 oz	50	1	0	0
Breast Skinless Honey Roasted	2 oz	60	3	2	0
Breast Skinless Oven Roasted	2 oz	50	1	0	0
Breast Skinless Rotisserie	2 oz	50	1	1	0
Breast Slices Hickory Smoked	1 slice (2 oz)	50	1	0	0
Breast Slices Honey Roasted	1 slice (2 oz)	60	3	2	0
Breast Slices Oven Roasted	1 slice (2 oz)	50	1	0	0
Breast Slices Rotisserie	1 slice (2 oz)	50	1	1	0
Carving Board Hickory Smoked	2 slices (1.6 oz)	40	0	0	0
Carving Board Oven Roasted Thin	6 slices (2.1 oz)	60	1	0	0
Carving Board Oven Roasted Traditional	2 slices (1.6 oz)	40	0	0	0
Carving Board Rotisserie	2 slices (1.6 oz)	40	0	0	0
Cotto Salami	1 slice (28 g)	40	0	0	0
Deli-Thin Oven Roasted	4 slices (1.8 oz)	50	2	0	0

FOOD	PORTION	CALS.	CARB.	SUG.	FIB.
Louis Rich (CONT.)					
Deli-Thin Smoked	4 slices (1.8 oz)	50	1	tr	0
Fat Free Hickory Smoked Breast	1 slice (1 oz)	25	1	0	0
Fat Free Oven Roasted Breast	1 slice (1 oz)	25	1	tr	0
Fat Free Oven Roasted Deli-Thin Breast	4 slices (1.8 oz)	45	2	tr	0
Fat Free Turkey Ham Honey	2 slices (1.7 oz)	35	2	1	0
Fat Free Turkey Ham Smoked	2 slices (1.7 oz)	35	1	tr	0
Hickory Smoked	1 slice (1 oz)	30	1	0	0
Oven Roasted	1 slice (1 oz)	30	1	0	0
Pastrami	1 slice (1 oz)	30	1	0	0
Salami	1 slice (28 g)	40	0	0	0
Smoked	1 slice (1 oz)	30	0	0	0
Turkey Ham	1 slice (1 oz)	30	1	0	0
Turkey Ham Chopped	1 slice (1 oz)	45	1	0	0
Turkey Ham Honey Cured	1 slice (1 oz)	30	1	tr	0
Mr. Turkey					
Deli Cuts Hardwood Smoked Breast	3 slices	30	1	—	—
Deli Cuts Honey Roasted Breast	3 slices	30	2	—	—
Deli Cuts Oven Roasted Breast	3 slices	30	2	—	—
Deli Cuts Turkey Ham	3 slices	35	1	—	—
Deli Cuts Turkey Pastrami	3 slices	35	1	—	—
Hardwood Smoked Breast	1 slice	30	2	—	—
Hardwood Smoked Turkey Ham	1 slice	35	0	0	0
Honey Cured Turkey Ham	1 slice	30	1	—	—
Oven Roasted Breast	1 slice	30	2	—	—
Smoked Breakfast Turkey Ham	1 oz	30	1	—	—
Turkey Bologna	1 slice	70	1	—	—
Turkey Cotto Salami	1 slice	50	1	—	—
Turkey Ham	1 slice	35	0	0	0
Turkey Pastrami	1 slice	30	1	—	—
Oscar Mayer					
Free Oven Roasted Breast	4 slices (1.8 oz)	40	2	tr	0
Free Smoked Breast	4 slices (1.8 oz)	40	2	tr	0
Lunchables Fun Pack Turkey/Pacific Cooler	1 pkg (11.2 oz)	460	53	39	tr

FOOD	PORTION	CALS.	CARB.	SUG.	FIB.
Oscar Mayer (CONT.)					
Lunchables Fun Pack Turkey/Surger Cooler	1 pkg (11.2 oz)	440	60	45	0
Lunchables Turkey/ Cheddar	1 pkg (4.5 oz)	360	20	5	1
Oven Roasted White	1 slice (1 oz)	30	1	tr	0
Smoked White	1 slice (1 oz)	30	1	0	0
Perdue					
Nuggets Dinosaur	3 (3 oz)	200	15	2	2
Sara Lee					
Hardwood Smoked Breast Of Turkey	2 oz	60	0	0	0
Hardwood Smoked Turkey Ham	2 oz	60	1	1	—
Honey Roasted Breast Of Turkey	2 oz	60	2	1	—
Honey Roasted Turkey Ham	2 oz	70	2	2	—
Mesquite Smoked Breast Of Turkey	2 oz	60	0	0	0
Oven Roasted Breast Of Turkey	2 oz	60	0	0	0
Peppered Breast Of Turkey	2 oz	50	2	—	—
Seasoned Breast Of Turkey Pastrami	2 oz	60	2	1	—
Shady Brook					
Meatballs Italian Style	3 oz	130	350	—	—
Tyson					
Breast	1 slice	20	tr	—	—
Ham	1 slice	23	1	—	—
Wampler Longacre					
Bologna	1 oz	60	tr	—	—
Breast Chops	1 serv (4 oz)	120	0	0	0
Breast Sliced	1 slice (1 oz)	35	1	—	—
Breast Sliced Smoked	1 slice (0.75 oz)	20	1	—	—
Burger	1 (3 oz)	170	0	0	0
Burger	1 (4 oz)	230	0	0	0
Burger Barbecue	1 (4 oz)	240	4	—	—
Chef Select Breast Skinless	1 oz	35	tr	—	—
Chef Select Breast Smoked	1 oz	35	1	—	—
Chunk Dark Smoked Cured	1 oz	45	1	—	—
Chunk Ham 12% Water Smoked	1 oz	45	tr	—	—
Chunk Ham 20% Water	1 oz	40	2	—	—

FOOD	PORTION	CALS.	CARB.	SUG.	FIB.
Wampler Longacre (CONT.)					
Chunk Pastrami	1 oz	35	tr	—	—
Cook-In-The-Bag Breast	1 oz	30	1	—	—
Cook-In-The-Bag Breast Mini	1 oz	30	tr	—	—
Cook-In-The-Bag Combo Roast	1 oz	35	tr	—	—
Cook-In-The-Bag Thigh Roast	1 oz	40	1	—	—
Dark Smoked Cured	1 oz	45	1	—	—
Deli Chef Breast And White Meat No Skin	1 oz	40	1	—	—
Gourmet Breast	1 oz	35	1	—	—
Gourmet Breast Mini	1 oz	35	1	—	—
Gourmet Breast Mini Smoked	1 oz	35	1	—	—
Gourmet Breast Smoked	1 oz	30	1	—	—
Gourmet Brown & Glazed Breast	1 oz	35	1	—	—
Gourmet Brown & Roasted Breast	1 oz	35	1	—	—
Gourmet Honey Cured Breast	1 oz	30	1	—	—
Lean-Lite Breast Skinless	1 oz	35	0	0	0
Lean-Lite Deli Breast	1 oz	35	0	0	0
Lean-Lite Deli Breast Smoked	1 oz	35	1	—	—
Old Fashioned Brown & Roasted Breast	1 oz	35	tr	—	—
Pastrami	1 oz	35	tr	—	—
Premium Breast Skinless	1 oz	30	1	—	—
Premium Brown & Roasted Breast Skinless	1 oz	16	1	—	—
Roll Combo	1 oz	44	tr	—	—
Roll Sliced Breast	1 slice (0.75 oz)	30	1	—	—
Roll White	1 oz	45	tr	—	—
Salami	1 oz	50	1	—	—
Salt Watchers Breast Skinless	1 oz	35	0	0	0
Seasoned Roast	1 oz	40	0	0	0
Sliced Salami	1 slice (0.8 oz)	45	1	—	—
Tenderlings BBQ	1 serv (4 oz)	110	0	0	0

FOOD	PORTION	CALS.	CARB.	SUG.	FIB.
Wampler Longacre (CONT.)					
Tenderlings Cajun	1 serv (4 oz)	110	0	0	0
Tenderlings Garlic & Pepper	1 serv (4 oz)	110	0	0	0
Tenderlings Original	1 serv (4 oz)	110	0	0	0
Turkey Ham 12% Water Baked	1 oz	45	tr	—	—
Turkey Ham 20% Water Baked	1 oz	40	1	—	—
Unseasoned Roast	1 oz	40	0	0	0
Whole Browned & Roasted	1 oz	60	tr	—	—
Weight Watchers					
Deli Thin Smoked Breast	5 slices (⅓ oz)	10	tr	—	—
Oven Roasted Breast	2 slices (¾ oz)	25	tr	—	—
Oven Roasted Turkey Ham	2 slices (¾ oz)	25	tr	—	—
Roasted & Smoked Breast	2 slices (¾ oz)	25	tr	—	—

TURKEY DISHES
(*see also* DINNER, TURKEY SUBSTITUTES)

CANNED

FOOD	PORTION	CALS.	CARB.	SUG.	FIB.
Dinty Moore					
Stew	1 cup (8.5 oz)	140	19	3	2
FROZEN					
gravy & turkey	1 cup (8.4 oz)	160	11	—	—
gravy & turkey	1 pkg (5 oz)	95	7	—	—
Hot Pocket					
Stuffed Sandwich Turkey & Ham With Cheese	1 (4.5 oz)	320	38	7	1
Lean Pockets					
Stuffed Sandwich Turkey & Ham With Cheddar	1 (4.5 oz)	260	35	6	4
Stuffed Sandwich Turkey Broccoli & Cheese	1 (4.5 oz)	260	35	7	4
Luigino's					
Gravy Dressing & Turkey	1 pkg (8 oz)	340	36	0	2
Ovenstuffs					
Turkey Turnover	1 (4.75 oz)	350	35	—	—
READY-TO-EAT					
Wampler Longacre					
Meatloaf Italian	1 serv (4 oz)	114	5	—	—
Meatloaf Mexican	1 serv (4 oz)	114	4	—	—
Meatloaf Original	1 serv (4 oz)	126	10	—	—
Salad	1 oz	60	3	—	—
Salad Turkey Ham	1 oz	50	3	—	—

FOOD	PORTION	CALS.	CARB.	SUG.	FIB.
Wampler Longacre (CONT.)					
Teriyaki	1 serv (4 oz)	112	14	—	—
SHELF-STABLE					
Dinty Moore					
Microwave Cup Stew	1 pkg (7.5 oz)	130	16	3	2
TURKEY SUBSTITUTES					
Harvest Direct					
TVP Poultry Chunks	3.5 oz	280	32	—	18
TVP Poultry Ground	3.5 oz	280	32	—	18
Soy Is Us					
Turkey Not!	½ cup (1.75 oz)	140	15	4	9
White Wave					
Meatless Sandwich Slices	2 slices (1.6 oz)	80	7	0	1
Worthington					
Smoked Turkey Meatless	3 slices (2 oz)	140	3	tr	2
Turkee Slices	3 slices (3.3 oz)	130	3	tr	2
TURNIPS					
CANNED					
greens	½ cup	17	3	—	—
Allen					
Chopped Greens And Diced Turnip	½ cup (4.2 oz)	30	5	1	tr
Greens	½ cup (4.2 oz)	25	3	tr	2
Sunshine					
Chopped Greens And Diced Turnip	½ cup (4.2 oz)	30	5	1	tr
Greens	½ cup (4.2 oz)	25	3	tr	2
FRESH					
cooked mashed	½ cup (4.2 oz)	47	10	—	—
cubed cooked	½ cup (3 oz)	33	7	—	—
greens chopped cooked	½ cup	15	3	—	2
greens raw chopped	½ cup	7	2	—	1
raw cubed	½ cup (2.4 oz)	25	6	—	—
FROZEN					
greens cooked	½ cup	24	4	—	2
Birds Eye					
Chopped Greens	1 cup (3.1 oz)	30	1	2	1
Greens w/ Diced Root	1 cup (3 oz)	25	2	1	2
TURTLE					
raw	3½ oz	85	0	0	0
TUSK FISH					
raw	3½ oz	79	0	0	0

FOOD	PORTION	CALS.	CARB.	SUG.	FIB.
VANILLA					
Hershey					
Vanilla Milk Chips	¼ cup	240	25	—	—
VEAL					
(*see also* DINNER, VEAL DISHES)					
cutlet lean only braised	3 oz	172	0	0	0
cutlet lean only fried	3 oz	156	0	0	0
ground broiled	3 oz	146	0	0	0
loin chop w/ bone lean & fat braised	1 chop (2.8 oz)	227	0	0	0
loin chop w/ bone lean only braised	1 chop (2.4 oz)	155	0	0	0
shoulder w/ bone lean only braised	3 oz	169	0	0	0
sirloin w/ bone lean & fat roasted	3 oz	171	0	0	0
sirloin w/ bone lean only roasted	3 oz	143	0	0	0
VEGETABLE JUICE					
vegetable juice cocktail	6 fl oz	34	8	—	—
vegetable juice cocktail	½ cup	22	6	—	—
Mott's					
Vegetable Juice as prep	8 fl oz	60	13	7	2
Muir Glen					
Organic	8 oz	70	15	11	3
Organic Reduced Sodium	8 oz	70	15	11	3
Odwalla					
Vegetable Cocktail	8 fl oz	70	18	14	2
Smucker's					
Vegetable Juice Hearty	8 fl oz	58	13	—	—
Vegetable Juice Hot & Spicy	8 fl oz	58	13	—	—
V8					
No Salt Added	6 fl oz	35	8	—	—
Original	6 fl oz	35	8	—	—
Spicy Hot	6 fl oz	35	8	—	—
Splash Tropical Blend	8 fl oz	120	30	27	—
VEGETABLES MIXED					
(*see also* VEGETABLE JUICE)					
CANNED					
mixed vegetables	½ cup	39	8	—	—
peas & carrots	½ cup	48	11	—	—

FOOD	PORTION	CALS.	CARB.	SUG.	FIB.
peas & carrots low sodium	½ cup	48	11	—	—
peas & onions	½ cup	30	5	—	—
succotash	½ cup	102	23	—	—
Allen					
Green Beans And Potatoes	½ cup (4.2 oz)	35	7	2	2
Okra & Tomatoes	½ cup (4 oz)	25	5	1	3
Okra Tomatoes & Corn	½ cup (4.1 oz)	30	6	1	4
Chi-Chi's					
Diced Tomatoes & Green Chilies	¼ cup (2.5 oz)	20	4	3	0
Del Monte					
Mixed	½ cup (4.4 oz)	40	8	3	2
Peas And Carrots	½ cup (4.5 oz)	60	11	4	2
Green Giant					
Garden Medley	½ cup (4.2 oz)	40	9	3	2
Mixed	½ cup (4.3 oz)	60	12	4	2
Sweet Peas & Carrots	½ cup (4.3 oz)	50	11	4	3
Sweet Peas & Tiny Pearl Onions	½ cup (4.4 oz)	60	11	3	4
House Of Tsang					
Vegetables & Sauce Cantonese Classic	½ cup (4.2 oz)	70	14	8	1
Vegetables & Sauce Hong Kong Sweet & Sour	½ cup (4.5 oz)	160	40	35	0
Vegetables & Sauce Szechuan Hot & Spicy	½ cup (4.2 oz)	70	14	8	1
Vegetables & Sauce Tokyo Teriyaki	½ cup (4.4 oz)	100	23	19	1
Ka-Me					
Stir Fry	½ cup (4.5 oz)	20	4	2	2
La Choy					
Chop Suey Vegetables	½ cup	10	2	—	tr
LeSueur					
Early Peas w/ Mushrooms & Pearl Onions	½ cup (4.3 oz)	60	11	4	2
S&W					
Garden Salad Marinated	½ cup	60	11	—	—
Mixed Vegetables Old Fashion Harvest Time	½ cup	35	6	—	—
Peas & Carrots Water Pack	½ cup	35	7	—	—
Succotash Country Style	½ cup	80	16	—	—
Sweet Peas & Diced Carrots	½ cup	50	9	—	—

FOOD	PORTION	CALS.	CARB.	SUG.	FIB.
S&W (CONT.)					
Sweet Peas w/ Tiny Pearl Onions	½ cup	60	10	—	—
Seneca					
Peas & Carrots	½ cup	60	9	—	4
Succotash	½ cup	90	18	—	2
Sunshine					
Green Beans And Potatoes	½ cup (4.2 oz)	35	7	2	2
Trappey					
Okra & Tomatoes	½ cup (4 oz)	25	5	1	3
Okra Tomatoes & Corn	½ cup (4.1 oz)	30	6	1	4
FROZEN					
mixed vegetables cooked	½ cup	54	12	—	2
peas & carrots cooked	½ cup	38	8	—	—
peas & onions cooked	½ cup	40	8	—	—
succotash cooked	½ cup	79	17	—	—
Amy's Organic					
Pocket Sandwich Mediterranean Vegetables	1 (4.5 oz)	220	33	5	3
Pocket Sandwich Roasted Vegetables	1 (4.5 oz)	220	35	5	4
Pocket Sandwich Vegetable Pie	1 (5 oz)	230	37	2	2
Big Valley					
California Blend	¾ cup (3 oz)	25	6	6	3
Italian Blend	¾ cup (3 oz)	30	5	3	2
Oriental Blend	¾ cup (3 oz)	25	5	2	3
Stew Vegetables	⅔ cup (3 oz)	40	10	3	2
Winter Blend	¾ cup (3 oz)	25	4	1	2
Birds Eye					
Baby Bean & Carrot Blend	1 cup (2.9 oz)	30	5	3	2
Broccoli Cauliflower Carrots w/ Cheese	½ cup (3.9 oz)	70	7	3	2
Brussels Sprouts Cauliflower Carrots	½ cup (3.1 oz)	30	7	3	3
Chicken Viola Garlic	2 cups (6.2 oz)	260	27	6	1
Chicken Viola Pesto	2¼ cups (6.6 oz)	250	25	5	1
Chicken Viola Three Cheese	1¾ cups (6.2 oz)	240	26	7	9
Chicken Voila Teriyaki	2⅓ cups (6.1 oz)	230	26	7	2
Farm Fresh Broccoli Carrots Water Chestnuts	½ cup (3.3 oz)	30	7	3	3
Farm Fresh Broccoli Cauliflower	½ cup (3.2 oz)	20	4	2	2

FOOD	PORTION	CALS.	CARB.	SUG.	FIB.
Birds Eye (CONT.)					
Farm Fresh Broccoli Cauliflower Carrots	½ cup (3.2 oz)	25	5	3	2
Farm Fresh Broccoli Cauliflower Red Peppers	½ cup (3.3 oz)	20	5	3	2
Farm Fresh Broccoli Corn Red Peppers	½ cup (3.6 oz)	50	12	3	3
Farm Fresh Broccoli Red Peppers Onions Mushrooms	½ cup (3.5 oz)	25	5	3	2
Farm Fresh Brussels Sprouts Cauliflower Carrots	½ cup (3.1 oz)	30	7	3	3
Farm Fresh Cauliflower Carrots Snow Peas Pods	½ cup (3.2 oz)	30	6	3	2
For Soup	⅔ cup (3 oz)	45	9	3	2
For Stew	¾ cup (2.9 oz)	40	9	2	1
Gumbo Blend	¾ cup (3 oz)	40	10	3	2
International Bavarian Style	1 cup (5.5 oz)	150	15	3	3
International California Style	½ cup (3 oz)	100	9	4	3
International French Country Style	⅔ cup (4.4 oz)	110	10	2	2
International Italian Style	1 cup (5.8 oz)	150	12	3	3
International New England Style	1 pkg (9 oz)	260	29	6	3
International Oriental Style	½ cup (3 oz)	60	4	3	2
International Stir Fry Style	½ cup 3.6 oz)	60	5	4	1
Peas & Carrots	⅔ cup (3 oz)	50	9	4	3
Peas & Pearl Onions	⅔ cup (4.2 oz)	90	18	9	5
Peas & Potatoes In Cream Sauce	½ cup (4.4 oz)	90	13	5	2
Seasoning Blend	¾ cup (2.9 oz)	20	5	4	1
Stir Fry Asparagus	2 cups (5.8 oz)	90	16	4	3
Stir Fry Broccoli	1 cup (3.3 oz)	30	5	3	2
Stir Fry Pepper	1 cup (2.9 oz)	25	5	4	2
Stir Fry Sugar Snap	¾ cup (2.6 oz)	35	5	3	1
Stir Fry Whole Green Bean	1¾ cup (5.3 oz)	100	19	4	2
Budget Gourmet					
Mandarin Vegetables	1 pkg (5.25 oz)	160	13	—	—
New England Recipe Vegetables	1 pkg (5.5 oz)	230	21	—	—
Spring Vegetables In Cheese Sauce	1 pkg (5 oz)	130	9	—	—

FOOD	PORTION	CALS.	CARB.	SUG.	FIB.
Fresh Like					
California Blend	3.5 oz	31	7	—	1
Chuckwagon Blend	3.5 oz	71	17	—	1
Italian Blend	3.5 oz	33	7	—	1
Midwestern Blend	3.5 oz	42	9	—	1
Mixed	3.5 oz	69	14	—	1
Oriental Blend	3.5 oz	26	5	—	1
Peas & Carrots	3.5 oz	63	12	—	1
Winter Blend	3.5 oz	26	5	—	1
Green Giant					
American Mixtures Broccoli Carrots Cauliflower	¾ cup (2.6 oz)	25	5	2	2
American Mixtures Broccoli Carrots Waterchestnuts	¾ cup (3 oz)	30	6	2	3
American Mixtures Carrots Green Bean Cauliflower	¾ cup (2.7 oz)	25	5	2	2
American Mixtures Cauliflower Broccoli Sugar Snap & Sweet Pea	¾ cup (2.8 oz)	35	7	2	3
American Mixtures Corn Broccoli Red Pepper	¾ cup (3.1 oz)	60	13	3	2
American Mixtures Green Beans Potatoes Onions Red Peppers	¾ cup (2.8 oz)	45	8	2	2
American Mixtures Sweet Peas Potatoes Carrots	⅔ cup (3 oz)	70	12	2	3
Butter Sauce Broccoli Cauliflower Carrots Corn Sweet Peas	¾ cup (3.6 oz)	60	8	3	2
Butter Sauce Broccoli Pasta Sweet Peas Corn Red Peppers	¾ cup (3.5 oz)	70	11	3	2
Butter Sauce Mixed	¾ cup (3.6 oz)	70	11	3	3
Cheese Sauce Broccoli Cauliflower Carrots	⅔ cup (4.3 oz)	80	11	5	2
Harvest Fresh Broccoli Cauliflower Carrots	1 cup (3.4 oz)	30	5	2	3
Harvest Fresh Mixed Vegetables	⅔ cup (3.1 oz)	50	10	3	3
Harvest Fresh Sweet Peas & Pearl Onions	½ cup (2.7 oz)	55	10	2	3
Mixed	¾ cup (2.9 oz)	50	11	1	3
Select Sweet Peas & Pearl Onions	⅔ cup (3.1 oz)	60	12	2	4

FOOD	PORTION	CALS.	CARB.	SUG.	FIB.
La Choy					
Mixed Fancy	½ cup	12	2	—	1
Ore Ida					
Stew Vegetables	⅔ cup (3 oz)	50	11	1	tr
Soglowek					
Golden Vegetarian Nuggets	4 pieces (2.5 oz)	190	9	1	1
Tree Of Life					
Mixed	½ cup (3 oz)	65	13	3	3
Veg-All					
Country Wisconsin Blend	3.5 oz	52	13	—	1
Scandinavian Blend	3.5 oz	48	9	—	1
Vegetables For Soup (Eight)	3.5 oz	34	12	—	1
Vegetables For Soup (Potatoes)	3.5 oz	53	12	—	1
Vegetables For Stew 4-Way	3.5 oz	51	12	—	1
Vegetables For Stew 5-Way	3.5 oz	54	12	—	1
SHELF-STABLE					
Pantry Express					
Corn Green Beans Carrots Pasta In Tomato Sauce	½ cup	80	17	—	3
Green Beans Potatoes And Mushrooms In A Seasoned Sauce	½ cup	50	9	—	2
Mixed Vegetables	½ cup	35	8	—	1
VENISON					
roasted	3 oz	134	0	0	0
Broken Arrow Ranch					
Antelope Chili Meat	3.5 oz	115	1	—	—
Antelope Ground Venison	3.5 oz	110	tr	—	—
Antelope Stew Meat	3.5 oz	110	2	—	—
Nilgai Chili Meat	3.5 oz	115	1	—	—
Nilgai Leg	3.5 oz	100	1	—	—
Nilgai Stew Meat	3.5 oz	110	2	—	—
Venison & Beef Smoked Sausage	6 oz	432	4	—	—
Venison Meat Chunks	6 oz	175	0	0	0
Venison Salami	6 oz	252	0	0	0
VINEGAR					
balsamic	1 tbsp (0.5 oz)	5	2	2	—
cider	1 tbsp	tr	1	—	—
Hain					
Cider	1 tbsp	2	4	—	—

FOOD	PORTION	CALS.	CARB.	SUG.	FIB.
Ka-Me					
Chinese Seasoned	1 tbsp (0.5 fl oz)	5	1	0	0
Rice Wine Chinese	1 tbsp (0.5 fl oz)	5	1	0	0
Rice Wine Japanese	1 tbsp (0.5 oz)	0	1	0	0
Seasoned Rice Japanese	1 tbsp (0.5 fl oz)	10	3	2	0
Nakano					
Rice	1 tbsp	0	0	0	0
Regina					
Red Wine	1 oz	4	0	0	0
Tree Of Life					
Apple Cider Organic	1 tbsp (0.5 oz)	0	tr	—	—
Brown Rice	1 tbsp (0.5 oz)	2	0	0	0
Victoria					
Balsamic	1 tbsp (0.5 oz)	5	2	2	—
White House					
Apple Cider	2 tbsp	2	1	—	0
Red Wine	2 tbsp	4	2	—	—

WAFFLES
FROZEN

FOOD	PORTION	CALS.	CARB.	SUG.	FIB.
buttermilk	1 4 in sq (1.2 oz)	88	14	—	1
plain	1 4 in sq (1.2 oz)	88	14	—	1
Aunt Jemima					
Blueberry	2 (2.5 oz)	190	28	—	1
Buttermilk	2 (2.5 oz)	170	27	—	1
Cinnamon	2 (2.5 oz)	180	28	—	1
Oatmeal	2 (2.5 oz)	170	27	—	3
Whole Grain	2 (2.5 oz)	170	24	—	2
Belgian Chef					
Belgian	2 (2.5 oz)	140	24	5	1
Downyflake					
Blueberry	2	180	32	—	—
Buttermilk	2	190	32	—	—
Multi-Grain	2	250	28	—	4
Oat Bran	2	260	30	—	3
Regular	2	120	20	—	—
Regular Jumbo	2	170	30	—	—
Rice Bran	2	210	25	—	4
Roman Meal	2	280	33	—	3
Waffles	2	180	27	—	—
Eggo					
Apple Cinnamon	2 (2.7 oz)	220	33	5	1
Banana Bread	2 (2.7 oz)	200	32	5	2
Blueberry	2 (2.7 oz)	220	32	6	1

FOOD	PORTION	CALS.	CARB.	SUG.	FIB.
Eggo (CONT.)					
Buttermilk	2 (2.7 oz)	220	31	3	1
Golden Oat	2 (2.7 oz)	150	29	3	3
Homestyle	2 (2.7 oz)	220	32	3	1
Minis Cinnamon Toast	12 (3.2 oz)	290	45	17	2
Minis Cinnamon Toast	12 (3.2 oz)	280	40	18	0
Minis Homestyle	12 (3.3 oz)	260	38	3	2
Nut & Honey	2 (2.7 oz)	240	31	5	2
Nutri-Grain	2 (2.7 oz)	190	30	4	4
Nutri-Grain Multi-Bran	2 (2.7 oz)	180	32	4	6
Nutri-Grain Raisin & Bran	2 (2.9 oz)	210	36	10	5
Special K	2 (2 oz)	120	26	4	1
Strawberry	2 (2.7 oz)	220	32	5	1
Great Starts					
Belgian Waffles And Sausage	2.85 oz	280	21	—	—
Belgian Waffles Strawberries And Sausage	3.5 oz	210	31	—	—
Waffle With Bacon	2.2 oz	230	19	—	—
Kellogg's					
Homestyle Low Fat	2 (2.7 oz)	180	34	5	1
Nutri-Grain Low Fat	2 (2.7 oz)	160	31	4	3
Nutri-Grain Low Fat Blueberry	2 (2.7 oz)	160	33	7	3
Van's					
7 Grain Belgain	2	152	9	3	8
Belgian Original	2	145	30	4	2
Belgian Original Toaster	2	145	24	4	2
Blueberry Toaster	2	157	24	4	2
Blueberry Wheat Free Toaster	2	225	32	7	5
Fat Free	2	155	30	3	7
Mini	4	107	18	4	6
Multigrain Toaster	2	160	25	4	6
Organic Whole Wheat	2	190	30	4	6
Organic Whole Wheat Blueberry	2	190	30	4	6
Wheat Free Cinnamon Apple Toaster	2	220	32	5	5
Wheat Free Toaster	2	220	32	4	5
HOME RECIPE					
plain	1 (7 in diam)	218	25	—	—

FOOD	PORTION	CALS.	CARB.	SUG.	FIB.
MIX					
plain as prep	1 7 in diam (2.6 oz)	218	26	—	1
WALNUTS					
black dried	1 oz	172	3	—	1
black dried chopped	1 cup	759	15	—	—
english dried	1 oz	182	5	—	1
english dried chopped	1 cup	770	22	—	6
Planters					
Black	1 pkg (2 oz)	340	8	2	3
Gold Measure Halves	1 pkg (2 oz)	380	8	3	2
Halves	⅓ cup (1.2 oz)	220	5	tr	1
Pieces	¼ cup (1 oz)	190	4	tr	1
WASABI					
root raw	1 (5.9 oz)	184	40	—	12
root raw sliced	1 cup (4.6 oz)	142	31	—	10
WATER					
(*see* MINERAL/BOTTLED WATER)					
Canada Dry					
Sparkling Water	8 fl oz	0	0	0	0
Crystal Geyser					
Sparkling Lemon	1 bottle (12 fl oz)	0	0	0	0
Sparkling Mineral	1 bottle (12 fl oz)	0	0	0	0
Sparkling Natural Cola Berry	1 bottle (12 fl oz)	0	0	0	0
Sparkling Natural Wild Cherry	1 bottle 12 fl oz	0	0	0	0
Sparkling Orange	1 bottle (12 fl oz)	0	0	0	0
Evian					
Water	1 liter	0	0	0	0
Glacier Springs					
Drinking Water	8 fl oz	0	0	0	0
LaCroix					
Spring	1 bottle (12 oz)	0	0	0	0
Mt Shasta					
Natural Spring	1 bottle (20 oz)	0	0	0	0
San Pellegrino					
Acqua Panna	8 fl oz	0	0	0	0
Mineral Water	1 liter (33.8 oz)	0	0	0	0
Saratoga					
Sparkling	1 liter	0	0	0	0
Snapple					
Natural Spring	8 fl oz	0	0	0	0

FOOD	PORTION	CALS.	CARB.	SUG.	FIB.
Water Joe					
Caffeine Enhanced	8 fl oz	0	0	0	0
WATER CHESTNUTS					
CANNED					
chinese sliced	½ cup	35	9	—	—
Empress					
Sliced	2 oz	14	3	—	—
Whole	2 oz	14	3	—	—
Ka-Me					
Whole In Water	½ cup (4.5 oz)	45	11	2	4
La Choy					
Sliced	¼ cup	18	4	—	tr
Whole	4	14	4	—	tr
FRESH					
sliced	½ cup	66	15	—	—
WATERCRESS					
(*see also* CRESS)					
raw chopped	½ cup	2	tr	—	tr
WATERMELON					
FRESH					
cut up	1 cup	50	11	—	1
wedge	1/16	152	35	—	2
SEEDS					
dried	1 oz	158	4	—	—
dried	1 cup	602	17	—	—
WATERMELON JUICE					
Kool-Aid					
Splash Drink	1 serv (8 oz)	110	30	30	0
WAX BEANS					
CANNED					
Del Monte					
Cut Golden	½ cup (4.3 oz)	20	4	2	2
S&W					
Golden Cut Premium	½ cup	20	5	—	—
Seneca					
Cuts Natural Pack	½ cup	25	6	—	2
Wax Beans	½ cup	25	6	—	2
WHALE					
raw	3.5 oz	134	0	0	0
WHEAT					
(*see also* BULGUR, BRAN, CEREAL, COUSCOUS, FLOUR, WHEAT GERM)					
sprouted	1 cup (3.8 oz)	214	46	—	1

FOOD	PORTION	CALS.	CARB.	SUG.	FIB.
starch	3½ oz	348	86	—	—
Arrowhead					
Kamut Grain	¼ cup (1.7 oz)	140	32	0	5
Seitan Quick Mix	⅓ cup (1.4 oz)	150	14	0	2
Hodgson Mill					
Vital Wheat Gluten Plus Ascorbic Acid	1 tbsp (0.3 oz)	30	2	0	1
Near East					
Taboule Salad Mix as prep	⅔ cup	120	23	1	3
Wheat Pilaf as prep	1 cup	220	42	1	5
Sonoma					
Wheat Nuts Salted	2 tbsp (0.5 oz)	60	8	0	1
White Wave					
Seitan	½ pkg (4 oz)	140	4	0	1
Seitan Fajita Strips	⅓ cup (1.8 oz)	60	2	0	1
Seitan Marinated Slices	3 slices (1.8 oz)	60	2	0	1

WHEAT GERM

FOOD	PORTION	CALS.	CARB.	SUG.	FIB.
plain toasted	¼ cup (1 oz)	108	14	—	4
plain toasted	1 cup	431	56	—	—
w/ brown sugar & honey toasted	1 oz	107	17	—	—
w/ brown sugar & honey toasted	1 cup	426	69	—	—
Arrowhead					
Wheat Germ	3 tbsp (0.5 oz)	50	10	0	2
Hodgson Mill					
Wheat Germ	2 tbsp (0.5 oz)	55	7	0	4
Kretschmer					
Honey Crunch	¼ cup	105	15	—	3
Original	¼ cup	103	12	—	3
Stone-Buhr					
Untoasted	2 tbsp (0.5 oz)	58	7	0	2

WHEY

FOOD	PORTION	CALS.	CARB.	SUG.	FIB.
acid dry	1 tbsp (3 g)	10	2	—	—
acid fluid	1 cup (8 fl oz)	59	13	—	—
sweet dry	1 tbsp (8 g)	26	6	—	—
sweet fluid	1 cup (8 fl oz)	66	13	—	—
whey cheese	3.5 oz	440	33	0	0

WHIPPED TOPPINGS

(*see also* CREAM)

FOOD	PORTION	CALS.	CARB.	SUG.	FIB.
cream pressurized	1 cup (2.1 oz)	154	7	—	—
cream pressurized	1 tbsp (3 g)	8	tr	—	—

FOOD	PORTION	CALS.	CARB.	SUG.	FIB.
nondairy frzn	1 tbsp	13	1	—	—
nondairy powdered as prep w/ whole milk	1 cup	151	13	—	—
nondairy powdered as prep w/ whole milk	1 tbsp (4 g)	8	1	—	—
nondairy pressurized	1 tbsp (4 g)	11	1	—	—
nondairy pressurized	1 cup	184	11	—	—
Cool Whip					
Extra Creamy	2 tbsp (0.3 oz)	25	2	2	0
Free	2 tbsp (0.3 oz)	15	3	1	0
Lite	2 tbsp (0.3 oz)	20	2	1	0
Original	2 tbsp (0.3 oz)	25	2	1	0
Dream Whip					
Mix as prep	2 tbsp (0.3 oz)	20	2	2	0
Estee					
Whipped Topping Sugar Free as prep	2 tbsp	10	1	0	—
Hood					
Instant	2 tbsp	20	1	tr	0
Light Instant	2 tbsp	15	1	tr	0
Kraft					
Dairy Whip Light Cream	2 tbsp (0.2 oz)	10	tr	tr	0
Fat Free	1 tbsp (0.3 oz)	15	2	2	0
La Creme					
Topping	1 tbsp	16	1	—	—
Pet					
Whip	1 tbsp	14	1	—	—
Reddiwip					
Lite	2 tbsp (8 g)	15	2	tr	—
Non-Dairy	2 tbsp (8 g)	20	2	0	—
Real Whipped Heavy Cream	2 tbsp (8 g)	30	tr	—	—
Real Whipped Light Cream	2 tbsp (8 g)	20	tr	tr	—
WHITE BEANS					
CANNED					
white beans	1 cup	306	58	—	—
Goya					
Spanish Style	7.5 oz	130	29	—	12
Progresso					
Cannellini	½ cup (4.6 oz)	100	18	0	5
DRIED					
regular cooked	1 cup	249	45	—	—
small cooked	1 cup	253	46	—	—
WHITEFISH					
baked	3 oz	146	0	0	0

FOOD	PORTION	CALS.	CARB.	SUG.	FIB.
smoked	1 oz	39	0	0	0
smoked	3 oz	92	0	0	0

WHITING
cooked	3 oz	98	0	0	0
raw	3 oz	77	0	0	0

WILD RICE
cooked	1 cup (5.7 oz)	166	35	—	3
Haddon House					
Extra Fancy	¼ cup (1.6 oz)	170	35	0	2

WINE
(*see also* CHAMPAGNE, WINE COOLERS)

FOOD	PORTION	CALS.	CARB.	SUG.	FIB.
madeira	3.5 oz	169	10	10	0
port	3.5 oz	156	11	11	0
red	3½ oz	74	2	—	—
rose	3½ oz	73	2	—	—
sherry	2 oz	84	5	—	—
sweet dessert	2 oz	90	7	—	—
vermouth dry	3½ oz	105	1	—	—
vermouth sweet	3½ oz	167	12	—	—
white	3½ oz	70	1	—	—
Boone's					
Country Kwencher	1 fl oz	24	3	—	—
Delicious Apple	1 fl oz	21	3	—	—
Sangria	1 fl oz	22	3	—	—
Snow Creek Berry	1 fl oz	18	3	—	—
Strawberry Hill	1 fl oz	22	3	—	—
Sun Peak Peach	1 fl oz	18	3	—	—
Wild Island	1 fl oz	18	3	—	—
Carlo Rossi					
Blush	1 fl oz	21	1	—	—
Burgundy	1 fl oz	22	tr	—	—
Chablis	1 fl oz	21	tr	—	—
Paisano	1 fl oz	23	tr	—	—
Red Sangria	1 fl oz	24	2	—	—
Rhine	1 fl oz	21	1	—	—
Vin Rose'	1 fl oz	21	1	—	—
White Grenache	1 fl oz	20	1	—	—
Fairbanks					
Cream Sherry	1 fl oz	42	4	—	—
Port	1 fl oz	44	4	—	—
Sherry	1 fl oz	34	2	—	—
White Port	1 fl oz	44	4	—	—

FOOD	PORTION	CALS.	CARB.	SUG.	FIB.
Gallo					
Blush Chablis	1 fl oz	22	1	—	—
Burgundy	1 fl oz	22	tr	—	—
Cabernet Sauvignon	1 fl oz	22	0	0	0
Chablis Blanc	1 fl oz	20	tr	—	—
Chardonnay	1 fl oz	23	tr	—	—
Classic Burgundy	1 fl oz	21	0	0	0
French Colombard	1 fl oz	21	1	—	—
Hearty Burgundy	1 fl oz	22	tr	—	—
Johannisbery Riesling '88	1 fl oz	20	1	—	—
Pink Chablis	1 fl oz	20	1	—	—
Red Rosé	1 fl oz	23	1	—	—
Rhine	1 fl oz	22	1	—	—
Sauvignon Blanc '90	1 fl oz	20	tr	—	—
White Grenache '92	1 fl oz	20	1	—	—
White Grenache New Vintage	1 fl oz	20	1	—	—
White Zinfandel '91	1 fl oz	18	tr	—	—
White Zinfandel New Vintage	1 fl oz	18	tr	—	—
Zinfandel '87	1 fl oz	23	0	0	0
Ka-Me					
Chinese Cooking	2 tbsp (1 fl oz)	20	5	0	0
Sheffield Cellars					
Sherry	1 fl oz	44	4	—	—
Tawny Port	1 fl oz	45	4	—	—
Vermouth Extra Dry	1 fl oz	28	1	—	—
Vermouth Sweet	1 fl oz	43	4	—	—
Very Dry Sherry	1 fl oz	32	1	—	—

WINE COOLERS
FOOD	PORTION	CALS.	CARB.	SUG.	FIB.
Bartles & Jaymes					
Berry	12 fl oz	210	32	29	—
Margarita	12 fl oz	260	46	39	—
Original	12 fl oz	190	28	23	—
Peach	12 fl oz	210	33	29	—
Pina Colada	12 fl oz	280	49	45	—
Planter's Punch	12 fl oz	230	36	32	—
Strawberry	12 fl oz	210	32	28	—
Strawberry Daquiri	12 fl oz	230	37	32	—
Tropical	12 fl oz	230	38	33	—

WINGED BEANS
FOOD	PORTION	CALS.	CARB.	SUG.	FIB.
dried cooked	1 cup	252	26	—	—

FOOD	PORTION	CALS.	CARB.	SUG.	FIB.
WOLFFISH					
atlantic baked	3 oz	105	0	0	0
YAM					
(see also SWEET POTATO*)*					
CANNED					
Allen					
Cut	⅔ cup (5.8 oz)	160	40	20	3
Bruce					
Cut	½ cup	139	20	—	—
Mashed	½ cup	130	29	—	—
Vacuum Pack	½ cup	122	28	—	—
Whole	½ cup	139	31	—	—
Princella					
Cut	⅔ cup (5.8 oz)	160	40	20	3
Royal Prince					
Whole	4 pieces (5.9 oz)	200	48	16	4
S&W					
Candied	½ cup	180	44	—	—
Southern Whole In Extra Heavy Syrup	½ cup	139	31	—	—
Sugary Sam					
Cut	⅔ cup (5.8 oz)	160	40	20	3
Trappey					
Whole	4 pieces (5.9 oz)	200	48	16	4
FRESH					
mountain yam hawaii cooked	½ cup	59	14	—	—
yam cubed cooked	½ cup	79	19	—	—
YAMBEAN					
cooked	¾ cup	38	9	—	—
YARDLONG BEANS					
dried cooked	1 cup	202	36	—	—
YAUTIA (TANNIER)					
raw sliced	1 cup (4.7 oz)	132	32	—	2
root raw	1 (10.7 oz)	299	72	—	5
YEAST					
baker's compressed	1 cake (0.6 oz)	18	3	—	2
baker's dry	1 pkg (¼ oz)	21	3	—	—
baker's dry	1 tbsp	35	5	—	3
brewer's dry	1 tbsp	25	3	—	—
Fleischmann's					
Active Dry	1 pkg (¼ oz)	20	3	—	—

FOOD	PORTION	CALS.	CARB.	SUG.	FIB.
Fleischmann's (CONT.)					
Fresh Active	1 pkg (0.6 oz)	15	2	—	—
Household Yeast	½ oz	15	2	—	—
RapidRise	1 pkg (¼ oz)	20	3	—	—
Red Star					
Yeast	4 tbsp (0.5 oz)	47	5	1	4
Yeast Flakes	3 tbsp (0.5 oz)	47	5	1	4
YELLOW BEANS					
canned	½ cup	13	3	—	1
canned low sodium	½ cup	13	3	—	1
dried cooked	1 cup	254	45	—	—
fresh cooked	½ cup	22	5	—	—
fresh raw	½ cup	17	4	—	—
frozen cooked	½ cup	18	4	—	—
YELLOWEYE BEANS					
CANNED					
B&M					
Baked	½ cup (4.6 oz)	170	28	7	7
YELLOWTAIL					
baked	3 oz	159	0	0	0
YOGURT					
(*see also* YOGURT FROZEN)					
coffee lowfat	8 oz	194	31	—	—
fruit lowfat	8 oz	225	42	—	—
fruit lowfat	4 oz	113	21	—	—
plain	8 oz	139	11	—	—
plain lowfat	8 oz	144	16	—	—
plain no fat	8 oz	127	17	—	—
vanilla lowfat	8 oz	194	31	—	—
Breyers					
Blended Blueberry	4.4 oz	130	25	23	0
Blended Peach	4.4 oz	130	26	22	0
Blended Strawberry	4.4 oz	130	26	23	0
Light Nonfat Apple Pie A La Mode	8 oz	120	22	16	0
Light Nonfat Berry Banana Split	8 oz	120	21	16	0
Light Nonfat Black Cherry Jubilee	8 oz	120	23	17	0
Light Nonfat Blueberries N' Cream	8 oz	120	23	17	0
Light Nonfat Cherry Bon-Bon	8 oz	120	22	17	0

FOOD	PORTION	CALS.	CARB.	SUG.	FIB.
Breyers (CONT.)					
Light Nonfat Cherry Vanilla Cream	8 oz	120	22	17	0
Light Nonfat Classic Strawberry	8 oz	120	22	17	0
Light Nonfat Key Lime Pie	8 oz	120	22	15	0
Light Nonfat Lemon Chiffon	8 oz	120	22	17	0
Light Nonfat Peaches N' Cream	8 oz	120	22	17	0
Light Nonfat Raspberries N' Cream	8 oz	120	22	17	0
Light Nonfat Strawberry Cheesecake	8 oz	120	22	17	tr
Lowfat Black Cherry	8 oz	240	44	43	0
Lowfat Blueberry	8 oz	230	43	42	0
Lowfat Mixed Berry	8 oz	320	43	42	0
Lowfat Peach	8 oz	240	43	43	0
Lowfat Pineapple	8 oz	240	45	44	0
Lowfat Red Raspberry	8 oz	230	43	42	2
Lowfat Strawberry	8 oz	230	43	43	0
Lowfat Strawberry Banana	8 oz	240	44	43	tr
Lowfat Vanilla	8 oz	220	38	38	0
Smooth & Creamy Apple Cobbler	8 oz	230	46	40	0
Smooth & Creamy Black Cherry Parfait	8 oz	240	46	41	0
Smooth & Creamy Black Cherry Parfait	4.4 oz	130	26	23	0
Smooth & Creamy Blueberries 'N Cream	8 oz	240	46	40	0
Smooth & Creamy Blueberries 'N Cream	4.4 oz	130	26	22	0
Smooth & Creamy Classic Strawberry	8 oz	230	45	39	0
Smooth & Creamy Classic Strawberry	4.4 oz	130	25	22	0
Smooth & Creamy Orange Vanilla Cream	8 oz	230	45	39	0
Smooth & Creamy Peaches 'N Cream	4.4 oz	130	25	22	0
Smooth & Creamy Peaches 'N Cream	8 oz	230	46	40	0
Smooth & Creamy Raspberries 'N Cream	8 oz	230	45	40	0

FOOD	PORTION	CALS.	CARB.	SUG.	FIB.
Breyers (CONT.)					
Smooth & Creamy Strawberry Banana Split	8 oz	240	48	41	tr
Smooth & Creamy Strawberry Cheesecake	8 oz	240	46	39	0
Cabot					
All Flavors	8 oz	220	42	—	—
Plain	8 oz	140	16	—	—
Colombo					
Banana Strawberry	8 oz	210	39	36	0
Black Cherry	8 oz	200	36	31	0
Blueberry	8 oz	200	36	32	0
Fat Free Apples 'n Spice	8 oz	190	39	33	0
Fat Free Apricot	8 oz	190	39	33	0
Fat Free Banana Strawberry	8 oz	200	42	36	0
Fat Free Blueberry	8 oz	190	39	33	0
Fat Free Cappuccino	8 oz	180	35	27	0
Fat Free Cherry	8 oz	190	39	33	0
Fat Free Cranberry Strawberry	8 oz	200	43	40	0
Fat Free French Roast	8 oz	180	35	29	0
Fat Free Fruit Cocktail	8 oz	190	39	33	0
Fat Free Lemon	8 oz	170	33	27	0
Fat Free Peach	8 oz	190	33	33	0
Fat Free Plain	8 oz	110	16	10	0
Fat Free Raspberry	8 oz	190	39	33	0
Fat Free Strawberry	8 oz	190	39	33	0
Fat Free Strawberry Pineapple Orange	8 oz	190	38	35	0
Fat Free Vanilla	8 oz	170	32	27	0
French Vanilla	8 oz	180	29	27	0
Light 100 Blueberry	8 oz	100	16	12	0
Light 100 Cherry Vanilla	8 oz	100	16	12	0
Light 100 Coffee & Cream	8 oz	100	16	12	0
Light 100 Creamy Vanilla	8 oz	100	16	10	0
Light 100 Fruit Medley	8 oz	100	16	12	0
Light 100 Juicy Peach	8 oz	100	16	12	0
Light 100 Lemon Creme	8 oz	100	16	11	0
Light 100 Mandarin Orange	8 oz	100	16	12	0
Light 100 Mixed Berries	8 oz	100	16	12	0
Light 100 Raspberry	8 oz	100	16	12	0
Light 100 Strawberry	8 oz	100	16	12	0
Peach Melba	8 oz	200	36	34	0
Plain	8 oz	120	12	11	0

FOOD	PORTION	CALS.	CARB.	SUG.	FIB.
Colombo (CONT.)					
Raspberry	8 oz	200	36	33	0
Strawberry	8 oz	200	36	33	0
Dannon					
Chunky Fruit Nonfat Apple Cinnamon	6 oz	160	33	29	0
Chunky Fruit Nonfat Blueberry	6 oz	160	32	29	0
Chunky Fruit Nonfat Cherry Vanilla	6 oz	160	31	28	0
Chunky Fruit Nonfat Peach	6 oz	160	33	29	0
Chunky Fruit Nonfat Strawberry	6 oz	160	32	28	0
Chunky Fruit Nonfat Strawberry Banana	6 oz	160	32	28	0
Daniamls Lowfat Tropical Punch	4.4 oz	130	25	22	0
Danimals Lowfat Blueberry	4.4 oz	130	24	21	0
Danimals Lowfat Grape Lemonade	4.4 oz	120	22	20	0
Danimals Lowfat Lemon Ice	4.4 oz	120	22	19	0
Danimals Lowfat Orange Banana	4.4 oz	130	24	21	0
Danimals Lowfat Strawberry	4.4 oz	130	24	21	0
Danimals Lowfat Vanilla	4.4 oz	120	23	21	0
Danimals Lowfat Wild Raspberry	4.4 oz	120	22	19	0
Double Delights Banana Creme Strawberry	6 oz	160	32	28	0
Double Delights Bavarian Creme Raspberry	6 oz	170	34	31	0
Double Delights Cheesecake Cherry	6 oz	170	34	30	0
Double Delights Cheesecake Strawberry	6 oz	170	33	39	0
Double Delights Chocolate Cheesecake	6 oz	220	45	42	0
Double Delights Chocolate Dipped Strawberry	6 oz	210	45	41	0
Double Delights Chocolate Eclair	6 oz	220	45	42	0
Double Delights Vanilla Strawberry	6 oz	170	33	29	0

FOOD	PORTION	CALS.	CARB.	SUG.	FIB.
Dannon (CONT.)					
Double Delights Vanilla Peach & Apricot	6 oz	170	33	29	0
Fruit On The Bottom Lowfat Apple Cinnamon	8 oz	240	46	45	1
Fruit On The Bottom Lowfat Blueberry	8 oz	240	46	44	1
Fruit On The Bottom Lowfat Boysenberry	8 oz	240	45	42	1
Fruit On The Bottom Lowfat Cherry	8 oz	240	46	44	1
Fruit On The Bottom Lowfat Minipack Mixed Berry	4.4 oz	130	25	24	tr
Fruit On The Bottom Lowfat Minipack Strawberry	4.4 oz	130	25	24	tr
Fruit On The Bottom Lowfat Mixed Berries	8 oz	240	45	43	1
Fruit On The Bottom Lowfat Orange	8 oz	240	45	44	0
Fruit On The Bottom Lowfat Peach	8 oz	240	45	44	1
Fruit On The Bottom Lowfat Raspberry	8 oz	240	45	43	1
Fruit On The Bottom Lowfat Strawberry	8 oz	240	46	44	1
Fruit On The Bottom Lowfat Strawberry Banana	8 oz	240	43	40	1
Light 'N Crunchy Mint Chocolate Chip	8 oz	140	27	14	0
Light 'N Crunchy Nonfat Caramel Apple Crunch	8 oz	140	26	14	0
Light 'N Crunchy Nonfat Lemon Blueberry Cobbler	8 oz	140	25	17	0
Light 'N Crunchy Nonfat Mocha Cappuccino	8 oz	140	26	14	0
Light 'N Crunchy Nonfat Raspberry w/ Granola	8 oz	140	26	13	2
Light 'N Crunchy Nonfat Vanilla Chocolate Crunch	8 oz	130	23	13	0
Light Duets Cherry Cheesecake	6 oz	90	18	12	0
Light Duets Peaches N' Cream	6 oz	90	18	13	0

FOOD	PORTION	CALS.	CARB.	SUG.	FIB.
Dannon (CONT.)					
Light Duets Raspberry Royale	6 oz	90	17	12	0
Light Duets Strawberry Cheesecake	6 oz	90	18	12	0
Light Nonfat Banana Cream Pie	8 oz	100	15	9	0
Light Nonfat Blueberry	8 oz	100	18	12	0
Light Nonfat Cappuccino	8 oz	100	16	9	0
Light Nonfat Cherry Vanilla	8 oz	100	18	13	0
Light Nonfat Coconut Cream Pie	8 oz	100	16	9	0
Light Nonfat Creme Caramel	8 oz	100	15	9	0
Light Nonfat Lemon Chiffon	8 oz	100	15	9	0
Light Nonfat Mint Chocolate Cream Pie	8 oz	100	17	9	0
Light Nonfat Peach	8 oz	100	16	11	0
Light Nonfat Raspberry	8 oz	100	17	11	0
Light Nonfat Strawberry	8 oz	100	16	10	0
Light Nonfat Strawberry Banana	8 oz	100	17	11	0
Light Nonfat Strawberry Kiwi	8 oz	100	16	10	0
Light Nonfat Tangerine Chiffon	8 oz	100	15	9	0
Light Nonfat Vanilla	8 oz	100	15	9	0
Lowfat Coffee	8 oz	210	36	34	0
Lowfat Cranberry Raspberry	8 oz	210	36	35	0
Lowfat Lemon	8 oz	210	36	35	0
Lowfat Vanilla	8 oz	210	36	34	0
Minipack Blended Nonfat Blueberry	4.4 oz	120	25	22	0
Minipack Blended Nonfat Cherry	4.4 oz	110	24	20	0
Minipack Blended Nonfat Peach	4.4 oz	120	23	21	0
Minipack Blended Nonfat Raspberry	4.4 oz	120	24	21	0
Minipack Blended Nonfat Strawberry	4.4 oz	120	23	20	0
Minipack Blended Nonfat Strawberry Banana	4.4 oz	120	23	20	0

FOOD	PORTION	CALS.	CARB.	SUG.	FIB.
Dannon (CONT.)					
Sprinkl'ins Cherry Vanilla	1 (4.1 oz)	130	24	20	0
Sprinkl'ins Strawberry	1 (4.1 oz)	130	24	20	0
Sprinkl'ins Strawberry Banana	1 (4.1 oz)	130	24	20	0
Sprinkl'ins Vanilla w/ Cherry Crystals	1 (4.1 oz)	110	21	19	0
Sprinkl'ins Vanilla w/ Orange Crystals	1 (4.1 oz)	110	21	19	0
Friendship					
Coffee	8 oz	210	30	29	0
Fruit Crunch Blueberry	6 oz	190	32	27	0
Fruit Crunch Peach	6 oz	190	31	27	0
Fruit Crunch Strawberry	6 oz	190	31	27	0
Fruit Crunch Strawberry Banana	6 oz	190	32	27	0
Plain	8 oz	150	13	12	0
Hood					
Fat Free Blueberry	1 (8 oz)	190	40	35	1
Fat Free Cherry	1 (8 oz)	190	40	35	1
Fat Free Peach	1 (8 oz)	190	40	35	1
Fat Free Plain	1 (8 oz)	130	18	18	0
Fat Free Raspberry	1 (8 oz)	190	40	36	1
Fat Free Strawberry	1 (8 oz)	190	39	36	1
Fat Free Strawberry Banana	1 (8 oz)	190	40	36	1
Fat Free Vanilla	1 (8 oz)	190	34	34	1
Fat Free Swiss Blueberry	1 (8 oz)	210	45	40	0
Fat Free Swiss Lemon	1 (8 oz)	210	45	41	0
Fat Free Swiss Raspberry	1 (8 oz)	210	45	40	0
Fat Free Swiss Strawberry	1 (8 oz)	210	45	40	0
Fat Free Swiss Strawberry Banana	1 (8 oz)	210	45	40	0
Fat Free Swiss Vanilla	1 (8 oz)	210	45	41	0
Jell-O					
Lowfat Cherry	4.4 oz	130	25	22	0
Lowfat Grape	4.4 oz	130	25	22	0
Lowfat Raspberry	4.4 oz	130	25	22	0
Lowfat Tropical Berry Twist	4.4 oz	130	25	22	0
Lowfat Tropical Punch	4.4 oz	130	25	22	0
Lowfat Watermelon	4.4 oz	130	25	22	0
Lowfat Wild Berry	4.4 oz	130	25	22	0
Lowfat Wild Strawberry	4.4 oz	130	25	22	0
La Yogurt					
French Style Banana	6 oz	180	32	29	0

FOOD	PORTION	CALS.	CARB.	SUG.	FIB.
La Yogurt (CONT.)					
French Style Blueberry	6 oz	180	32	29	1
French Style Cherry	6 oz	180	32	29	0
French Style Cherry Vanilla	6 oz	190	35	32	0
French Style Guava	6 oz	180	32	29	1
French Style Key Lime	6 oz	180	32	29	0
French Style Mango	6 oz	180	32	29	0
French Style Mixed Berry	6 oz	180	32	29	0
French Style Nonfat Blueberry	6 oz	70	12	8	0
French Style Nonfat Cherry	6 oz	75	13	8	0
French Style Nonfat Raspberry	6 oz	70	12	8	0
French Style Nonfat Strawberry	6 oz	70	12	8	0
French Style Nonfat Strawberry Banana	6 oz	70	12	8	0
French Style Peach	6 oz	180	32	28	0
French Style Pina Colada	6 oz	180	32	29	0
French Style Raspberry	6 oz	180	32	29	1
French Style Strawberry	6 oz	180	32	29	0
French Style Strawberry Banana	6 oz	180	32	27	0
French Style Strawberry Fruit Cup	6 oz	180	32	29	0
French Style Tropical Orange	6 oz	180	32	29	0
French Style Vanilla	6 oz	170	28	25	0
Latin Style Banana	6 oz	190	34	31	0
Latin Style Guava	6 oz	190	34	31	0
Latin Style Mango	6 oz	190	34	31	0
Latin Style Papaya	6 oz	190	34	31	0
Latin Style Passion Fruit	6 oz	190	34	31	0
Latin Style Strawberry Kiwi	6 oz	180	32	30	0
Light N'Lively					
Free Blueberry	4.4 oz	70	13	10	0
Free Peach	4.4 oz	70	12	9	0
Free Strawberry	4.4 oz	70	12	9	0
Free Strawberry Banana Cream	4.4 oz	70	13	10	0
Free Strawberry Fruit Cup	4.4 oz	70	13	10	0
Lowfat Blueberry	4.4 oz	130	25	23	0
Lowfat Peach	4.4 oz	130	26	22	0
Lowfat Pineapple	4.4 oz	130	26	22	0

FOOD	PORTION	CALS.	CARB.	SUG.	FIB.
Light N'Lively (CONT.)					
Lowfat Red Raspberry	4.4 oz	120	23	20	0
Lowfat Strawberry	4.4 oz	130	26	23	0
Lowfat Strawberry Banana Cream	4.4 oz	130	25	22	0
Lowfat Strawberry Fruit Cup	4.4 oz	130	25	22	0
Lite Line					
Swiss Style Cherry Vanilla	1 cup	240	45	—	—
Swiss Style Peach	1 cup	230	42	—	—
Swiss Style Plain	1 cup	140	16	—	—
Swiss Style Strawberry	1 cup	240	46	—	—
Meadow Gold					
Plain	1 cup	160	16	—	—
Sundae Style Raspberry	1 cup	250	42	—	—
Mountain High					
Blueberry	1 cup	220	31	—	—
Plain	1 cup	200	16	—	—
Weight Watchers					
Ultimate 90 Blueberries 'n Creme	1 cup	90	14	9	3
Ultimate 90 Cappuccino	1 cup	90	14	7	0
Ultimate 90 Cherries Jubilee	1 cup	90	14	8	3
Ultimate 90 Cranberry Raspberry	1 cup	90	14	7	0
Ultimate 90 Lemon Chiffon	1 cup	90	14	7	1
Ultimate 90 Plain	1 cup	90	14	7	0
Ultimate 90 Raspberries 'n Creme	1 cup	90	14	7	0
Ultimate 90 Strawberry	1 cup	90	14	7	2
Ultimate 90 Strawberry Banana	1 cup	90	14	7	2
Ultimate 90 Vanilla	1 cup	90	14	7	0
Utlimate 90 Peach	1 cup	90	14	7	0
Yoplait					
Custard Style Banana	6 oz	190	32	—	—
Custard Style Blueberry	6 oz	190	32	—	—
Custard Style Cherry	6 oz	180	30	—	—
Custard Style Lemon	6 oz	190	32	—	—
Custard Style Mixed Berry	6 oz	180	30	—	—
Custard Style Raspberry	6 oz	190	32	—	—
Custard Style Strawberry	6 oz	190	32	—	—
Custard Style Strawberry	4 oz	130	21	—	—

FOOD	PORTION	CALS.	CARB.	SUG.	FIB.
Yoplait (CONT.)					
Custard Style Strawberry Banana	6 oz	190	32	—	—
Custard Style Strawvberry Banana	4 oz	130	21	—	—
Custard Style Vanilla	4 oz	130	20	—	—
Custard Style Vanilla	6 oz	180	30	—	—
Fat Free Blueberry	6 oz	150	31	—	—
Fat Free Cherry	6 oz	150	31	—	—
Fat Free Mixed Berry	6 oz	150	31	—	—
Fat Free Peach	6 oz	150	31	—	—
Fat Free Raspberry	6 oz	150	31	—	—
Fat Free Strawberry	6 oz	150	31	—	—
Fat Free Strawberry Banana	6 oz	150	31	—	—
Light Blueberry	4 oz	60	9	—	—
Light Blueberry	6 oz	80	13	—	—
Light Cherry	4 oz	60	9	—	—
Light Cherry	6 oz	80	13	—	—
Light Peach	6 oz	80	13	—	—
Light Peach	4 oz	60	9	—	—
Light Raspberry	4 oz	60	9	—	—
Light Raspberry	6 oz	80	13	—	—
Light Strawberry	4 oz	60	9	—	—
Light Strawberry	6 oz	80	13	—	—
Light Strawberry Banana	6 oz	80	13	—	—
Light Strawberry Banana	4 oz	60	9	—	—
Nonfat Plain	8 oz	120	18	—	—
Nonfat Vanilla	8 oz	180	35	—	—
Original Apple	6 oz	190	32	—	—
Original Blueberry	4 oz	120	21	—	—
Original Blueberry	6 oz	190	32	—	—
Original Boysenberry	6 oz	190	32	—	—
Original Cherry	6 oz	190	32	—	—
Original Lemon	6 oz	190	32	—	—
Original Mixed Berry	6 oz	190	32	—	—
Original Orange	6 oz	190	32	—	—
Original Peach	6 oz	190	32	—	—
Original Peach	4 oz	120	21	—	—
Original Pina Colada	6 oz	190	32	—	—
Original Pineapple	6 oz	190	32	—	—
Original Plain	6 oz	130	15	—	—
Original Raspberry	4 oz	120	21	—	—
Original Raspberry	6 oz	190	32	—	—
Original Strawberry	4 oz	120	21	—	—

FOOD	PORTION	CALS.	CARB.	SUG.	FIB.
Yoplait (CONT.)					
Original Strawberry	6 oz	190	32	—	—
Original Strawberry Banana	6 oz	190	32	—	—
Original Strawberry Rhubarb	6 oz	190	32	—	—
Original Vanilla	6 oz	180	29	—	—
YOGURT FROZEN					
chocolate soft serve	½ cup (4 fl oz)	115	18	—	—
vanilla soft serve	½ cup (4 fl oz)	114	17	16	—
Bee-Lite					
Chocolate	4 oz	100	23	—	—
Vanilla	4 oz	110	23	—	—
Ben & Jerry's					
Cherry Garcia	½ cup (3.7 oz)	170	31	30	0
Chocolate Fudge Brownie	½ cup (3.7 oz)	190	35	26	2
Coffee Almond Fudge	½ cup (3.7 oz)	200	30	29	1
English Toffee Crunch	½ cup (3.7 oz)	190	32	32	0
No Fat Cappuccino	½ cup (3.3 oz)	140	32	23	0
Pop Cherry Garcia	1 (3.8 oz)	290	34	30	2
Borden					
Strawberry	½ cup	100	19	—	—
Bresler's					
All Flavors	5 oz	145	28	—	—
All Flavors Lite	5 oz	135	30	—	—
Breyers					
Chocolate	½ cup (2.6 oz)	130	23	18	tr
Fat Free Chocolate	½ cup (2.6 oz)	100	23	17	0
Fat Free Cookies N Cream	½ cup (2.6 oz)	110	25	18	tr
Fat Free Peach	½ cup (2.6 oz)	90	20	16	0
Fat Free Strawberry	½ cup (2.6 oz)	100	22	15	0
Fat Free Take Two Vanilla Chocolate	½ cup (2.6 oz)	100	23	18	tr
Fat Free Vanilla	½ cup (2.6 oz)	100	23	18	tr
Fat Free Vanilla Fudge Twirl	½ cup (2.6 oz)	110	25	19	0
Vanilla	½ cup (2.6 oz)	120	22	17	0
Vanilla Chocolate Strawberry	½ cup (2.6 oz)	120	22	17	0
Dannon					
Light Cappuccino	½ cup (2.8 oz)	80	20	6	0
Light Cherry Vanilla Swirl	½ cup (2.8 oz)	90	21	5	0
Light Chocolate	½ cup (2.7 oz)	80	21	5	tr
Light Mint Chocolate Fudge	½ cup (2.8 oz)	90	23	5	0
Light Peach Raspberry Melba	½ cup (2.8 oz)	90	20	6	0

FOOD	PORTION	CALS.	CARB.	SUG.	FIB.
Dannon (CONT.)					
Light Strawberry Cheesecake	½ cup (2.8 oz)	90	21	5	0
Light Vanilla	½ cup (2.8 oz)	80	20	6	0
Light 'N Crunchy Carmel Toffee Crunch	½ cup (2.8 oz)	110	26	13	0
Light 'N Crunchy Rocky Road	½ cup (2.8 oz)	110	27	12	tr
Light 'N Crunchy Vanilla Streusel	½ cup (2.8 oz)	110	25	11	0
Light Duets Strawberry Sundae	6 oz	90	18	12	0
Light Nonfat Cappuccino	8 oz	100	17	13	0
Light'N Crunchy Banana Cream Pie	½ cup (2.8 oz)	110	23	11	0
Light'N Crunchy Mocha Chocolate Chunk	½ cup (2.8 oz)	110	23	9	0
Light'N Crunchy Peanut Chocolate Crunch	½ cup (2.8 oz)	110	24	11	0
Light'N Crunchy Triple Chocolate	½ cup (2.8 oz)	110	25	11	tr
Desserve					
All Flavors	4 oz	70	16	—	—
Dutch Chocolate	4 oz	80	18	—	—
Edy's					
Banana Strawberry	3 oz	80	15	—	—
Blueberry	3 oz	80	15	—	—
Cherry	3 oz	80	15	—	—
Chocolate	3 oz	80	15	—	—
Chocolate Chip	3 oz	100	20	—	—
Citrus Heights	3 oz	80	15	—	—
Cookies'N'Cream	3 oz	100	20	—	—
Marble Fudge	3 oz	100	20	—	—
Perfectly Peach	3 oz	80	15	—	—
Raspberry	3 oz	80	15	—	—
Raspberry Vanilla Swirl	3 oz	80	15	—	—
Strawberry	3 oz	80	15	—	—
Vanilla	3 oz	80	15	—	—
Elan					
Blueberry	4 oz	130	23	—	—
Caramel Almond Praline	4 oz	150	26	—	—
Chocolate	4 oz	130	24	—	—
Chocolate Almond	4 oz	160	22	—	—
Coffee	4 oz	130	22	—	—

FOOD	PORTION	CALS.	CARB.	SUG.	FIB.
Elan (cont.)					
Coffee Decaffeinated	4 oz	130	22	—	—
Peach	4 oz	130	23	–	—
Rum Raisin	4 oz	135	25	–	—
Strawberry	4 oz	125	22	—	—
Vanilla	4 oz	130	22		-
Fi-Bar					
Chocolate	1	190	26	–	4
Strawberry	1	190	26	-	4
Vanilla	1	190	26	—	4
Friendly's					
Apple Bettie	½ cup (2.6 oz)	140	25	21	J
Fabulous Fudge Swirl	½ cup (2.6 oz)	140	23	15	0
Fudge Berry Swirl	½ cup (2.6 oz)	150	25	18	0
Lowfat Perfectly Peach	½ cup (2.6 oz)	110	21	17	0
Lowfat Purely Chocolate	½ cup (2.6 oz)	120	20	16	0
Lowfat Raspberry Delight	½ cup (2.6 oz)	120	21	17	0
Lowfat Simply Vanilla	½ cup (2.6 oz)	120	19	15	0
Lowfat Strawberry Patch	½ cup (2.6 oz)	110	20	17	0
Mint Chocolate Chip	½ cup (2.6 oz)	130	21	17	0
Strawberry Cheesecake Blast	½ cup (2.6 oz)	140	22	18	0
Toffee Almond Crunch	½ cup (2.6 oz)	160	24	18	tr
Good Humor					
Creamsicle Raspberry	1 (2.8 oz)	100	23	22	0
Frista Cup	1 (6.2 oz)	220	38	32	1
Haagen-Dazs					
Banana Nut Blast	½ cup (3.5 oz)	220	29	21	1
Bars Cherry Chocolate Fudge	1 (2.6 oz)	240	26	20	1
Bars Peach	1 (2.5 oz)	90	19	16	0
Bars Pina Colada	1 (2.5 oz)	100	19	14	0
Bars Raspberry & Vanilla	1 (2.5 oz)	90	19	16	0
Bars Strawberry Daiquiri	1 (2.5 oz)	90	18	14	0
Chocolate	½ cup (3.4 oz)	160	26	18	tr
Coffee	½ cup (3.4 oz)	160	26	18	0
Fat Free Bar Raspberry & Vanilla	1 (2.5 oz)	90	20	14	0
Fat Free Cherry Vanilla	½ cup (3.3 oz)	140	30	19	0
Fat Free Chocolate	½ cup (3.3 oz)	140	28	17	tr
Fat Free Coffee	½ cup (3.3 oz)	140	29	17	0
Fat Free Vanilla	½ cup (3.3 oz)	140	29	17	0
Fat Free Vanilla Fudge	½ cup (3.3 oz)	160	34	22	0
Orange Tango	½ cup (3.5 oz)	130	26	21	0

FOOD	PORTION	CALS.	CARB.	SUG.	FIB.
Haagen-Dazs (CONT.)					
Pina Colada	½ cup (3.4 oz)	130	26	21	0
Raspberry Randevous	½ cup (3.5 oz)	130	26	21	1
Strawberry Cheesecake Craze	½ cup (3.6 oz)	220	31	23	0
Strawberry Duet	½ cup (3.4 oz)	130	26	22	tr
Vanilla	½ cup (3.4 oz)	160	26	19	0
Hood					
Bavarian Truffle & Twist	½ cup (2.6 oz)	150	26	25	0
Coffee Toffee Chunk Sundae	½ cup (2.6 oz)	150	27	26	0
Combo Bars	1 (2.2 oz)	90	17	17	0
Cookies & Cream	½ cup (2.6 oz)	140	25	22	0
Grandma's Raisin Oatmeal Cookie Dough	½ cup (2.6 oz)	140	25	24	0
Mixed Berry Swirl	½ cup (2.6 oz)	120	24	24	0
Natural Strawberry	½ cup (2.6 oz)	110	21	20	0
Natural Strawberry Banana	½ cup (2.6 oz)	110	21	21	0
Natural Vanilla	½ cup (2.6 oz)	120	22	22	0
Nonfat Caramel & Brownie Sundae	½ cup (2.6 oz)	120	28	26	0
Nonfat Chocolate Marshmallow	½ cup (2.6 oz)	110	26	24	0
Nonfat Double Raspberry	½ cup (2.6 oz)	120	26	24	0
Nonfat Mocha Fudge	½ cup (2.6 oz)	120	27	25	0
Nonfat Olde Fashioned Vanilla	½ cup (2.6 oz)	110	24	23	0
Nonfat Peach Cobbler A La Mode	½ cup (2.6 oz)	110	25	24	0
Nonfat Strawberry	½ cup (2.6 oz)	100	23	22	0
Nonfat Vanilla Fudge	½ cup (2.6 oz)	120	27	26	0
Raspberry Swirl	½ cup (2.6 oz)	130	25	23	0
Sundae Cups Chocolate & Strawberry	1 (2.2 oz)	110	24	23	1
Vanilla Chocolate Strawberry	½ cup (2.6 oz)	120	22	21	0
Vanilla Swiss Almond Sundae	½ cup (2.6 oz)	150	25	24	0
Just 10					
All Flavors	1 oz	10	3	—	—
Kissed With Honey					
Chocolate	3.5 oz	100	18	—	—
Nonfat Chocolate	3.5 oz	85	19	—	—

FOOD	PORTION	CALS.	CARB.	SUG.	FIB.
Kissed With Honey (CONT.)					
Nonfat Vanilla	3.5 oz	85	18	—	—
Vanilla	3.5 oz	100	17	—	—
Meadow Gold					
Strawberry	½ cup	100	19	—	—
Sealtest					
Chocolate	½ cup (2.7 oz)	120	24	17	tr
Mocha Fudge	½ cup (2.6 oz)	130	25	17	tr
Vanilla	½ cup (2.6 oz)	120	24	17	0
Tofutti					
Better Than Yogurt Chocolate Fudge	4 fl oz	120	25	18	0
Better Than Yogurt Coffee Marshmallow Swirl	4 fl oz	100	24	14	0
Better Than Yogurt Passion Island Fruit	4 fl oz	100	21	14	0
Better Than Yogurt Peach Mango	4 fl oz	100	23	16	0
Better Than Yogurt Strawberry Banana	4 fl oz	100	23	17	0
Better Than Yogurt Vanilla Fudge	4 fl oz	120	24	16	0
Turkey Hill					
Chocolate Cherry Cordial	½ cup (2.6 oz)	130	22	21	0
Chocolate Chip Cookie Dough	½ cup (2.6 oz)	140	23	21	0
Death By Chocolate	½ cup (2.6 oz)	150	25	22	0
Nonfat Chocolate Cherry Cordial	½ cup (2.4 oz)	100	24	21	0
Nonfat Chocolate Marshmallow	½ cup (2.4 oz)	130	30	21	0
Nonfat Coffee Cappuccino	½ cup (2.4 oz)	110	23	20	0
Nonfat Mint Cookie 'N Cream	½ cup (2.4 oz)	110	24	18	0
Nonfat Neapolitan	½ cup (2.4 oz)	100	22	19	0
Nonfat Raspberry Chocolate Bliss	½ cup (2.4 oz)	110	25	22	0
Nonfat Southern Lemon Pie	½ cup (2.4 oz)	110	25	22	0
Nonfat Vanilla Fudge	½ cup (2.4 oz)	110	24	21	0
Peach Raspberry	½ cup (2.6 oz)	110	20	20	0
Strawberry	½ cup (2.6 oz)	110	20	20	0
Tin Roof Sundae	½ cup (2.6 oz)	140	21	20	0
Vanilla & Chocolate	½ cup (2.6 oz)	110	19	18	0

FOOD	PORTION	CALS.	CARB.	SUG.	FIB.
Turkey Hill (CONT.)					
Vanilla Bean	½ cup (2.6 oz)	110	17	17	0
ZUCCHINI					
CANNED					
italian style	½ cup	33	8	—	—
Del Monte					
With Italian Tomato Sauce	½ cup (4.2 oz)	30	7	1	1
Progresso					
Italian Style	½ cup (4.2 oz)	40	7	4	2
S&W					
Italian Style	½ cup	45	7	—	—
FRESH					
baby raw	1 (0.5 oz)	3	1	—	tr
raw sliced	½ cup	9	2	—	1
sliced cooked	½ cup	14	4	—	1
FROZEN					
cooked	½ cup	19	4	—	—
Big Valley					
Zucchini	¾ cup (3 oz)	10	2	3	1
Empire					
Breaded	1 (2.9 oz)	100	18	4	1

PART TWO

RESTAURANT

AND

TAKE-OUT FOODS

FOOD	PORTION	CALS.	CARB.	SUG.	FIB.
ASIAN FOOD					
cha siu bao steamed buns w/ chicken filling	1 (2.3 oz)	160	26	4	tr
chicken teriyaki	¾ cup	399	7	—	—
chicken teriyaki w/ rice	1 serv (11 oz)	430	77	10	1
chop suey w/ beef & pork	1 cup	300	13	—	—
chop suey w/ pork	1 cup	375	29	—	2
chow mein chicken	1 cup	255	10	—	—
chow mein pork	1 cup	425	21	—	3
chow mein shrimp	1 cup	221	21	—	3
chow mein vegetable	1 serv (8 oz)	90	15	2	4
fried rice	6.6 oz	249	48	—	2
fried rice w/ egg	6.7 oz	395	49	—	2
spring roll	1 (3.5 oz)	112	37	—	5
sweet & sour pork	1 serv (8 oz)	250	37	30	2
szechuan chicken w/ lo mein	1 cup (5.3 oz)	190	35	3	0
wonton fried	½ cup (1 oz)	111	8	—	1
wonton soup	1 cup	205	26	—	1
BEANS					
baked beans	½ cup	190	27	—	—
barbecue beans	3.5 oz	120	26	—	—
four bean salad	3.5 oz	100	20	—	—
refried beans	½ cup	43	5	—	—
three bean salad	¾ cup	230	31	—	1
BEEF					
beef bouriguignon	1 serv (7 oz)	254	3	—	1
roast beef medium	2 oz	70	0	0	0
roast beef rare	2 oz	70	0	0	0
BEEF DISHES					
bubble & squeak	5 oz	186	16	—	3
bulgoghi korean grilled beef	1 serv (5.2 oz)	256	5	3	tr
cornish pasty	1 (8 oz)	847	79	—	3
irish stew	1 cup (7 oz)	280	10	—	—
kebab indian	1 (5.4 oz)	553	2	—	—
kheena	6.7 oz	781	1	—	tr
koftas	5	280	3	—	tr
samosa	2 (4 oz)	652	20	—	2
shepherds pie	1 serv (7 oz)	282	20	—	2
steak & kidney pie w/ top crust	1 slice (5 oz)	400	23	—	1
stew	6 oz	208	6	—	1
stew w/ vegetables	1 cup	220	15	—	—

FOOD	PORTION	CALS.	CARB.	SUG.	FIB.
stroganoff	¾ cup	260	43	—	—
swiss steak	4.6 oz	214	10	—	2
toad in the hole	1 (4.7 oz)	383	23	—	1
BISCUIT					
buttermilk	1	127	17	—	—
plain	1 (35 g)	276	13	—	—
tea biscuit	1 (3 oz)	210	30	12	1
w/ egg	1	315	24	—	—
w/ egg & bacon	1	457	29	—	—
w/ egg & sausage	1	582	41	—	—
w/ egg & steak	1	474	37	—	—
w/ egg cheese & bacon	1	477	33	—	—
w/ ham	1	387	44	—	—
w/ sausage	1	485	40	—	—
w/ steak	1	456	44	—	—
BLINTZE					
cheese	1 (2.7 oz)	160	15	4	tr
BREAD					
chapatis as prep w/ fat	1 bread (1.6 oz)	95	18	1	3
chapatis as prep w/o fat	1 (2½ oz)	141	31	—	5
cornbread	2 in x 2 in (1.4 oz)	107	18	—	—
cornstick	1 (1.3 oz)	101	13	—	tr
focaccia onion	1 piece (4.6 oz)	282	43	2	2
focaccia rosemary	1 piece (3.5 oz)	251	40	1	2
focaccia tomato olive	1 piece (4.7 oz)	270	42	1	2
garlic bread	2 slices (2 oz)	190	27	1	1
naan	1 bread (3.5 oz)	286	43	3	2
papadums fried	2 (1.5 oz)	81	9	—	2
paratha	1 bread (2.1 oz)	201	23	1	2
CABBAGE					
stuffed cabbage	1 (6 oz)	373	18	—	—
sweet & sour red cabbage	4 oz	61	8	—	3
CAKE					
angelfood	½12 cake (1 oz)	73	16	—	1
apple crisp	½ cup (5 oz)	230	46	—	—
baklava	1 oz	126	10	—	1
boston cream pie	⅙ cake (3.3 oz)	293	43	—	1
carrot w/ cream cheese icing	½12 cake (3.9 oz)	484	52	—	—
cheesecake w/ cherry topping	½12 cake (5 oz)	359	33	—	—
chocolate w/ chocolate frosting	⅛ cake (2.2 oz)	235	35	—	2

FOOD	PORTION	CALS.	CARB.	SUG.	FIB.
coffeecake cheese	1/6 cake (2.7 oz)	258	38	—	1
coffeecake crumb topped cheese	1/6 cake (2.7 oz)	258	38	—	1
coffeecake crumb topped cinnamon	1/9 cake (2.2 oz)	263	29	—	2
cream puff w/ custard filling	1 (4.6 oz)	336	30	—	—
french apple tart	1 (3.5 oz)	302	37	15	2
fruitcake	1/36 cake (2.9 oz)	302	54	—	3
gingerbread	1/9 cake (2.6 oz)	264	36	—	2
panettone dal forno	1/9 cake (1.9 oz)	212	31	20	0
petit fours	2 (0.9 oz)	120	15	12	0
pineapple upside down	1/9 cake (4 oz)	367	58	—	—
pound fat free	1 oz	80	17	—	—
pound cake	1 slice (1 oz)	120	15	—	—
sheet cake w/ white frosting	1/9 cake	445	77	—	—
strudel apple	1 piece (2½ oz)	195	29	—	2
tiramisu	1 piece (5.1 oz)	409	31	17	tr
trifle w/ cream	6 oz	291	34	—	1
yellow w/ vanilla frosting	1/8 cake (2.2 oz)	239	38	—	—
CALZONE					
cheese	1 (12 oz)	1020	86	26	8
CHEESE DISHES					
cheese omelette as prep w/ 2 eggs	1 (6.8 oz)	519	tr	—	0
fondue	1 cup (7.5 oz)	492	8	—	—
fondue	½ cup (3.8 oz)	247	4	—	—
souffle	1 serv (7 oz)	504	18	5	1
CHICKEN					
boneless breaded & fried w/ barbecue sauce	6 pieces (4.6 oz)	330	25	—	—
boneless breaded & fried w/ honey	6 pieces (4 oz)	339	27	—	—
boneless breaded & fried w/ mustard sauce	6 pieces (4.6 oz)	323	21	—	—
boneless breaded & fried w/ sweet & sour sauce	6 pieces (4.6 oz)	346	29	—	—
breast & wing breaded & fried	2 pieces (5.7 oz)	494	20	—	—
drumstick breaded & fried	2 pieces (5.2 oz)	430	16	—	—
oven roasted breast of chicken	2 oz	60	0	0	0
thigh breaded & fried	2 pieces (5.2 oz)	430	16	—	—
CHICKEN DISHES					
chicken & dumplings	¾ cup	256	12	—	tr

FOOD	PORTION	CALS.	CARB.	SUG.	FIB.
chicken & noodles	1 cup	365	26	—	—
chicken a la king	1 cup	470	12	—	—
chicken cacciatore	¾ cup	394	9	—	2
chicken pie w/ top crust	1 slice (5.6 oz)	472	32	—	1

CHILI
con carne w/ beans	8.9 oz	254	22	—	—

CLAMS
breaded & fried	20 sm	379	19	—	—

COFFEE
cafe au lait	1 cup (8 fl oz)	77	6	7	—
cafe brulot	1 cup (4.8 fl oz)	48	3	3	—
cappuccino	1 cup (8 fl oz)	77	6	7	—
coffee con leche	1 cup (8 fl oz)	77	6	7	—
espresso	1 cup (3 fl oz)	2	tr	0	—
irish coffee	1 serv (9 fl oz)	107	3	0	—
latte w/ skim milk	13 oz	88	12	11	0
latte w/ whole milk	13 oz	152	12	11	0
mocha	1 mug (9.6 fl oz)	202	17	12	—

COLESLAW
coleslaw w/ dressing	½ cup	42	7	—	—
vinegar & oil coleslaw	3.5 oz	150	16	—	—

COOKIES
biscotti with nuts chocolate dipped	1 (1.3 oz)	117	16	11	1
black & white	1 lg (3 oz)	302	52	31	1

CORN
fritters	1 (1 oz)	62	9	—	1
scalloped	½ cup	258	43	—	—

CORNMEAL
hush puppies	5 (2.7 oz)	256	35	—	4
hush puppies	1 (0.75 oz)	74	10	—	1

CRAB
baked	1 (3.8 oz)	160	4	—	—
cake	1 (2 oz)	160	5	—	—
soft-shell fried	1 (4.4 oz)	334	31	—	—

CROISSANT
w/ egg & cheese	1	369	24	—	—
w/ egg cheese & bacon	1	413	24	—	—
w/ egg cheese & ham	1	475	24	—	—
w/ egg cheese & sausage	1	524	25	—	—

FOOD	PORTION	CALS.	CARB.	SUG.	FIB.
CUCUMBER					
cucumber salad	3.5 oz	50	11	—	—
kimchee	½ cup (1.8 oz)	36	4	3	tr
tzatziki	½ cup (3.4 oz)	72	4	3	1
CUSTARD					
baked	½ cup (5 oz)	148	15	—	—
flan	½ cup (5.4 oz)	220	35	—	—
zabaione	½ cup (57.2 g)	135	13	—	0
DANISH PASTRY					
almond	1 (4¼ in) (2.3 oz)	280	30	—	2
apple	1 (4¼ in) (2.5 oz)	264	34	—	1
cheese	1 (3 oz)	353	29	—	—
cheese	1 (4¼ in) (2.5 oz)	266	26	—	—
cinnamon	1 (3 oz)	349	47	—	—
cinnamon	1 (4¼ in) (2.3 oz)	262	29	—	1
cinnamon nut	1 (4¼ in) (2.3 oz)	280	30	—	2
fruit	1 (3.3 oz)	335	45	—	—
lemon	1 (4¼ in) (2.5 oz)	264	34	—	1
raisin	1 (4¼ in) (2.5 oz)	264	34	—	1
raisin nut	1 (4¼ in) (2.3 oz)	280	30	—	2
raspberry	1 (4¼ in) (2.5 oz)	264	34	—	1
strawberry	1 (4¼ in) (2.5 oz)	264	34	—	1
DELI MEATS/COLD CUTS					
corned beef	2 oz	70	0	0	0
corned beef brisket	2 oz	90	0	0	0
EGG DISHES					
deviled	2 halves	145	1	—	—
salad	½ cup	307	2	—	—
scotch egg	1 (4.2 oz)	301	16	—	2
scrambled	2 eggs	202	2	—	—
sunny side up	1	91	1	—	—
EGG ROLLS					
lobster	1 (4.8 oz)	270	43	4	6
meat & shrimp	1 (4.8 oz)	320	41	3	4
pork & shrimp	1 (5 oz)	300	41	6	7
shrimp	1 (3 oz)	170	24	5	5
spicy pork	1 (3 oz)	200	23	3	3
vegetable	1 (3 oz)	170	28	4	4
EGGPLANT					
baba ghannouj	¼ cup	55	5	—	—
caponata	2 tbsp (1 oz)	30	3	2	—
indian eggplant runi	1 serv	180	13	1	1

FOOD	PORTION	CALS.	CARB.	SUG.	FIB.
ENGLISH MUFFIN					
w/ butter	1	189	30	—	—
w/ cheese & sausage	1	394	29	—	—
w/ egg cheese & bacon	1	487	31	—	—
w/ egg cheese & canadian bacon	1	383	31	—	—
FALAFEL					
falafel	1 (1.2 oz)	57	5	—	—
FISH					
fish cake	1 (4.7 oz)	166	6	—	—
jamaican brown fish stew	1 serv	426	9	—	2
kedgeree	5.6 oz	242	15	—	1
mousse	1 serv (3.5 oz)	185	3	tr	tr
stew	1 cup (7.9 oz)	157	10	—	—
taramasalata	3.5 oz	446	4	—	—
FLOUNDER					
battered & fried	3.2 oz	211	15	—	—
breaded & fried	3.2 oz	211	15	—	—
FRENCH TOAST					
w/ butter	2 slices	356	36	—	—
HADDOCK					
breaded & fried	1 piece (3.5 oz)	187	3	0	tr
HAM DISHES					
croquettes	1 (3.1 oz)	217	11	—	tr
salad	½ cup	287	5	—	tr
HAMBURGER					
double patty w/ bun	1 reg	544	43	—	—
double patty w/ cheese & bun	1 reg	457	22	—	—
double patty w/ cheese & double bun	1 reg	461	44	—	—
double patty w/ cheese ketchup mayonnaise onion pickle tomato & bun	1 reg	416	35	—	—
double patty w/ ketchup mayonnaise onion pickle tomato & bun	1 reg	649	53	—	—
double patty w/ ketchup cheese mayonnaise mustard pickle tomato & bun	1 lg	706	40	—	—

FOOD	PORTION	CALS.	CARB.	SUG.	FIB.
double patty w/ ketchup mustard mayonnaise onion pickle tomato & bun	1 lg	540	40	—	—
double patty w/ ketchup mustard onion pickle & bun	1 reg	576	39	—	—
single patty w/ bacon ketchup cheese mustard onion pickle & bun	1 lg	609	37	—	—
single patty w/ bun	1 lg	400	25	—	—
single patty w/ bun	1 reg	275	31	—	—
single patty w/ cheese & bun	1 reg	320	32	—	—
single patty w/ cheese & bun	1 lg	608	47	—	—
single patty w/ ketchup cheese ham mayonnaise pickle tomato & bun	1 lg	745	38	—	—
single patty w/ ketchup mustard mayonnaise onion pickle tomato & bun	1 reg	279	27	—	—
triple patty w/ cheese & bun	1 lg	769	27	—	—
triple patty w/ ketchup mustard pickle & bun	1 lg	693	29	—	—

HERRING

atlantic kippered	1 fillet (1.4 oz)	87	0	0	0
atlantic pickled	½ oz	39	1	—	—
fried	1 serv (3.5 oz)	233	2	—	0

HOT DOG

corndog	1	460	56	—	—
w/ bun chili	1	297	31	—	—
w/ bun plain	1	242	18	—	—

HUMMUS

hummus	⅓ cup	140	17	—	—

ICE CREAM AND FROZEN DESSERTS

cone vanilla light soft serve	1 (4.6 oz)	164	24	—	—
gelato chocolate hazelnut	½ cup (5.3 oz)	370	26	21	2
gelato vanilla	½ cup (3 oz)	211	18	18	0
sundae caramel	1 (5.4 oz)	303	49	—	—
sundae hot fudge	1 (5.4 oz)	284	48	—	—
sundae strawberry	1 (5.4 oz)	269	45	—	—

KNISH

cheese & blueberry	1 (7 oz)	378	40	—	—
cheese & cherry	1 (7 oz)	378	40	—	—

FOOD	PORTION	CALS.	CARB.	SUG.	FIB.
everything	1 (7 oz)	221	34	—	—
kashe	1 (7 oz)	270	45	—	—
potato	1 med (3.5 oz)	166	25	2	tr
potato	1 lg (7 oz)	332	49	5	1
potato w/ broccoli & cheese	1 (7 oz)	312	33	—	—
potato w/ spinach & mushroom	1 (7 oz)	214	32	—	—

LAMB DISHES

FOOD	PORTION	CALS.	CARB.	SUG.	FIB.
curry	¾ cup	345	22	—	—
moussaka	5.6 oz	312	16	—	1
stew	¾ cup	124	11	—	2

LENTILS

FOOD	PORTION	CALS.	CARB.	SUG.	FIB.
indian sambar	1 serv	236	37	—	9

LOBSTER

FOOD	PORTION	CALS.	CARB.	SUG.	FIB.
newburg	1 cup	485	13	—	—

MOUSSE

FOOD	PORTION	CALS.	CARB.	SUG.	FIB.
chocolate	½ cup (7.1 oz)	447	33	—	—

NOODLE DISHES

FOOD	PORTION	CALS.	CARB.	SUG.	FIB.
noodle pudding	½ cup	132	11	—	—

ONION

FOOD	PORTION	CALS.	CARB.	SUG.	FIB.
fried	½ cup (7.5 oz)	176	17	—	—
rings breaded & fried	8 to 9	275	31	—	—

OYSTERS

FOOD	PORTION	CALS.	CARB.	SUG.	FIB.
battered & fried	6 (4.9 oz)	368	40	—	—
breaded & fried	6 (4.9 oz)	368	40	—	—
eastern breaded & fried	6 med (88 g)	173	10	—	—
eastern breaded & fried	3 oz	167	10	—	—
oysters rockefeller	3 oysters	66	5	—	—
stew	1 cup	278	15	—	tr

PANCAKES

FOOD	PORTION	CALS.	CARB.	SUG.	FIB.
blueberry	1 (4 in diam)	84	11	—	—
buckwheat	1 (4 in diam)	55	6	—	—
potato	1 (4 in diam)	78	4	—	tr
w/ butter & syrup	3	519	91	—	—

PASTA DINNERS

FOOD	PORTION	CALS.	CARB.	SUG.	FIB.
lasagna	1 piece (2.5 in x 2.5 in)	374	25	—	2
macaroni & cheese	1 cup	230	26	—	—
manicotti	¾ cup (6.4 oz)	273	28	—	2
rigatoni w/ sausage sauce	¾ cup	260	28	—	3

FOOD	PORTION	CALS.	CARB.	SUG.	FIB.
spaghetti w/ meatballs & cheese	1 cup	407	38	—	—
PASTA SALAD					
elbow macaroni salad	3.5 oz	160	26	—	—
italian style pasta salad	3.5 oz	140	15	—	—
mustard macaroni salad	3.5 oz	190	23	—	—
pasta salad w/ vegetables	3.5 oz	140	21	—	—
PEAS					
pea & potato curry	1 serv (7 oz)	284	19	—	6
pea curry	1 serv (4.4 oz)	438	11	—	4
PIE					
apple	⅛ of 9 in pie (5.4 oz)	411	58	—	3
banana cream	⅛ of 9 in pie (5.2 oz)	398	49	—	—
blueberry	⅛ of 9 in pie (5.2 oz)	360	49	—	—
butterscotch	⅛ of 9 in pie (4.5 oz)	355	42	—	—
cherry	⅛ of 9 in pie (6.3 oz)	486	69	—	—
coconut creme	⅛ of 9 in pie (4.7 oz)	396	46	—	—
coconut custard	⅙ of 8 in pie (3.6 oz)	271	32	—	—
custard	⅛ of 9 in pie (4.5 oz)	262	34	—	2
lemon meringue	⅛ of 9 in pie (4.5 oz)	362	50	—	2
mince	⅛ of 9 in pie (5.8 oz)	477	79	—	—
pecan	⅙ of 8 in pie (4 oz)	452	65	—	4
pumpkin	⅙ of 8 in pie (3.8 oz)	229	30	—	3
vanilla cream	⅛ of 9 in pie (4.4 oz)	350	41	—	—
PIZZA					
cheese	12 in pie	1121	164	—	—
cheese	⅛ of 12 in pie	140	21	—	—
cheese deep dish individual	1 (5.5 oz)	460	47	4	2
cheese meat & vegetables	⅛ of 12 in pie	184	21	—	—
cheese meat & vegetables	12 in pie	1472	170	—	—

FOOD	PORTION	CALS.	CARB.	SUG.	FIB.
pepperoni	⅛ of 12 in pie	181	20	—	—
pepperoni	12 in pie	1445	157	—	—

PLANTAINS
ripe fried	2.8 oz	214	38	—	4

PORK DISHES
pork roast	2 oz	70	0	0	0
tourtiere	1 piece (4.9 oz)	451	21	—	—

POT PIE
beef	⅓ of 9 in pie (7.4 oz)	515	39	—	—
chicken	⅓ of 9 in pie (8.1 oz)	545	42	—	—

POTATO
au gratin w/ cheese	½ cup	178	17	—	—
baked topped w/ cheese sauce	1	475	47	—	—
baked topped w/ cheese sauce & bacon	1	451	44	—	—
baked topped w/ cheese sauce & broccoli	1	402	47	—	—
baked topped w/ cheese sauce & chili	1	481	56	—	—
baked topped w/ sour cream & chives	1	394	50	—	—
curry	1 serv (6 oz)	292	36	—	4
french fried	1 lg	358	44	—	—
french fried	1 reg	237	29	—	—
hash brown	½ cup	163	17	—	2
indian yogurt potatoes	1 serv	315	52	—	0
mashed	½ cup	111	18	—	—
mustard potato salad	3.5 oz	120	16	—	—
o'brien	1 cup	157	30	—	—
potato dumpling	3½ oz	334	74	—	3
potato pancakes	1 (1.3 oz)	101	11	—	—
potato salad	½ cup	179	14	—	—
potato salad	⅓ cup	108	13	—	—
potato salad w/ vegetables	3.5 oz	120	20	—	—
scalloped	½ cup	127	18	—	—

PUDDING
blancmange	1 serv (4.7 oz)	154	25	—	tr
bread pudding	1 serv (6.7 oz)	564	94	—	6

FOOD	PORTION	CALS.	CARB.	SUG.	FIB.
bread w/ raisins	½ cup	180	31	—	—
chocolate	½ cup (5.5 oz)	206	41	—	—
queen of puddings	1 serv (4.4 oz)	266	41	—	tr
rice pudding	1 serv (3 oz)	110	17	—	tr
rice w/ raisins	½ cup	246	42	—	4
tapioca	½ cup (5.3 oz)	189	26	—	—
vanilla	½ cup (4.3 oz)	130	20	—	—
QUICHE					
cheese	1 slice (3 oz)	283	16	—	1
lorraine	⅛ of 8 in pie	600	29	—	—
mushroom	1 slice (3 oz)	256	17	—	1
RICE					
nasi goreng indonesian rice & vegetables	1 cup (4.9 oz)	130	28	1	1
paella	1 serv (7 oz)	308	17	—	3
pilaf	½ cup	84	11	—	3
risotto	6.6 oz	426	65	—	3
spanish	¾ cup	363	19	—	—
SALAD					
caesar	2 cups (5 oz)	235	11	3	1
chef w/o dressing	1½ cups	386	9	—	—
tossed w/o dressing	¾ cup	16	3	—	—
tossed w/o dressing	1½ cups	32	7	—	—
tossed w/o dressing w/ cheese & egg	1½ cups	102	5	—	—
tossed w/o dressing w/ chicken	1½ cups	105	4	—	—
tossed w/o dressing w/ pasta & seafood	1½ cups (14.6 oz)	380	32	—	—
tossed w/o dressing w/ shrimp	1½ cups	107	7	—	—
waldorf	½ cup	79	6	—	1
SALMON					
salmon cake	1 (3 oz)	241	6	—	—
SANDWICH					
chicken fillet plain	1	515	39	—	—
chicken fillet w/ cheese lettuce mayonnaise & tomato	1	632	42	—	—
croque monsieur	1 (12.4 oz)	765	43	9	2
fish fillet w/ tartar sauce	1	431	41	—	—
fish fillet w/ tartar sauce & cheese	1	524	48	—	—
fried egg w/ cheese	1	340	26	—	—
fried egg w/ cheese & ham	1	348	31	—	—

FOOD	PORTION	CALS.	CARB.	SUG.	FIB.
ham w/ cheese	1	353	33	—	—
roast beef submarine sandwich w/ tomato lettuce & mayonnaise	1	411	44	—	—
roast beef w/ cheese	1	402	27	—	—
roast beef plain	1	346	33	—	—
steak w/ tomato lettuce salt & mayonnaise	1	459	52	—	—
submarine w/ salami ham cheese lettuce tomato onion & oil	1	456	51	—	—
tuna salad submarine sandwich w/ lettuce & oil	1	584	55	—	—

SAUCE

bearnaise	1 oz	177	1	—	tr

SAUSAGE

pork	1 link (0.5 oz)	48	tr	—	—
pork	1 patty (1 oz)	100	tr	—	—

SAUSAGE DISHES

sausage roll	1 (2.3 oz)	311	22	—	1

SCALLOP

breaded & fried	6 (5 oz)	386	38	—	—

SCONE

cheese	1 (1.75 oz)	182	22	—	1
fruit	1 (1.75 oz)	158	27	—	2
orange poppy	1 (3 oz)	260	47	12	2
plain	1 (1.75 oz)	181	27	—	1
raisin	1 (3 oz)	270	50	15	2

SHRIMP

breaded & fried	3 oz	206	10	—	—
breaded & fried	6 to 8 (6 oz)	454	40	—	—
jambalaya	¾ cup	188	26	—	8

SOLE

battered & fried	3.2 oz	211	15	—	—
breaded & fried	3.2 oz	211	15	—	—

SOUP

beef stew soup	1 cup (8.8 oz)	221	20	—	—
black bean turtle soup	1 cup	241	45	—	—
brunswick stew soup	1 cup (8.5 oz)	232	17	—	—
corn & cheese chowder	¾ cup	215	21	—	3
gazpacho	1 cup	46	5	—	—

FOOD	PORTION	CALS.	CARB.	SUG.	FIB.
greek	¾ cup	63	7	—	2
hot & sour	1 serv (14 oz)	173	8	1	1
onion soup gratinee	1 serv	492	38	6	4
oxtail	5 oz	64	7	—	—
pasta e fagioll	1 cup (8.8 oz)	194	30	—	—
ratatouille	1 cup (7.5 oz)	266	12	—	—
SPAGHETTI SAUCE					
bolognese	5 oz	195	4	—	tr
SPANISH FOOD					
burrito w/ apple	1 sm (2.6 oz)	231	35	—	—
burrito w/ apple	1 lg (5.4 oz)	484	73	—	—
burrito w/ beans	2 (7.6 oz)	448	71	—	—
burrito w/ beans & cheese	2 (6.5 oz)	377	55	—	—
burrito w/ beans & chili peppers	2 (7.2 oz)	413	58	—	—
burrito w/ beans & meat	2 (8.1 oz)	508	66	—	—
burrito w/ beans cheese & beef	2 (7.1 oz)	331	40	—	—
burrito w/ beans cheese & chili peppers	2 (11.8 oz)	663	85	—	—
burrito w/ beef	2 (7.7 oz)	523	59	—	—
burrito w/ beef & chili peppers	2 (7.1 oz)	426	49	—	—
burrito w/ beef cheese & chili peppers	2 (10.7 oz)	634	64	—	—
burrito w/ cherry	1 sm (2.6 oz)	231	35	—	—
burrito w/ cherry	1 lg (5.4 oz)	484	73	—	—
chimichanga w/ beef	1 (6.1 oz)	425	43	—	—
chimichanga w/ beef & cheese	1 (6.4 oz)	443	39	—	—
chimichanga w/ beef & red chili peppers	1 (6.7 oz)	424	46	—	—
chimichanga w/ beef cheese & red chili peppers	1 (6.3 oz)	364	38	—	—
enchilada w/ cheese	1 (5.7 oz)	320	29	—	—
enchilada w/ cheese & beef	1 (6.7 oz)	324	30	—	—
enchirito w/ cheese beef & beans	1 (6.8 oz)	344	34	—	—
frijoles w/ cheese	1 cup (5.9 oz)	226	29	—	—
nachos w/ cheese	6 to 8 (4 oz)	345	36	—	—
nachos w/ cheese & jalapeno peppers	6 to 8 (7.2 oz)	607	60	—	—
nachos w/ cheese beans ground beef & peppers	6 to 8 (8.9 oz)	568	56	—	—
nachos w/ cinnamon & sugar	6 to 8 (3.8 oz)	592	63	—	—
taco	1 sm (6 oz)	370	27	—	—

FOOD	PORTION	CALS.	CARB.	SUG.	FIB.
taco salad	1½ cups	279	24	—	—
taco salad w/ chili con carne	1½ cups	288	27	—	—
tostada w/ beans & cheese	1 (5.1 oz)	223	27	—	—
tostada w/ beans beef & cheese	1 (7.9 oz)	334	30	—	—
tostada w/ beef & cheese	1 (5.7 oz)	315	23	—	—
tostada w/ guacamole	2 (9.2 oz)	360	32	—	—
SPINACH					
indian saag	1 serv	28	2	—	1
spanakopita spinach pie	1 cup (6 oz)	196	35	4	4
STUFFING/DRESSING					
bread	½ cup (3½ oz)	195	26	—	3
sausage	½ cup	292	40	—	1
SUSHI					
california roll	1 piece (0.8 oz)	28	4	tr	—
kim chi	⅓ cup (5.8 oz)	18	4	1	—
sashimi	1 serv (6 oz)	198	4	1	—
tuna roll	1 piece (0.7 oz)	23	3	tr	—
vegetable roll	1 piece (1.2 oz)	27	5	tr	—
vinegared ginger	⅓ cup (1.6 oz)	48	12	4	—
wasabi	2 tsp (0.3 oz)	5	1	—	—
yellowtail roll	1 piece (0.6 oz)	25	3	tr	—
SWEET POTATO					
candied	3½ oz	144	29	—	—
TOMATO					
stewed	1 cup	80	13	—	—
TUNA DISHES					
tuna salad	3 oz	159	8	—	—
tuna salad	1 cup	383	19	—	—
VEAL DISHES					
parmigiana	4.2 oz	279	6	—	2
VEGETABLES MIXED					
curry	1 serv (7.7 oz)	398	22	—	—
gyoza potstickers vegetable	8 (4.9 oz)	210	34	7	5
pakoras	1 (2 oz)	108	12	—	3
ratatouille	1 serv (3.5 oz)	96	7	7	4
samosa	2 (4 oz)	519	25	—	3
succotash	½ cup	111	23	—	—
ZUCCHINI					
indian paalkora	1 serv	46	7	—	2

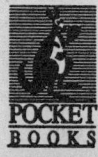

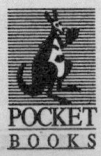